PROGRESS IN BRAIN RESEARCH

VOLUME 106

CURRENT NEUROCHEMICAL AND PHARMACOLOGICAL ASPECTS OF BIOGENIC AMINES

Their Function, Oxidative Deamination and Inhibition

EDITED BY

PETER M. YU

Neuropsychiatry Research Unit, University of Saskatchewan, Saskatoon, Saskatchewan, Canada

KEITH F. TIPTON

Department of Biochemistry, Trinity College, Dublin, Ireland

ALAN A. BOULTON

Neuropsychiatry Research Unit, University of Saskatchewan, Saskatoon, Saskatchewan, Canada

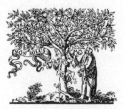

ELSEVIER
AMSTERDAM – LAUSANNE – NEW YORK – OXFORD – SHANNON – TOKYO
1995

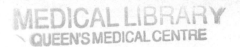
ISBN 0-444-81938-X (volume)
ISBN 0-444-80104-9 (series)

Published by:
Elsevier Science B.V.
P.O. Box 211
1000 AE Amsterdam
The Netherlands

Library of Congress Cataloging-in-Publication Data

Current neurochemical and pharmacological aspects of biogenic amines: their function, oxidative deamina-
    tion, and inhibition/edited by Peter M. Yu, Alan A. Boulton, and Keith F. Tipton.
        p. cm. --(Progress in brain research; v. 106)
    Includes bibliographical references and index.
    ISBN 0-444-81938-X   1000620399

1. Biogenic amines--Physiological effect. 2. Biogenic amines--Metabolism. 3. Monoamine oxidase. 4. Monoamine oxidase--Inhibitors. I. Yu, Peter M. II. Boulton, A. A. (Alan A.) III. Tipton, Keith F. IV. Series.
    [DNLM: 1. Biogenic Amines--metabolism. 2. Brain--metabolism. 3. Brain Chemistry--drug effects. 4. Monoamine Oxidase. W1 Pr667J v. 106 1995/WL 300 C977]
QP376.P7 vol. 106
[QP801.B66]
612.8'2 s--dc20
[612.8'22]
DNLM/DLC
for Library of Congress   95-23747
                                                                                  CIP

Printed in The Netherlands on acid-free paper

List of Contributors

G. Alton, Department of Food Science and Nutrition, University of Alberta, Edmonton, Alberta, T6G 2G2, Canada

Y. Arai, Department of Pharmacology, School of Medicine, Showa University, Tokyo 141, Japan

P. Arányi, Chinoin Pharmaceutical and Chemical Works, Budapest, Hungary

G.B. Baker, Neurochemical Research Unit, Department of Psychiatry, University of Alberta, Edmonton, Alberta, T6G 2B7, Canada

C. Beedham, Pharmaceutical Chemistry, School of Pharmacy, University of Bradford, Bradford, BD7 1DP, UK

E.E. Billett, Department of Life Sciences, The Nottingham Trent University, Clifton Lane, Nottingham, NG11 8NS, UK

A.A. Boulton, Neuropsychiatry Research Unit, Department of Psychiatry, University of Saskatchewan, Saskatoon, Saskatchewan, S7N 5E4, Canada

X.O. Breakefield, Department of Neurology, Massachusetts General Hospital, Boston, MA 02114 and Department of Neurology, Harvard Medical School, Boston, MA 02115, USA

D.S. Bruyette, Department of Clinical Sciences, College of Veterinary Medicine, Kansas State University, Manhattan, KS 66502, USA

F. Buffoni, Department of Preclinical and Clinical Pharmacology of the University of Florence, Florence, Italy

R.F. Butterworth, Neuroscience Research Unit, Hôpital St-Luc (University of Montréal), Montréal, Quebec, H2X 3J4, Canada

B.A. Callingham, Veterinary Pharmacology Unit, Department of Pharmacology, University of Cambridge, Cambridge, CB2 1QJ, UK

H. Carter, Pharmaceutical Chemistry, School of Pharmacy, University of Bradford, Bradford, BD7 1DP, UK

T.R. Cheek, The Babraham Institute Laboratory of Molecular Signalling, Department of Zoology, University of Cambridge, Cambridge, CB2 3EJ, UK

K. Chen, Department of Molecular Pharmacology and Toxicology, School of Pharmacy, University of Southern California, Los Angeles, CA 90033, USA

C.W. Cotman, Department of Psychobiology, University of California, Irvine, CA, USA

A.E. Crosbie, Veterinary Pharmacology Unit, Department of Pharmacology, University of Cambridge, Cambridge, CB2 1QJ, UK

B.J. Cummings, Department of Psychobiology, University of California, Irvine, CA, USA

B.A. Davis, Neuropsychiatry Research Unit, Department of Psychiatry, University of Saskatchewan, Saskatoon, Saskatchewan, S7N 5E4, Canada

J. Degen, University of Hamburg, Zoologisches Institut, Neurophysiology, Martin-Luther-King-Platz 3, 20146 Hamburg, Germany

R.M. Denney, Department of Human Biological Chemistry and Genetics, University of Texas Medical Branch, Galveston, TX 77555, USA

A. DePaoli, Deprenyl Animal Health, Inc., 10955 Suite 710, Overland Park, KS, 66210, USA

P. Dostert, Pharmacia, Via Per Pogliano, 20014 Nerviano, Milan, Italy

C. Dyczkowski, University of Hamburg, Zoologisches Institut, Neurophysiology, Martin-Luther-King-Platz 3, 20146 Hamburg, Germany

P.D. Evans, The Babraham Institute Laboratory of Molecular Signalling, Department of Zoology, University of Cambridge, Cambridge, CB2 3EJ, UK

J. Fang, Neuropsychiatry Research Unit, Department of Psychiatry, University of Saskatchewan, Saskatoon, Saskatchewan, S7N 5E4, Canada

C.C. Finch, Department of Life Sciences, The Nottingham Trent University, Clifton Lane, Nottingham, NG11 8NS, UK

T. Fujita, Laboratory of Biological Chemistry, Faculty of Science and Engineering, Ishinomaki Senshu University, Ishinomaki 986, Japan

J. Gaál, Chinoin Pharmaceutical and Chemical Works, Budapest, Hungary

M. Gewecke, University of Hamburg, Zoologisches Institut, Neurophysiology, Martin-Luther-King-Platz 3, 20146 Hamburg, Germany

M. Hadjiconstantinou, Departments of Pharmacology and Psychiatry, The Ohio State University College of Medicine, Columbus, Ohio 43210, USA

K.D. Hagele, Marion Merrell Dow Research Centre, 16, rue d'Ankara, 67080 Strasbourg Cédex, France

L.M. Hall, Department of Biochemical Pharmacology, School of Pharmacy, State University of New York, Buffalo, NY 14260, USA

J. Hallman, Department of Psychiatry, University Hospital. 7551 85 Uppsala, Sweden

F.L. Hannan, The Babraham Institute Laboratory of Molecular Signalling, Department of Zoology, University of Cambridge, Cambridge, CB2 3EJ, UK

J. Harris, Department of Chemistry and Biochemistry, Arizona State University, Tempe, AS, 85287-1604, USA

L. Head, Department of Psychology and Physiology, University of Toronto, Toronto, Canada

C. Hinze, Marion Merrell Dow Research Centre, 16, rue d'Ankara, 67080 Strasbourg Cédex, France

S.L. Ho, Department of Clinical Neurology, Birmingham University, Birmingham B15 2TH, UK

A. Holt, Neurochemical Research Unit, Department of Psychiatry, University of Alberta, Edmonton, Alberta, T6G 2B7, Canada

Y. -P.P. Hsu, Departments of Pharmacology and Psychiatry, The Ohio State University College of Medicine, Columbus, Ohio 43210, USA

N.D. Huebert, Marion Merrell Dow Research Centre, 16, rue d'Ankara, 67080 Strasbourg Cédex, France

A.V. Juorio, Neuropsychiatry Research Unit, Department of Psychiatry, University of Saskatchewan, Saskatoon, Saskatchewan, S7N 5E4, Canada

V. Kardos, Institute for Drug Research, Budapest, Hungary

H. Kinemuchi, Laboratory of Biological Chemistry, Faculty of Sciences and Engineering, Ishinomaki Senshu Univ., Ishinomaki 986, Japan

I. Király, Institute for Drug Research, Budapest, Hungary

K. Kisara, Department of Pharmacology, Tohoku College of Pharmacy, Aobaku, Sendai 981, Japan

M.E. Knight, Departmernt of Physiology and Biophysics, University of Illinois at Chicago, Chicago, IL. 60612-7342, USA

E. Kollár, Institute for Drug Research, Budapest, Hungary

C.T. Lai, Neuropsychiatry Research Unit, Department of Psychiatry, University of Saskatchewan, Saskatoon, Saskatchewan, S7N 5E4, Canada

J. Lengyel, Central Isotope Laboratory, Semmelweis University of Medicine, Budapest, Hungary

X.M. Li, Neuropsychiatry Research Unit, Department of Psychiatry, University of Saskatchewan,

Saskatoon, Saskatchewan, S7N 5E4, Canada

G.A. Lyles, Department of Pharmacology and Clinical Pharmacology, University of Dundee, Ninewells Hospital and Medical School, Dundee, DD1 9SY, U.K.

K. Magyar, Department of Pharmacodynamics, Semmelweis University of Medicine, Budapest, Hungary

K.S. Manhattan, Deprenyl Animal Health, Inc., 10955 Suite 710, Overland Park, KS 66210, USA

P. Marrari, Pharmacia, Via Per Pogliano, 20014 Nerviano, Milan, Italy

M. Martignoni, Pharmacia, Via Per Pogliano, 20014 Nerviano, Milan, Italy

W. Maruyama, Department of Neurology, Nagoya University School of Medicine, Tsurumai-cho 65, Showa-ku, Nagoya 466, Japan

J.M. Midgley, Department of Pharmaceutical Sciences, University of Strathclyde, Royal College, Glasgow, G1 1XW, UK

N.W. Milgram, Department of Psychology and Physiology, University of Toronto, Toronto, Canada

D.D. Mousseau, Neuroscience Research Unit, Hôpital St-Luc (University of Montréal), Montréal, Quebec, H2X 3J4, Canada

D.L. Murphy, Laboratory of Clinical Science, NIMH, Bethesda, MD 20892, USA

M. Naoi, Department of Biosciences, Nagoya Institute of Technology, Gokiso-cho, Showa-ku, Nagoya 466, Japan,

N.H. Neff, Departments of Pharmacology and Psychiatry, The Ohio State University College of Medicine, Columbus, OH 43210, USA

L. Oreland, Department of Medical Pharmacology, POB 593, BMC, University of Uppsala, 751 24 Uppsala, Sweden

K. Oyama, Department of Pharmacology, Tohoku College of Pharmacy, Aobaku, Sendai 981, Japan

M.M. Palcic, Department of Chemistry, University of Alberta, Edmonton, Alberta, T6G 2G2, Canada

G.I. Panoutsopoulos, Pharmaceutical Chemistry, School of Pharmacy, University of Bradford, Bradford, BD7 1DP, UK

T.M. Paslawski, Neurochemical Research Unit, Department of Psychiatry, University of Alberta, Edmonton, Alberta, T6G 2B7, Canada

I.A. Paterson, Neuropsychiatry Research Unit, Department of Psychiatry, University of Saskatchewan, Saskatoon, Saskatchewan, S7N 5E4, Canada

M. Patthy, Institute for Drug Research, Budapest, Hungary

C.F. Peet, Pharmaceutical Chemistry, School of Pharmacy, University of Bradford, Bradford, BD7 1DP, UK

I. Poggesi, Pharmacia, Via Per Pogliano, 20014 Nerviano, Milan, Italy

R.R. Ramsay, School of Biological and Medical Sciences, University of St. Andrews, St. Andrews KY 16 9AL, Scotland, and Department of Biochemistry and Biophysics University of California San Francisco, San Francisco, CA 94143, USA.

M.M. Rasenick, Department of Physiology and Biophysics, University of Illinois at Chicago, Chicago, IL 60612-7342, USA

V. Reale, The Babraham Institute Laboratory of Molecular Signalling, Department of Zoology, University of Cambridge, Cambridge, CB2 3EJ, UK

S. Robb, The Babraham Institute Laboratory of Molecular Signalling, Department of Zoology, University of Cambridge, Cambridge, CB2 3EJ, UK

M. Rocchetti, Pharmacia, Via Per Pogliano, 20014 Nerviano, Milan, Italy

T. Roeder, University of Hamburg, Zoologisches Institut, Neurophysiology, Martin-Luther-King-Platz 3, 20146 Hamburg, Germany

B.A. Rous, Veterinary Pharmacology Unit, Department of Pharmacology, University of Cambridge, Tennis Court Road, Cambridge, CB2 1QJ, UK

W.W. Ruehl, Deprenyl Animal Health, Inc., 10955 Suite 710, Overland Park, KS 66210, USA

S.O. Sablin, Department of Biochemistry and Biophysics, University of California San Francisco, San Francisco, CA 94143, USA

C.H. Scaman, Department of Chemistry, University of Alberta, Edmonton, Alberta, T6G 2G2, Canada

D.E. Schuback, Department of Neurology, Massachusetts General Hospital, Boston, MA 02114, USA

V. Schwach, Marion Merrell Dow Research Centre, 16, rue d'Ankara, 67080 Strasbourg Cédex, France

N. Seiler, Groupe de Recherche en Thérapeutique Anticancéreuse, Laboratoire de Biologie Cellulaire, Facult de Médecine, Université de Rennes, 35043 RENNES, Cédex, France

C. Shalish, Department of Neurology, Massachusetts General Hospital, Boston, MA 02114, USA

J.C. Shih, Department of Molecular Pharmacology and Toxicology, School of Pharmacy, University of Southern California, Los Angeles, CA 90033, USA

R.B. Silverman, Department of Chemistry, Northwestern University, Evanston, IL 60208-3113, USA

T.P. Singer, Molecular Biology Division, Department of Veteran Affairs Medical Center, 4150, Street, San Francisco, CA 94121, USA

B.D. Sloley, Department of Zoology, University of Alberta, Edmonton, T6G 2B7 Alberta, Canada

T.L. Smidberg, Deprenyl Animal Health, Inc., 10955 Suite 710, Overland Park, KS 66210, USA

J.A. Smith, Pharmaceutical Chemistry, School of Pharmacy, University of Bradford, Bradford, BD7 1DP, UK

M. Strolin Benedetti, Pharmacia, Via Per Pogliano, 20014 Nerviano, Milan, Italy

L.S. Swales, The Babraham Institute Laboratory of Molecular Signalling, Department of Zoology, University of Cambridge, Cambridge, CB2 3EJ, UK

I. Szatmári, Chinoin Pharmaceutical and Chemical Works Co. Ltd., Budapest, Hungary

I. Sziráki, Institute for Drug Research, Budapest, Hungary

T. Tadano, Department of Pharmacology, Tohoku College of Pharmacy, Aobaku, Sendai 981, Japan

E.A. Tivol, Department of Neurology, Massachusetts General Hospital, Boston, MA 02114, USA

P. Tocchetti, Pharmacia, Via Per Pogliano, 20014 Nerviano, Milan, Italy

M. Togashi, Laboratory of Biological Chemistry, Faculty of Sciences and Engineering, Ishinomaki Senshu Univ., Ishinomaki 986, Japan

Z. Tömöskozi, Chinoin Pharmaceutical and Chemical Works Co. Ltd., Budapest, Hungary

A.C. Williams, Department of Clinical Neurology, Birmingham University, B15 2TH, UK

A. Yonezawa, Department of Pharmacology, Tohoku College of Pharmacy, Aobaku, Sendai 981, Japan

P.H. Yu, Neuropsychiatry Research Unit, Department of Psychiatry, University of Saskatchewan, Saskatoon, Saskatchewan, S7N 5E4, Canada

X. Zhang, Neuropsychiatry Research Unit, Department of Psychiatry, University of Saskatchewan, Saskatoon, Saskatchewan, S7N 5E4, Canada

Q.-S. Zhu, Department of Molecular Pharmacology and Toxicology, School of Pharmacy, University of Southern California, Los Angeles, CA 90033, USA

D.M. Zuo, Neuropsychiatry Research Unit, Department of Psychiatry, University of Saskatchewan, Saskatoon, Saskatchewan, S7N 5E4, Canada

Preface

In August 1994, a distinguished group of scientists gathered in Saskatoon, Canada to participate in an international joint meeting, the 6th Amine Oxidase Workshop and the 5th Trace Amine Conference; this joint meeting was sponsored as an IUPHAR satellite meeting. New developments in both basic and applied studies related to monoamine oxidases (MAO), semicarbazide-sensitive amine oxidase (SSAO) and the trace amines were addressed. Following the meeting several participants were invited to contribute chapters which after anonymous peer review are presented in this volume.

New data concerning the reaction mechanism of oxidative deamination including redox potentials, radicals, and stereospecificity was presented. The latest advances in the molecular biology of MAO i.e. related to structure, function and transcription factors and the promoters of both types of MAO's, were reviewed as well as MAO-A gene deletion and its relationship to illness and the relationship of platelet MAO-B activity to personality, neuropsychological traits and Parkinson's disease. The potential neurotoxicity of tetrahydro-isoquinolines was discussed along with the metabolism of deprenyl and the side effects of phenelzine and of several new groups of selective MAO inhibitors. Discussions concerning the possible mechanisms of action obtaining in neuroprotection and neurorescue in several in vitro and in vivo models with respect to deprenyl and the aliphatic propargylamines engendered a great deal of interest.

With respect to SSAO, diamine oxidase and polyamine oxidase new data concerning their biochemistry, function and potential relevance to some pathological disorders was discussed as were recent findings concerning the pathological and pharmacological implications of the trace amines; trace amine receptors and the role of L-aromatic amino acid decarboxylase in the regulation of biogenic amines. The relevance of these latter studies to deprenyl's mechanisms of action was also discussed.

We wish to express our gratitude to the International Society for Neurochemistry, Burroughs Wellcome (Canada), Ciba-Geigy Canada, Ciba-Geigy Ltd. (Basel), Chiesi Pharmaceuticals (Italy), Eli Lilly Canada, Nordic Merrell Dow (Canada), Orion Corporation (Finland), Rhone-Poulenc Pharma (Canada), Synthelabo Research (France), Upjohn Canada, whose generous support made the meeting possible and most enjoyable. We also wish to thank all the participants and contributors; the science was exciting, the discussions stimulating and the social interactions enjoyable. Finally we thank Elsevier for publishing this volume.

Peter H. Yu and Alan A. Boulton
Saskatoon 1995

Contents

Peter M. Yu, Keith F. Tipton and Alan A. Boulton (Eds.)
Progress in Brain Research, Vol 106

CHAPTER 1

The colorful past and bright future of monoamine oxidase research*

Thomas P. Singer

Molecular Biology Division, Department of Veteran Affairs Medical Center, 4150 Clement Street, San Francisco, CA 94121, USA, and Department of Biochemistry and Biophysics and Division of Toxicology, University of California, San Francisco, CA 94143, USA

When the organizers of this workshop asked me to give a talk on a subject of my choice, I wondered what would be appropriate. Finally, I decided on an anecdotal history of monoamine oxidase research, joshing the great, the nearly great, and the would be great, and trying to show how, despite all their efforts, the field has flourished, solid knowledge has accrued, and exciting problems for the future have arisen.

My first plunge into MAO research was over 50 years ago, when, as a graduate student, I tried to assess the importance of the -SH group in enzymes (Barron and Singer, 1943). My major professor, E.S. Guzman Barron, suggested three enzymes for in-depth study, succinate dehydrogenase, monoamine oxidase, and what he called "pyruvate oxidase". I opted for the first two enzymes, the study of which occupied much of my career, because my chief's favorite test subject for the third one was a virulent strain of *Gonococci*, a culture of which was always on hand, because he loved to shake them in Warburg vessels and at the end of the experiment splashed them with gay

abandon into the sink, sending sprays of the bacteria all over the lab. And I could think of more pleasurable ways of getting a G.C. infection than having my incredibly messy professor splash it into my eyes.

By then Mary Hare Bernheim's "tyramine oxidase" (Hare, 1928) was known as "monoamine oxidase". During the next 20 to 25 years research on mitochondrial MAO was centered on problems of pharmacological and physiological importance, such as its role in the inactivation of catecholamines and of 5-HT, with Blaschko's laboratory playing a dominant role, while Zeller's laboratory was exploring the substrate specificity, kinetics, and inhibitors of what most people still considered one enzyme.

By the mid 1960s several laboratories began studying the molecular properties of the enzyme. Reports began appearing at an increasing pace about its purification from beef liver (Igaue et al., 1967), kidney (Erwin and Hellerman, 1967), and somewhat later from rat liver (Youdim and Sourkes, 1972) and recognition of the fact that it contained a flavin dinucleotide in covalently bound form. Concurrently, a plethora of papers from Gorkin's laboratory appeared about the "transformation" of MAO with a puzzling change in substrate specificity (e.g., Gorkin and Tatyanenko, 1967), and from a multitude of laborato-

---

*This article is dedicated to the memory of Richard E. Heikkila, a scientist of vision, a man of great wit and compassion, forever missed by his friends, of whom I am proud to have been one.

ries about reversible and irreversible inhibitors, several of clinical interest. But perhaps the most significant development in the late 1960s was a growing awareness that there must be more than one form of MAO in mitochondria.

The existence of two forms of MAO in mitochondria was clearly recognized as early as 1961 by Hardegg and Heilbron, on the basis of the different inhibitory effects of iproniazid on the oxidation of serotonin (an A substrate) and tyramine (an A-B substrate) in rat liver mitochondria. Others considered the same possibility in the 1960s but these suggestions were obscured by later reports of five or more electrophoretically separable forms of MAO, with different kinetic properties (Youdim, 1972). To my lights, as an enzymologist, the first unmistakable clue to the existence of the two forms of MAO, which we now call A and B, was the fundamental discovery by Knoll and Magyar (1972) that deprenyl inhibits the oxidation of benzylamine and phenylethylamine at very low concentrations, while in the same tissues the oxidation of serotonin is blocked only at much higher concentrations, and Johnston's report (1968) that clorgyline selectively inhibits serotonin oxidation at low concentrations, but blocks the oxidation of benzylamine and phenylethylamine only at much higher concentrations. The conclusion was inevitable that two different forms of MAO may co-exist in the same tissue, such as rat and human liver or brain. The fact that some tissues, such as bovine liver or human platelets, contain practically exclusively the deprenyl-sensitive or B form, whereas human placenta only the clorgyline-sensitive or A form, clinched the issue. Therefore, I could not quite understand the polemics that raged in the field for the next 20 years about what I believed to be a somewhat artificial question, good only for a few more papers and as a filler in research grants.

But the question would not go away. Even some highly experienced biochemists got trapped into coming up with notions which might explain all the findings without having to involve two separate proteins. In what follows I'd like to show a few examples of the seeming immortality of

misconceptions in the field of MAO of which many of us, myself included, have been guilty.

One of the notions that emerged concerned the possibility that MAO was a single protein with two active sites, one of which catalyzes the oxidation of A substrates, the other of B substrates, and both A-B substrates (Mantle et al., 1975). To me, the argument seemed illogical, because while MAO B was known by then to be dimeric, it was thought to have a single flavin and, thus, possessed a single catalytic site. The remarkably unorthodox notion of dual binding sites for A and B substrates on the same protein was laid to rest years ago but not for the reasons I had given, for it became evident later, through the work of Weiler (1989), that both MAO A and B had two identical subunits, hence, each had two catalytic sites.

There was another notion, which would have it that MAO A and B are the same protein but with different lipids attached and these determine its specificity. This concept arose as a result of misinterpretations of Houslay and Tipton's demonstration (1973) that the treatment of membranous preparations with chaotropic agents, such as perchlorate, which tend to break hydrophobic lipid-protein bonds and yield relatively delipidated preparations, dampens the differences in the sensitivities of the two forms of MAO to clorgyline. This observation cannot be taken as evidence for the differences between MAO A and B being due to different lipids attached. A more likely interpretation is that clorgyline, a relatively hydrophobic molecule, tends to be partitioned into the lipid phase of mitochondria, so that the actual concentration of the inhibitor in which MAO is exposed is much higher in membranes than the concentration in the aqueous phase, whereas in purified, lipid-free preparations the concentration of clorgyline around the enzyme is close to the average concentration in the reaction vessel (Krueger and Singer, 1993). The concept that MAO A and B differ only in the nature of the lipids attached to a common protein seemed to be supported by the report of Ekstedt and Oreland (1976), showing that the treatment of pig liver mitochondria with aqueous methyl ethyl ketone results in the extraction of part of the MAO activity but with an apparent change in specificity, so that the solvent-treated preparation oxidized only what we now know are B or A-B substrates, having lost reactivity with MAO A substrates. Since the extraction procedure removes some 90% of the phospholipids, several workers interpreted the results to suggest that methyl ethyl ketone causes a change in specificity because it strips off the phospholipids which determine it. In their excellent paper Ekstedt and Oreland (1976) emphasized that their "results do not support the hypothesis that the multiple functional forms of monoamine oxidase are explained by the binding of different amounts of membrane material [lipids] to one single enzyme..." and suggested that a more likely explanation was differential inactivation of MAO A by the organic solvent in the mixture of the two enzymes

A further argument against the role of lipids in determining the specificity of MAO is that highly purified MAO B from bovine kidney and MAO A from human placenta contain no phospholipids and MAO B from bovine liver, very little, most of which can be removed with only a small loss of activity, yet they are fully active (Erwin and Hellerman, 1967; Husain et al., 1981). Moreover, the turnover number of essentially lipid-free preparations per mol of cysteinyl flavin is the same in the isolated enzyme as in mitochondria: if it were not for that, we could not have used the turnover number to calculate the MAO B content for estimating the enzyme concentration in tissues. Finally, phospholipase A_2, carefully freed from proteolytic contaminants, does not inactivate MAO B from bovine liver, bovine kidney or MAO A from placenta (Singer, 1991); in fact, it is applied as an essential step in widely used methods for the isolation of MAO A and B (Salach, 1979; Weyler and Salach,1985).

These observations, however, failed to lay to rest the mystique that MAO is a phospholipid-requiring enzyme. Thus the fallacy that MAO A and B are a single protein, like a well-fed amoeba, started budding and generated a second and third

fallacies, namely that lipids are essential for the activity of MAO and that the nature of the lipids present determines the differences in specificity of the two forms of MAO. But let me try to deal with these one at a time.

Evidence that MAO A and B are immunologically distinct proteins was reported by McCauley and Racker as early as 1973. Additional evidence that MAO A and B activities are catalyzed by different proteins accrued steadily in the years to follow from differences in subunit molecular weights and peptide pattern (Smith et al., 1985; Castro Costa and Breakefield, 1980; Brown et al., 1980).

The question of the interrelation of monoamine oxidases A and B came into sharp focus at a MAO Symposium that Dick Van Korff and I organized in Midland, MI, in 1979. Both Peter Yu and Keith Tipton gave important talks, emphasizing the limitations and complexities of delipidation experiments and the fallacy of interpreting these to suggest that MAO A and B are one protein, and Keith aptly summarized the problems inherent in the various approaches used to settle the question (Yu, 1979; Tipton and Della Corte, 1979). To my mind, however, the most impressive evidence presented at that meeting for two different proteins being involved was Xandra Breakefield's demonstration that different labelled peptides arise on proteolysis from the two forms of MAO (Pintar et al., 1979). Together with the fact that by then highly purified preparations of MAO B from liver (Salach, 1979) and of MAO A from human placenta (Zeller, 1979; Salach and Detmar, 1979) were available, each free from cross-contamination with the other enzyme but each retaining full activity and specificity, left little room for doubt. And yet, even then, the notion of a single enzyme with different subunits and active sites for MAO A and B activity was revived (White and Tansik, 1979), on the basis of inability to separate the two activities in brain preparations by subcellular location and in soluble samples by conventional procedures. In retrospect, that careful study was doomed to failure a priori, because both enzymes are located in the mitochondrial outer membrane and despite the extensive knowledge of the properties of the pure enzymes, to this day the only known way to separate them is using immunoaffinity columns (Denney et al., 1982).

Subsequent events, of course, yielded irrefutable proof that MAO A and B are different proteins. Monoclonal antibodies against MAO B from human platelets and against human MAO A from placenta (Kochersperger et al., 1985) were shown not to cross-react with the other form of MAO. Similar conclusions were reached by Xandra Breakefield's group using antibodies to bovine liver MAO B (Pintar et al., 1983). The final evidence came from the isolation of cDNA clones for MAO A and B and determination of the deduced amino acid sequences of the two enzymes from human liver, showing that only 70% of the sequences are identical (Bach et al., 1988). The conserved regions include the amino acids around the covalently bound flavin, which we had earlier shown to be the same in MAO A and B (Nagy and Salach, 1981).

The question of the multiplicity of MAO was interwoven and possibly obscured by earlier reports of several eletrophoretically separable forms of MAO with different substrate specificities and sensitivities to inhibitors (Youdim, 1972). This fourth fallacy concerning MAO should have been laid to rest by the elegant work of Houslay and Tipton (1973), who treated similar MAO preparations with sodium perchlorate, which, being a chaotropic agent, strips off phospholipids and other membrane material from the enzyme and disaggregates it as well. After the perchlorate treatment the enzyme had lost no activity and it migrated as a single band in gel electrophoresis. The multiple electrophoretically detectable forms were therefore concluded to be preparative artifacts.

Let us, then, examine the basis of the claim that lipids are essential for the activity monoamine oxidase. The most vocal advocates of this idea have been Naoi and Yagi. In their initial excursion into this field they isolated various ill-defined enzyme fractions from bovine heart mitochondria,

none of which resembled either in subunit molecular weight or specificity either MAO A or B (Naoi and Yagi, 1980). Their partial "delipidation" was accomplished with sodium dodecyl sulfate, a protein denaturant, so that the ensuing loss of activity was more likely due to unfolding or inhibition by this detergent, and what was interpreted as a reactivation by phospholipids may have been explained by partial refolding or displacement of the inhibitory detergent. Their later studies became even more bizarre, since they claimed to crystallize the enzyme from pig liver mitochondria and found it to be flavin-free and not inhibited by either deprenyl or clorgyline (Yagi and Naoi, 1982). To this day I have not a clue what enzyme they were working with.

Perhaps in response to such criticisms, Yagi's group repeated their studies with Salach's widely used procedure (Salach, 1979) for the isolation of MAO B from bovine liver but applied it to pig liver, which, in contrast to bovine liver, contains both MAO A and B, producing thereby yet another strange enzyme preparation, reported to oxidize serotonin rapidly in a clorgyline-insensitive manner (Inagaki et al., 1986). They also replaced the sodium dedecyl sulfate with sodium cholate in the delipidation step, seemingly unaware that cholate is also a powerful inhibitor of the enzyme. The ensuing restoration of activity by added lipids could have been again nothing more than displacement of the inhibitory detergent. A personally troubling facet of this latest opus is that in the discussion they claimed that Navarro-Welch and McCauley (1982) and our group (Husain et al., 1981) had proposed that the phospholipid environment is an important factor in MAO activity. In actual fact, both of these papers vigorously question that conclusion.

Although by 1981 an impressive body of evidence had accrued showing that MOA A and B are different proteins, rather than a single protein modulated by different lipids, some investigators were loathe to give up the beguiling idea that lipids determined the substrate specificity of MAO. Among these was Huang, who published a long series of papers arguing the point without ever presenting any unambiguous evidence. One example is a study (Huang and Faulkner, 1981) employing phospholipase A_2 to delipidate MAO preparations and measuring the changes in kinetic parameters on subsequent relipidation. Unfortunately, the assay method used was entirely unsuitable for kinetic studies, with the result that these authors reached the erroneous conclusion that they had demonstrated the reversible resolution of a lipoprotein into inactive components. Navarro-Welch and McCauley (1982) published an important paper which gives a thought-provoking, alternative explanation. They showed that depletion of the phospholipids and subsequent replacement with pure lipids does not change the V_{max} either of MAO A or of B if one uses a proper, kinetic assay, nor does it change the substrate specificity. Instead, the phospholipids may lower the apparent K_m for the amine substrates. However, this effect on K_m was shown to be an indirect one, because added lipids similarly lowered the K_m in intact, non-delipidated mitochondria. They viewed the effect as an artifact and suggested that the added phospholipids do not combine with the protein, as an essential cofactor would, but with the amine substrate and that the resulting complex may be more readily acted upon by the enzyme.

I should like to offer an alternative possibility. I am not sure that I have seen convincing proof that phospholipids are essential for the activity of any enzyme in the usual sense. I should think that many instances of the apparent stimulation of catalytic activity of an enzyme, particularly K_m effects, might result from the phospholipids creating a microenvironment around proteins in which hydrophobic substrates would be concentrated, resulting in an apparent lowering of the K_m. Negatively charged phospholipids might also attract positively charged amines. The resulting effect on catalytic parameters would, if this is true, vary with the degree of hydrophobicity and pK of the amine substrate, yielding the appearance of changed specificity.

As I noted earlier, fallacies seem to generate still other fallacies. The studies on pig liver MAO referred to (Yagi and Naoi, 1982) claimed crystallization of the enzyme. It seems that pig liver is a favorite source for producing crystalline MAO with peculiar properties. As early as 1974 Carper et al. reported the crystallization of MAO from this source, with an absolute requirement for copper. I might mention that 20 years later no one has succeeded in crystallizing a genuine preparation of either form of MAO, including ourselves, in collaboration with Scott Mathews, one of the foremost protein crystallographers in the country.

The next durable fallacy is that the flavin-dependent MAO contains a metal. Although the inhibition of MAO by metal chelators had been reported earlier, the first claim that copper is an essential component of mitochondrial MAO came from Yasunobu's laboratory (Nara et al., 1966). That copper is not a component of the enzyme but an accidental contaminant was shown soon thereafter by Erwin and Hellerman (1967) and Oreland (1971). Nevertheless, as mentioned above, Carper et al. (1974) revived the notion that copper is an essential component several years later.

The fact that the oxidation of monoamines is depressed in iron-deficient animals (Symes et al., 1969) and its presence in purified preparations from rat, pig, and bovine liver (Youdim and Sourkes, 1966; Oreland, 1971; Salach, 1979) added to the wide-spread belief that iron may be a component of the enzyme, although Sourkes (1979) reminded us that there are other possible explanations for the decreased MAO activity in iron deficiency. I then suggested to Walter Weyler that he use gradient centrifugation at alkaline pH to remove iron-containing impurities, tenaciously bound to MAO. The method had worked many years earlier in removing FAD-containing impurities tenaciously held to NADH-Q oxidoreductase. It also worked with purified MAO B from bovine liver and the resulting preparation contained only trivial amounts of iron, but retained full activity (Weyler and Salach, 1981). Ichinose et al. (1982) also concluded that MAO B is not an iron-dependent enzyme (Ichinose et al., 1982). Nevertheless, to this day I keep receiving manuscripts for refereeing claiming that MAO is an iron- or copper-containing enzyme.

Turning to the flavin prosthetic group of MAO, the elucidation of its structure was what aroused my interest in this fascinating enzyme and represented our first major contribution to the MAO field. By the late 1960s several laboratories reported on the presence of flavin in covalently bound form in the enzyme (Igaue et al., 1967; Oreland, 1971; Erwin and Hellerman, 1967). The last of these papers was a particularly important contribution, characteristic of Hellerman's meticulous studies, bringing much-needed chemical reasoning and approaches into a field till then dominated by biologists. By then our laboratory had nearly 15 years experience with covalently bound flavins, starting with their discovery in 1955 as a component of succinate dehydrogenase (Kearney and Singer, 1955) through the elucidation of its structure as 8α-[(N-3)-histidyl]-FAD (Fig. 1) (Walker et al., 1972) and its chemical

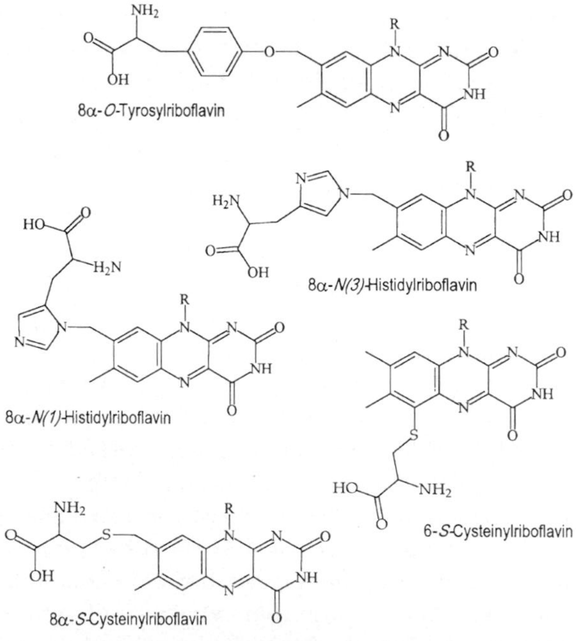

Fig. 1. Structure of the five known covalently bound flavins. Succinate dehydrogenase contains 8α-[N(3)]-histidylriboflavin in the dinucleotide form.

synthesis in collaboration Peter Hemmerich's lab. This was the first of the five known types of covalently bound flavins our laboratory characterized and synthesized over the years (Fig. 1). Having finished the studies on succinate dehydrogenase, we turned our attention to MAO, again in collaboration with the late Peter Hemmerich and Sandro Ghisla.

Collaboration with Peter was a roller-coaster ride. A brilliant chemist, primarily responsible for bringing the use of modern biophysical tools and the concepts of mechanistic organic chemistry into the flavoenzyme field, he was also given to fierce outbursts of temper and unshakable prejudices, one of which was the notion that biochemists are not "real" chemists. Thus, in the 1960s he sent an assistant and a postdoctoral fellow to our laboratory to... teach us chemistry. He saw as my role the large-scale isolation of enzymes containing covalently bound flavin, leaving it to his laboratory to work out their structure. During those days both of our laboratories were trying to decide which isomer of histidyl-riboflavin, N(3) or N(1), was present in succinate dehydrogenase (Fig. 2). One morning I suggested to the German postdoctoral, Wolfram Walker, that he carry out a simple synthetic procedure to decide the question: it worked and in a few days we had the answer. Peter was furious. He kept calling us, collect, from Germany, lambasting us for our arrogance in having carried out this "unauthorized experiment". Then, when we came up with the first direct evidence that MAO B contains 8α-S-cysteinyl-FAD (Fig. 1), he was so upset that he dissolved the collaboration and decided to compete with us instead. Yet all our subsequent discoveries concerning flavin structure were based on what we had learned from Peter.

Thus, by mid-1971 we had determined the structure of the flavin component of MAO B as 8α-S-cysteinyl-FAD and the peptide sequence to which it is attached (Kearney et al., 1971; Walker et al., 1971). Shortly thereafter Ghisla and Hemmerich (1971) synthesized cysteinyl riboflavin. Knowledge of its structure laid the basis for the fluorometric determination of MAO B

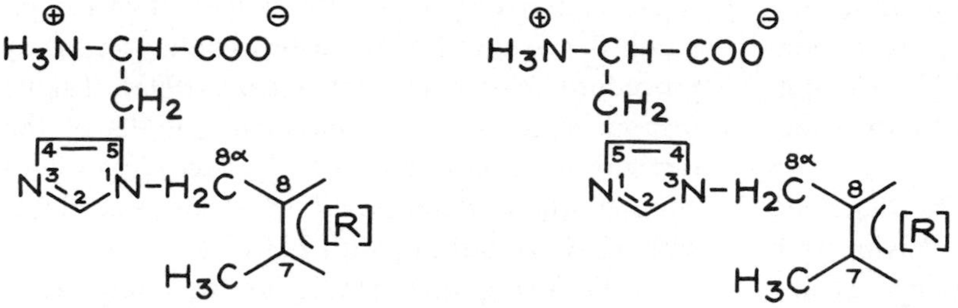

Fig. 2. Structure of the isomeric 8α-histidylriboflavins.

content of mitochondria and impure preparations and providing a method for estimating its turnover number. This came in very handy later.

Our entry into the MAO field was not greeted with boundless enthusiasm by the prevailing Establishment. When, in 1971, we learned that a prestigious meeting on MAO would be held later that year in Sardinia and asked if I could come and show a slide on the structure of the flavin coenzyme of MAO and its surrounding amino acids, I was politely told that Moussa Youdim had already agreed to discuss the flavin of MAO. Even my old friend Albert Zeller could not get us an invitation. We had the same experience a few years later. When in 1984, together with Castagnoli and Trevor, we obtained the first hard evidence that MPTP is bioactivated in the brain by glial MAO B and that the process is blocked by deprenyl and other selective inhibitors of MAO B, we thought that these findings were sufficiently important to present at a forthcoming Parkinson symposium. I called the organizer of the meeting, asking if I could briefly present these exciting new findings. I was told that "Moussa will tell us all the biochemistry we care to know". It was obvious that Moussa had a direct pipeline to the movers and shakers in the pharmacological and neurological communities and was the accepted Boswell of all things biochemical. So, if we ever hoped to participate in a MAO-related symposium, we would either have to organize it ourselves or team up with Moussa. I decided to try both.

The opportunity came a few years later when we came across a paper by Tipton (1968), reporting that MAO purified from pig brain contains non-covalently bound flavin. It seemed unlikely to us that, in contrast to all other animal tissues examined, including pig liver, pig brain contained the flavin moiety in non-covalent linkage. Had it been anyone other than Tipton, I would have probably ignored that paper, but one could not ignore the work of a man who was by then recognized as an outstanding kineticist and whose elegant papers over the years brought order into the chaotic world of MAO inhibition and specificity studies.

We attempted, therefore, to repeat the observations but encountered difficulties in trying to reproduce Tipton's preparative procedure. We then formed a consortium with Moussa Youdim and Kerry Yasunobu to settle the problem. This collaboration had its amusing moments. Since we could not get fresh pig brain in the San Francisco area while it was plentiful in Honolulu, we asked Kerry Yasunobu to prepare and ship to us pig brain mitochondria for purification and analysis of the enzyme. The first shipment arrived a few months later in a huge box of dry ice, containing nearly a kilo of pig brain "mitochondria". Considering the size of a pig brain and its content of mitochondria, if the bottle had contained mostly mitochondria, its preparation would have decimated the porcine population of Oahu.

After much effort, all three of our laboratories concluded that the turnover number of pig brain MAO, based on [14C]pargyline binding or covalently bound flavin, is well in the range reported for the bovine liver and kidney enzymes. At the CIBA symposium, where the results were presented (Salach et al., 1976), Tipton accepted the results graciously, starting nearly 20 years of delightful scientific interaction with us. The notion of non-covalently bound flavin in MAO was not abandoned, however: it kept popping up over the years, as I had feared.

Our laboratory has contributed its share to misconceptions. Along with others (Erwin and Hellerman, 1967; Youdim, 1976; Oreland et al., 1971; Minamiura and Yasunobu, 1978), we have underestimated the flavin content of MAO B to correspond to 1 mol FAD per mol of enzyme (110–120 kDa) (Salach, 1979). Since the enzyme is dimeric, this meant that only one of the two subunits could contain flavin. A careful reexamination of the question with improved preparative and analytical methods, showed that, in fact, 1 mol of cysteinyl flavin was present in each subunit of both MAO A and B (Weyler, 1989). It had been earlier shown that the peptide sequence around the flavin is the same in the two forms of MAO (Nagy and Salach, 1981). Although the amino acids attached to the flavin are well known and readily identified in the deduced sequences, the substrate-binding region remains to be identified, despite major efforts in two laboratories.

Turning to the specificities of MAO A and B and their inhibitors, the number of publications is so vast that I can only discuss a few relatively recent studies, selecting them not according to the importance of the work but because they paved the way toward future research. Before doing so, however, I must dwell on some problems and misconceptions.

Even a brief survey of the literature shows that widely varying values have been published for the relative rates of oxidation of substrates by the enzyme from the same source, as well as their K_m values. Similar, large divergences can be found for the inhibition constants. As Tipton has emphasized (Tipton, 1978), the underlying reason in virtually all cases is the use of assay conditions unsuited for the determination of kinetic parameters.

Thus, for instance, discontinuous assays, like the radiochemical procedure, can only with difficulty be adapted to the measurement of initial rates (Tipton and Singer, 1993). Recently we compared this method with various continuous assay procedures (Krueger and Singer, 1993). Taking extreme care to avoid the many pitfalls of the method, we could arrive at V_{max} and K_m values close to those determined by other procedures with MAO B, but not with MAO A.

In discussing divergences in the literature I refer to major ones, such as the fact that the ratio of the rates of oxidation of benzylamine to serotonin by bovine liver MAO B varies nearly 2 orders of magnitude depending on which paper you read. Some variation in the K_m value for a substrate from the same tissues but at different stages of purification is not unexpected, since K_m is not a physical constant but a ratio of rates, which could readily vary with the purity and, hence, the lipid content of the preparation. We have recently reported such findings and suggested that somewhat lipophilic substrates might be concentrated in the lipid milieu of the mitochondria, giving rise to a lower apparent K_m in mitochondria than in the pure enzyme (Krueger and Singer, 1993). The same is, of course, true of highly lipophilic inhibitors, with the result that the K_i value, which, in contrast to K_m, should be a constant independent of the purity of the preparation, may also appear to be lower in mitochondria than in highly purified preparations. Further, the K_m as well as the K_i values might vary for the same compound in different sources of MAO with differences in the amino acid sequences at the substrate binding sites. We have found that to be the case for the K_m values of MAO B in human, rat, and bovine liver mitochondria for benzylamine.

In principle, such problems do not arise with tightly bound irreversible inhibitors, such as the mechanism-based inhibitors pargyline, clorgyline, and deprenyl, if the determination of the amount of inhibitor required is carried out under valid assay conditions and sufficient time of contact is allowed to complete the interaction of the inhibitor with the enzyme prior to assay.

Nevertheless, there are reports in the literature claiming that the I_{50} value for the inactivation of

MAO by clorgyline is a function of what substrate is used to measure the residual activity. Even Tipton, an expert kineticist, fell into the trap of reporting such data for the I_{50} of clorgyline for MAO B, stating that the value was significantly different when serotonin, instead of a typical B substrate, was used to measure the activity (Tipton and Della Corte, 1979), although he recognized that the problem might be the result of using too low a concentration of substrate. Indeed, Salach et al. (1979) showed that when all substrates are used at concentrations much above their K_m value, the titration curves for clorgyline or deprenyl inhibition of purified and crude bovine liver MAO B are superimposable in assays with benzylamine, dopamine, and serotonin. This is, of course, how it must be, for with a tightly bound, irreversible inhibitor what one is measuring is how much active enzyme is left, which is in reality a titration.

Our studies on the specificity of MAO A and B started when in 1984 Neal Castagnoli and A. Trevor invited me to join them to prove that the enzymatic processing of MPTP to the neurotoxic MPP^+ by brain mitochondria, which they had just discovered (Chiba et al., 1984), was indeed catalyzed by MAO. We found right away that both highly purified MAO A and MAO B oxidized MPTP quite well, but whilst the oxidation by the B enzyme was quite fast (about 40% of the rate on benzylamine) the A enzyme acted relatively slowly on MPTP (Salach et al., 1984; Singer et al., 1986). Further, the oxidation products, both $MPDP^+$ and MPP^+, were competitive inhibitors of the enzyme, but whereas MAO A was quite sensitive to these inhibitors, MAO B was rather insensitive (Singer et al., 1985). Together with the fact the processing of MPTP by MAO A is rather slow, this accounts for the fact that in vivo deprenyl or pargyline alone can block the toxic effects of MPTP administration (Langston et al., 1984; Heikkila et al., 1984). We also noted in these initial studies that MPTP and $MPDP^+$ were mechanism-based, irreversible inhibitors of both forms of MAO.

I was intrigued by the fact that a tertiary amine should turn out to be such an excellent substrate of MAO B, when, up till then, tertiary amines were thought to be oxidized only very slowly or not at all by either type of MAO. So while pursuing the exciting possibilities that the first animal model for Parkinsonism offered and unravelling the biochemistry of events subsequent to the formation of MPP^+, we also started an intensive effort to characterize the structural features required for the rapid oxidation of MPTP analogs by MAO. It soon became apparent that whereas substitution on the pyridine ring or lengthening the alkyl chain at N(1) decreased or abolished activity as a substrate, substitution on the benzene ring did not; in fact it often enhanced the activity (Trevor et al., 1987). Several other laboratories, such as Sayre's (Sayre, 1989) pursued the same quest. What we needed was a series of systematically varied MPTP analogs.

The opportunity for this came in 1987 while in Luteren, Holland, at the first meeting of the International Neurotoxicology Association, an event punctuated by some hilarious episodes, too risqué to recount here. There I had the pleasure of getting to know Dick Heikkila, laying the foundation of a few short years of intensive, pleasurable, and exciting collaboration until his untimely and tragic death. Besides being an outstanding neurochemist and pharmacologist, Heikkila also had the good fortune of having a gifted organic chemist, Steve Youngster, in his laboratory who synthesized dozens of interesting MPTP analogs for us, in labelled and unlabelled form.

Our collaboration turned out to be even more productive than either of us anticipated. Within a short time the broad outlines of the substrate specificity of MAO A and B for tertiary amines became apparent (Table 1). As seen here, several MPTP analogs were excellent substrates of MAO A or B or both, some as good as or even better than any previously used substrate, particularly in the case of MAO B (Youngster et al., 1989). Moreover, the longer the alkyl chain substituted at the 2'-position of the aromatic ring, the better a substrate of MAO A it became and the less it was oxidized by MAO B (Heikkila et al., 1988). This was in accord with the fact that in black mice the neurotoxicity of MPTP was prevented by deprenyl alone, that of 2'-Me-MPTP by a combination of deprenyl and clorgyline, whereas clorgyline alone prevented the neurotoxicity of 2'-ethyl-MPTP. Taken together, it became clear that rapid oxidation by either A or B MAO is a necessary but not sufficient condition for a tetrahydropyridine derivative to be neurotoxic.

Another interesting outcome of our joint study was that, like MPP$^+$, all of its analogs tested are powerful inhibitors of MAO A but not of B. Of

TABLE 1

Oxidation of MPTP and its analogs by pure MAO

Substrate	Turnover number/K_m	
	MAO A	MAO B
Control	1,283	1,064
MPTP	143	523
2'-Methyl-MPTP	593	1,275
2'-Ethyl-MPTP	688	295
2'-n-Propyl-MPTP	658	86
2'-Methoxy-MPTP	511	233
2'-Fluoro-MPTP	100	1,054
2'-Chloro-MPTP	400	1,353
2'-Isopropyl-MPTP	1,131	51
2'-6'-Dimethyl-MPTP	490	209
3'-Methyl-MPTP	76	650
3'-Fluoro-MPTP	391	900
3'-Chloro-MPTP	567	1,132
3'-Bromo-MPTP	300	2,036
3'-Methoxy-MPTP	—	944
4'-Methyl-MPTP	58	345
4'-Fluoro-MPTP	—	423
4'-Chloro-MPTP	69	595
4'-Amino-MPTP	12	54
4'-Nitro-MPTP	185	16
EPTP	28	200
MCTP	270	688
M(4Bz)TP	100	2,675
M(4tBu)TP	—	92
PPTP	73	31
2'-Trifluoromethyl-MPTP	169	520
3'-Trifluoromethyl-MPTP	214	514
MTHIQ[a]	0	0
1-methyl-4(2pyridinyl)-TP	19	41
1-methyl-4(1-CH3−2-pyrroyl)-TP	534	347

The control substrates were kynuramine for MAO A and benzylamine for MAO B. Polarographic assays at 30°C.
[a]Although this isoquinoline is not oxidized, it is a competitive inhibitor of both enzymes.
EPTP, 1-ethyl-4-phenyl-1,2,3,6-tetrahydropyridine; MCTP, 1-methyl-4-cyclohexyl-1,2,3,4-tetrahydropyridine; M(4Bz)TP, 1-methyl-4-benzyl-tetrahydropyridine; M(4tBu)TP, 1-methyl-4-t-butyl-1,2,3,6-tetrahydropyridine; PPTP, 1-propyl-4-phenyl-1,2,3,6-tetrahydropyridine; MTHIQ, 1-methyl-tetrahydroisoquinoline.

particular importance was the behavior of 4'-alkyl substituted MPP⁺ analogs: the longer the alkyl chain, the lower was the K_i value for MAO A (Table 2). This fact led to the synthesis of 4'-azido-MPP⁺, a compound with all the properties needed for photoaffinity labelling of the substrate site. The 4'alkyl-MPP⁺ analogs also enabled us later to show that MPP⁺, rotenone, and piericidin combine at the same site in Complex I (Ramsay et al., 1991a,b).

The discovery of the rapid oxidation of MPTP by MAO B was a potential gold mine for the biochemist. For example, it had been thought (Husain et al., 1982) that, depending on the substrate, MAO B either operates by a bimolecular or ping-pong mechanism (Fig. 3, upper path) or by a tertiary complex mechanism (Fig. 3, lower path), involving reduced enzyme-product-O_2, but never both concurrently. By comparing the rates of re-oxidation of the free reduced enzyme with and without MPTP present in stopped-flow experiments Ramsay et al. (1987) showed that the reduced enzyme product complex was not reoxidized, at least for tertiary amines, contrary to a recent paper (Walker and Edmondson, 1994). Instead, the reduced enzyme combines with substrate and O_2 and these two pathways operate

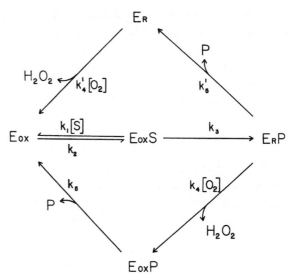

Fig. 3. The binary complex (upper path) and ternary complex (lower path) kinetic mechanisms of MAO as visualized in 1982.

concurrently with a given substrate (Fig. 4). This pathway has been shown to be the predominant one with some substrates (Ramsay and Singer, 1991).

TABLE 2

K_i values for competitive inhibition of MAO A and B by MPP⁺ analogs at 30°C

Compound	$K_i (\mu M)$	
	MAO A	MAO B
MPP⁺	3.0	230
4'-Me-MPP⁺	1.6	~ 1000
4'-Propyl-MPP⁺	0.2	100
4'-t-Butyl-MPP⁺	0.32	35
4'-Pentyl-MPP⁺	0.13	43
4'-Heptyl-MPP⁺	0.59	32
4'-Decyl-MPP⁺	3.1	51
4'-Azido-MPP⁺	0.70	374
4'-Pentyl-azido-MPP⁺	0.075	59
4'-Pentyl-4-phenylpyridine	35	38

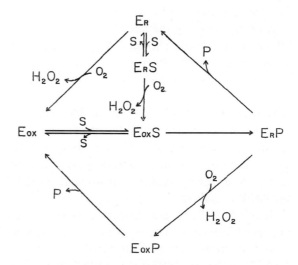

Fig. 4. The reduced enzyme-substrate-O_2 ternary complex and the binary complex kinetic mechanism of MAO A and B, as elucidated in 1987. The reduced enzyme-product-O_2 complex does not play a role in the kinetic mechanism of MAO A or B.

Our initial observations on the time-dependent, irreversible inactivation of MAO by MPTP (Singer et al., 1984) were confirmed by others (Tipton et al., 1986; Arai et al., 1986; Brossi et al., 1986). Like ourselves, they found a logarithmic decline of MAO activity on incubation with MPTP. We suspected that this might actually be an artifact, observed only at high concentrations of enzyme and MPTP. At lower concentrations a break in the curve appeared (Fig. 5), in accord with the expectation that the inactivation occurs during each of the two sequential oxidation steps. In fact, the second phase gave the same rate constant as did inactivation during the oxidation of $MPDP^+$, which yielded, of course, a monophasic decay curve. It thus became clear that MPTP and its analogs offered a unique opportunity to describe the events of mechanism-based inactivation in a situation where the inactivation of the enzyme occurred in sequential steps. Although beset by formidable difficulties, such as the fast chemical dismutation of $MPDP^+$ to MPTP and MPP^+, by using a rapid scan spectrophotometer and a multicomponent analysis program we succeed in deconvoluting the observed spectra, yielding clear progress curves of the course of events (Fig. 6). By applying this technique to a series of MPTP analogues, we showed that the inactivation of MAO A and B involves the reactive species generated in both oxidation steps (Krueger et al., 1990).

The untimely death of Richard Heikkila, besides its devastating personal impact on us, put our future studies on MAO in jeopardy, since we had no synthetic facilities, and depended entirely on the New Jersey group to provide the MPTP and MPP^+ analogs.

Help came from unexpected sources. Simon Efange at the University of Minnesota, originally from Cameroon, synthesized for us a series of flexible analogs of MPTP and MPP^+, while S.O. Bachurin in Chernogolovka, Russia, made some rigid tetrahydrostibasole analogs and their oxidation products available to us.

The oxidation of some of the flexible analogs

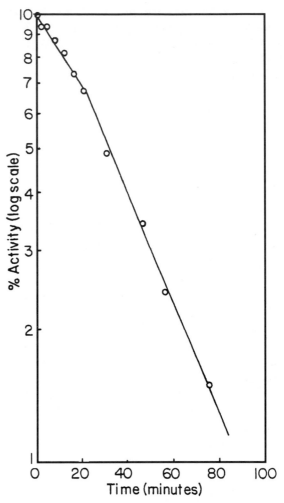

Fig. 5. Time course of the inactivation of MAO B by MPTP (from Krueger et al., 1990).

by MAO A and B (Krueger et al., 1992; Efange et al., 1993) is shown in Fig. 7 and Table 3. It is clear that several of these are superb substrates of both types of MAO, particularly of MAO A. Analysis of the results offered an insight into the factors determining the specificities of MAO A and B and were fitted into a computer simulation of the active sites of the two enzymes (Efange and Boudreau, 1991). Collaboration with him has always been rewarding. Whenever I hesitantly inquired how long it would take him to make a particularly difficult analog, he was apt to say: "how about a

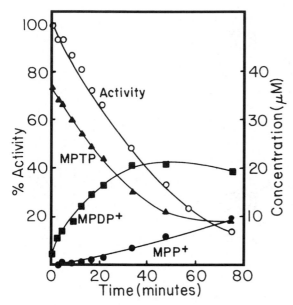

Fig. 6. Multicomponent analysis by rapid-scan spectrophotometry of the products formed during the inactivation of MAO B by MPTP (from Kruger et al., 1990).

couple of weeks? Why don't you ever ask me to make something difficult?"

By then, Sergey Bachurin and S. Tkachenko had published some papers on the synthesis of stilbazole analogs of MPTP and their processing by MAO, but using an enzyme preparation which contained both forms of MAO, so that it was difficult to sort out which enzyme was responsible for the oxidation. We suggested a collaboration, using our pure preparations of MAO A and B in order to reexamine the question if they could supply the compounds. After many months of silence, explained by the fact that mail in Russia, apart from in the center of Moscow, is as unpredictable as the weather, that telephones don't work and Federal Express does not deliver to Chernoglovka, though only an hour's drive from Moscow, there appeared Sergey Sablin in San Francisco, one of the speakers of this symposium, bringing the compounds in his baggage, and advising me that he has no intention of going back.

Our collaboration with our Russian friends has been rocky, to say the least. Pressed by the primary need to survive after the collapse of the Soviet Union and to support one's family in a crisis situation, where stellar institutes of the Russian Academy of Sciences were shut down because they could not pay the electric bill, they could ill afford the luxury of making the compounds we needed but had to concentrate on commercial activities. So we learned to adapt our research program to using compounds they chose to supply. Nevertheless, the stilbazole derivatives sent to us were invaluable, because they not only provided a much better insight into the factors determining the different specificities of MAO A and B, but also led to two important findings. One was the fact that MAO B, but not A, was highly stereospecific. We prepared stereoisomers of the compounds shown in Fig. 8 and found that in all but one case the *cis* isomer is a far better substrate than the *trans* (Table 4) (Sablin et al., 1994). The other was a downward curvature at high substrate concentrations in double reciprocal plot of MAO A activity on tetrahydrostilbazoles (Fig. 9). This turned out to be due to the fact that at low substrate concentrations the rate of reoxidation of the free enzyme predominates, but at high substrate concentrations the dominant reaction is reoxidation within the tertiary complex of the reduced enzyme, substrate and O_2, providing thereby the first direct evidence for the importance of the alternative pathways in the steady-state turnover of MAO A (Ramsay et al., 1993).

The plethora of papers dealing with MAO inhibitors which continue appearing prevents me from even trying to discuss trends in the field. The reader is referred to a review (Singer, 1991) and to the proceedings of the last MAO workshop (Tipton et al., 1994). I would like to call attention though to two important studies, since they are relevant to the still open question of identifying the substrate sites of MAO A and B. The first of these is a series of elegant papers from Silverman's laboratory on mechanism-based inhibitors of MAO. It was shown (Silverman and Zieske, 1986) that the inactivation of MAO B by

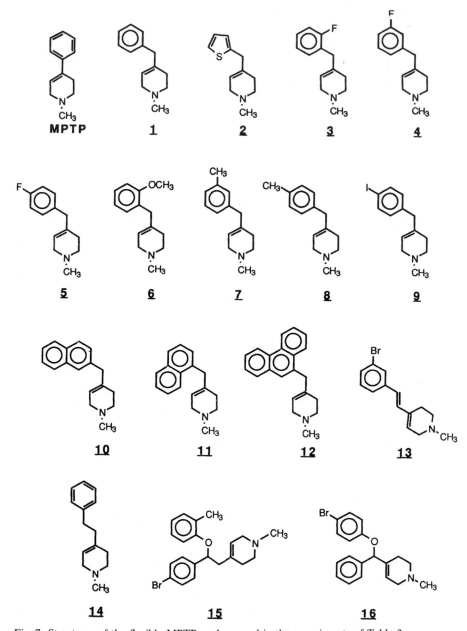

Fig. 7. Structures of the flexible MPTP analogs used in the experiments of Table 3.

1-phenylcyclopropylamine involves a reversible adduct formation with a cysteine residue, as predicted earlier in our studies (Paech et al., 1980), although the structure we had envisioned for the adduct was incorrect. This adduct could be stabilized by reduction with borohydride.

Since the -SH involved is very probably at the substrate site, this offered the possibility of radiolabelling that particular thiol group and identifying the labelled peptide following proteolysis. In a joint study with Silverman's laboratory designed to test this idea, several labelled peptides were

TABLE 3

Oxidation of novel MPTP analogs by highly purified MAO A and B

Compound[a]	MAO A			MAO B		
	TN[b]	K_m (mM)	TN/K_m	TN[b]	K_m (mM)	TN/K_m
Kynuramine	146	0.17	860			
Benzylamine				283	0.29	963
MPTP	20	0.14	143	204	0.39	523
1	9.2	0.066	139	193	0.154	1250
2	8.4	0.048	175	337	0.102	3270
3	20.2	0.034	594	182	0.126	1440
4	30.8	0.208	148	191	0.082	2330
5	27.7	0.14	198	142	0.124	1140
6	28.8	0.0725	398	106	0.735	145
7	58.7	0.122	480	158	0.262	603
8	17.6	0.0181	973	150	0.244	615
9	76	0.042	1830	144	0.121	1190
10	121	0.036	3340	276	0.892	310
11	433	0.167	2590	89	0.847	105
12	365	0.48	759	> 53[c]		
13	(113)[d]	(4)	(28)	24.6	4.16	6
14	137	0.123	1120	61	0.054	1130
15	33.6	0.462	73	16.5	1.49	11
16	19.2	0.73	26	2.3	0.068	34

[a] The structures of the compounds are given in Fig. 7. [b] TN, turnover number from double-reciprocal plots at 30°C expressed as micromoles of substrate oxidized per minute per micromole of enzyme. [c] Activity at solubility limit. [d] Lineweaver-Burk plots are biphasic, possibly because of the presence of *cis* and *trans* isomers.

found, indicating that the radiolabel had migrated after denaturation. This was not surprising, for in MAO research nothing comes easily and the simple answer is seldom the right one.

Mazouz et al. (1990, 1993) reported on a series of highly potent reversible inhibitors for MAO B from rat liver, with virtually no effect on the A enzyme. Following up these reports, we found that their K_i values toward pure MAO B from bovine liver were several orders of magnitude higher (Fig. 10 and Table 5). In order to eliminate the possibility that the differences were due to the tendency of these highly lipophilic compounds to be concentrated in the membranes, we compared their effect on MAO B in mitochondria from rat, human, and bovine liver. The inhibition constants for the rat and human liver enzymes

were very similar, whereas the values for the enzyme in bovine liver mitochondria were strikingly different, considering that the sequences of the human and rat liver enzymes differ only by 11.8%, but the sequence of the bovine liver appears to differ from both to a greater extent. Of the 41% of the sequence of the bovine liver enzyme so far determined, an 18.2% difference from the rat liver enzyme has been found. It would be highly desirable to complete the sequencing of bovine liver MAO B. That would permit identifying the regions of difference. By eliminating the peptide regions which are also present in MAO A from the same species, one could narrow down the possible regions where the substrate site may be located. A further selection could be made of those parts of the sequence

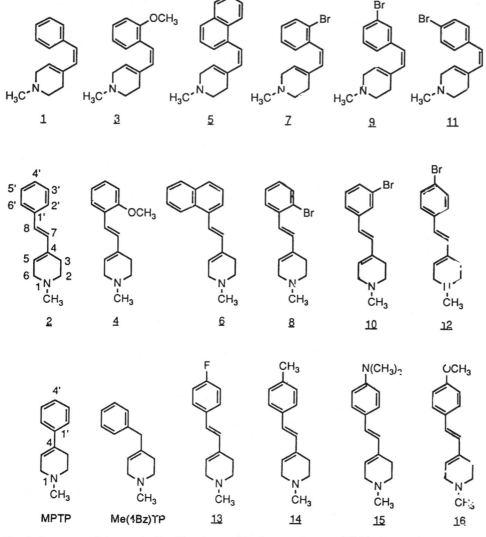

Fig. 8. Structures of the tetrahydrostilbazoles used in the experiments of Table 4.

which contain the -SH group, which mutagenesis studies have shown to be essential for activity (Wu et al., 1993).

In order to keep this paper from becoming excessively long, I have neglected discussing several aspects of MAO research in which important discoveries have occurred in recent years, such as the chemical mechanism, site-directed mutagenesis, the redox potential and its dramatic alteration by substrates, and especially the biological and

medical aspects. However, other speakers at this symposium have dealt with developments in these areas.

Instead, I would like to mention in closing my thoughts on important questions for future research to resolve.

Of paramount importance is the crystallization and determination of the three-dimensional structures of MAO A and B. With techniques now at hand, the fact that MAO is membrane-

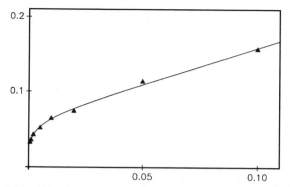

Fig. 9. Lineweaver-Burke plot of reciprocal rate of oxidation (ordinate) vs. reciprocal concentration of tetrahydrostilbazole (abscissa) using highly purified MAO A (from Ramsay et al., 1993).

bound is no longer a deterrent, as several membrane enzymes have been crystallized (e.g., Allen et al., 1988). The successful overexpression of MAO A from human liver by Weyler (Weyler et al., 1990) permits the isolation of several hundred milligrams of pure MAO A. Thus, efforts to crystallize it are well on the way. As to MAO B from human liver, although two laboratories have reported its successful expression in yeast, the quantities available have been minuscule. Recently, our collaboration with P. Urban in Gif-sur-Yvette has yielded expression of the active enzyme in much larger amounts, sufficient for kinetic studies but still well below the amount needed for crystallization. Once the tertiary and quaternary structure of these enzymes is established, localization of the substrate site will be facilitated from the computer models of these sites in the A and B enzymes developed by Efange (Efange and Boudreau, 1991). In the meantime,

TABLE 4

Oxidation of 1-methyl-1,2,3,6-tetrahydrostilbazoles of highly purified MAO A and B

Compound[a]	Isomer	MAO A				MAO B		
		TN[b]	K_{m1}^c (mM)	K_{m2}^c (mM)	TN/K_{m2}	TN[b]	K_m (mM)	TN/K_m
MPTP		20	0.14	143	204	0.39	523	
1	cis	5	0.014	0.47	81	73	0.080	912
2	trans	35	0.010	0.40	88	35	1.8	19
3	cis	37	0.025	0.49	75	25	0.27	93
4	trans	31	0.029	0.48	65	33	2.1	16
5	cis	31	0.013	0.22	141	19	0.39	49
6	trans	31	0.015	0.24	129	13	0.63	21
7	cis	27	0.010	0.28	96	30	0.28	107
8	trans	11	0.009	0.23	48	74	0.12	617
9	cis	150	0.012	0.63	238	169	0.16	1,056
10	trans	132	0.018	0.70	189	25	4.2	6.0
11	cis	5	0.005	0.30	17	98	0.11	890
12	trans	20	0.003	0.38	53	40	0.41	98
13	trans	47	0.005	0.30	157	83	0.60	138
14	trans	34	0.008	0.60	57	10	0.17	59
15	trans	27	0.008	0.35	77	7.4	0.11	67
16	trans	20	0.01	0.42	48	20	0.32	63

[a]The structures of the compounds are given in Fig. 8. [b]TN, turnover number at 30°C from double reciprocal plots expressed as micromoles of substrate oxidized per minute per micromole of enzyme. [c]K_{m1} and K_{m2} derived from biphasic Lineweaver-Burk plots represent the values corresponding to the low and high substrate concentration ranges, respectively.

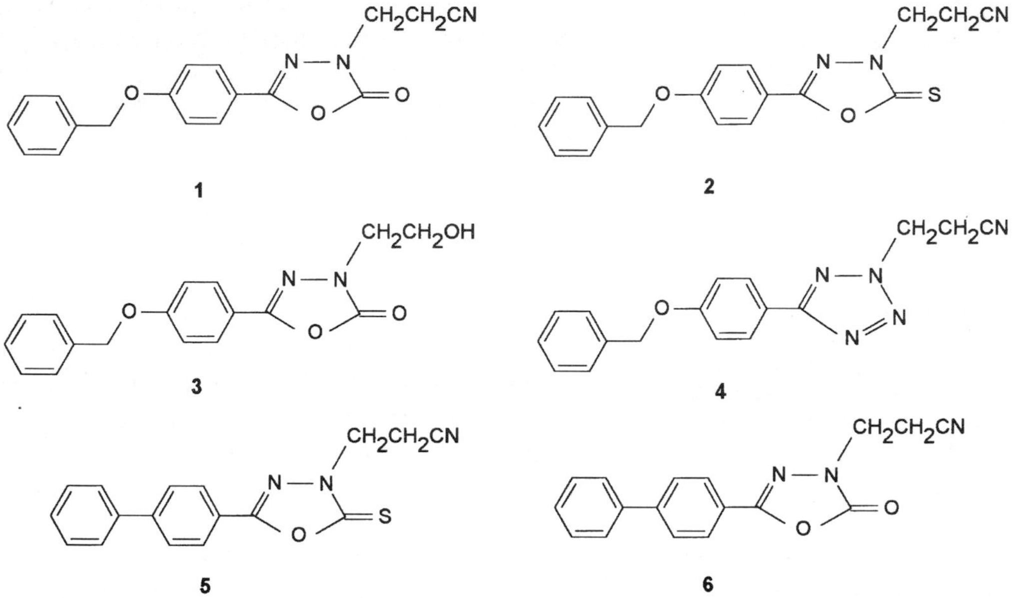

18

Fig. 10. Structures of the potent reversible MAO-B inhibitors used in the experiments of Table 5.

the best hope for locating it in the A enzyme is probably photoaffinity labelling with 4'-azido-MPP$^+$.

Identification of the region where the substrates are bound will, of course, permit site-directed mutagenesis, so as to explore what amino acids, other than cysteine, play a role in these

TABLE 5

Inhibition constants for the oxadiazolones and oxadiazathiones on the oxidation of benzylamine by monoamine oxidase B activity of liver mitochondria from different species

Compound[a]	K_i (nM)		
	Rat	Human	Bovine
1	0.6	0.5	480
2	0.5	0.8	1800
3	1.2	1.1	1300
4	0.9	2.4	3900
5	4.8	2.4	5400
6	5.3	3.2	83000

[a] The structures of the compounds are given in Fig. 10.

sites. In this context, the role, if any, which the -SH group plays at the catalytic site remains to be clarified. Perhaps then an explanation will emerge for the curious "transformations" reported by Gorkin's group involving dramatic changes in specificity they observed on oxidation of the -SH group and treatment with inhibitors which react with thiols (Gorkin, 1976; Gorkin and Tatyanenko, 1967).

The processing of pro-drugs by MAO and inhibition or potentiation of MAO activity will surely remain an active field. Perhaps the most exciting area in further research on deprenyl and other highly selective MAO B inhibitors is the prolongation of life, improvement of CNS function in aged animals, and the still debated question of its clinical use in delaying the progression of Parkinson's disease and perhaps even preventing its onset. If Parkinsonism is the result of "oxidative stress", i.e., damage to the nigrostriatal cells by excessive formation of oxygen radicals, as appears to be the case, then deprenyl would be expected to be beneficial, because of its selective inactivation of MAO B, since the primary source of oxyradicals in the brain is MAO B, which increases hugely on proliferation on aging of the glial cells where most of it is localized.

The mechanism of the neuroprotective effect of deprenyl is still a matter of intensive discussion, since, besides inhibiting MAO B, it is known to inhibit the uptake of monoamines in catecholaminergic neurons and on prolonged treatment has been reported to increase superoxide dismutase (SOD) activity in rats (Knoll, 1993; Gerlach et al., 1994). It would be important to sort out the relative importance of these and other factors, such as the fact that deprenyl is metabolized to amphetamine, in the neuroprotective action.

I find the claim (Knoll, 1988) that 1-deprenyl produces a large increase in SOD particularly interesting. It has been confirmed by some workers (Carillo et al., 1992; Clow et al., 1990), but Lai et al. (1994) found no increase in either type of SOD on chronic administration of deprenyl. If the observation could be confirmed in rigorous trials, it would be of great interest to elucidate the mechanism involved. And much remains to be done to explain the life-prolonging effects of this MAO B inhibitor (Knoll, 1983, 1988).

References

Allen, J.P., Feher, G., Yeates, T.O. Komiya, H. and Rees, D.C. (1988) Structure of the reaction center from *Rhodobacter sphaeroides* R-26: Protein-cofactor (quinones and Fe^{+2}) interactions. *Proc. Natl. Acad. Sci. USA,* 85: 8487–8491.

Arai, Y., Hamamichi, N. and Kinemuchi, H. (1986) Time-dependent inhibition of rat brain monoamine oxidase by an analogue of 1-methyl-4-phenyl-1,2,3,6-tetrahydropyridine (MPTP). *Neurosci. Letts.,* 70: 255–260.

Bach, A.W.J., Lan, N.C., Johnson, D.L., Abell, C.W., Bembenek, M.E., Kwan, S.W., Seeburg, P.H. and Shih, J.C. (1988) cDNA cloning of human liver monoamine oxidase A and B: Molecular basis of differences in enzymatic properties. *Proc. Natl. Acad. Sci. USA,* 85: 4934–4938.

Barron, E.S.G. and Singer, T.P. (1943) Enzyme systems containing active sulfhydryl groups. *Science,* 97: 356–358.

Brossi, A., Gessner, W.P., Fritz, R.R., Bembenek, M.E. and Abell, C.W. (1986) Interaction of monoamine oxidase B with analogues of 1-methyl-4-phenyl-1,2,3,6-tetrahydropyridine derived from prodine-type analgesics. *J. Med.,* 29: 444–445.

Carillo, M.C. Kitani, K., Kanai, S., Sato, Y., Ivy, G.O. (1992) The ability of (-)deprenyl to increase superoxide dismutase activities in the rat tissue and brain region selective. *Life Sci.,* 50: 1985–1992.

Carper, W.R., Stoddard, D.D. and Martin, D.F. (1974) Pig liver monoamine oxidase 1: Isolation and characterization. *Biochim. Biophys. Acta,* 334: 287–296.

Chiba, K., Trevor, A. and Castagnoli, N., Jr. (1984) Metabolism of the neurotoxic tertiary amine, MPTP, by brain monoamine oxidase. *Biochem. Biophys. Res. Commun.,* 120: 574–578.

Clow, A., Hussain, T., Glover, V., Sandler, M., Dexter, D.T. and Walker, M. (1990) (-) Deprenyl can induce soluble superoxide dismutase in rat striata. *J. Neural. Transm. [Gen. Sect.],* 86: 77–80.

Denney, R.M., Fritz, R.R., Patel, N.T. and Abell, C.W. (1982) Human Liver MAO-A and MAO-B separated by immunoaffinity chromatography with MAO-B specific monoclonal antibody. *Science,* 215: 1400–1403.

Efange, S.M.N. and Boudreau, R.J. (1991) Molecular determinants in the bioactivation of the dopaminergic neurotoxin N-methyl-4-phenyl-1,2,3,6-tetrahydropyridine (MPTP). *J. Computer-Aided Molec. Design.,* 5: 405–417.

Efange, S.M.N., Michelson, R.H., Tan, A.K., Krueger, M.J. and Singer, T.P. (1993) Molecular size and flexibility as determinants of selectivity in the oxidation of N-methyl-4-phenyl-1,2,3,6-tetrahydropyridine analogs by monoamine oxidase A and B. *J. Med. Chem.,* 36: 1278–1283.

Ekstedt, B. and Oreland, L. (1976) Effect of lipid depletion on different forms of monoamine oxidase in rat liver mitochondria. *Biochem. Pharmacol.,* 25: 119–124.

Erwin, V.G. and Hellerman, L. (1967) Mitochondrial monoamine oxidase I. Purification and characterization of the bovine liver enzyme. *J. Biol. Chem.,* 242: 4230–4238.

Gerlach, M., Youdim, M.B.H. and Riederer, P. (1994) Is selegeline neuroprotective in Parkinson's disease? *J. Neural. Transm. Suppl.,* 41: 177–188.

Ghisla, S. and Hemmerich, P. (1971) Synthesis of the flavocoenzyme of monoamine oxidase. *FEBS. Letts.,* 16: 229–232.

Gorkin, V.Z. (1976) Monoamine oxidase inhibitors and the transformation of monoamine oxidase. In: J. Knight (Ed.), *Monoamine Oxidase and its Inhibition,* Elsevier, Amsterdam, pp. 61–79.

Gorkin, V.Z. and Tatyanenko, L.V. (1967) "Transformation" of mitochondrial monoamine oxidase into a diamine oxidase-like enzyme in vitro. *Biochem. Biophys. Res. Commun.,* 27: 613–617.

Hardegg, W. and Heilbron E. (1961) Oxydation von Serotonin und Tyramin durch Rattenlebermitochondrien. *Biochim. Biophys Acta,* 51: 553–560.

Hare, M.L.C. (1928) Tyramine oxidase I. A new enzyme system in liver. *Biochem. J.,* 22: 968–979.

Heikkila, R.E., Manzino, L., Cabbat, F.S. and Duvoisin, R.C. (1984) Protection against the dopaminagic neurotoxicty of

1-methyl-4-phenyl-1,2,3,6-tetrahydropyridine by mono-amine oxidase inhibitors. *Nature,* 311:467−469.

Heikkila, R.E., Kindt, M.V., Sonsalla, P.K., Youngster, S.K., McKeown, K.A. and Singer, T.P. (1988) The importance of MAO-A in the bioactivation of neurotoxic MPTP analogs. *Proc. Natl. Acad. Sci. USA,* 85: 6172−6179.

Houslay, M.D. and Tipton, K.F. (1973) The nature of the electrophoretically separable forms of rat liver monoamine oxidase. *Biochem. J.,* 135: 173−186.

Huang, R.H. and Faulkner, R. (1981) The role of phospholipid in the multiple functional forms of brain monoamine oxidase. *J. Biol. Chem.,* 256: 9211−9215.

Husain, M., Edmondson, D.E. and Singer, T.P. (1981) Catalytic mechanism of MAO from liver. In: E. Usdin, N. Weiner and M.B.H. Youdim, (Eds.), *Function and Regulation of Monoamine Enzymes,* Macmillan, London, pp. 477−487.

Husain, M., Edmondson, D.E. and Singer, T.P. (1982) Kinetic studies on the catalytic mechanism of liver monoamine oxidase. *Biochemistry,* 21: 595−600.

Ichinose, M., Gomes, B., Sanimori, H. and Yasunobu, K.T. (1982) Bovine liver mitochondrial monoamine oxidase is not an iron-dependent enzyme. *J. Biol. Chem.,* 257: 887−888.

Igaue, I., Gomes, B. and Yasunobu, K.T. (1967) Beef mitochondrial monoamine oxidase, a flavin dinucleotide enzyme. *Biochem. Biophys. Res. Commun.,* 29: 562−570.

Inagaki, T., Rao, N.A. and Yagi, K. (1986) Modulation by phospholipids of the activity of monoamine oxidase purified from pig liver. *J. Biochem. (Jap.),* 100: 597−603.

Johnston, J.P. (1968) Some observations upon a new inhibitor of monoamine oxidase in brain tissue. *Biochem. Pharmacol.,* 17: 1285−1297.

Kearney, E.B. and Singer, T.P. (1955) On the prosthetic group of succinic dehydrogenase. *Biochim. Biophys. Acta,* 17: 596−597.

Knoll, J. (1983) (−)-Deprenyl (selegiline): the history of its development and pharmacological action. *Acta Neurol. Scand. Suppl.,* 95: 57−80.

Knoll, J. (1988) The striatal dopamine dependency of lifespan in male rats. Longevity study with (−)-deprenyl. *Mech. Ageing Dev.,* 46: 237−262.

Knoll, J. (1993) The pharmacological basis of the beneficial effects of (−)-deprenyl (selegeline) in Parkinson's and Alzheimer's disease. *J. Neural. Transm. Suppl.,* 40: 69−91.

Knoll, J. and Magyar, K. (1972) Some puzzling effects of monoamine oxidase inhibitors. *Adv. Biochem. Psychopharm.,* 5: 393−408.

Kochersperger, L.M., Waguespack, A., Patterson, J.C., Hsieh, C.C.W., Weyler, W., Salach, J.I. and Denney, R.M. (1985) Immunological uniqueness of human monoamine oxidases A and B: new evidence from studies with monoclonal antibodies to human monoamine oxidase A. *J. Neurosci.,* 5: 2874−2881.

Krueger, M. and Singer, T.P. (1993) An examination of the reliability of the radiochemical assay for monoamine oxidase A and B. *Anal. Biochem.,* 214: 116−123.

Krueger, M.J., McKeown, K., Ramsay, R.R., Youngster, S.K. and Singer, T.P. (1990) Mechanism-based inactivation of monoamine oxidase A and B by tetrahydropyridines and dihydropyridines. *Biochem. J.,* 268: 219−224.

Krueger, M.J., Efange, S.M.N., Michelson, R.H. and Singer, T.P. (1992) Interaction of flexible analogs of *N*-methyl-4-phenyl-1,2,3,6-tetrahydro-pyridine and of *N*-methyl-4-phenylpyridinium with highly purified monoamine oxidase A and B. *Biochemistry,* 31: 5611−5615.

Lai, C.T., Zuo, D.M. and Yu, P.H. (1994) Is brain superoxide dismutase activity increased following chronic treatment with l-deprenyl? *J. Neural. Transm. Suppl.,* 41: 221−229.

Langston, S.W., Irwin, I. and Langston, E.B. (1984) Pargyline prevents MPTP-induced Parkinsonism in primates. *Science,* 225: 1480−1482.

Mantle, T.J., Wilson, K. and Long, R.F. (1975) Studies on the selective inhibition of membrane-bound monoamine oxidase. *Biochem. Pharmacol.,* 24: 2031−2038.

Mazouz, F., Lebreton, L., Milcent, R. and Burnstein, C. (1990) 5-aryl-1,3,4-oxadiazol-2(3*H*)-one derivatives and sulfur analogues as new selective and competitive monoamine oxidase type B inhibitors. *Eur. J. Med. Chem.,* 25: 659−671.

Mazouz, F., Gueddari, S., Burstein, C., Mansuy, D. and Milcent, R. (1993) [4-(benzyloxy)phenyl]-1,3,4-oxadiazol-2(3*H*)-one derivatives and related analogues: New reversible, highly potent and selective monoamine oxidase type B inhibitors. *J. Med. Chem.,* 36: 1157−1167.

McCauley, R. and Racker, E. (1973) Separation of two monoamine oxidases from bovine brain. *Mol. Cell. Biochem.,* 1: 73−81.

Minamiura, N. and Yasunobu, K.T. (1978) Bovine liver monoamine oxidase. A modified purification procedure and preliminary evidence for two subunits and one FAD. *Arch. Biochem. Biophys.,* 189: 481−489.

Nagy, J. and Salach, J.I. (1981) Identity of the active site flavin-peptide fragments from the human "A"-form and the bovine "B"-form of monoamine oxidase. *Arch. Biochem. Biophys.,* 208: 388−394.

Naoi, M. and Yagi, K. (1980) Effect of phospholipids in beef heart mitochondrial monoamine oxidase. *Arch. Biochem. Biophys.,* 205: 18−26.

Nara, S., Gomes, B. and Yasunobu, K.T. (1966) Beef liver mitochondrial monoamine oxidase, a copper-containing protein. *J. Biol. Chem.,* 241: 2774−2780.

Navarro-Welch, C. and McCauley, R.B. (1982) An evaluation of phospholipids as regulators of monoamine oxidase A and monoamine oxidase B activities. *J. Biol. Chem.,* 257: 13645−13649.

Oreland, L. (1971) Purification and properties of pig liver

mitochondrial monoamine oxidase. *Arch. Biochem. Biophys.,* 146: 410–421.

Paech, C., Salach, J.I. and Singer, T.P. (1980) Suicide inactivation of monoamine oxidase by *trans*-phenylcyclopropylamine. *J. Biol. Chem.,* 255: 2700–2704.

Pintar, J.E., Cawthon, R.M., Castro Costa, M.R. and Breakefield, X.O. (1979) A search for structural differences in MAO: Electrophoretic analysis of ^{3}H-pargyline labelled proteins. In: T.P. Singer, R.W. Von Korff and D.L. Murphy (Eds.), *Monoamine Oxidase: Structure, Function and Altered Functions,* Academic Press, New York, pp. 185–196.

Pintar, J.E., Levitt, P. Salach, J.I., Weyler, W., Rosenberg, M.B. and Breakefield, X.O. (1983) Specificity of antisera prepared against pure bovine MAO B. *Brain Res.,* 276: 127–139.

Ramsay, R.R. and Singer, T.P. (1991) The kinetic mechanism of monoamine oxidases A and B. *Biochem. Soc. Trans.,* 19: 219–233.

Ramsay, R.R., Koerber, S.C. and Singer, T.P. (1987) Stopped-flow studies on the mechanism of the oxidation of N-methyl-4-phenyl-tetrahydropyridine (MPTP) by bovine liver monoamine oxidase B. *Biochemistry,* 26: 3045–3050.

Ramsay, R.R., Krueger, M.J., Youngster, S.K. and Singer, T.P. (1991a) Evidence that the inhibition sites of the neurotoxic amine, 1-methyl-4-phenylpyridinium (MPP$^+$) and if the respiratory chain inhibitor, piericidin A, are the same. *Biochem. J.,* 273: 481–484.

Ramsay, R.R., Krueger, M.J., Youngster, S.K., Gluck, M.R., Cassida, J.E. and Singer, T.P. (1991b) Interactions of 1-methyl-4-phenylpyridinium ion (MPP$^+$) and its analogs with the rotenone/piericidin binding site of NADH dehydrogenase. *J. Neurochem.,* 56: 1189–1190.

Ramsay, R.R., Sablin, S.O., Bachurin, S.O. and Singer, T.P. (1993) Oxidation of tetrahydrostilbazole by monoamine oxidase A demonstrates the effect of alternate pathways in the kinetic mechanism. *Biochemistry,* 32: 9025–9030.

Sablin, S.O., Krueger, M.J., Singer, T.P., Bachurin, S.O., Khare, A.B., Efange, S.M.N. and Tkachenko, S.E. (1994) Interaction of tetrahydro-stilbazoles with monoamine oxidase A and B. *J. Med. Chem.,* 37: 151–157.

Salach, J.I. (1979) Monoamine oxidase from beef liver mitochondria. Simplified isolation procedure, properties and determination of its cysteinyl flavin content. *Arch. Biochem. Biophys.,* 192: 128–137.

Salach, J.I. and Detmer, K. (1979) Chemical characterization of monoamine oxidase A from human placental mitochondria. In: T.P. Singer, R.W. Von Korff and D.L. Murphy, (Eds.), *Monoamine Oxidase: Structure, Function and Altered Functions,* Academic Press, New York, pp. 121–128.

Salach, J.I., Singer, T.P., Yasunobu, K.T., Minamiura, N. and Youdim, M.B.H. (1976) Cysteinyl flavin in monoamine oxidase from the central nervous system. In: J. Knight (Ed.),

Monoamine Oxidase and its Inhibition, Elsevier, Amsterdam, pp. 49–56.

Salach, J.I., Detmer, K. and Youdim, M.B.H. (1979) The reaction of bovine and rat liver monoamine oxidase with [^{14}C]-clorgyline and [^{14}C]-deprenyl. *Mol. Pharmacol.,* 16: 234–241.

Salach, J.I., Singer, T.P., Castagnoli, N. Jr. and Trevor, A. (1984) Oxidation of the neurotoxic amine 1-methyl-4-phenyl-1,2,3,6-tetra-hydr opyridine (MPTP) by monoamine oxidases A and B and suicide inactivation of the enzyme by MPTP. *Biochem. Biophys. Res. Commun.,* 125: 831–835.

Sayre, L.M. (1989) Biochemical mechanism of action of the dopaminergic neurotoxin 1-methyl-4-phenyl-1,2,3,6-tetrahydropyridine (MPTP). *Toxicol. Letts.,* 48: 128–149.

Silverman, R.B. and Zieske, P.A. (1986) Identification of the amino acid bound to the labile adduct formed during inactivation of monoamine oxidase by phenyl-cyclopropylamine. Biochem. Biophys. Res. Commun., 135: 154–159.

Singer, T.P. (1991) Monoamine Oxidases. In: F. Müller (Ed.), *Chemistry and Biochemistry of Flavoenzymes,* Vol. II, CRC Press, Boca Raton, pp. 437–470.

Singer, T.P., Salach, J.I. and Crabtree, D. (1985) Reversible inhibition and mechanism-based irreversible inactivation of monoamine oxidases by 1-methyl-4-phenyl-1,2,3,6-tetrahydropyridine. *Biochem. Biophys. Res. Commun.,* 127: 707–712.

Singer, T.P., Salach, J.I., Castagnoli, N., Jr. and Trevor, A. (1986) Interactions of the neurotoxic amine, MPTP, with monoamine oxidases. *Biochem. J.,* 235: 785–789.

Sourkes, T. (1979) Influences of hormones, vitamins and metals on monoamine oxidase activity. In: T.P. Singer, R.W. Von Korff and D.L. Murphy, *Monoamine Oxidase: Structure, Function and Altered Functions,* Academic Press, New York, pp. 291–307.

Symes, A.L., Sourkes, T.L., Youdim, M.B.H., Gregoriadis, G. and Birnbaum, H. (1969) Decreased monoamine oxidase activity in liver of iron deficient rats. *Can. J. Biochem. Physiol.,* 47: 999–1002.

Tipton, K. (1968) Prosthetic group of pig brain mitochondrial amine oxidase. *Biochim. Biophys. Acta,* 159: 451–459.

Tipton, K.F. (1978) Enzyme assay and kinetic studies. In: H.L. Kornberg, J.C. Metcalf, D.H. Northcote, C.I. Pogson and K.F. Tipton (Eds.), *Techniques in The Life Sciences—Biochemistry,* Vol. BI/II, Elsevier/North Holland, Amsterdam, pp. B112/1–56.

Tipton, K.F. and Della Corte, L. (1979) Problems concerning the two forms of monoamine oxidase. In: T.P. Singer, R.W. Von Korff and D.L. Murphy, (Eds.), *Monoamine Oxidase: Structure, Function and Altered Functions,* Academic Press, New York, pp. 87–100.

Tipton, K.F. and Singer, T.P. (1993) The radiochemical assay for monoamine oxidase activity. Problems and pitfalls. *Biochem. Pharmacol.,* 46: 1311–1316.

Tipton, K.F., McCrodden, J.M. and Youdim, M.B.H. (196) Oxidation and enzyme-activated irreversible inhibition of rat liver monoamine oxidase-B by1-methyl-4-phenyl-1,2,3,6-tetrahydropyridine (MPTP). *Biochem. J.,* 240: 379–383.

Tipton, K.F., Youdim, M.B.H., Barwell, C.J., Callingham, B.A. and Lyles, G.A. (Eds.) (1994) Amine oxidases: function and dysfunction. *J. Neural. Transm. Suppl.,* 41.

Trevor, A.J., Singer, T.P., Ramsay, R.R. and Castagnoli, N., Jr. (1987) Processing of MPTP by monoamine oxidases: implications for molecular toxicology. *J. Neural. Transm. Suppl.,* 23: 73–89.

Walker, M.C. and Edmondson, D.E. (1994) Structure-activity relationships in the oxidation of benzylamine analogues by bovine liver mitochondrial monoamine oxidase B. *Biochemistry,* 33: 7088–7098.

Walker, W.H., Singer, T.P., Ghisla, S., Hemmerich, P., Hartmann, V. and Zeszotek, E. (1972) Studies on succinate dehydrogenase XVII. 8 α-histidyl-FAD at the active center of succinate dehydrogenase. *Eur. J. Biochem.,* 26: 279–289.

Weyler, W. (1989) Monoamine oxidase A from human placenta and monoamine oxidase B from bovine liver both have one FAD per subunit. *Biochem. J.,* 260: 725–729.

Weyler, W. and Salach, J.I. (1981) Iron content and structural properties of highly purified bovine liver monoamine oxidase. *Arch. Biochem. Biophys.,* 212: 147–153.

Weyler, W. and Salach, J.I. (1985) Purification and properties of mitochondrial monoamine oxidase type A from human placenta. *J. Biol.Chem.,* 260: 13199–13207.

Weyler, W., Titlow, C.C. and Salach, J.I. (1990) Catalytically active monoamine oxidase type A from human liver expressed in *Saccharomyces cerevisiae* contains covalent FAD. *Biochem. Biophys. Res. Commun.,* 173: 1205–1211.

White, H. and Tansik, R.L. (1979) Characterization of multiple substrate binding sites of MAO. In: T.P. Singer, R.W. Von Korff and D.L. Murphy, (Eds.), *Monoamine Oxidase: Structure, Function and Altered Functions*, Academic Press, New York, pp. 129–144.

Wu, H.F., Chen, K. and Shih, J.C. (1993) Site-directed mutagenesis of monoamine oxidase A and B: role of cysteines. *Mol. Pharmacol.,* 43: 888–893.

Yagi, K. and Naoi, M. (1982) Crystallization of a monoamine oxidase purified from pig liver mitochondria. *Biochem. Int.,* 4: 457–463.

Youdim, M.B.H. (1972) Multiple forms of monoamine oxidase and their properties. *Adv. Biochem. Psychopharm.,* 5: 67–77.

Youdim, M.B.H. (1976) Rat liver mitochondrial monoamine oxidase — an iron requiring flavoprotein. In: T.P. Singer, (Ed.), *Flavins and Flavoproteins*, Elsevier, Amsterdam, pp. 593–604.

Youdim, M.B.H. and Sourkes, T.L. (1972) The flavin prosthetic group of purified rat liver mitochondrial monoamine oxidase. *Adv. Biochem. Psychopharm.,* 5: 167–180.

Youngster, S.K., McKeown, K.A., Jin, Y.Z., Ramsay, R.R., Heikkila, R.E. and Singer, T.P. (1989) The oxidation of analogs of 1-methyl-4-phenyl-1,2,3,6-tetrahydropyridine by monoamine oxidases A and B and the inhibition of monoamine oxidases by the oxidation products. *J. Neurochem.,* 53: 1837–1842.

Yu, P.H. (1979) Effect on lipid depletion on Type-A and Type-B monoamine oxidase of rat heart and beef liver mitochondria. In: T.P. Singer, R.W. Von Korff and D.L. Murphy, (Eds.), *Monoamine Oxidase: Structure, Function and Altered Functions*, Academic Press, New York, pp. 233–244.

Zeller, E.A., Arora, K.L., Gurne, D.H. and Huprikar, S.V. (1979) On the topochemistry of the active site of monoamine oxidases types A and B. In: T.P. Singer, R.W. Von Korff and D.L. Murphy, (Eds.), *Monoamine Oxidase: Structure, Function and Altered Functions*, Academic Press, New York, pp.101–120.

Peter M. Yu, Keith F. Tipton and Alan A. Boulton (Eds.)
Progress in Brain Research, Vol 106
© 1995 Elsevier Science BV. All rights reserved.

CHAPTER 2

Radical thoughts about the life of MAO

Richard B. Silverman

*Department of Chemistry, Department of Biochemistry, Molecular Biology, and Cell Biology, and the Institute for
Neuroscience, Northwestern University, Evanston, IL 60208-3113, USA*

Introduction

Monoamine oxidase (MAO; EC 1.4.3.4), a flavoenzyme that oxidatively deaminates a variety of biogenic and xenobiotic amines, plays an important role in the regulation of the intracellular concentrations of these monoamine neurotransmitters (Haefely et al., 1992). Two different isozymes of MAO, known as MAO A and MAO B (Johnston, 1968), have been identified; MAO A selectively oxidizes norepinephrine and serotonin and MAO B oxidizes phenylethylamine and benzylamine (Strolin Benedetti and Dostert, 1992). Compounds that selectively inhibit MAO A exhibit antidepressant activity (Ives and Heym, 1989), whereas selective inhibitors of MAO B are used in the treatment of Parkinson's disease (Tetrud and Langston, 1989). Because of the importance of MAO in the treatment of neurological diseases, we have been interested in the elucidation of its catalytic mechanism so that we could use this information in the design of new classes of inactivators for this enzyme. One approach that we have taken is to design new mechanism-based inactivators (Silverman, 1988) that may give information about the catalytic mechanism. Mechanism-based enzyme inactivators are unreactive compounds that bear a structural similarity to the substrate or product for a target enzyme. Once inside the active site they are converted by the normal catalytic mechanism into species that inactivate the enzyme. These inactivators are important to the study of enzyme mechanisms because they are substrates for the target enzyme that are converted via the normal catalytic mechanism into products that inactivate the enzyme. From the inactivation mechanism, then, information about the catalytic mechanism can be gleaned. Much of the discussion will be based on this principle.

The reaction catalyzed by MAO is shown in Fig. 1. The flavin adenine dinucleotide cofactor is covalently attached at the 8α-position to a cysteine residue at the active site. The flavin is the electron acceptor, undergoing a two-electron reduction with concomitant oxidation of the substrate amine to the corresponding imine. The reduced flavin is oxidized by molecular oxygen, which is reduced to hydrogen peroxide. Amine oxidations to imines is relatively common in solution; they can be oxidized by chemical oxidizing agents (Hull et al., 1969; Lindsay Smith and Mead, 1973), electrochemically (Mann and Barnes, 1970) and photochemically (Cohen et al., 1973; Lewis and Ho, 1980). Because all of these chemical oxidations proceed by one-electron oxidation mechanisms, we (Silverman et al., 1980) and Krantz et al. (1979) proposed a single-electron mechanism for MAO, shown in a modified form in Fig. 2. All of the pathways are initiated by a single-electron transfer from the amine to the flavin to give an aminyl radical (or radical cation). Pathways a and b involve deprotonation; pathway a then proceeds by second-electron transfer and pathway b involves radical coupling of the α-radical to an active-site radical (either the flavin semiquinone or an amino acid radical) to give a covalent adduct, which breaks down by β-elimination to the imine. Pathway c combines deprotonation and electron transfer into one step as a hydrogen atom transfer, bypassing the intermediate α-radical.

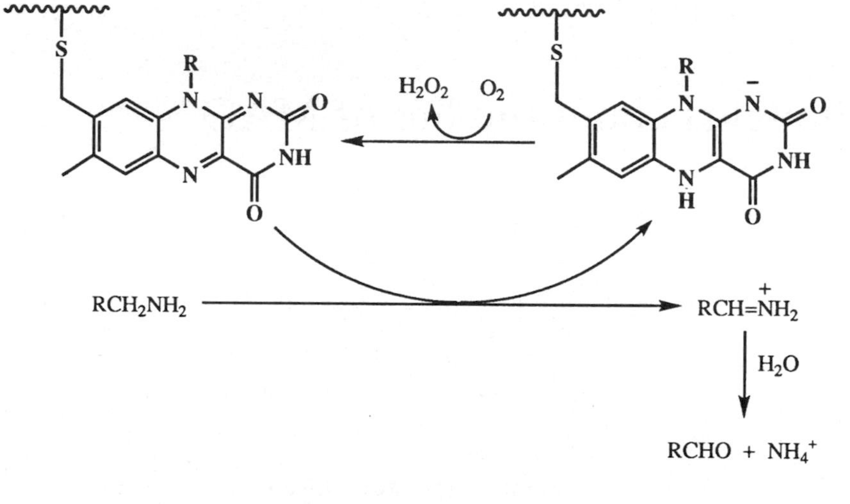

Early evidence for the first electron transfer

A radical mechanism was tested by attaching a substituent to the substrate for MAO that would divert the chemistry and, by identification of the product, would indicate that a radical intermediate could have been involved. Because of the known rapid cleavage of cyclopropylaminyl radicals (Maeda and Ingold, 1980), a series of cyclopropylamine-containing substrate molecules were synthesized and their reactions with MAO investigated (Silverman, 1992). If the first step involves single-electron transfer to give an aminyl radical (or radical cation), then the cyclopropylaminyl radical formed would very rapidly break open to give a carbon radical, which would combine with an active-site radical to give a covalent

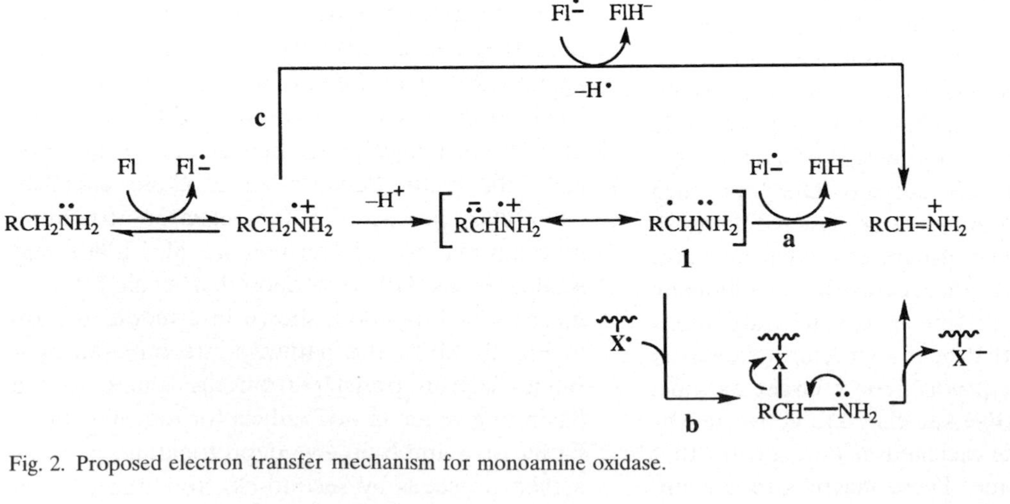

Fig. 2. Proposed electron transfer mechanism for monoamine oxidase.

adduct (Fig. 3 shows a generic reaction for many of the compounds studied). By radioactively labeling these mechanism-based inactivators at different sites, inactivating, then denaturing the enzyme, the stoichiometry of inactivation could be determined. The structures of the released amines were identified, the radioactive adduct was chemically cleaved from the protein, and the structures of the released moieties were identified. The mechanism shown in Fig. 3 is consistent with the results of these studies.

Evidence for deprotonation to a second radical intermediate

Recently, we took a chemical approach to determine whether deprotonation (Fig. 2, pathway a or b) or hydrogen atom transfer (pathway c) is more relevant. The difference between these pathways is that pathways a and b proceed via radical intermediate 1, whereas pathway c bypasses that intermediate. As a test for intermediate 1, (aminomethyl)cubane (2, Fig. 4) was synthesized and studied as a substrate and inactivator of MAO. If the reaction proceeds via intermediate 3, then, because of the rapid rate of decomposition of cubylcarbinyl radical (Choi et al., 1992), ring cleavage should occur (pathway a) and either

a metabolite without an intact cubane ring should be generated or inactivation should occur (e.g., 4). If second-electron transfer occurs prior to ring cleavage (pathway b), turnover to product (5) would result, and cubanecarboxaldehyde (6) would be isolated. Hydrogen atom transfer (pathway c) would go directly to 5 and no non-cubane-containing metabolites or inactivation would be observed. The reaction was carried out on a large scale (14 mg, 0.12 μmol of homogeneous MAO B), the products were isolated by extraction, and NMR and GC–mass spectrometry were carried out. The mass spectrum indicated the formation of a non-cubane-containing metabolite and NMR spectroscopy showed the presence of protons at about 7 ppm, indicating vinyl or aromatic hydrogens (cubane decompositions often result in the formation of cyclooctatetraenes, which have protons that resonate close to 7 ppm). Both of these results are consistent with the intermediacy of radical 3 (Fig. 4). In addition to this metabolite, cubanecarboxaldehyde (6) was also formed. It is not clear whether this metabolite comes from a rapid second-electron transfer (pathway b) or from hydrogen atom transfer (pathway c), but it seems chemically more appealing for an enzyme to utilize one mechanistic pathway for a given substrate, and, therefore, pathway b is favored. The

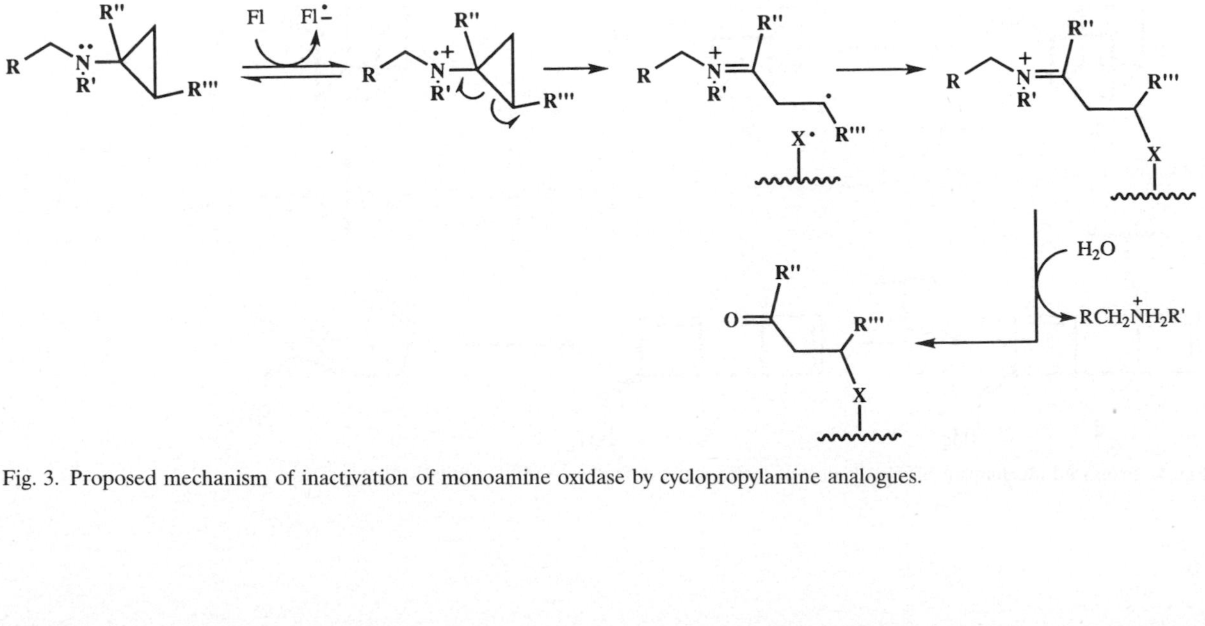

Fig. 3. Proposed mechanism of inactivation of monoamine oxidase by cyclopropylamine analogues.

results of this approach are consistent with the formation of an α-radical in the MAO-catalyzed oxidation of amines. Therefore, pathways a or b via intermediate **1** (Fig. 2) are reasonable.

Spectral studies on the resting state of MAO

Three types of spectroscopy were studied with resting-state MAO B: fluorescence, electron paramagnetic resonance (EPR), and electron nuclear double resonance (ENDOR) spectroscopies.

Fluorescence spectroscopy

The fluorescence spectrum of resting-state MAO B exhibited two chromophores with $\lambda_{ex} = 450$ nm (Fig. 5A) and 412 nm (Fig. 5B). Excitation at 450 nm produced an emission at $\lambda_{em} = 530$ nm (Fig. 6A), and excitation at 412 nm resulted in an emission at 480 nm (Fig. 6B). MAO B is a homodimer, each subunit containing a FAD cofactor

covalently bound (Weyler, 1989). These results suggest that there may be a difference in the two flavin cofactors. The excitation spectrum at 450 nm and the corresponding emission at 530 nm are consistent with an enzyme-bound oxidized flavin (Ghisla et al., 1974); the excitation at 412 nm and emission at 480 nm correspond well to the spectrum for a red anionic flavin semiquinone (Yue et al., 1993; Igaue et al., 1967). Denaturation of the enzyme resulted in loss of the excitation at 412 nm and emission at 480 nm, consistent with the presence of a flavin semiquinone. Inactivation of MAO with pargyline, a compound known to attach to the active-site flavin and exhibit half-sites reactivity (Chuang et al., 1974; Oreland et al., 1973), has no effect on the excitation at 412 nm or the emission at 480 nm, but causes a dramatic change in the 450 nm excitation and 530 nm emission spectra. These results are consistent with the two flavins in the subunits of MAO B having

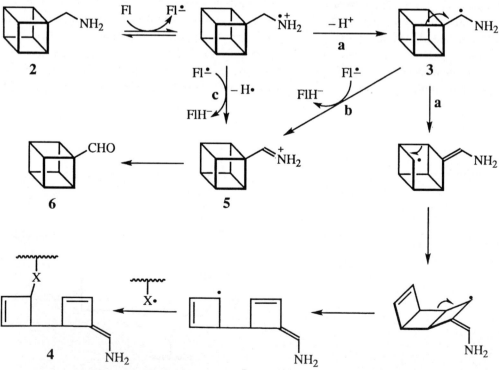

Fig. 4. Proposed mechanism of inactivation of monoamine oxidase by (aminomethyl)cubane.

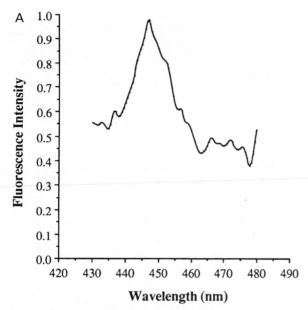

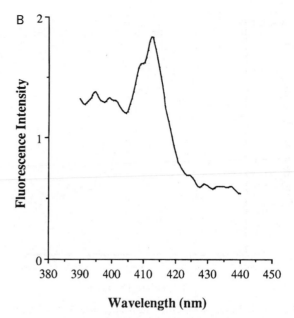

Fig. 5. (A) Excitation spectrum of resting state MAO B (0.58 μM), pH 7.2 (430–480 nm).

Fig. 5. (B) Excitation spectrum of resting state MAO B (0.58 μM), pH 7.2 (390–440 nm).

two different oxidation states, the active-site flavin being fully oxidized and the other subunit having semiquinone character.

Electron paramagnetic resonance spectroscopy

To characterize the chromophores further, EPR spectroscopy was carried out on the resting-state enzyme. A preliminary X-band (9 GHz) spectrum (Fig. 7A) has the appearance of a π-radical with resolved hyperfine coupling to a single nitrogen; the simulated spectrum (Fig. 7B) is virtually identical. The preliminary Q-band (35 GHz) EPR spectrum is shown in Fig. 8A. Simulation using the same parameters used for Fig. 7B except with the field set at 35 GHz gave a spectrum similar to the experimental spectrum (Fig. 8B). The abnormalities in the linewidth may be the result of unusual relaxation effects at this higher field (Palmer et al., 1971). Inactivation of the enzyme with pargyline had no effect on the EPR spectra, but the resonances disappear upon denaturation of the enzyme. Both of these results are consistent with those obtained in the fluorescence spec-

tral studies and support a flavin semiquinone in a site other than the active site of MAO.e

Another experiment was carried out to confirm that the EPR resonance was arising from a site other than the active site. Photochemical reduction of the active-site flavin of MAO in the presence of EDTA (Igaue et al., 1967) gives the X-band spectrum shown in Fig. 9. It is apparent, by comparison of this spectrum with that for the resting-state enzyme (Fig. 7A), that these spectra are different. The photochemically reduced spectrum does not have the hyperfine coupling to nitrogen. Likewise, the preliminary Q-band spectrum of the enzyme treated with light and EDTA (Fig. 10) lacks hyperfine coupling. This indicates that the resting-state radical is not the active-site semiquinone.

Electron nuclear double resonance spectroscopy

To characterize the radical further, ENDOR spectroscopy was carried out. The couplings in the preliminary spectrum obtained (Fig. 11) are consistent with reported values for an anionic

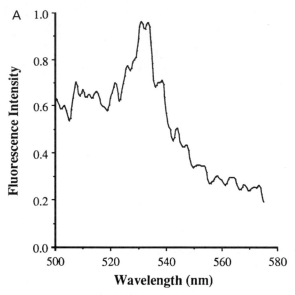

Fig. 6. (A) Emission spectrum of resting state MAO B (0.58 μM), pH 7.2, upon excitation at 450 nm.

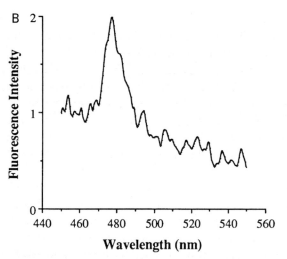

Fig. 6. (B) Emission spectrum of resting state MAO B (0.58 μM), pH 7.2, upon excitation at 412 nm.

flavin semiquinone radical (Kurreck et al., 1984; Ehrenberg et al., 1968).

Conclusions from spectral studies

The reasonable conclusion from these preliminary spectral studies is that there are two distinct

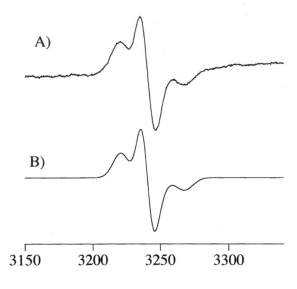

Magnetic Field (Gauss)

Fig. 7. X-band EPR spectrum of (A) resting-state MAO B (98 μM) at pH 7.2. Spectrometer conditions: 9.093 GHz microwave frequency, 0.25 mW microwave power, 125 K, 10 G modulation amplitude, 4 min scan time, 10 transients. (B) Simulation with $g\perp = 2.0047$, $g\| = 2.0014$, $A\perp\ ^{14}N = 3.0$ MHz, $A\|\ ^{14}N = 67$ MHz.

flavins in the dimeric enzyme. On the basis of the fluorescence spectra and the observation that pargyline does not affect the EPR spectrum, it appears that the active-site flavin is in the oxidized state and the flavin in the other subunit is in the semiquinone form. However, the intensity of the resting-state signal corresponds to only 0.02 spins per dimer. Yue et al. (1993) have suggested that the low semiquinone concentration may be the result of spin-spin coupling to another radical present in the enzyme.

The function of the flavin semiquinone is not clear, but one possibility is shown in Fig. 12. According to this mechanism the active-site flavin is involved in the oxidation of the substrate and the flavin semiquinone catalyzes the transfer of electrons from the active-site flavin to oxygen. Since oxygen does not interact with the flavin semiquinone site in the resting state, there may

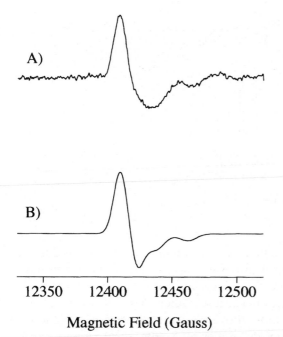

A)

B)

12350   12400   12450   12500

Magnetic Field (Gauss)

Fig. 8. (A) Q-band EPR spectrum of resting state MAO B (600 μM) at pH 7.2. Spectrometer conditions: 34.76 GHz microwave frequency, 1.3 mW microwave power, 77 K, 4.2 G modulation amplitude, 1 min scan time, 5 transients. (B) Simulation with $g\perp = 2.0047$, $g\parallel = 2.0014$, $A\perp\ ^{14}N = 3.0$ MHz, $A\parallel\ ^{14}N = 67$ MHz.

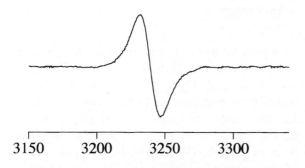

3150   3200   3250   3300

Magnetic Field (Gauss)

Fig. 9. X-band EPR spectrum of photoreduced MAO B (82 μM). Spectrometer conditions: 9.095 GHz microwave frequency, 0.5 mW microwave power, 125 K, 10 G modulation amplitude, 4 min scan time, 10 transients. $g = 2.0065$, peak to peak width = 15 gauss (spectrum is attenuated 40-times relative to Fig. 7A).

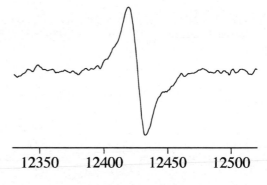

12350   12400   12450   12500

Magnetic Field (Gauss)

Fig. 10. Q-band EPR spectrum of photoreduced MAO B (88 μM). Spectrometer conditions: 34.88 GHz microwave frequency, 0.05 mW microwave power, 77K, 3.3 G modulation amplitude, 1 min. scan time, 5 transients. $g = 2.0033$, peak to peak width = 15 gauss (spectrum is attenuated 40-times relative to Fig. 8A).

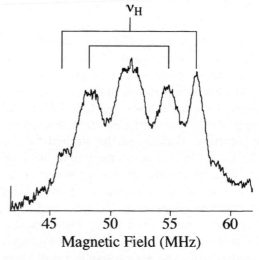

45   50   55   60

Magnetic Field (MHz)

Fig. 11. Proton ENDOR spectrum of resting state MAO B (600 μM). Spectrometer conditions: 35.04 GHz microwave frequency, 2 mW microwave power, 2 K, 53.21 MHz field center, 20 MHz sweep width, 1 MHz/s sweep rate, 2 gauss modulation amplitude, 12510 field set, 630 gain, 100 transients.

be a conformational change after substrate oxidation occurs that allows oxygen to interact with the second subunit. The flavins could communicate

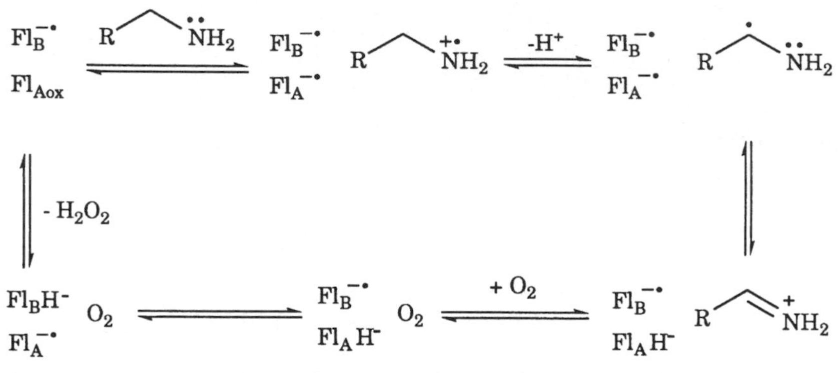

Fig. 12. Possible function for the flavin semiquinone in monoamine oxidase.

via electron-transfer reactions, possibly mediated by an amino acid residue in the active site.

Evidence against a direct hydrogen atom mechanism

Recently, it was reported (Walker and Edmondson, 1994) that, on the basis of steady-state and reductive half-reaction stopped-flow kinetics of *para*- and *meta*-substituted benzylamines, an electron transfer mechanism was not favored; instead they suggest a direct hydrogen atom abstraction of the substrate. Because of the strength of the benzylic C-H bond, it was noted that the only possible species capable of this hydrogen atom abstraction would be the hypothetical amino acid radical that was proposed to be spin-coupled to the flavin semiquinone (Yue et al., 1993); oxidized flavin would not be capable of such a hydrogen atom abstraction. The spectroscopic results presented here, however, indicate that the resting-state paramagnetic species is not in the active site, and is not directly involved in substrate oxidation. Therefore, if such an amino acid radical is present, it is not located in the active site, and, therefore, the hydrogen atom mechanism is highly improbable. Furthermore, a hydrogen atom mechanism is not consistent with the numerous reactions of MAO B with cyclopropylamines and cyclobutylamines (Silverman, 1992; Silverman et al., 1993) in which ring cleavage and attachment

to either the flavin or a cysteine residue was shown to occur; these reactions cannot be rationalized in terms of a direct hydrogen atom abstraction because either there is no α-hydrogen atom to abstract or ring cleavage to the observed products would not result. Furthermore, several flavin adducts which were isolated (Silverman, 1992) could not arise from direct cyclopropyl or cyclobutyl cleavage by oxidized flavin; they must arise from some electron-deficient nitrogen species, such as an amine radical.

Acknowledgments

I am grateful to Dr. Jianping Zhou, Dr. Xingliang Lu, Dr. Victoria J. DeRose, Jonathan C.G. Woo and William P. Hawe for carrying out the research described here, to Prof. Brian M. Hoffman for invaluable discussions about the EPR and ENDOR spectroscopy, and to the National Institutes of Health (GM32634) for financial support of this research (R.B.S.) and for a postdoctoral fellowship (GM14259) to V.J.D.

References

Choi, S.-Y., Eaton, P.E., Newcomb, M. and Yip, Y.C. (1992) Picosecond radical kinetics. Bond cleavage of the cubyl-carbinyl radical. *J. Am. Chem. Soc.*, 114: 6326–6329.

Cohen, S.G., Parola, A. and Parsons, G.H. (1973) Photoreduction by amines. *Chem. Rev.*, 73: 141–161.

Cook, M., Hares, O., Johns, A., Murphy, J.A. and Patterson, C.W. (1986) Novel synthesis of vinyl ethers induced by carbon-halogen bond homolysis. *J. Chem. Soc. Chem. Commun.*,: 1419–1420.

Dickinson, J.M., Murphy, J.A., Patterson, C.W. and Wooster, N.F. (1990) A novel probe for free radicals featuring epoxide cleavage. *J. Chem. Soc. Perkin Trans.*, 1: 1179–1184.

Ehrenberg, A., Eriksson, J.E.G. and Hyde, J.S. (1968) Electron-nuclear double resonance from flavin free radicals in NADPH dehydrogenase ('old yellow enzyme'). *Biochim. Biophys. Acta*, 167: 482–484.

Ghisla, S., Massey, V., Lhoste, J.-M. and Mayhew, S.G. (1974) Fluorescence and optical characteristics of reduced flavines and flavoproteins. *Biochemistry*, 13: 589–597.

Haefely, W.E., Burkard, W.P., Cesura, A.M., Kettler, R., Lorez, H.P., Martin, J.P., Richards, J.G., Scherschlicht, R. and Da Prada, M. (1992) Biochemistry and pharmacology of moclobemide, a prototype RIMA. *Psychopharmacology*, 106 (Suppl.): 6–14.

Hull, L.A., Davis, G.T. and Rosenblatt, D.H. (1969) Oxidation of amines. IX. Correlation of rate constants for reversible one-electron transfer in amine oxidation with reactant potentials. *J. Am. Chem. Soc.*, 91: 6247–6250.

Igaue, I., Gomes, B. and Yasunobu, K.T. (1967) Beef mitochondrial monoamine oxidase, a flavin dinucleotide enzyme. *Biochem. Biophys. Res. Commun.*, 29: 562–570.

Ives, J.L. and Heym, J. (1989) Antidepressant agents. *Annu. Rep. Med. Chem.*, 24: 21–29.

Johnston, J.P. (1968) Some observations upon a new inhibitor of monoamine oxidase in brain tissue. *Biochem. Pharmacol.*, 17: 1285–1297.

Krantz, A., Kokel, B., Sachdeva, Y.P., Salach, J., Detmer, K., Claesson, A. and Sahlberg, C. (1979) Inactivation of mitochondrial monoamine oxidase by $\beta\gamma\delta$-allenic amines. In: T.P. Singer, R.W. Von Korff and D.L. Murphy (Eds.), *Monoamine Oxidase: Structure, Function, and Altered Functions*, Academic Press, New York, p. 51.

Kurreck, H., Bock, M., Bretz, N., Elsner, M., Kraus, H., Lubitz, W., Müller, F., Geissler, J. and Kroneck, P.M.H. (1984) Fluid and solid-state electron nuclear double resonance studies of flavin model compounds and flavoenzymes. *J. Am. Chem. Soc.*, 106: 737–746.

Lewis, F.D. and Ho, T. (1980) On the selectivity of tertiary amine oxidations. *J. Am. Chem. Soc.*, 102: 1751–1752.

Lindsay Smith, J.R. and Mead, L.A.V. (1973) Amine oxidation. Part VII. The effect of structure on the reactivity of alkyl tertiary amines towards alkaline potassium hexacyanoferrate(III). *J. Chem. Soc., Perkin Trans.*, 2: 206–210.

Maeda, Y. and Ingold, K.U. (1980) Kinetic applications of electron paramagnetic resonance spectroscopy. 35. The search for a dialkylaminyl rearrangement. Ring opening of *N*-cyclobutyl-*N-n*-propylaminyl. *J. Am. Chem. Soc.*, 102: 328–331.

Mann, C.K. and Barnes, K.K. (1970) *Electrochemical Reactions in Non-Aqueous Systems*, Marcel Dekker, New York, Chapter 9.

Palmer, G., Müller, F. and Massey, V. (1971) Electron paramagnetic resonance studies on flavoprotein radicals. In: H. Kamin (Ed.), *Flavins and Flavoproteins*, University Park Press, Baltimore, pp. 123–140.

Silverman, R.B. (1988) *Mechanism-Based Enzyme Inactivation: Chemistry and Enzymology*, CRC Press, Boca Raton, FL.

Silverman, R.B. (1992) Electron transfer chemistry of monoamine oxidase. In: P.S. Mariano (Ed.), *Advances in Electron Transfer Chemistry*, Vol. 2, JAI Press, Greenwich, CT, pp. 177–213.

Silverman, R.B., Hoffman, S.J. and Catus, W.B., III (1980) A mechanism for mitochondrial monoamine oxidase-catalyzed amine oxidation. *J. Am. Chem. Soc.*, 102: 7126–7128.

Silverman, R.B., Cesarone, J.M. and Lu, X. (1993) Stereoselective ring opening of 1-phenylcyclopropylamine catalyzed by monoamine oxidase B. *J. Am. Chem. Soc.*, 115: 4955–4961.

Strolin Benedetti, M. and Dostert, P. (1992) Monoamine oxidase: from physiology and pathophysiology to the design and clinical application of reversible inhibitors. In: B. Testa (Ed.), *Advances in Drug Research*, Vol. 23, Academic Press, London, pp. 65–125.

Tetrud, V.W. and Langston, J.W. (1989) The effect of deprenyl (selegine) on the natural history of Parkinson's disease. *Science (Wash. DC)*, 245: 519–522.

Walker, M.C. and Edmondson, D.E. (1994) Structure-activity relationships in the oxidation of benzylamine analogues by bovine liver mitochondrial monoamine oxidase B. *Biochemistry*, 33: 7088–7098.

Weyler, W. (1989) Monoamine oxidase A from human placenta and monoamine oxidase B from bovine liver both have one FAD per subunit. *Biochem. J.*, 260: 725–729.

Yue, K.T., Bahattacharyya, A.K., Zhelyaskov, V.R. and Edmondson, D.E. (1993) Resonance Raman spectroscopic evidence for an anionic flavin semiquinone in bovine liver monoamine oxidase. *Arch. Biochem. Biophys.*, 300: 178–185.

Peter M. Yu, Keith F. Tipton and Alan A. Boulton (Eds.)
Progress in Brain Research, Vol 106

CHAPTER 3

Redox properties of the flavin cofactor of monoamine oxidases A and B and their relationship to the kinetic mechanism

Rona R. Ramsay*, Sergey O. Sablin and Thomas P. Singer

*Department of Biochemistry and Biophysics, University of California San Francisco, San Francisco, CA 94143, USA, and
Molecular Biology Division, Department of Veterans Affairs Medical Center 151-S, 4150 Clement Street,
San Francisco, CA 94121, USA*

Introduction

Monoamine oxidases catalyze the oxidation of primary, secondary and tertiary amines and are important in regulating the level of biogenic amines. MAO A and MAO B are encoded by different genes (Bach et al, 1988) and are expressed in different proportions in the various regions and cell types of the central nervous system. The A form predominates in catecholaminergic neurons and the B form predominates in astrocytes and serotonergic neurons (Fowler et al., 1987; Thorpe et al., 1987). The two forms of MAO show 73% sequence homology (Weyler et al., 1990a) and have overlapping but distinct substrate and inhibitor specificity (Singer, 1991). They follow the same kinetic mechanism (Ramsay et al., 1987; Ramsay, 1991) and chemical mechanism (Silverman, 1992).

Our previous work has established the branched pathway mechanism for MAO in which the reoxidation of the covalently bound FAD cofactor is realized by either direct oxidation of the free enzyme or by reoxidation of the enzyme-substrate

complex. The rate of reoxidation by these two pathways affects the flux through the enzyme in the cell. The free enzyme is reoxidized at a rate of only 6000 M^{-1} s^{-1}, whereas the enzyme-substrate complex is reoxidized at a rate 2- to 120-fold faster depending on the substrate (Tan and Ramsay, 1993).

From the kinetic properties which characterize the isolated enzymes (summarized in Table 1), we can draw conclusions about the flux through each enzyme under various conditions likely to occur in vivo. The net effect of these properties is that flux through MAO A responds to the concentration and type of amine present whereas the flux through MAO B responds more to the oxygen concentration than to that of the amine. Table 2 illustrates what this means physiologically for various levels of amine and oxygen. At low oxygen concentration and high amine, MAO A is important in the oxidative process but under normoxic conditions MAO B would be the main catalyst of amine oxidation. The different substrate specificity of MAO A and B and their different localization in specific brain regions enhanced by oxygen variation may be a way of regulating the level and type of biogenic amines in brain compartments.

Two major kinetic questions remain. First, a great problem in MAO catalysis is the vast dif-

---

*Present address: School of Biological and Medical Sciences, University of St. Andrews, St. Andrews KY 16 9AL, Scotland.

TABLE 1

Summary of the kinetic properties of MAO A and MAO B

MAO A	MAO B
Reduction is rate-limiting.	Reduction not always rate-limiting.
Oxidation strongly stimulated by substrate.	Oxidation stimulated only slightly by certain substrates.
Flavin mostly oxidized in steady-state.	Flavin reduced to various degrees in steady-state.
Variations in $[O_2]$ have little effect on rate.	Variation in $[O_2]$ have significant effect on rate.

ference between the redox potentials of flavin, amine, and oxygen. An explanation for the ability of MAO to oxidize amines despite the thermodynamically unfavorable difference in the redox potentials of the amine (around $+1$ V) and the flavin (-208 mV) has long been sought. Second, how does the substrate simulate the oxidation of the reduced flavin and why is it different in MAO A and B? To seek answers to these questions, we studied the redox properties of the flavin in both enzymes.

Methods

The purified enzyme preparations used were human liver MAO A expressed in yeast (Tan et al., 1991) and bovine liver MAO B (Salach, 1979). The redox potentials in the absence of substrate were determined by the method developed by Massey (1991). Briefly, the xanthine/urate couple

(-350 mV at pH 7) is used to reduce xanthine oxidase, which equilibrates rapidly with methyl viologen, which in turn reacts rapidly with other dyes and flavoproteins.

MAO A or B in 50 mM potassium phosphate, pH 7.2, containing 0.02% Brij-35, 30 mM glucose, 1–2 μM methylviologen, 5–15 μM dye and 200 μM xanthine is placed in an anaerobic cuvette with 1 unit/ml glucose oxidase and 24 units/ml catalase in a drop at the top of the cuvette and mixed anaerobically with xanthine oxidase (to give 12–96 μM). From the spectral changes recorded, the concentrations of the reduced and oxidized enzyme and dye are either determined at given wavelengths or calculated using NONLIN (nonlinear regression program from Phillip H. Sherrod, Nashville, TN).

For the determination of the redox potential in the presence of a substrate ($50 \times K_m$), substrate is used as the source of electrons instead of

TABLE 2

Flux through MAO A and B at different amine and oxygen levels

	Fixed low O_2		Fixed high O_2	
	Low S	High S	Low S	High S
A substrate	Most A	Most A	A and B	A > B
B substrate	B > A	A > B	Most B	Most B
Mixed substrate	A > B	A >> B	Most B	Most B

xanthine oxidase reaction. No semiquinone formation is observed. The influence of the normal substrates for MAO A and MAO B on the redox potential of the covalently bound flavin cannot be assessed by this method because they reduce the enzyme too rapidly to permit equilibrium with the dye. To ensure equilibrium among the redox species, only relatively slow substrates can be used. All the experiments were carried out at 25°C.

Results and discussion

The redox potentials of the cysteinyl-FAD in unliganded MAO A and B have been determined. The spectral changes observed in a mixture of MAO B and the reference dye, indigo disulfonate, are shown in Fig. 1. Reduction of the dye is characterized by the disappearance of the peak at 610 nm observed for the oxidized dye and the appearance of an equally prominent peak at 370

nm for the reduced dye. These changes are superimposed on the decrease at 456 nm observed for the reduction of the cysteinyl-FAD from the oxidized form to the semiquinone. The concomitant increase at 412 nm appears as a shoulder on the reduced dye peak. The calculated ratios of oxidized/semiquinone FAD are plotted against those for the oxidized/reduced dye in Fig. 1 (inset). The difference between the potential of the reference dye and the enzyme is determined from the value when ln(oxidized/reduced dye) is zero.

After the yield of flavin semiquinone had stabilized at its maximum value and the reduction of the first dye was completed, a second reference dye was added anaerobically. The concomitant reduction of enzyme and dye was followed spectrophotometrically as before. Selected spectra for the second electron reduction of MAO B (semiquinone to fully reduced) are shown in Fig. 2. Here, the spectra of the fully reduced indigo disulfonate and the increasing amounts of re-

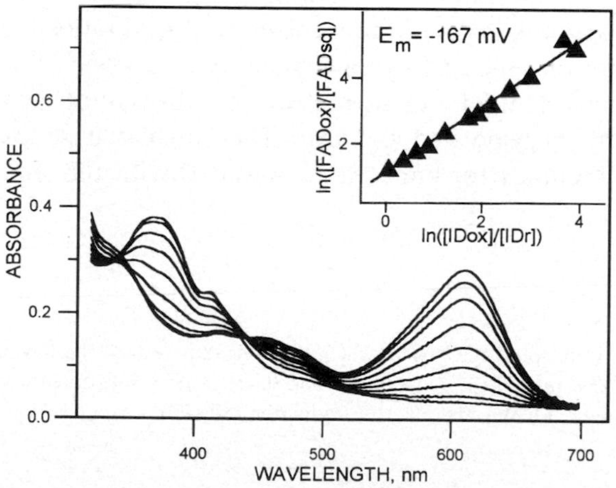

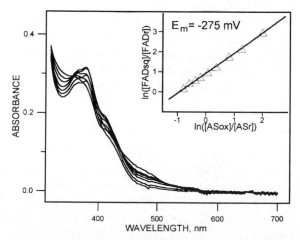

Fig. 1. Determination of the redox potential for the reduction of MAO B from the oxidized to semiquinone form. MAO B (7 μM) and indigo disulfonate (ID) (8 μM) were reduced with xanthine oxidase as described in Methods. In the course of the reaction the peak at 610 nm (oxidized dye) disappears, the peak at 456 nm (oxidized FAD), and decreases new bands of absorbance at 380 nm (reduced dye) and 412 nm (flavin semiquinone) appear. Ratios of $[FAD_{ox}]/[FAD_{sq}]$ and $[ID_{ox}]/[ID_r]$ for the plot in the inset were calculated as described in text.

Fig. 2. Determination of the redox potential for the reduction of MAO B from the semiquinone to the fully reduced form. At the end point of the reaction of Fig. 1, anthraquinone-2-sulfonate (AS) (7 μM) was added. In this reaction there is significant bleaching of the absorbance at 330 nm (oxidized dye), and increase at 390 nm (reduced dye), as well as disappearance of the flavin semiquinone peak (412 nm) on the shoulder of the peak of the reduced dye. Ratios of $[FAD_{ox}]/[FAD_{sq}]$ and $[AS_{ox}]/[AS_r]$ for the plot in the inset were calculated using linear regression analysis.

duced anthraquinone-2-sulfonate are superimposed in the 400 nm region so that the decreasing absorbance at 412 nm and at 456 nm due to the conversion of the semiquinone to the reduced flavin is obscured. However, molar fractions of the individual species can be calculated using linear regression analysis. Fig. 2 (inset) is the double logarithmic plot for the semiquinone/reduced FAD ratio against the ratio of oxidized/reduced dye. To ensure equilibrium, the determinations were repeated with various concentrations of xanthine oxidase to regulate the rate of electron generation.

From the midpoint potentials relative to the dyes and the absolute values (relative to the standard hydrogen electrode) determined for the dyes from cyclic voltametry, values for the redox potentials for MAO A and MAO B in the absence of substrate were obtained. From the data in Figs. 1 and 2 and repeated experiments, the potentials for MAO B were -167 ± 4 mV and -275 ± 3 mV for the first and second electron, respectively. From similar experiments the potentials obtained for MAO A were -159 ± 4 mV and -262 ± 3 mV. From the single-electron redox potentials, the calculated two-electron potential for the unliganded enzyme would be -210 mV for MAO A and -221 mV for MAO B. These values are close to those obtained for free FAD in solution at pH 7.2 (-208 mV) (Draper and Ingraham, 1968).

Although the anionic flavin semiquinone is formed during partial reduction of MAO by dithionite (Weyler and Salach, 1985) or by the xanthine oxidase method used here, reduction by substrate always yields fully reduced flavin. We determined the potentials of both MAO A and B in the presence of both substrates and inhibitors (Table 3). For the inhibitors, the xanthine oxidase method was used as for the free enzyme. However, substrates reduce the flavin so no external source of electrons is required, but the rate of reduction must be slow enough that the redox state of the MAO flavin remains in equilibrium with the reporter dye. The concentration of substrate was set at > 50 K_m to ensure that all the enzyme was complexed with substrate at equilibrium, so that the redox potentials determined are those for the enzyme-substrate complex.

Figure 3 shows the reduction of MAO B and indigo disulfonate by α-methylbenzylamine over a period of 150 min. As expected, there is no sign of semiquinone formation. The double logarithmic plots of the oxidized/reduced ratios for the enzyme and dye are linear with a slope of 1, consistent with the two-electron reduction of both the enzyme and the dye. The calculated redox potentials for both MAO A and B with this and

TABLE 3

Redox potentials for MAO A and B in the absence and presence of ligands and the rate at which these ligands reduce the flavin. The redox potentials (E_m) were determined as described in the text. The rate of the reduction of the flavin (k_3) by substrates was determined anaerobically. The potentials in the presence of inhibitors are for the first electron reduction only (*).

Ligand	MAO A		MAO B	
	E_m (mV)	k_3 (min^{-1})	E_m (mV)	k_3 (min^{-1})
None	-210	–	-221	–
Serotonin	–	–	$+194 \pm 9$	5.82
Benzylamine	$+263 \pm 15$	3.6	–	–
α-Methyl-BA	-116 ± 4	0.012	$+281 \pm 12$	0.042
Amphetamine	-176 ± 5	~ 0	–	–
1-Methyl-4-styrylpyridinium	-158 ± 4*	–	–	–

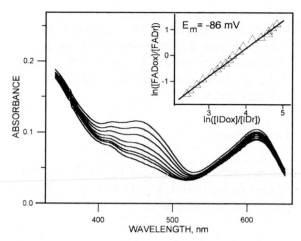

Fig. 3. Reduction of MAO B and indigo disulfonate by α-methylbenzylamine and the determination of the two-electron redox potential of flavin in the presence of saturating concentration of the substrate. Ratios of $[FAD_{ox}]/[FAD_{sq}]$ and $[ID_{ox}]/[ID_r]$ for the plot in the inset were calculated at 440 nm and at 610 nm, respectively.

other substrates are shown in Table 3. Each substrate raises the potential of the flavin but the values obtained are different for each substrate and for each enzyme. Thus, α-methylbenzylamine-saturated MAO A has a redox potential of -116 mV but α-methylbenzylamine-saturated MAO B has a redox potential of -86 mV.

The redox potentials for MAO A and B in the presence of saturating concentrations of inhibitors were also determined. 1-Methyl-4-styrylpyridinium (MS^+) is the four-electron oxidation product of 1-methyltetrahydrostilbazole and is a competitive inhibitor of the steady-state turnover of both MAO A ($K_i = 2.7\ \mu M$) and B ($K_i = 100\ \mu M$) (Sablin et al., 1994). It has no effect on the redox potentials for the first electron for either enzyme (Table 3) nor does it prevent the formation of the semiquinone in the xanthine oxidase-based procedure. The slopes of the double logarithmic plots in this case are 0.5 as expected for one-electron reduction of the enzyme in the presence of a two-electron reporter dye (indigo disulfonate). The other inhibitor used was D-amphetamine, which inhibits the oxidation of kynuramine by MAO A with a K_i of 14 μM

(Weyler et al., 1990b) and of benzylamine by MAO B with a K_i of 3.1 μM (Weyler and Salach, 1984). Amphetamine is, in fact, a slow substrate (Weyler and Salach, 1984) but reduction of the flavin was extremely slow under anaerobic conditions so the xanthine oxidase method was used to provide reducing equivalents. The redox potentials are given in Table 3. Unlike true substrates, amphetamine does not increase the redox potential of the cysteinyl-FAD in MAO. Indeed, the values obtained are marginally lower than those obtained for the unliganded enzyme.

From Table 3 we can see the first indication of an explanation for the ability of MAO to oxidize amines despite the thermodynamically unfavorable difference in the redox potentials of the amine and the flavin. For both MAO A and B, a poor substrate (slow k_3) increases the potential only modestly but the better substrate increases it by more. If one extrapolates from these points, kynuramine might be expected to increase the redox potential of MAO A to about 0 mV and benzylamine to increase that of MAO B to about $+10$ mV. More data are required to establish this. We can also speculate that binding of the amine to MAO might decrease the redox potential of the amine, so that the barrier to the transfer of electrons from the more positive amine to the flavin is substantially reduced.

In contrast, the effect of substrate binding on the potential does not seem to explain the substrate stimulation of the rate of reoxidation of the reduced flavin. On the whole, the greater the difference between the flavin and oxygen, the faster should be the rate of transfer of electrons, but the unliganded enzyme has the greatest difference and the slowest rate of reoxidation. If indeed the redox potential correlates with k_3 as is indicated by the data above, we can compare k_3 and k_{ox} to see if there is a trend. From the few examples shown in Table 4, there is clearly no correlation. This lack of correlation holds for all the substrates studied with both MAO A and B (Tan and Ramsay, 1993). The explanation of the distinct effect of substrate, as opposed to product, on the reoxidation must lie elsewhere. As an

TABLE 4

The enhancement by substrate of the rate of reoxidation of MAO A does not correlate with the rate of reduction by that substrate. The values for the rates of the reductive and oxidative half-reactions are taken from Tan and Ramsay (1993).

Substrate	MAO A		MAO B	
	k_3 (s^{-1})	k_{ox} (s^{-1})	k_3 (s^{-1})	k_{ox} (s^{-1})
Kynuramine	3.1	120	13.6	2.17
Serotonin	2.1	5.7	0.097	1.7
MPTP	0.2	40	3.7	6.0
Benzylamine	0.06	23	10.9	7.6

additional point, it should be noted that the only stable products (the quaternary amines, such as MPP$^+$ or MS$^+$) do not stimulate reoxidation (Tan and Ramsay, 1993), nor do they affect the redox potential (Table 3). It seems unlikely that the imine products, which have been suggested to be responsible for the stimulation of the reoxidation by others (Walker and Edmondson, 1994), do so either.

Conclusions

1. The redox potentials of the cysteinyl-FAD in unliganded MAO A and B are close to that for free flavin.
2. The redox potential in the enzyme-substrate complex is positively shifted towards the potential of the amine substrate. This shift is different for each substrate. The values for the redox potentials for MAO in the presence of physiological substrates remain to be determined.
3. The rate of reduction of the flavin by substrate correlates with the redox potential, i.e., an increase in the potential of the flavin favors electron transfer from amine to flavin, resolving the conundrum of the transfer of electrons from the high potential amines to the much lower potential flavin which has puzzled MAO researchers for decades.

4. The substrate site influences the flavin very specifically depending on the ligand, in both MAO A and B. The amino acids involved in the binding of substrate remain unknown and provide the challenge for the next advances in understanding MAO.

Ackowledgements

This research was supported by the National Institutes of Health (HL-16251) and by the Department of Veterans Affairs.

References

Bach, A.W.J., Lan, N.C., Johnson, D.L., Abell, C.W., Bembenek, M.E., Kwan, S.-W., Seeburg, P.H. and Shih, J.C. (1988) cDNA cloning of human liver monoamine oxidase A and B: molecular basis of differences in enzymatic properties. *Proc. Natl. Acad. Sci. USA*, 85: 4934–4938.

Draper, R. and Ingraham, L. (1968) A potentiometric study of the flavin semiquinone equilibrium. *Arch. Biochem. Biophys.*, 125: 802–808.

Fowler, J.S., Macgregor, R.R., Wolf, A.P., Arnett, C.D., Dewey, S.L., Schlyer, D., Christman, D., Logan, J., Smith, M., Sachs, H., Aquilonius, S.M., Bjurling, P., Halldin, C., Hartvig, P., Leeders, K.L., Lundqvist, H., Oreland, L., Stalnacke, C.-G. and Langstrom, B. (1987) Mapping human brain monoamine oxidase A and B with C^{11}-labelled suicide inactivators and PET. *Science*, 235: 481–485.

Husain, M., Edmundson, D.E. and Singer, T.P. (1982) Kinetic studies on the catalytic mechanism of liver monoamine oxidase. *Biochemistry*, 21: 595–600.

Massey, V. (1991) A simple method for the determination of redox potentials. In: B.Curti, S. Ronchi, G. Zanett (Eds.), *Flavins and Flavoproteins* 1990, Walter de Gruyter, New York. pp. 59–66.

Ramsay, R.R. (1991) The kinetic mechanism of monoamine oxidase A. *Biochemistry*, 30: 4624–4629.

Ramsay, R.R., Koerber, S.C. and Singer, T.P. (1987) Stopped-flow studies on the mechanism of the oxidation of N-methyl-4-phenyltetrahydropyridine (MPTP) by bovine liver monoamine oxidase B. *Biochemistry*, 26: 3045–3050.

Sablin, S.O., Krueger, M.J., Singer, T.P., Bachurin, S.O., Kharei, A.B., Efange, S.M.N. and Tkachenko, S.E. (1994) Interaction of tetrahydrostilbazoles with monoamine oxidase A and B. *J. Med. Chem.*, 37: 151–157.

Salach, J.I. (1979) Monoamine oxidase from beef liver mitochondria: simplified isolation procedure, properties, and determination of its cysteinyl flavin content. *Arch. Biochem. Biophys.*, 192: 128–137.

Silverman, R.B. (1992) Electron transfer chemistry of monoamine oxidase. *Adv. Electron Transfer Chem.*, 2: 177–213.

Singer, T.P. (1991) Monoamine oxidases. In: F. Muller (Ed.), *Chemistry and Biochemistry of Flavoenzymes*, Vol. III, CRC Press, Boca Raton, FL, pp. 437–470.

Tan, A.K. and Ramsay, R.R. (1993) Substrate-specific enhancement of the oxidative half-reaction of monoamine oxidase. *Biochemistry*, 32: 2137–2143.

Tan, A.K., Weyler, W., Salach, J.I. and Singer, T.P. (1991) Differences in substrate specificities of monoamine oxidase A from human liver and placenta. *Biochem. Biophys. Res. Commun.*, 181: 1084–1088.

Thorpe, L.W., Westlund, K.N., Kochersperger, L.M., Abell, C.W. and Denney, R.M. (1987) Immunocytochemical localization of monoamine oxidases A and B in human peripheral tissues and brain. *J. Histochem. Cytochem.*, 35: 23–32.

Walker, M.C. and Edmundson, D.E. (1994) Structure-activity relationships in the oxidation of benzylamine analogues by bovine liver mitochondrial monoamine oxidase B. *Biochemistry*, 33: 7088–7098.

Weyler, W. and Salach, J.I. (1984) Non-stereospecific reduction of monoamine oxidase from bovine liver by analogs of amphetamine. In: R. C. Bray, P. C. Engel, S. G. Mayhew (Eds.), *Flavins and Flavoproteins* 1984, Walter de Gruyter, Berlin—New York, pp. 595–598.

Weyler, W. and Salach, J.I. (1985) Purification and properties of mitochondrial monoamine oxidase type A from human placenta. *J. Biol. Chem.*, 260: 13199–13207.

Weyler, W., Hsu, Y.-P.P. and Breakefield, X.O. (1990a) Biochemistry and genetics of monoamine oxidase. *Pharmacol. Ther.*, 47: 391–417.

Weyler, W., Titlow, C. C. and Salach, J.I. (1990b) Catalytically active monoamine oxidase type A from human liver expressed in *Saccharomyces cerevisiae* contains covalent FAD. *Biochem. Biophys. Res. Commun.*, 173: 1205–1211.

Peter M. Yu, Keith F. Tipton and Alan A. Boulton (Eds.)
Progress in Brain Research, Vol 106
© 1995 Elsevier Science BV. All rights reserved.

CHAPTER 4

Stereochemistry and cofactor identity status of semicarbazide-sensitive amine oxidases

Monica M. Palcic[1], Christine H. Scaman[1] and Gordon Alton[2]

[1]*Department of Chemistry, University of Alberta, Edmonton, Alberta, Canada T6G 2G2, and* [2]*Department of Food Science and Nutrition, University of Alberta, Edmonton, Alberta, Canada T6G 2G2*

Introduction

Several classes of enzymes catalyze the oxidative deamination of amines, converting them to their corresponding aldehydes with the release of ammonia and hydrogen peroxide. These include the flavin-containing monoamine oxidases (EC 1.4.3.4), copper amine oxidases (EC 1.4.3.6), lysyl oxidases (EC 1.4.3.13) and semicarbazide-sensitive amine oxidases (SSAOs) (Mondovi, 1985). The flavin monoamine oxidases (MAOs) have been the subject of intensive investigation following the observation that certain inhibitors of MAO can be used clinically to alleviate depression. The flavin enzymes are a distinct class, since they are not inhibited by semicarbazide and other carbonyl reagents that inactivate the other three types of enzyme.

The relationship between the SSAOs and copper amine oxidase enzymes, however, is unclear. The copper enzymes are ubiquitous, they are found in bacteria, fungi, yeast, plants, mammalian serum and tissues (McIntire and Hartmann, 1992). In addition to copper, these soluble enzymes contain a redox cofactor, the quinone of 2,4,5-trihydroxyphenylalanine (topa) which is reduced and reoxidized during the catalytic cycle (Janes et al., 1990, 1992). The cofactor arises by a post- or co-translational modification of a tyrosine in the protein backbone with the consensus sequence Asn-Tyr-Asp/Glu (Janes et al., 1992; Mu et al., 1992). Membrane-bound semicarbazide-sensitive amine oxidases are found in many tissues, including smooth muscle tissue, adipose tissue, and aorta (Coquil et al., 1973; Lewinsohn, 1981; Barrand and Callingham, 1984; Callingham and Barrand, 1987; Hysmith and Boor, 1987; Precious and Lyles, 1988; Raimondi et al., 1993). Their copper dependence has not been shown and they generally have a greater affinity (lower K_m) for the nonphysiological amine benzylamine compared to the copper amine oxidases. Both classes are glycoproteins with subunit molecular weights of approx. 90 kDa (Callingham and Barrand, 1987).

The overall kinetic reaction scheme for these enzymes is similar. After amine binding to oxidized enzyme and formation of an $E_{ox} \cdot S$ complex, proton abstraction from C-1 of substrate occurs concomitant with enzyme cofactor reduction. The imine formed is hydrolyzed by water, giving an aldehyde product and ammonia. Reoxidation of the reduced enzyme by molecular oxygen completes the catalytic cycle.

$$E_{ox} + {}^+NH_3 - CH_2 - R$$
$$\rightleftharpoons E_{ox} \cdot {}^+NH_3 - CH_2 - R$$
$$\rightleftharpoons E_{red}^+ NH = CH - R + H_2O$$
$$\rightarrow E_{red} NH_2 + O = CH\text{-}R$$
$$E_{red} NH_2 + O_2 \rightarrow E_{ox} + H_2O_2 + NH_3$$

In this article we will compare and contrast the spectral properties of the cofactors and stereochemical studies of substrate oxidation for the soluble copper amine oxidases and membrane associated SSAO.

Stereochemical studies on amine oxidases

The copper topaquinone amine oxidases are a unique class of enzyme since all possible modes of proton abstraction from C-1 of substrates have been observed (Table 1). The pea seedling, soybean seedling, chick pea seedling and porcine kidney enzymes remove the pro-S hydrogen from C-1 of tyramine, dopamine or phenethylamine substrates, while the porcine and horse plasma enzymes are pro-R specific. Sheep, bovine and rabbit plasma enzymes exhibit mirror-image binding and catalysis with net nonstereospecific proton removal (Table 1). The membrane-bound semicarbazide-sensitive amine oxidases and lysyl oxidase react with abstraction of the pro-S hydrogen, while the flavin monoamine oxidases, (MAO A and MAO B) from all sources exhibit pro-R specificity.

In addition to the main catalytic pathway, a side-reaction of imine-enamine tautomerization has been found to occur in some of the enzymes

TABLE 1

Summary of stereochemistry of proton abstraction and solvent exchange with tyramine, dopamine or phenethylamine substrates by amine oxidases

Enzyme source	C-1 proton abstraction	C-2 solvent exchange	Reference
Copper amine oxidases (EC 1.4.3.6)			
Porcine plasma	pro-R	Yes	a,b
Horse plasma	pro-R	Yes	c
Beef plasma	nonstereospecific	Yes a,b,d,e,f	
Sheep plasma	nonstereospecific	Yes	b
Rabbit plasma	nonstereospecific	Yes	b
Pea seedling	pro-S	No	a,f,g,h
Soybean seedling	pro-S	No	b
Chick pea seedling	pro-S	No	b
Pig kidney	pro-S	No	b,f
Semicarbazide-sensitive amine oxidases			
Porcine aorta	pro-S	Yes	i
Beef aorta	pro-S	Yes	i
Rat aorta	pro-S	not determined	f
Lysyl oxidase (EC 1.4.3.13)			
Beef aorta	pro-S	Yes	j
Flavin monoamine oxidases (EC 1.4.3.4)			
Beef liver (MAO B)	pro-R	No	f,k
Human placenta (MAO A)	pro-R	not determined	l
Rat liver (MAO A and B)	pro-R	not determined	h,l,m

Studies quoted: (a) Coleman et al. (1989); (b) Coleman et al. (1991); (c) this report; (d) Summers et al. (1979); (e) Farnum and Klinman (1986); (f) Yu (1988); (g) Battersby et al. (1979); (h) Battersby et al. (1980); (i) Scaman and Palcic (1992); (j) Shah et al. (1993); (k) Lovenberg and Beaven (1971); (l) Yu et al. (1986); (m) Belleau et al. (1960).

whereby a proton at the β-position of the substrate exchanges with a proton from solvent (Lovenberg and Beaven, 1971).

$$E_{red}^{+}NH = CH\text{-}CH_2 \rightleftharpoons E_{red}NH\text{-}CH = CH\text{-}R$$

Within the different classes there is a strong correlation between the solvent exchange pathway and the stereochemical course of proton abstraction at C-1. For the copper amine oxidases, the pro-R and nonstereospecific enzymes catalyze the exchange process, while the pro-S enzymes do not (Table 1). The stereochemical course of the exchange process is identical for all of the copper topaquinone enzymes; loss of the proton is nonstereospecific, while reprotonation occurs mainly with pro-R specificity (Farnum and Klinman, 1986; Scaman et al., unpublished results).

Lysyl oxidase and SSAO both exhibit the solvent exchange pathway. In contrast to the copper amine oxidases, exchange occurs in a stereospecific manner, with loss and reprotonation exhibiting pro-R specificity (Scaman and Palcic, 1992; Shah et al., 1993). To date, none of the flavin monoamine oxidases have been shown to catalyze solvent exchange. These stereochemical studies suggest that lysyl oxidase and the membrane-associated semicarbazide-sensitive amine oxidases are closely related mechanistically in a manner distinct from the copper topaquinone enzymes.

Quinoid nature of the SSAO cofactor

The organic cofactor in tissue-bound SSAO has long been recognized to contain a carbonyl functional group. In this manuscript we confirm that SSAO is a quinoprotein by using the specific redox-cycling staining method of Paz et al. (1991). In this method quinones oxidize glycine at alkaline pH. The superoxide anion released in the reaction reduces nitroblue tetrazolium (NBT) to formazan, yielding a distinct blue-purple color. The method will detect all quinoids, including topaquinone and pyrroloquinoline quinone. Protein samples are first separated by sodium dodecyl sulfate polyacrylamide gel electrophoresis. The separated proteins are electrophoretically transferred from the polyacrylamide gel onto nitrocellulose paper which can be stained with NBT/glycinate or a protein-specific stain. Paz et al. (1991) have used this procedure to demonstrate that lysyl oxidase and bovine plasma amine oxidase are quinoproteins. This method has been

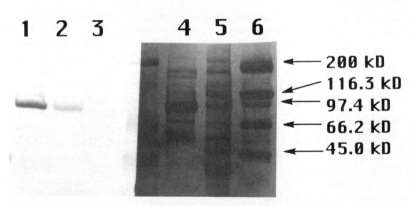

Fig. 1. NBT/glycinate and protein staining of pea seedling amine oxidase and bovine semicarbazide-sensitive amine oxidase on a SDS-PAGE electroblot. Lanes 1 and 4, bovine plasma amine oxidase obtained from Sigma; lanes 2 and 5, partially purified bovine aorta semicarbazide-sensitive amine oxidase; lanes 3 and 6, molecular weight standard proteins. Lanes 1–3 were stained for quinoproteins with NBT/glycinate, lanes 4–6 for protein with Coomassie R-250. Equal amounts of protein were used for protein and quinoprotein staining for bovine plasma amine oxidase and the standards; for SSAO 5-times more protein was required for quinoprotein detection.

used to confirm the quinoprotein nature of SSAO partially purified from bovine aorta by detergent extraction, ion-exchange and lentil lectin chromatography to a final specific activity of 0.07 units/mg protein (Scaman and Palcic, 1992). Figure 1 shows the quinoprotein staining of electroblotted samples of commerical bovine plasma amine oxidase and bovine aorta semicarbazide-sensitive amine oxidase in lanes 1 and 2. There is one quinoprotein-positive band at a molecular weight of approx. 90 kDa for both of the samples. Staining for protein with Coomassie R-250 (lanes 4 and 5) gives multiple bands. Protein standards are run in lanes 3 and 6. Treatment of SSAO with *p*-nitrophenylhydrazine or semicarbazide completely abolishes all catalytic activity and these samples no longer give a quinoprotein positive band.

UV-visible spectral properties of derivatized copper amine oxidases and SSAO

Topaquinone is readily derivatized in native proteins by reaction with phenylhydrazine or *p*-nitrophenylhydrazine (Janes et al., 1992; Palcic and Janes, in press). The visible spectral properties of the *p*-nitrophenylhydrazine adducts are unique to topaquinone and can be used to identify the cofactor. These spectral characteristics are demonstrated for the soluble copper amine oxidase obtained from pea seedlings in Fig. 2C. At neutral pH (7.2), the derivative is a bright yellow color with an absorbance peak maximum at 463 nm (Fig. 2C). In basic solution (2 M KOH) there is a shifting of the absorbance spectrum to 581 nm with the generation of a new purple chromophore (Fig. 2C). This spectral shift is attributed to the ionization of the azo group of the derivatized cofactor as shown in Fig. 3. A pK_a of 12.2 has been measured by titration of the *p*-nitrophenylhydrazine adduct of a model topaquinone hydantoin (Mure and Klinman, 1993) thus deprotonation is essentially complete at pH values of 14.3 used for the characterization of the cofactor. All topaquinone enzymes examined thus far exhibit similar spectral properties. These in-

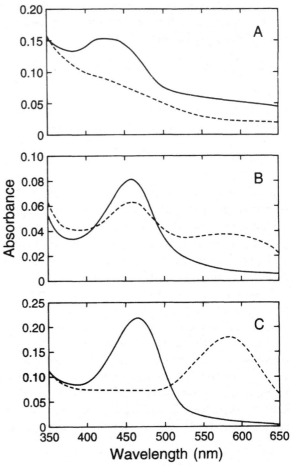

Fig. 2. Visible absorbance spectra of *p*-nitrophenylhydrazine or phenylhydrazine-derivatized amine oxidases. A. Spectra of the phenylhydrazone adduct of bovine aorta semicarbazide-sensitive amine oxidase in 0.1 M potassium phosphate buffer, pH 7.2 (—) and in 2.8 M KOH solution (----). B. Spectra of *p*-nitrophenylhydrazone adduct of bovine aorta semicarbazide-sensitive amine oxidase in 0.1 M potassium phosphate buffer, pH 7.2 (—) and in 2 M KOH solution (----). C. Spectra of pea seedling copper topaquinone amine oxidase in 0.1 M potassium phosphate buffer, pH 7.2 (—) and in 2 M KOH solution (----).

clude mammalian, plant and bacterial sources (Palcic and Janes, in press) with maxima at neutral pH found at 457–472 nm with a 120 nm shift in basic solution to 578–587 nm.

The spectra of *p*-nitrophenylhydrazine-derivatized bovine aorta semicarbazide-senstive amine

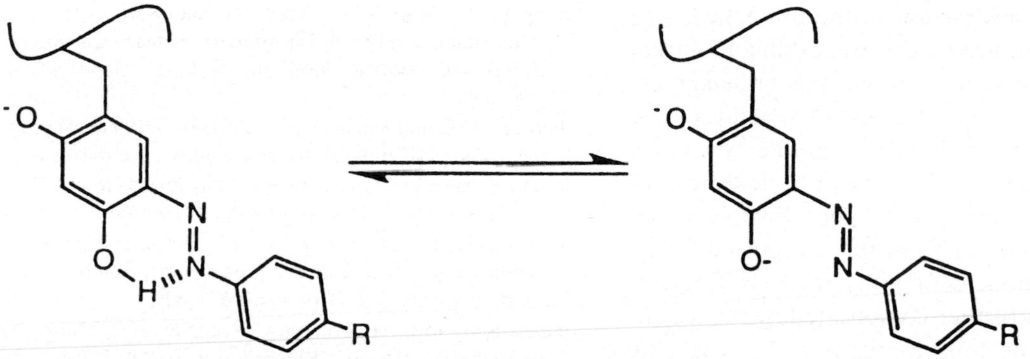

R = H   phenylhydrazine adduct

R = NO$_2$ *p*-nitrophenylhydrazine adduct

Fig. 3. Proposed structures for the phenylhydrazine and *p*-nitrophenylhydrazine derivatives of topaquinone at pH 7 (left) and pH 14 (right).

oxidase is shown in Fig. 2B. The spectrum at pH 7.2 has an absorbance maximum of 456 nm, similar to that of topaquinone-containing enzymes. However, unlike the topa enzymes the spectral shift in 2 M KOH is incomplete, suggesting that the pK_a of the carbonyl cofactor of bovine SSAO is greater than 12.2.

The spectrum of phenylhydrazine-derivatized bovine aorta SSAO is shown in Fig. 2A. The maximal wavelength at neutral pH is 428 nm; however, in basic solution (1–2.8 M KOH) the spectrum bleaches. This is unlike the pattern observed for topaquinone enzymes. These have absorbance maxima at 437–447 nm (Janes et al., 1992) which shift about 50 nm to 480–490 nm in basic solution. There was no evidence for a spectral shift for SSAO, only bleaching is observed. It should also be noted that there is some difficulty in reproducibly derivatizing SSAO, and some preparations of the enzyme do not yield the characteristic chromophores shown in Fig. 2A and B.

The spectral properties of SSAO derivatives do not provide conclusive evidence for topaquinone as the organic cofactor in these enzymes. As well, all topaquinone enzymes characterized to date have the consensus sequence of Asn-Tyr-Asp/Glu

where the tyrosine is further oxidized to generate the cofactor (Mu et al., 1992; Janes et al., 1992). While no sequence information is available for any SSAO, the stereochemically closely related enzyme lysyl oxidase has been cloned and sequenced and does not contain this topaquinone motif (Trackman et al., 1990). Work is continuing in our laboratory to sequence bovine aorta semicarbazide-sensitive amine oxidase and to isolate derivatized active-site peptides to elucidate the cofactor structure.

Summary

The relationship between the soluble copper topaquinone amine oxidases, the membrane bound semicarbazide-sensitive amine oxidases and lysyl oxidase remains unclear. The stereochemical course of substrate oxidation has been determined for each enzyme type and these studies suggest that SSAO and lysyl oxidase are closely related mechanistically, and that they are distinct from the copper amine oxidases. Both lysyl oxidase and SSAO catalyze the oxidation of tyramine with removal of the pro-*S* hydrogen from C-1 of this substrate. The copper amine oxidase enzymes that react with abstraction of the pro-*S* hydrogen from C-1 of substrates do not exhibit a solvent exchange pathway. In contrast, this exchange occurs in lysyl oxidase and SSAO reactions. The organic cofactor in all three enzyme types is a quinone; however, the spectral features of phenylhydrazine and *p*-nitrophenylhydrazine-derivatized SSAO differ from those reported for all known topaquinone-containing enzymes. Cofactor identification is further complicated by the lack of the characteristic topa motif, Asn-Tyr-Asp/Glu, in lysyl oxidase and the absence of any sequence information for SSAO.

Acknowledgements

This work was funded by the Natural Sciences and Engineering Research Council of Canada and the Alberta Heritage Foundation for Medical Research.

References

Barrand, M.A. and Callingham, B.A. (1984) Solubilization and some properties of a semicarbazide-sensitive amine oxidase in brown adipose tissue of the rat. *J. Biochem.*, 222: 467–475.

Battersby, A.R., Staunton, J., and Summers, M.C. (1979) Stereochemistry of oxidative ring cleavage adjacent to nitrogen during the biosynthesis of chelidonine. *J. Chem. Soc. Perkin Trans.*, 1: 45–52.

Battersby, A.R., Chrystal, E.J. T. and Staunton, J. (1980) Studies of enzyme-mediated reactions Part 12. Stereochemical course of the decarboxylations of (2*S*)-tyrosine to tyramine by microbial, mammalian and plant systems. *J. Chem. Soc. Perkin Trans.*, 1: 31–42.

Belleau, B., Fang, M., Burba, J. and Moran, J. (1960) Absolute optical specificity of monoamine oxidase. *J. Am. Chem. Soc.*, 82: 5752–5754.

Callingham, B.A. and Barrand M.A. (1987) Some properties of semicarbazide-sensitive amine oxidases. *J. Neural. Transm. [Suppl.]*, 23: 37–54.

Coleman, A.A., Hindsgaul, O. and Palcic, M.M. (1989) Stereochemistry of copper amine oxidase reactions. *J. Biol. Chem.*, 264: 19500–19505.

Coleman, A.A., Scaman, C.H., Kang, Y.J. and Palcic, M.M. (1991) Stereochemical trends in copper amine oxidase reactions. *J. Biol. Chem.*, 266: 6795–6800.

Coquil, J.F., Goridis, C., Mack, G. and Neff, N.H. (1973) Monoamine oxidase in rat arteries: evidence for different forms and selective localization. *Br. J. Pharmacol.*, 48: 590–599.

Farnum, M.F. and Klinman, J.P. (1986) Stereochemical probes of bovine plasma amine oxidase: evidence for mirror image processing and a syn abstraction of hydrogens from C-1 and C-2 of dopamine. *Biochemistry*, 25: 6028–6036.

Hysmith, R.M. and Boor, P.J. (1987) Purification of benzylamine oxidase from cultured porcine aortic smooth muscle cells. *Biochem. Cell. Physiol.*, 66: 821–829.

Janes, S.M., Mu., D., Wemmer, D., Smith, A.J., Maltby, D., Burlingame, A.L. and Klinman, J.P. (1990) A new redox cofactor in eukaryotic enzymes: 6-hydroxydopa at the active site of bovine serum amine oxidase. *Science*, 248: 981–987.

Janes, S.M., Palcic, M.M., Scaman, C.H., Smith, A.J., Brown, D.E., Dooley, D.M., Mure, M. and Klinman, J.P. (1992) Identification of topaquinone and its consensus sequence in copper amine oxidases. *Biochemistry*, 31: 12147–12154.

Lovenberg, W. and Beaven, M.A. (1971) The release of tritium upon deamination of 3,4-dihydroxy[2-^{3}H]phenethylamine by plasma amine oxidase. *Biochim. Biophys. Acta*, 251: 452–455.

Lewinsohn, R. (1981) Amine oxidase in human blood vessels and non-vascular smooth muscle. *J. Pharm. Pharmacol.*, 33: 569–575.

McIntire, W.S. and Hartmann C. (1992) Copper containing amine oxidases. In: V.L. Davidson (Ed.), *Principles and Applications of Quinoproteins*, Marcel Dekker, New York, pp. 97–171.

Mondovi, B. (Ed.) (1985) *Structure and Functions of Amine Oxidases*, CRC Press, Boca Raton, 284 pp.

Mu, D., Janes, S.M., Smith, A.J., Brown, D.E., Dooley, D.M. and Klinman, J.P. (1992) Tyrosine codon corresponds to topa quinone at the active site of copper amine oxidases. *J. Biol. Chem.*, 267: 7979–7982.

Mure, M. and Klinman, J.P. (1993) Synthesis and spectroscopic characterization of model compounds for the active site cofactor in copper amine oxidases. *J. Am. Chem. Soc.*, 115: 7117–7127.

Palcic, M.M. and Janes, S.M. (1994) Spectrophotometric detection of topaquinone. *Methods Enzymol.*, in press.

Paz, M.A., Fluckiger, R., Boak, A., Kagan, H.M. and Gallop, P.M. (1991) Specific detection of quinoproteins by redox-cycling staining. *J. Biol. Chem.*, 266: 689–692.

Precious, E. and Lyles, G.A. (1988) Properties of a semicarbazide-sensitive amine oxidase in human umbical artery. *J. Pharm. Pharmacol.*, 40: 627–633.

Raimondi, L., Conforti, L., Banchelli, G., Ignesti, G., Pirisino, R. and Buffoni, F. (1993) Histamine lipolytic activity and semicarbazide-sensitive amine oxidase (SSAO) of rat white adipose tissue (WAT). *Biochem. Pharmacol.*, 46: 1369–1376.

Scaman, C.H. and Palcic, M.M. (1992) Stereochemical course of tyramine oxidation by semicarbazide-sensitive amine oxidase. *Biochemistry*, 31: 6829–6841.

Shah, M.A., Scaman, C.H., Palcic, M.M. and Kagan, H.M. (1993) Kinetics and stereospecificity of the lysyl oxidase reaction. *J. Biol. Chem.*, 268: 11573–11579.

Summers, M.C., Markovic, R. and Klinman, J.P. (1979) Stereochemistry and kinetic isotope effects in the bovine plasma amine oxidase catalyzed oxidation of dopamine. *Biochemistry*, 18: 1969–1979.

Trackman, P.C., Pratt, A.M., Wolanski, A., Tang, S.-S., Offner, G. D., Troxler, R.F. and Kagan, H.M. (1990) Cloning of rat aorta lysyl oxidase cDNA: complete codons and predicted amino acid sequence. *Biochemistry*, 29: 4863–4870.

Yu, P.H., Bailey, B.A., Durden, D.A. and Boulton, A. (1986) Stereospecific deuterium substitution at the α-carbon position of dopamine and its effect on oxidative deamination catalyzed by MAO-A and MAO-B from different tissues. *Biochem. Pharmacol.*, 35: 1027–1036.

Yu, P.H. (1988) Three types of stereospecificity and the kinetic deuterium isotope effect in the oxidative deamination of dopamine as catalyzed by different amine oxidases. *Biochem. Cell. Biol.*, 66: 853–861.

Peter M. Yu, Keith F. Tipton and Alan A. Boulton (Eds.)
Progress in Brain Research, Vol 106
© 1995 Elsevier Science BV. All rights reserved.

CHAPTER 5

Expression of human monoamine oxidase (MAO) A gene controlled by transcription factor Sp1

Jean C. Shih, Qin-shi Zhu and Kevin Chen

*Department of Molecular Pharmacology and Toxicology, School of Pharmacy, University of Southern California,
1985 Zonal Avenue, PSC 528, Los Angeles, CA 90033, USA*

Introduction

Monoamine oxidase (MAO) A and B (amine:oxygen oxidoreductase, EC 1.4.3.4) play important roles in regulating levels of biogenic and dietary amines. They catalyze an oxidative deamination and produce ammonia, aldehyde and hydrogen peroxide. The latter product may cause oxidative stress and neuron degeneration. MAO A inhibitors have been used for the treatment of mental depression (Youdim et al., 1988; Tipton, 1989) and the MAO B inhibitor, deprenyl, has been used for Parkinson disease (Parkinson Study Group, 1989, 1993). Recently, aggressive behavior in affected males of a Dutch family was found to be associated with MAO A deficiency (Brunner et al., 1993a,b).

MAO A and B are distinguished by their different substrate preference and inhibitor sensitivities. MAO A preferentially oxidizes serotonin and is sensitive to the inhibitor clorgyline (Johnston, 1968), whereas MAO B preferentially oxidizes phenylethylamine and is sensitive to the inhibitors pargyline and deprenyl (Knoll and Magyar, 1972). Dopamine and tyramine are common substrates for both types of the enzyme. The cloning of cDNAs for human liver MAO A and B (Bach et al., 1988; Hsu et al., 1988) and subsequent expression of the cDNAs in COS cells (Lan et al., 1989) demonstrated that the two types of

enzyme are coded by different genes. The deduced amino acid sequences of human brain, platelet and liver MAO B are the same (Chen et al., 1993). Genomic studies with MAO A and B cDNA as probes showed that both MAO A and B genes consist of 15 exons and exhibit identical exon-intron organizations, suggesting that the two genes are derived from duplication of a common ancestral gene (Grimsby et al., 1991). Systematic mutagenesis of the cysteine residues in MAO A and B proteins has demonstrated the essential role of specific cysteine residues for MAO catalytic activity (Wu et al., 1993).

MAO A and B are co-expressed in most human tissues examined (Grimsby et al., 1990). However, human placenta expresses mainly MAO A (Egashira and Yamanaka, 1981; Grimsby et al., 1990), and human platelets and lymphocytes contain only MAO B (Donnelly and Murphy, 1977). Different expression patterns of MAO A and B are observed in primate brain (Westlund et al., 1985). In human brain, MAO B is found in astrocytes and serotonergic neurons, while MAO A is expressed in catecholaminergic neurons (Fowler et al., 1987; Thorpe et al., 1987). Differential expression of MAO A and B is also observed in cultured cells (Yu and Hertz, 1982; Youdim et al., 1986). The expression of MAO A and B differs during development. MAO A activity appears before MAO B activity in fetal brain (Lewinsohn et al., 1980), whereas MAO B activity is higher than that of MAO A in adult human brain (Garrick and Murphy, 1982). Furthermore, significant variations of MAO A and B activities are observed among different individuals (Murphy et al., 1976; Costa et al., 1980). The molecular basis for these variations is not clear.

In order to understand the mechanisms for MAO gene expression, it is essential to characterize the promoter region of these two genes. We have previously determined the location of promoter for MAO A and B genes (Zhu et al., 1992). MAO A promoter activity is found in a 0.24 kb *Pvu*II/*Dra*II fragment, 62 basepairs (bp) 5′ of the translation start codon ATG. The DNA sequence upstream of this fragment down regulates MAO A promoter activity. Transcription initiation site determined by 5′ RACE PCR is located in the 3′ end of this fragment, 73 bp upstream of the ATG codon (Zhu et al., 1994). Sequence analysis of the 0.24 kb fragment reveals two 90 bp repeats, each containing two binding sites for the transcription factor Sp1. MAO B promoter is found in a 0.15 kb *Pst*I/*Nae*I fragment, 99 bp 5′ of the ATG codon. The DNA sequence upstream of this fragment also down-regulates the promoter activity. Primer extension experiments defined multiple transcription initiation sites, 117 to 169 bp upstream of the ATG. Sequence analysis of this fragment reveals two clusters of overlapping Sp1 binding sites, separated by a CACCC element and followed by a 3′ TAATATA box. Deletion assay shows that all these elements are necessary for maximal promoter activity. The sequences of these two promoters share approx. 60% identity, suggesting that MAO A and B promoters may be derived from a common ancestral promoter. However, none of the transcription factor binding sites is conserved at their corresponding positions, indicating that these two promoters have functionally diverged during evolution. The different promoter organization of MAO A and B genes provides the basis for their different tissue- and cell-specific expression. Our recent progress on the promoter of the human MAO A gene is reported here.

Sp1 site-containing repeats are found in MAO A promoter

The promoter of human MAO A gene is unique in that it consists of two 90 bp repeats with 81% sequence identity (Fig. 1A, the two long arrows I and II; 1B, repeat I is from nucleotide −268 to −179 and repeat II is from nucleotide −178 to −89. The A of the translation start codon ATG is defined as +1; the negative signs indicate positions 5′ of the ATG codon). Four potential Sp1 binding sites are located at the corresponding positions in these two repeats (Fig. 1B, boxed and numbered sequentially from 3′ to 5′). Sequence similarities can also been found in upstream (from −310 to −269, Fig. 1B) and downstream (from −88 to −41) sequences, but no Sp1 site is found in these sequences.

Further analysis of the two 90 bp repeats shows that each repeat can be further divided into two repeats of 42 and 48 bp in length, each containing an Sp1 binding site at corresponding locations (Fig. 1C, repeat 1–4). Sequence homology can also be found in both upstream and downstream sequences.

Sequence homology between the four short repeats is lower than between the two 90 bp repeats. The numbers of nucleotides in the short repeats are different (42 and 48), the identity between the four short repeats is lower (74% of the nucleotides in at least three out of the four repeats are considered conserved; 50% of the nucleotides in all four repeats are considered conserved; the extra six nucleotides in the 48 bp repeats are not included in homology calculation). These repeats increased the number of Sp1 sites in the promoter, and thus created a more efficient promoter. The promoter activity of the two 90 bp repeats (53% for the A0.24 fragment) is twice as great as one repeat (25% for A0.12 fragment; Zhu et al., 1992; Fig. 2).

Sp1 is the major transcription factor interacting with the MAO A promoter

Sequence analysis has revealed four potential Sp1 binding sites in the MAO A promoter. However,

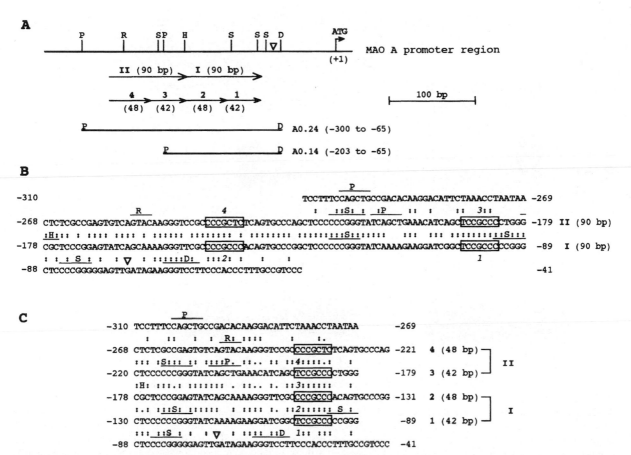

Fig. 1. Direct repeats in MAO A promoter region. A: restriction enzyme map of MAO A promoter region. ATG represents translation start codon. The locations of the two 90 bp repeats (I and II) and the four shorter repeats (1–4) are marked by arrows. The positions of MAO A 0.24 kb *Pvu*II/*Dra*II (A0.24) and 0.14 kb *Pvu*II/*Dra*II (A0.14) fragment are also shown. The transcription initiation site is marked by a triangle (also in B and C). The restriction enzyme sites are represented with a single letter: D, *Dra*II; H, *Hin*pI; P, *Pvu*II; R, *Rsa*I; S, *Sma*I. B: sequence homology between the two 90 bp repeats (I and II). The basepairs conserved in the two repeats are double-dotted (":"). The homology of the upstream (from −310 to −269) and downstream (from −88 to −41) sequences with both repeats is also marked. The four Sp1 binding sites are boxed and numbered sequentially from 3′ to 5′. Restriction enzyme sites are overlined and marked by a single letter as in A. C: the repeats 1–4, which are derived from the two 90 bp repeats I and II. The basepairs conserved in at least three of the four repeats are double-dotted. The single dots represent the conservation interrupted by a not-conserved basepair. For the upstream and downstream sequences, only the basepairs identical to the conserved basepairs in repeats 1–4 are marked. The Sp1 sites and the restriction enzyme sites are marked as in B.

it is not clear whether Sp1 is the major transcription factor binding to the MAO A promoter, since a number of other transcription factors also bind to Sp1 sites. In addition, the MAO A promoter may contain other transcription factor binding sites.

In order to see whether there are additional transcription factor binding sites, a DNase1 footprinting experiment was performed. DNase1 di-

gests the DNA fragment at random positions. In the presence of nuclear extract which contains various transcription factors, the DNA sequences bound by proteins are protected from DNase1 digestion and appear as "bleached" areas in the DNA ladder. The 0.24 kb MAO A promoter fragment (A0.24), radiolabeled at one end, was partially digested with DNase1 in the presence and absence of nuclear proteins from SHSY-5Y

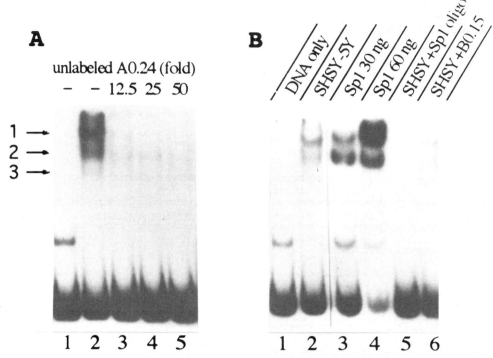

A

unlabeled A0.24 (fold)

−   − 12.5 25 50

1 →
2 →
3 →

1   2   3   4   5

B

DNA only / SHSY-5Y / Sp1 30 ng / Sp1 60 ng / SHSY+Sp1 oligo / SHSY+B0.15

1   2   3   4   5   6

Fig. 2. Gel retardation showing Sp1 binding to MAO A promoter fragment. A: the specificity of nuclear protein binding. The A0.24 kb *Pvu*II/*Dra*II fragment (A0.24) was ^{32}P-end-labeled and incubated with nuclear proteins extracted from SHSY-5Y cells (lane 2). Three retarded bands are numbered and indicated by arrows. The binding was competed with 12.5 (lane 3), 25 (lane 4) and 50 (lane 5) fold excess of unlabeled A0.24 fragment. Lane 1 shows free DNA without nuclear proteins. B: binding of Sp1 to the A0.24 fragment. Lane 1 shows free labeled A0.24 DNA. Lane 2, SHSY-5Y nuclear proteins are the same as in A. The same retarded bands were observed when the A0.24 fragment was incubated with 30 ng (lane 3) and 60 ng (lane 4) purified Sp1. The binding of SHSY-5Y nuclear proteins was competed with Sp1 consensus oligonucleotides (lane 5) or 50-fold excess of the 0.15 kb *Pst*I/*Nae*I MAO B promoter fragment (B0.15, lane 6).

(human neuroblastoma) cells which express MAO A. We found that only the four Sp1 binding sites are protected (Zhu et al., 1994), suggesting that these four sites are the major DNA sequences interacting with transcription factors.

To see whether the transcription factor interacting with the four sites is Sp1, we performed gel retardation experiments, in which a radiolabeled A0.24 fragment was incubated with SHSY-5Y nuclear proteins: the mixture was then separated on a non-denaturing polyacrylamide gel. The protein-DNA complexes, due to their higher molecular weight, were retarded behind the free (unbound) DNA during electrophoresis. The extent of retardation is mainly determined by the total

mass of proteins bound to the DNA fragment. Since the nuclear extract contained a large amount of proteins which bind to DNA without sequence specificity, excess (more than 5000-fold the radiolabeled A0.24) competitive DNA (poly[dI · dC][dI · dC]) was included in the incubation mixture to prevent non-specific DNA-binding proteins interacting with the A0.24 fragment. Under these conditions, only the proteins with high affinity to specific DNA sequences in the A0.24 fragment can bind.

Figure 2A, lane 1, shows the electrophoresis profile of labeled A0.24 fragment in the absence of nuclear proteins. In addition to the free A0.24 DNA band, a slower-moving DNA band can be seen. The nature of this band is not clear. It may represent A0.24 DNA molecules with secondary structures. When SHSY-5Y nuclear proteins were added, two strong (bands 1, 2) and a weaker (band 3) retarded bands could be seen. These bands may represent the A0.24 fragment with different numbers of Sp1 sites occupied by nuclear proteins. These bindings are specific, because unlabeled A0.24 fragment, in amounts less than 1% of the nonspecific competitive DNA, competed effectively with labeled A0.24 fragment for nuclear protein binding (lanes 3, 4, 5, with 12.5-, 25- and 50-fold excess unlabeled A0.24). On the other hand, competition with the MAO B promoter fragment (the 0.15 kb PstI/NaeI fragment, B0.15) was not efficient. A 50-fold excess of B0.15 reduced nuclear protein binding only partially (Fig. 2B, lane 6). This result suggests that the MAO B promoter has lower affinity for Sp1 than A0.24 and may interact with additional transcription factors.

Competition with synthetic oligonucleotides containing a consensus Sp1 binding sequence effectively eliminated Sp1 binding to the labeled A0.24 fragment (lane 5). Furthermore, purified Sp1 formed retarded bands at the same position as the two major bands (compare lanes 3 and 4 with lane 2). These results strongly suggest that Sp1 is the major transcription factor interacting with the MAO A promoter. The nature of the weaker band (band 3) is not clear. It was sensitive to the competition of Sp1 consensus oligonucleotides but was not observed with purified Sp1 under our experiment conditions. It could still be an Sp1-A0.24 complex with fewer Sp1 sites bound than in bands 1 and 2, but at relatively high Sp1 concentrations, as in lanes 3 and 4, more Sp1 sites will occupied, so the concentration of such a complex would be low. At the same time, this band may also represent another factor which interacts with A0.24.

There are a number of other transcription factors that also bind to Sp1 sequences, such as AP-2 (Mitchell et al., 1987), ETF (Kageyama et al., 1988), EGR-1 (Cao et al., 1990) and BTEB (Ohe et al., 1993), but the molecular weights of these factors are different from that of Sp1, so complexes of them with A0.24 DNA should be retarded to different positions in gel retardation experiments, which was not observed. The molecular weight of GCF is similar to that of Sp1, but it is a negative regulator (Kageyama and Pastan, 1989), so is unlikely to be the major protein factor binding to MAO A promoter. Furthermore, AP-2, ETF and EGR-1 are induced by phorbol esters, but the activity of the MAO A promoter is not.

However, our results cannot rule out the possibility that other transcription factors may bind to the Sp1 sites in the MAO A promoter in a way indistinguishable from Sp1 binding in gel retardation and DNase1 footprinting experiments. An Sp1-specific antibody should be able to discriminate these factors. Sp1 contains zinc fingers as its DNA binding motif. Since many transcription factors contain similar zinc fingers and possibly similar activating domains, it is essential that this antibody does not cross-react with these transcription factors. In addition, since we have so far tested only a limited number of cell lines, it is possible that different transcription factors may activate MAO A gene expression in other cells or tissues. Nonetheless, from our experimental results, Sp1 seems to be the major transcription factor interacting with the MAO A promoter.

MAO A promoter and catalytic activity is associated with cellular Sp1 concentration

Different cells vary widely in their MAO A catalytic activity. For example, SHSY-5Y cells have much higher MAO A catalytic activity (3.36 nmol/20 min per mg protein) than Caco2 (human colon carcinoma) cells (0.26 nmol/20 min per mg protein). To see whether this different expression is regulated at the transcription level, Northern analysis was performed. Fig. 3A shows that the level of MAO A mRNA (marked by an arrow) in SHSY-5Y cells (lane 1) is much higher than in Caco2 cells (lane 2), confirming that the MAO A promoter activity in these cells is the main determinant of its expression. In accordance with this, different promoter activities are observed when MAO A promoter fragment is transfected into different cell lines in the expression vector pOGH (Selden et al., 1986), which contains human growth hormone as the reporter gene. For example, a 0.14 kb *Pvu*II/*Dra*II fragment (derived from A0.24 by a 5′ deletion and showing the highest promoter activity; see Zhu et al., 1992) exhibited much higher promoter activity in SHSY-5Y cells (4356 cpm, or 88% of the control metallothionein promoter; Zhu et al., 1992) than in NIH3T3 (mouse fibroblast) cells (332 cpm, or 2% of the control promoter). Since the MAO A promoter in SHSY-5Y and Caco2 cell genome is the same, and the same MAO A promoter fragment (A0.14) was transfected into SHSY-5Y and NIH3T3 cells, the observed difference in MAO A

catalytic and promoter activity is very probably due to the difference in concentration of the transcription factor necessary for MAO A expression.

To test this hypothesis, nuclear proteins were extracted from these three cell lines and their Sp1 concentrations were compared in a gel retardation assay. Fig. 3B shows that the Sp1-A0.24 bands with SHSY-5Y nuclear proteins (lane 1) are much stronger than in NIH3T3 (lane 2) and Caco2 (lane 3) cells. A gel retardation assay with radiolabeled Sp1 consensus oligonucleotides also showed that the Sp1 concentration is higher in the SHSY-5Y nuclear extract (Fig. 3C, lane 1) than in NIH3T3 (lane 2) and Caco2 (lane 3) cells. These results coincide nicely with the difference

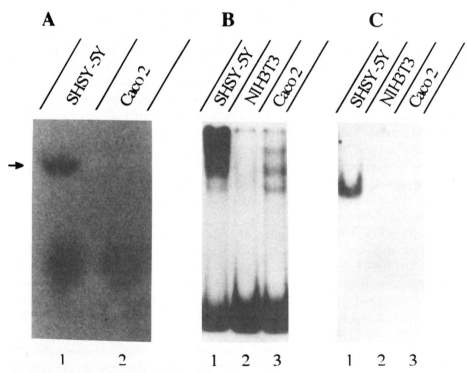

Fig. 3. Correlation of MAO A mRNA and Sp1 concentration in different cell lines. A: Northern blot showing that MAO A mRNA (approx. 5 kb, indicated by an arrow) in SHSY-5Y cells (lane 1) is significant, but is undetectable in Caco2 cells (lane 2). The lower band is 18S rRNA as an internal control for the total RNA in each lane. B and C: gel retardation assays comparing Sp1 concentration in SHSY-5Y (lane 1), NIH3T3 (lane 2) and Caco2 (lane 3) cells. The same amount of nuclear extracts from each cell line was incubated with radiolabeled A0.24 fragment (B) or Sp1 consensus oligonucleotides (C).

in MAO A catalytic and promoter activities measured in these cell lines and suggest that cellular Sp1 is an important controlling factor for MAO A gene expression.

Sp1 is a general transcription factor found in all cells of higher animals and is required for GC-box-containing promoters. Since many housekeeping gene promoters are GC-rich and contain Sp1-binding sites, the existence of Sp1 should be universal. On the other hand, the concentration of Sp1 varies dramatically (as high as 100-fold) from tissue to tissue and during development (Saffer et al., 1991), suggesting that Sp1 has a regulatory role. In other words, Sp1 might be a limiting factor for many promoters. This hypothesis is supported by the elevated transcription of Sp1-dependent genes when the cellular Sp1 concentration becomes higher (Saffer et al., 1990). The positive association between cellular Sp1 concentration and MAO A promoter activity, mRNA level and catalytic activity we observed in cultured cells also suggests an important role for Sp1 in MAO A expression. It would be interesting to investigate further whether the different MAO A catalytic activity in different tissues and development stages or in diseased states is also caused by variation in cellular Sp1 concentration.

We have reported previously that NIH3T3 cells have very high intrinsic MAO A catalytic activity (15.6 nmol/20min per mg protein; Zhu et al., 1992). The low promoter activity exhibited by human MAO A promoter fragment and the low Sp1 concentration in NIH3T3 cells indicate that mouse MAO A promoter is different from human and different transcription factors may be used by mouse cells in activation of MAO A gene expression.

Acknowledgments

The authors wish to thank Ms. Hui Xu for her technical assistance. This work was supported by grant R01 MH37020, R37 MH39085 (Merit Award), and Research Scientist Award K05 MH00796, from the National Institute of Mental Health. Support from the Boyd and Elsie Welin Professorship is also appreciated.

References

Bach, A.W.J., Lan, N.C., Johnson, D.L., Abell, C.W., Bembenek, M.E., Kwan, S-W., Seeberg, P.H. and Shih, J.C. (1988) cDNA cloning of human monoamine oxidase A and B: molecular basis of differences in enzymatic properties. *Proc. Natl. Acad. Sci. USA*, 85: 4934–4938.

Brunner, H.G., Nelen, M.R., van Zandvoort, P., Abeling, N.G.G.M., van Gennip, A.H., Wolters, E.C., Kuiper, M.A., Ropers, H.H. and van Oost, B.A. (1993a) X- linked borderline mental retardation with prominent behavioral disturbance: phenotype, genetic localization, and evidence for disturbed monoamine oxidase metabolism. *Am. J. Hum. Genet.*, 52: 1032–1039.

Brunner, H.G., Nelen, M., Breakefield, X.O., Ropers, H.H. and van Oost, B.A. (1993b) Abnormal behavior associated with a point mutation in the structure gene for monoamine oxidase A. *Science*, 262: 578–580.

Cao, X., Koshi, R.A., Gashler, A., McKieman, M., Morris, C.F., Gaffney, R., Hay, R.V. and Sukhatme, V.P. (1990) Identification and characterization of the EGR-1 product, a DNA binding Zinc finger protein induced by differentiation and growth signals. *Mol. Cell. Biol.*, 10: 1931–1939.

Chen, K., Wu, H.F. and Shih, J.C. (1993) The deduced amino acid sequences of human platalet and frontal cortex monoamine oxidase B are identical. *J. Neurochem.*, 61: 187-190.

Costa, M.R.C., Edelstein, S.B., Castiglione, C.M., Chao, H and Breakefield, X.O. (1980) Properties of monoamine oxidase in control and Lesch-Nyhan fibroblasts. *Biochem. Genet.*, 18: 577–590.

Donnelly, C.H and Murphy, D.L. (1977) Substrate- and inhibitor-related characteristics of human platelet monoamine oxidase. *Biochem. Pharmacol.*, 26: 853–858.

Egashira, T. and Yamanaka, Y. (1981) Further studies on the synthesis of A-form of MAO. *Jpn. J. Pharmacol.*, 31: 763–770.

Fowler, J.B., Macgregor, R.R., Wolf, A.P., Arnett, C.D., Dewey, S.L., Schlyer, D., Christman, D., Logan, J., Smith, M., Sachs, H., Aquilonius, S.M., Bjjurling, P., Halldin, C., Hartvig, P., Leenders, K.L., Lundqvist, H., Oreland, L., Stalnacke, C.-G. and Langstrom, B. (1987) Mapping human brain monoamine oxidase A and B with ^{11}C-labeled suicide inactivators and PET. *Science*, 235: 481–485.

Garrick, N.A. and Murphy, D.L. (1982) Monoamine oxidase type A: differences in selectivity towards norepinephrine compared to serotonin. *Biochem. Pharmacol.*, 31: 4061–4066.

Grimsby, J., Lan, N.C., Neve, R., Chen, K. and Shih, J.C. (1990) Tissue distribution of human monoamine oxidase A and B mRNA. *J. Neurochem.*, 55: 1166–1169.

Grimsby, J., Chen K., Wang, L.J., Lan N.C and Shih, J.C. (1991) Human monoamine oxidase A and B genes exhibit identical exon-intron organization. *Proc. Natl. Acad. Sci. USA*, 88: 3637–3641.

Hsu, Y.P., Weyler, W., Chen, S., Sims, K.B., Rinehart, W.B., Utterback, M., Powell, J.F. and Breakefield, X.O. (1988) Structural features of human monoamine oxidase elucidated from cDNA and peptide sequences. *J. Neurochem.*, 51: 1321–1324.

Johnston, J.P. (1968) Some observations upon a new inhibitor of monoamine oxidase in brain tissue. *Biochem. Pharmacol.*, 17: 1285–1297.

Kageyama, R., Merlino, G.T. and Pastan, I. (1988) A transcription factor active on the epidermal growth factor receptor gene. *Proc. Natl. Acad. Sci. USA*, 85: 5016–5020.

Kageyama, R. and Pastan, I. (1989) Molecular cloning and characterization of a human DNA binding factor that represses transcription. *Cell*, 59: 815–825.

Knoll, J. and Magyar, K. (1972) Some puzzling pharmacological effects of monoamine oxidase inhibitors. In: E. Costa and M. Sandler (eds.), *Advances in Biochemical Psychopharmacology, vol. 5, Monoamine Oxidase—New Vista*, Raven Press, New York, pp. 393–408.

Lan, N.C., Chen, C.H. and Shih, J.C. (1989) Expression of functional human monoamine oxidase A and B cDNAs in mammalian cells. *J. Neurochem.*, 52: 1652- 1654.

Lewinsohn, R., Glover, W. and Sandler, M. (1980) Development of benzylamine oxidase and monoamine oxidase A and B in men. *Biochem Pharmacol.*, 29: 1221–1230.

Mitchell, P.J., Wang, C. and Tjian, R. (1987) Positive and negative regulation of transcription in vitro: enhancer-binding protein AP-2 is inhibited by SV 40 T antigen. *Cell*, 50: 847–861.

Murphy, D.L., Wright, C., Buchsbaum, M., Nichols, A., Costa, J.L. and Wyatt, R.J. (1976) Platelet and plasma amine oxidase activity in 680 normals: sex and age differences and stability over time. *Biochem. Med.*, 16: 254–265.

Ohe, N., Yamasaki, Y., Sogawa, K., Inazawa, J., Ariyama, T., Oshimura, M. and Fujii-Kuriyama, Y. (1993) Chromosomal localization and cDNA sequence of human BTEB, a GC box binding protein. *Somat. Cell Mol. Genet.*, 19: 499–503.

Parkinson Study Group (1989) Effect of deprenyl on the progression of disability in early Parkinson's disease. *N. Engl. J. Med.*, 321: 1364–1371.

Parkinson Study Group (1993) Effects of tocopherol and deprenyl on the progression of disability in early Parkinson's disease. *N. Engl. J. Med.*, 328: 176–183.

Saffer, J.D, Jackson, S.J. and Thurston, S.J. (1990) SV40 stimulates expression of the trans-act factor Sp1 at the mRNA level. *Genes Dev.* , 4: 659–666.

Saffer, J.D., Jackson, S.P. and Annarella, M.B. (1991) Developmental expression of Sp1 in the mouse. *Mol. Cell. Biol.*, 11: 2189–2199.

Selden, R.F., Burke Howie, K., Rowe, M.E., Goodman, H.M. and Moore, D.D. (1986) Human growth hormone as a reporter gene in regulation studies employing transient gene expression. *Mol. Cell. Biol.*, 6: 3173–3179.

Thorpe, L.W., Westlund, K.N., Kochersperger, L.M., Abell, C.W. and Denney, R.M. (1987) Immunocytochemical localization of monoamine oxidase A and B in human peripheral tissues and brain. *J. Histochem. Cytochem.*, 35: 217–236.

Tipton, K.F. (1989) Monoamine oxidase inhibitors as antidepressants. In: K.F. Tipton and M.B.H. Youdim (eds.), *Biochemical and Pharmacological Aspects of Depression.*, Taylor and Francis, London, pp. 1–24.

Westlund, K.N., Denney, R.M., Kochersperger, L.M., Rose, R.M. and Abell, C.W. (1985) Distinct monoamine oxidase A and B populations in primate brain. *Science*, 230: 181–183.

Wu, H.F., Chen, K. and Shih, J.C. (1993) Site-directed mutagenesis of monoamine oxidase A and B: role of cysteine. *Mol. Pharmacol.*, 43: 888–893.

Youdim, M.B.H., Finberg, J.P.M., Tipton, K.F. (1988) Monoamine oxidase. In: U. Trendelendim and N. Weiner (eds.), *Handbook of Experimental Pharmacology*, Vol. 90, Springer Verlag, Berlin, pp. 119–192.

Youdim, M.B.H., Heldman, E., Pollard, H.B., Fleming, P and McHugh, E. (1986) Contrasting monoamine oxidase activity and tyramine induced catecholamine release in PC12 chromaffin cells. *Neuroscience*, 19: 1311–1318.

Yu, P.H. and Hertz, L. (1982) Differential expression of type A and B monoamine oxidase of mouse astrocytes in primary cultures. *J . Neurochem.*, 39: 1492–1495.

Zhu, Q.S., Grimsby, J., Chen K. and Shih, J.C. (1992) Promoter organization and activity of human monoamine oxidase (MAO) A and B genes. *J. Neurosci.*, 12: 4437–4446.

Zhu, Q.S., Chen, K. and Shih, J.C. (1994) Bidirectional promoter of human monoamine oxidase A (MAO A) controlled by transcription factor Sp1. *J. Neurosci.*, 14: 7393–7403.

Peter M. Yu, Keith F. Tipton and Alan A. Boulton (Eds.)
Progress in Brain Research, Vol 106
© 1995 Elsevier Science BV. All rights reserved.

CHAPTER 6

The promoter of the human monoamine oxidase A gene

Richard M. Denney

Department of Human Biological Chemistry and Genetics, Graduate School of Biomedical Sciences, University of Texas Medical Branch, Galveston, TX 77555, USA

Introduction

The human genes for monoamine oxidases (MAO) A and B each span nearly 100 kb (Grimsby et al., 1991; Chen et al., 1991) between Xp11.23 and Xp11.4 (Levy et al., 1989; Ozelius et al., 1988; Lan et al., 1989). They are arranged tail-to-tail on the human X chromosome, separated by about 40–45 kb (Chen et al., 1991). Each has 15 exons, and the exon/intron boundaries in each gene occur at homologous positions in the protein-coding sequences (Grimsby et al., 1991), consistent with their origin by gene duplication. Characterization of the human genes was made possible by prior cloning of cDNAs for human MAO A and B (Bach et al., 1988; Hsu et al., 1988; reviewed in Hsu et al., 1989). These cDNAs were isolated by a "reverse genetic" strategy in which short segments of protein sequence from MAO A and MAO B were used to design and synthesize screening oligonucleotides capable of encoding the respective peptide sequences.

Inhibitors of MAO A have antidepressant effects, and total, irreversible inhibition of the enzyme is associated with hypertensive episodes (the so-called "cheese effect"). The importance of MAO A is underscored by the striking behavioral abnormalities associated with MAO A deficiency in affected male members of a large Dutch kindred (Brunner et al., 1993a,b). Females heterozygous for MAO A deficiency exhibited no clinical phenotype, while MAO A deficient males exhibited mild mental retardation and histories of extreme impulsive-aggressive behavior. The mutation responsible for MAO A deficiency in this kindred is a single nucleotide substitution in exon 8 of the MAO A gene (Brunner ct al., 1993a).

Zhu et al. (1992) initiated studies of the human MAO A and B promoters by cloning and sequencing the DNA flanking the 5′ end of the human MAO A and B genes. Using a standard primer extension assay, these authors inferred three major transcription initiation sites 235, 225 and 189 nucleotides 5′ from the A of the ATG initiation codon, plus a number of minor initiation sites, the most proximal of which was 138 nucleotides 5′ from the ATG codon. With these data in hand, genomic DNA segments extending upstream from 64 nucleotides 5′ to the ATG codon were then tested for promoter activity by transient expression assays.

It is essential in studies of a new promoter to establish beyond doubt where transcription is initiated, a task which requires corroborative data from primer extension assays to establish the length of the 5′-untranslated end of the mRNA, and nuclease protection assays to pinpoint the first discontinuity in sequence between genomic DNA and mRNA (i.e., the first exon/intron boundary 5′ to the region of the gene which encodes the N-terminal end of the protein). Primer extension assays of the type used by Zhu et al. (1992) proved in our hands to be insufficiently sensitive and specific to identify transcription initiation sites for the human MAO A promoter. Accordingly, we reported in Denney et al. (1994) additional transcription site mapping data for the human MAO A gene derived from a more sensitive and specific primer extension assay: Rapid Amplification of cDNA Ends (5'-RACE; Frohman et al, 1988; Frohman and Martin, 1989, as modified by Delort et al., 1989, and Edwards et al., 1991). The reliability of the primer extension data was then confirmed by RNase protection assays. These studies revealed unambiguously that the earlier transcription initiation site mapping data had failed to detect the correct transcription initiation sites of the human MAO A gene (Denney et al., 1994).

The newer data show that most MAO A mRNA is initiated at one or a few closely spaced sites between 30 and 40 nucleotides 5' to the ATG translation initiation codon, i.e., much nearer the protein-coding segment of exon 1 than had previously been thought. The DNA sequence between 30 and 40 nucleotides 5' to the polypeptide initiation codon resembles pyrimidine-rich initiator elements (*Inr*) seen in many, but by no means all, eukaryotic promoters (Corden et al., 1980; Smale and Baltimore, 1989). The sequence requirement for activity of eukaryotic *Inr* elements is not stringent (PyPyCAPyTPyPyPy; Smale and Baltimore, 1989). Initiation generally occurs primarily at the underlined A residue immediately following a C. Based on experiments reported in Denney et al. (1994), I propose that the primary transcription initiation site of the MAO A gene (hereafter designated +1) is an A residue 40 nucleotides 5' to the ATG initiation codon. The sequence of the 5' flanking region of the MAO A gene is shown in Table 1, with the putative *Inr* sequence indicated.

Our independent sequencing data have confirmed the sequence of Zhu et al. (1992) for the immediate 5'-flanking region of the MAO A gene. The region between about −40 and −220 consti-

tutes two 90 bp, GC-rich repeats, each containing two inverted consensus sequences which might bind the widespread general transcription factor Sp1 (Table 1). The sequence of the MAO A promoter region resembles GC-rich housekeeping promoters, even though MAO A is not expressed by all cells and tissues. Therefore, it is not clear how the MAO A gene is regulated, or to what extent the tissue- and cell-type specificity of MAO A expression is controlled at the level of transcription initiation versus mRNA processing, transport, or stability.

There is a large body of older literature concerning the regulation of MAO activity in animals by hormones (for example, Holzbauer and Youdim, 1983; Dailey et al., 1981; Knopp and Tiorda, 1983; reviewed by Sourkes, 1979). Relatively few cell culture studies have examined short-term regulation of MAO activity by hormones. Edelstein and Breakefield (1986) first showed that MAO A activity and protein content increase in diploid human fibroblasts treated with the synthetic glucocorticoid, dexamethasone. This effect is associated with an increase in the steady-state level of MAO A mRNA, and dexamethasone treatment increases yields of MAO A mRNA for structural studies (Hotamisligil and Breakefield, 1991; Brunner et al., 1993a). Glucocorticoids regulate many promoters at the level of transcription initiation (Beato, 1989), though their regulatory effects are by no means limited to promoters. Glucocorticoid regulation of promoters is mediated by binding to a glucocorticoid receptor (GR). The GR-hormone complex is specifically transported to the nucleus, where the complex binds defined DNA sequences (glucocorticoid response elements or GREs), thereby modulating transcriptional initiation frequency. GR binding can increase or decrease initiation frequency, depending upon the promoter. Although the transcription of some genes is modulated directly by GR binding, in many more cases glucocorticoids modulate transcription indirectly. Glucocorticoids may alter expression of other transcription factors, thereby influencing the expression of the genes regulated by these secondary factors. Glucocorticoids can also have a profound effect on mRNA stability. There is as yet no evidence that the effect of glucocorticoids

Table 1

Sequence of the MAO A promoter region. +1 is the predicted primary transcription initiation site based upon primer extension and RNase protection data (Denney et al., 1994) and the presence of a consensus sequence for a putative eukaryotic initiator element. The restriction sites corresponding to the 5′ ends of MAO A promoter segments in pGL Sst-Pfl, Kpn-Pfl and Pvu-Pfl (Sst I, Kpn I and Pvu I) are underlined. The 3′ end of MAO A promoter segments in all constructs was +36, derived from a blunted Pfl MI site, which overlaps the ATG initiation codon (underlined CAANNNNTGG). The sequence presented here incorporates minor corrections from the sequence published in Denney et al. (1994). Note the symmetrically arranged series of four potential SP1 sites and the 8 bp CRE-like segment (underlined).

```
                          10          20          30          40          50          60
         Sst I            |           |           |           |           |           |
     -901 GAGCTCCGCA TACACTCCCC AATCAGCACT ACCGGTCTTA GCGAGAGTAC TGACTCCGAC

     -841 TCCAAGAGTG GCCTCCGGGG TTTCAGCGCT TACAACCCGA GCAGTCGGAT CCCCAAGTCT

     -781 ACCACCAGCT CGAACTCCTC CGATGGGGCC GTCACAGCCT CCAATCAGGA CACCGGCATT

     -721 CCCTGGGTAT TAGTAACAGG ACCTACCCCG CCCCGTAAAC TCCCCCGTAG AGTCATTGCA

     -661 AGGGTCTGCC TTCTCCTCAG GGTTCAGCAC CCCACGGGTT TGGTAAAAGG ACCGACCCTG

                              CRE?
     -601 CCCCCGGATT CCAACCTGAC CTCAGTGTCC GACTACACTT GGATATTTGT ACGGGGACCT

     -541 CCTATACCCA ATGACCTTTG AAGTGTAATA CAAGACTCAC ACCAGTAACA CCCCCGAGTG

                                                                           Kpn I
     -481 TCAGTACAAG GGTCTGCCGC ATCCTCAGTG TCCAGCTTCC CCTGGGGTTT GGTACCAGGA

     -421 CCACCTCTAC CCAATAACAT TTCCCCAGTG TCGCCACAAG CACCTCCTGC ACCCCATAAC

     -361 ATCCCCCCAG TGTCAAGGCA GGCGTCTACC CCCACCTCAG TGCCTGACAC TCCGCGGGGC

                                                        Pvu II
     -301 TTCAATACAA GAACCTCCTG CACCCAGTAA TCCTTCCAGC TGCCGACACA AGGACATTCT

                                                SP1
     -241 AAACCTAATA ACTCTCGCCG AGTGTCAGTA CAAGGGTCCG CCCCGCTCTC AGTGCCCAGC

               Pvu II*               SP1
     -181 TCCCCCCGGG TATCAGCTGA AACATCAGCT CCGCCCCTGG GCGCTCCCGG AGTATCAGCA

               SP1
     -121 AAAGGGTTCG CCCCGCCCAC AGTGCCCGGC TCCCCCCGGG TATCAAAAGA AGGATCGGCT

         SP1                                                              Inr
      -61 CCGCCCCCGG GCTCCCCGGG GGAGTTGATA GAAGGGTCCT TCCCACCCTT TGCCGTCCCC

         +1                                       Pfl MI   Translation start >
      +1 ACTCCTGTGC CTACGACCCA GGAGCGTGTC AGCCAAAGCA TGGAGAATCA AGAGAAGGCG

      +61 AGTATCGCGG GCCACATGTT CGACGTAGTC GTGATCGGAG GTGGCATTTC AGGTCAGGTG
```

on steady-state levels of MAO A mRNA is mediated at the transcriptional level. The availability of the MAO A promoter and luciferase reporter constructs under its control provides an opportunity to look for regulatory effects of glucocorticoids on MAO A promoter activity.

Yu and Hertz (1988) reported that cyclic AMP analogues altered the expression of MAO A and B activities in rodent astrocytes in culture. In analyzing the DNA sequence flanking the 5' end of the human MAO A gene, Zhu et al. (1992) noted a sequence which matched seven of eight nucleotides of the consensus for a cyclic AMP response element TGACGTCA (CRE; Montminy, 1986; the second G is a C in the MAO A promoter region). Below we present a test of the possible role of this sequence in regulating expression of the MAO A promoter.

Materials and methods

Cells and culture conditions

The mouse L cell line A9 was grown in Dulbecco's modified Eagle Minimal Essential Medium (DMEM) supplemented with 10% newborn calf serum at 37°C in a humidified atmosphere of 10% CO_2 in air.

Luciferase reporter constructs

The MAO A-luciferase constructs were derived from the promoterless luciferase reporter plasmid pGL Basic (Promega Corporation, Madison, WI), and contained segments of human genomic DNA which extended from +36 upstream to −169 (pGL Pvu-Pfl), −431 (pGL Kpn-Pfl) or −901 (pGL Sst-Pfl). Construction of the reporters is described in Denney et al. (1994). Note that here the numbering of bases in the 5' flanking region is from the A(+1) of the putative initiator, 40 nucleotides 5' to the ATG initiation codon, while the numbering in Denney et al. (1994) was designated +1 as the A of the ATG initiation codon. An additional luciferase construct, containing the genomic segment from 4 to approximately 3500 nucleotides 5' to the initiation codon (pGL −3.5), was constructed by linearizing pGLSst-Pfl with

Sst I and ligating in the 2.5 kb Sst I-Sst I genomic DNA fragment which extends 5' from the Sst I site in pGL Sst-Pfl. Plasmids with the 2.5 kb Sst I fragment in its natural orientation with respect to the promoter were identified by restriction mapping of minipreps. Insert structures and insert-vector boundaries for all constructs but pGL −3.5 have been verified by dideoxy sequence analysis. All DNA preparations used here were purified by centrifugation in CsCl density gradients.

Transient expression of luciferase

Mouse A9 cells (2×10^5 cells/35 mm well of 6-well culture plates) were grown overnight in DMEM medium containing 10% newborn calf serum. After 20–22 h, triplicate wells were exposed to 3 μg of DNA/well complexed with 15 μg of Transfectam lipofection reagent (Promega Corporation, Madison, WI) overnight in serum-free DMEM. In some experiments, medium was replaced the following day with 2 ml of DMEM plus or minus 10% serum and plus or minus potential regulatory molecules, and the cells were grown for an additional 24 h before harvest. Cells were harvested in 350 μl of luciferase lysis buffer (Promega Corporation, Madison, WI), and extracts were assayed in duplicate for luciferase activity as described in Denney et al. (1994). Luciferase activity is expressed as cpm of luminescence/μg protein. Protein was measured in triplicate by the method of Bradford (1976) with bovine serum albumin as standard.

Results

As a first step toward determining whether the glucocorticoid dexamethasone affected MAO A promoter activity, A9 cells were transfected with a series of luciferase reporter constructs and incubated for 24 h in serum-free medium plus or minus 10^{-7} M dexamethasone before harvest. The positive control was "pGL Control", which contains the SV40 early promoter and enhancer (designated "SV" in figures). The negative control was the promoterless "pGL Basic", designated "B" in the figures. The MAO A promoter con-

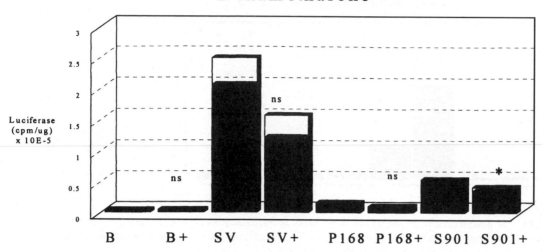

Fig. 1. Non-specific dexamethasone inhibition of luciferase expression in A9 cells transfected with luciferase constructs and grown continuously for 24 h in serum-free medium. B, pGL Basic; SV, pGL Control; P168, pGL Pvu-Pfl; S901, pGL Sst-Pfl. Transparent bars above filled bars: standard deviations of replicate transfections ($n = 3$).

structs were pGL Pvu-Pfl and pGL Sst-Pfl (designated respectively "P168" and "P901" in the figures). The results in Fig. 1 show that dexamethasone treatment inhibited the specific activity of luciferase (expressed as cpm/g protein) from all transfected constructs (∗ indicates $P < 0.01$). There was no evidence of a specific effect of dexamethasone on the MAO A promoter constructs, and no obvious difference in the effect of dexamethasone as a function of the length of the MAO A promoter region in the MAO A promoter constructs (168 nucleotides in P168, 901 nucleotides in S901).

Since dexamethasone inhibited luciferase expression from all reporter constructs, including background expression from the promoterless construct (B in Fig. 1), we investigated whether dexamethasone inhibited the transfection process itself, rather than expression of the transfected DNA. In the experiment in Fig. 2, A9 cells were transfected overnight in serum-free medium without hormone, then treated for an additional 24 h in serum-containing medium with 10^{-7} M dexamethasone (Fig. 2). Longer cultivation before harvested (48 versus 24 h) dramatically increased

the luciferase specific activity, but generalized inhibition of luciferase expression by dexamethasone was still seen. The data provided no evidence for specific dexamethasone effects on luciferase expression driven by MAO A promoter constructs (Fig. 2).

To test for possible effects of serum factors on MAO A promoter activity, we transfected cells for 24 h in serum-free medium and compared luciferase activities in cells harvested after an additional 24 h of growth in either serum-free or serum-containing media. Serum-grown cultures contained approximately 2-fold more protein and total luciferase activity ($P < .001$). However, the results in Fig. 3 show that the specific activities of luciferase in the serum-grown and serum-free cultures were similar (Fig. 3). The small increase seen in luciferase activity in the serum-grown culture transfected with pGL Sst-Pfl (designated S901 + in Fig. 3) was statistically significant.

A similar experiment tested the effect of 24 h of growth in serum-free versus serum-containing medium after transfection in serum-free medium for only 4 h. Though the difference in total protein and luciferase content per culture was less

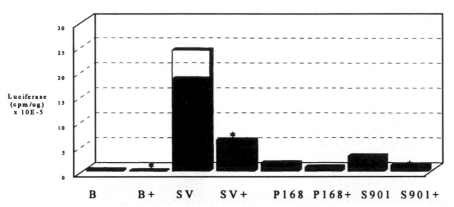

Fig. 2. Effect of 10^{-7} M dexamethasone on expression of luciferase in transfected A9 cells. Cells were transfected overnight in serum-free medium, then grown for an additional 24 h in serum- and dexamethasone-containing medium before assay for luciferase expression. The constructs are as in Fig. 1. Transparent bars: standard deviations as in Fig. 1.

marked in the serum-grown versus serum-free cultures compared to the cells grown for 48 h (Fig. 3), the specific activities of luciferase were similar for each construct regardless of the presence of serum (not shown). We conclude that the MAO A promoter region from -901 to $+36$ does not respond to the presence of serum when transfected into A9 cells.

The experiment in Fig. 4 demonstrates the lack of a specific effect of dibutyryl cyclic-AMP on expression of luciferase activity in transfected A9 cells. All constructs exhibited reduced luciferase

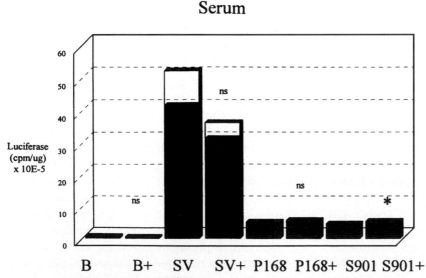

Fig. 3. Negligible specific effect of serum on expression of luciferase from MAO A promoter constructs transfected into A9 cells. Cells were transfected overnight in serum-free medium and incubated for an additional 24 h in either serum-free or serum-containing medium before luciferase assay. The constructs tested are as in Figs. 1 and 2. Transparent bars: standard deviations as in Fig. 1.

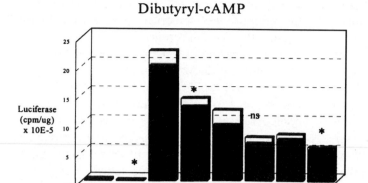

Fig. 4. Effect of dibutyryl cyclic-AMP on luciferase reporter activity in transfected A9 cells. Cells were transfected overnight in serum-free medium and grown for an additional 24 h in serum-containing medium supplemented with or without 10^{-3} M dibutyryl cyclic-AMP. Constructs are as in Figs. 1–3. Transparent bars: standard deviations as in Fig. 1.

specific activity ($P < .05$), except for pGL Pvu-Pfl, where the reduced activity was not statistically significant. The data reveal no specific effect of dibutyryl cyclic-AMP on the MAO A promoter, and in particular, no evidence for a specific effect of the this agent on the longer MAO A promoter construct (pGL Sst-Pfl), which contains a candidate CRE-like sequence element. We conclude that the CRE-like sequence does not function as a cyclic-AMP response element in transiently transfected A9 cells.

Discussion

Fine-scale mapping of the 5′ ends of mRNAs by PCR-assisted primer extension and RNase protection assays has detected one or a small number of major transcription initiation sites in a pyrimidine-rich segment located 29 to 45 nucleotides 5′ to the ATG initiation and minor initiation sites in the proximal GC-rich, 90 bp repeat codon (Denney et al., 1994). The agreement between data from PCR-assisted primer extension and RNase protection assays in this work strongly suggests that these results are more reliable than previously published transcription site mapping (Zhu et al., 1992). The correspondence in sequence between the major, proximal initiation region de-

tected in the newer data and previously described pyrimidine initiator (*Inr*) consensus sequences $(Py)_5CA(Py)_5$ also argues strongly in favor of the newer data. That there is a consensus sequence at many transcription initiation sites was first recognized by sequence comparisons of carefully mapped transcription initiation sites in TATA box-containing eukaryotic promoters (Corden et al., 1980). Subsequently it was shown that the *Inr* element from the lymphocyte-specific, murine terminal deoxyribonucleotidyltransferase (TdT) gene can specify accurate but low-frequency initiation in in vitro transcription assays and transfected cells, even without a TATA box or other *cis* activating element (Smale and Baltimore, 1989). The presence of an Sp1 site in either orientation (Smale et al., 1990) amplifies accurate transcription initiation from an *Inr* element, and sub-optimal spacing between an Sp1 binding site and an *Inr* element results in increased heterogeneity of initiation near the preferred initiation site (Smale and Baltimore, 1989). These observations are probably relevant to the MAO A promoter, which has four Sp1 consensus sequences immediately upstream from the principal transcription initiation site, the nearest centered on the G residue at −63. There is no TATA box-like sequence 25–30 nucleotides upstream from the primary transcription initiation site of the MAO A gene, suggesting that this is a TATA box-independent promoter.

One potential argument against our finding that most transcription initiation at the MAO A promoter occurs approximately 40 bp 5′ to the ATG codon is that the first published cDNA for MAO A has a 5′ leader which extends upstream 77 bp from the ATG initiation codon (Bach et al., 1988). This cDNA clearly was not derived from an mRNA initiated only 40 bp from the ATG codon. However, a small proportion of MAO A mRNA does appear to be initiated farther upstream in the proximal GC-rich 90 bp repeat approximately 95 and 136 nucleotides 5′ to the ATG initiation codon (Denney et al., 1994). We therefore suggest that the Bach et al. (1988) cDNA, with its 77 bp 5′-untranslated region, was derived from one of these longer, rarer transcripts. These minor, more distal initiation sites are located near the proximal two of the four, inverted Sp1 consensus sequences (Dynan and Tjian, 1983; Lee et al., 1987; CTCCGCCC, CCCGCCC). Dr. Shih reported at this meeting and in a published abstract (Zhu et al., 1993) that these sites are capable of binding Sp1, at least in vitro. It is interesting that despite the high sequence homology between the proximal and distal 90 bp GC-rich repeats, we detected no transcription initiation within the more distal of the two 90 bp repeats.

Based on our earlier observation that luciferase constructs containing DNA segments extending from 4 to 200, 4 to 465 and 4 to 935 nucleotides 5′ to the ATG initiation codon drove robust luciferase transient expression in transfected A9 cells, we investigated possible effects of dexamethasone, serum and dibutyryl cyclic-AMP on transiently expressed luciferase activity. The results revealed no specific effect of these agents on transiently expressed luciferase activity in A9 cells. These data must be interpreted cautiously, however, since A9 is a mouse L cell line, chosen primarily for its expression of high MAO A activity and easy transfectability. We had already defined basic conditions required for obtaining good luciferase expression from the control (SV40) promoter and low non-specific expression from the promoterless construct (pGL Basic). In this regard, the fold difference in luciferase expression between the pGL Control and pGL Basic is very high with these vectors in this system, as can be seen in Figs. 1–4. We have not tested the effects of serum, dexamethasone or dibutyryl cyclic-AMP on endogenous (mouse) MAO A activity or mRNA in A9 cells. Therefore, it remains possible that one or more of these agents might modulate MAO A promoter activity from a promoter transfected into other cells. We are particularly interested in assaying possible regulatory effects of dexamethasone in the luciferase constructs transfected into diploid human fibroblasts, whose MAO A activity increases several-fold when continuously exposed to dexamethasone. Experience with other systems has shown that it is impossible to predict how a promoter will be regulated merely by identifying consensus sequences. Furthermore, there may well be important regulatory elements farther upstream or downstream from the sequences tested in the luciferase reporter constructs to date. In this regard, we have expressed luciferase from a construct containing approx. 3.5 kb of 5′-flanking sequence of the MAO A gene (3′ endpoint, +36 as in the other constructs discussed here). Luciferase activity expressed from this construct is approx. 50% that of the activity expressed from the −901 to +36 construct (data not shown). Luciferase expression from this construct has not yet been tested for sensitivity to hormones. Of course, regulatory elements could also occur in the body of the gene. Since the first intron is extremely large (> 10 kb), devising schemes for finding and defining such intragenic elements is not trivial.

In conclusion, PCR-assisted primer extension and RNase protection assays have permitted unambiguous assignment of transcription initiation sites of the human MAO A gene. The relative utilization of the minor, GC-rich and major, proximal pyrimidine-rich initiation sites appears to vary among a colon tumor cell line and several normal tissues tested, but in all cases, the predominant initiation occurred at a putative *Inr* element centered 40 bp 5′ to the ATG initiation codon. Fragments of the 5′-flanking region of the MAO A gene which extend upstream from +36 to at least −168 exhibit promoter activity in transiently transfected A9 and HeLa cells, and sequences extending 5′ from −168 to at least −901 have relatively minor additional effect on promoter activity. These studies provide a sound basis for further studies of the human MAO A promoter. The CRE-like sequence TGACCTCA, reported first by Zhu et al. (1992) as similar to a cAMP response element, does not confer cAMP-sensitivity in transiently transfected mouse L cells. Though dexamethasone induces MAO A activity in human fibroblasts (Edelstein and Breakefield, 1986), there is currently no evidence that this effect is mediated at the transcriptional level. We have not detected any specific effect of dexamethasone on luciferase expression from MAO A promoter constructs in transiently transfected A9 cells. Continuing studies of the MAO A promoter should define sequences which are important in regulating the MAO A promoter and determining its cell type-specific expression.

Summary

Monoamine oxidase (MAO) A (EC 1.4.3.4) oxidizes norepinephrine and serotonin and is expressed in a cell type-specific manner. Evidence that MAO A deficient males in a large Dutch kindred suffer from mild mental retardation and occasional episodes of impulsive-aggressive behavior makes it important to understand how the human MAO A promoter is regulated. Workers in multiple laboratories have isolated and characterized protein-coding sequences of the human MAO A gene and the DNA region where mRNA synthesis is initiated. After summarizing our published findings concerning where transcription of the human MAO A gene is initiated, I summarize representative results of transient expression assays aimed at assessing whether some potential gene regulatory agents affect the expression of luciferase from MAO A promoter reporter constructs when transfected into a mouse L cell line which expresses MAO A. These studies revealed no specific regulatory effects of serum, dexamethasone or a stable cyclic-AMP analogue on the human MAO A promoter introduced.

Acknowledgments

This work was supported by NIH grant NS19543. I thank Ann Waguespack, who is supported by funds from the State of Texas administered by the Cancer Center of the University of Texas Medical Branch, and Sanat Dave for excellent technical assistance.

References

Bach, A.W.J., Lan, N.C., Johnson, D.L., Abell, C.W., Bembenek, M.E., Kwan, S.-W., Seeberg, P.H. and Shih, J.C. (1988) cDNA cloning of human monoamine oxidase A and B: molecular basis of differences in enzymatic properties. *Proc. Natl. Acad. Sci. USA*, 85: 4934–4938.

Beato, M. (1989) Gene regulation by steroid hormones. *Cell*, 56: 335–344.

Bradford, M.M. (1976) A rapid and sensitive method for the quantitation of microgram quantities of protein utilizing the principle of protein-dye binding. *Anal. Biochem.*, 72: 248–254.

Brunner, H.G., Nelen, M.R., Breakefield, X.O., Ropers, H.H. and van Oost, B.A. (1993a) Abnormal behavior associated with a point mutation in the structural gene for monoamine oxidase A. *Science*, 262: 578–580.

Brunner, H.G., Nelen, M.R., van Zandvoort, P., Abeling, N.G.G.M., van Gennip, A.H., Wolters, E.C., Kuiper, M.A., Ropers, H.H. and van Oost, B.A. (1993b) X-linked borderline mental retardation with prominent behavioral disturbance: Phenotype, genetic localization and evidence for disturbed monoamine metabolism. *Am. J. Hum. Genet.*, 42: 1032–1039.

Chen, Z.-Y., Hotamisligil, G.S., Huang, J.K., Wen, L., Ezzeddine, D., Aydin-Muderrisoglu, N., Powell, J.F., Huang, R.H., Breakefield, X.O., Craig, I.W. and Hsu, Y.-P.P. (1991) Structure of the human gene for monoamine oxidase type A. *Nucl. Acids Res.*, 19: 4537–4541.

Chen, Z.-Y., Hendriks, R.W., Jobling, M.A., Powell, J.F., Breakefield, X.O., Sims, K.B. and Craig, I.W. (1992a) Isolation and characterization of a candidate gene for Norrie disease. *Nature Genet.*, 1: 204–208.

Chen, Z.-Y., Powell, J.F., Hsu, Y.-P., Breakefield, X.O. and Craig, I. W. (1992b) Organization of the human monoamine oxidase genes and long-range physical mapping around them. *Genomics,* 14: 75–82.

Corden, J., Wasylyk, B., Buchwalder, A., Sassone-Corsi, P., Kedinger, C. and Chambon, P. (1980) Promoter sequences of eukaryotic protein-coding genes. *Science,* 209: 1405–1414.

Dailey, J.W., Battarbee, H.D. and McNatt, L. (1982). Mineralocorticoid treatment and the adrenalectomy-induced increase in monoamine oxidase activity. *Experientia,* 38: 953–955.

Delort, J., Dumas, J.B., Darmon, M.C. and Mallet, J. (1989) An efficient strategy for cloning 5′ extremities of rare transcripts permits isolation of multiple 5′-untranslated regions of rat tryptophan hydroxylase mRNA. *Nucl. Acids Res.,* 17: 6439–6448.

Denney, R.M., Sharma, A., Dave, S.K. and Waguespack, M.A. (1994) A new look at the promoter of the human monoamine oxidase A gene. Mapping transcription initiation sites and capacity to drive luciferase expression. *J. Neurochem.,* 63,843–856.

Dynan, W.S. and Tjian, R. (1983) The promoter-specific transcription factor Sp1 binds to upstream sequences in the SV40 early promoter. *Cell,* 35,79–87.

Edelstein, S.B. and Breakefield, X.O. (1986) Monoamine oxidases A and B are differentially regulated by glucocorticoids and "aging" in human skin fibroblasts. *Cell. Molec. Neurobiol.,* 6: 121–150.

Edwards, J.B., Delort, J. and Mallet, J. (1991) Oligodeoxyribonucleotide ligation to single-stranded cDNAs: a new tool for cloning 5′ ends of mRNAs and for constructing cDNA libraries by in vitro amplification. *Nucl. Acids Res.,* 19: 5227–5232.

Frohman, M.A., Dush, M.K.and Martin, G.R. (1988) Rapid production of full-length cDNAs from rare transcripts: Amplification using a single gene-specific oligonucleotide primer. *Proc. Natl. Acad. Sci. USA,* 85: 8998–9002.

Frohman, M.A. and Martin, G.R. (1989) Rapid amplification of cDNA ends using nested primers. *Technique,* 1: 165–170.

Grimsby, J., Chen, K., Wang, L.-J., Lan, N.C. and Shih, J.C. (1991) Human monoamine oxidase A and B genes exhibit identical exon-intron organization. *Proc. Natl. Acad. Sci. USA,* 88: 3637–3641.

Holzbauer, M. and Youdim, M.B.H. (1983) Specific changes in type A and B monoamine oxidase activity in different tissues of hypophysectomized rats. *Biochem. Pharmacol.,* 32: 469–473.

Hsu, Y.-P.P., Weyler, W., Chen, S., Sims, K.B., Rinehart, W.B., Utterback, M., Powell, J.F. and Breakefield, X.O. (1988) Structural features of human monoamine oxidase A elucidated from cDNA and peptide sequences. *J. Neurochem.,* 51: 1321–1324.

Hsu, Y.-P., Powell, J.F., Sims, K.B. and Breakefield, X.O. (1989) Molecular genetics of the monoamine oxidases. *J. Neurochem.,* 53: 12–18.

Knopp, J. and Torda, T. (1983) Effect of hypophysectomy and administration of TSH on the activity of monoamine oxidase in the thyroid gland of rats. *Hormone Metab. Res.,* 15: 191–193.

Lan, N.C., Heinzmann, C., Gal, A., Klisak, I., Orth, U., Lai, E., Grimsby, J., Sparkes, R.S., Mohandas, T. and Shih, J.C. (1989) Human monoamine oxidase A and B genes map to Xp11.23 and are deleted in a patient with Norrie disease. *Genomics,* 4: 552–559.

Levy, E.R., Powell, J.F., Buckle, V.J., Hsu, Y.-P.P., Breakefield, X.O. and Craig, I.W. (1989) Localization of human monoamine oxidase-A gene to Xp11.23-11.4 by in situ hybridization: implications for Norrie disease. *Genomics,* 5: 368–370.

Montminy, M.R., Sevarino, K.A., Wagner, J.A., Mandel, G., Goodman, R.H. (1986) Identification of a cyclic-AMP-responsive element within the rat somatostatin gene. *Proc. Natl. Acad. Sci. USA,* 83: 6682–6686.

Ozelius, L., Hsu, Y.-P.P., Bruns, G., Powell, J.F., Chen, S., Weyler, W., Utterback, M., Zucker, D., Haines, J., Trofalter, J.A., Conneally, P. M., Gusella, J.F. and Breakefield, X.O. (1988) Human monoamine oxidase gene (MAOA): chromosome position (Xp21-p11) and DNA polymorphism. *Genomics,* 3: 53–58.

Sims, K.B., de la Chapelle, A., Norio, R., Sankila, E.-M., Hsu, Y.-P.P., Rinehart, W.B., Corey, T.J., Ozelius, L., Powell, J.F., Bruns, G., Gusella, J.F., Murphy, D.L. and Breakefield, X.O. (1989) Monoamine oxidase deficiency in males with an X chromosome deletion. *Neuron,* 2: 1069–1076.

Smale, S.T. and Baltimore, D. (1989) The "Initiator" as a transcription control element *Cell,* 57: 103–113.

Smale, S.T., Schmidt, M.C., Berk, A.J. and Baltimore, D. (1990) Transcriptional activation by Sp1 as directed through TATA or initiator: Specific requirement for mammalian transcription factor IID *Proc. Natl. Acad. Sci. USA,* 87: 4509–4513.

Sourkes, T.L. (1979) Influence of hormones, vitamins and metals on monoamine oxidase activity. In: Singer, T.P., Von Korff, R.W. and Murphy, D.L. (Eds.), *Monoamine Oxidase: Structure, Function and Altered Functions,* Academic Press, New York, pp. 291–307.

Yu, P.H. and Hertz, L (1982) Differential expression of type A and type B monoamine oxidase of mouse astrocytes in primary culture. *J. Neurochem.,* 39. 1492–1495.

Zhu, Q.-S., Grimsby, J., Chen, K. and Shih, J.C. (1992) Promoter organization and activity of human monoamine oxidase (MAO) A and B genes. *J. Neurosci.,* 12: 4437–4446

Zhu, Q.-S., Chen, K. and Shih, J.C. (1993) Bidirectional promoter activity of the human monoamine oxidase (MAO) A gene differentially controlled by Sp1 binding to 4 tandem repeats. *Soc. Neurosci. Abs.,* 19: 696.

Peter M. Yu, Keith F. Tipton and Alan A. Boulton (Eds.)
Progress in Brain Research, Vol 106
© 1995 Elsevier Science BV. All rights reserved.

CHAPTER 7

Analysis of *MAOA* mutations in humans

Y.-P.P. Hsu[1], D.E. Schuback[2], E.A. Tivol[2], C. Shalish[2], D.L. Murphy[4] and
X.O. Breakefield[2,3]

[1]*Research, VA Medical Center, West Roxbury, MA 02132, USA,* [2]*Department of Neurology, Massachusetts General Hospital,
Boston, MA 02114, USA,* [3]*Department of Neurology, Harvard Medical School, Boston, MA 02115, USA, and* [4]*Laboratory
of Clinical Science, NIMH, Bethesda, MD 20892, USA*

Monoamine oxidase (MAO) catalyzes the oxidative deamination of a broad range of biogenic amines, including amine neurotransmitters, such as dopamine, norepinephrine and serotonin (for reviews see Breakefield et al., 1994; Kwan et al., 1992; Shih, 1991; Weyler et al., 1990). The two forms of the enzyme, MAO-A and MAO-B, are isozymes with extensive amino acid homologies, but exhibit distinctive substrate specificity, inhibitor sensitivity, and tissue distribution.

The activities of MAO can be measured in living humans using platelets or lymphocytes, which express mostly MAO-B activity (Bond and Bond, 1977; Murphy et al., 1976), and cultured skin fibroblasts, which express primarily MAO-A activity (Edelstein et al., 1978). Each isozyme shows more than 50-fold variations in activity levels among normal humans (Hotamisligil and Breakefield, 1991; Murphy et al., 1976). This variation may be tolerated due to the fact that these two isozymes have overlapping substrates and tissue distribution, and hence can compensate for each other to some extent. Furthermore, other degradative enzymes, such as catechol-*O*-methyltransferase and phenylsulfotransferase, also act on MAO substrates. Therefore, there may be little selection pressure exerted by mutations that result in different activity levels of one or the other isozyme of MAO. However, it is still possible that genetic variations associated with deficiency of a particular isozyme may confer susceptibility to some disease. This is exemplified by studies on the role of aldehyde dehydrogenase in alcoholism (Crabb et al., 1989), and *N*-acetyltransferase in isoniazid-induced nerve damage (Deguchi et al., 1990).

The role of MAO-B has been studied in a variety of psychiatric and neurological disorders (for reviews see Fowler et al., 1982; Giller et al., 1982; Sandler et al., 1981; von Knorring et al., 1985; Zureick and Meltzer, 1988). Since these studies are mostly based on measurements of MAO-B activities in platelets, secondary effects of drugs or physiological conditions are difficult to rule out. The literature on MAO-B and disease is vast and frequently contradictory. However, it may be noteworthy that a variant of MAO-B, with altered sensitivity to ethanol, which presumably could result from altered enzyme structure, has been associated with type II alcoholism (Tabakoff et al., 1988). The role of MAO-A in human disease has been less frequently studied because of difficulties in measuring the enzyme activity, which requires skin biopsy and culturing of fibroblasts. In the small numbers of patients studied so far, no loss of MAO-A activity was noted in some patients with the following diseases: Lesch-Nyhan syndrome (Costa et al., 1980), manic-depressive illness (Breakefield et al., 1980), schizophrenia (Giller et al., 1982), autism, Gilles de la Tourette syndrome (Giller et al., 1980), and torsion dystonia (Giller et al., 1980). However, a recent study has demonstrated deficiency of MAO-A activity in males with a syndrome of mild mental retardation and a decrease in impulse control (Brunner et al., 1993a; see below).

The cloning of *MAOA* and *MAOB* cDNAs (Bach et al., 1988; Hsu et al., 1988, 1989) has opened new avenues for studying the molecular basis of variations in MAO activities and their roles in genetic diseases. The human *MAOA* and *MAOB* genes are located in a tail-to-tail (3′ to 3′) fashion adjacent to each other (Chen et al., 1992a) in band p11.3 of the X chromosome (Lan et al., 1989; Levy et al., 1989). This location in the X chromosome may explain the somewhat higher level of MAO-B activity measured in females than in males, because one of the two copies of the X-linked genes may not be completely inactivated. Thus the summed activity of MAO from the two alleles in female cells would be higher than those in male cells which have only one allele of the gene. This also predicts a higher frequency of male patients if low activity of one or the other MAO isozymes does contribute to a disease state.

The first clues to an MAO deficiency state came from studies of males carrying deletions in the *MAO* region of the X chromosome. The *MAO* genes are located next to the Norrie disease gene (Berger et al., 1992; Chen et al., 1992b; Sims et al., 1992), the disruption of which causes an X-linked recessive disease characterized by congenital blindness, progressive deafness, mental retardation, and sometimes psychosis. A more severe phenotype, including severe mental retardation, seizures, hypotonic crises, and poor growth is manifested by the "atypical" patients with Norrie disease (Warburg, 1966), who have chromosomal deletions encompassing the Norrie disease gene, the *MAO* genes and possibly a few other genes in the region (de la Chapelle et al., 1985; Donnai et al., 1988; Gal et al., 1986; Sims et al., 1989; Zhu et al., 1989). Some of these patients

have lived to be more than 20 years of age, which demonstrates that complete loss of MAO activity is not incompatible with life. The question is then: what is the phenotype of persons missing either MAO-A or MAO-B because of discrete mutations in these genes? Based on comparison of symptoms of Norrie disease with or without deletions of *MAO* genes, as well as in human and animal studies using MAO inhibitors, one can predict that mental retardation, psychiatric problems, hypertensive crises related to intake of exogenous amines, seizures, and hyperactivity might be phenotypes resulting from defects in either of the *MAO* genes.

A direct correlation between an *MAOA* mutation and a phenotype has been provided by recent studies of a pedigree in the Netherlands (Brunner et al., 1993a; Brunner et al., 1993b). Eight males in the pedigree, who are mildly retarded and show episodic aggressive behavior, including attempted murder, attempted rape, exhibitionism, attempted suicide and arson, were found to carry a point mutation which converts a glutamine codon into a stop codon in the eighth exon. This mutation completely disrupts MAO-A activity (Brunner et al., 1993a). The common feature shared by these males of an apparent episodic loss of impulse control suggests it may reflect physiological changes resulting from MAO-A deficiency, but could also be related to mild retardation. In the search for other genetic MAO-A deficiencies, it may be helpful to keep in mind that the effects of temporary and partial inhibition of MAO activities may be quite different from those resulting from the complete absence of MAO activity throughout development and life, because biogenic amines have been proposed (Lauder, 1985) to serve as guiding molecules during the development of the nervous system. In addition to looking for mental retardation, behavioral problems, or episodic hypertension, one should be open-minded about symptoms which may be related to defects in *MAOA*. It may be helpful to prescreen patients and controls for dramatically altered levels of amines or their metabolites in urine, cerebrospinal fluid (CSF), or plasma which have been associated with MAO deficiency states (Brunner et al., 1993b; Murphy et al., 1990). Abnormally low levels of MHPG in concert with elevated normetanephrine levels appear to be the most predictive change associated with MAO-A deficiency (Murphy et al., 1990).

Mutations causing complete loss of MAO activities are most likely to involve coding sequences. To screen for such "null mutations" which disrupt the enzyme structure, we have developed the following "exon-scanning" method. This is based on results from detailed mapping of the exons and from sequencing introns in the flanking regions (Chen et al., 1991; Grimsby et al., 1991; Tivol et al., in press). There are 15 exons with similar intron/exon junctions for the *MAOA* and *MAOB* genes. The exons range from about 50 bp to 150 bp in the translated regions. Fifteen sets of PCR primers, mostly derived from intron sequences, have been developed for the amplification of each of the exons from genomic DNA (Tivol et al., in press). The amplified DNA fragments can be analyzed by the technique of SSCP (single-strand conformational polymorphisms) (Orita et al., 1989a,b). This is based on the fact that conformational changes of single-stranded DNA (in the range of 50–300 bases) resulting from a single base change, as well as more extensive changes in sequence, can be detected by electrophoresis in nondenaturing polyacrylamide gels. A "shift" in the mobility of the DNA indicates the presence of a sequence variation. This method can detect 70–90% of single base changes depending on the conditions used. One can then do "asymmetric PCR" to generate sufficient amounts of the single-stranded DNA for sequencing (Gibbs et al., 1989).

Figure 1 shows the sequencing results from a number of control fibroblast cell lines which varied over 50-fold in MAO-A activity levels (Tivol et al., in press). Of the five single basepair changes found in 11 lines examined, four do not change the deduced amino acid sequence, and the only change, Lys to Arg (which corresponds to a difference between human and bovine sequences at that position (Powell et al., 1989), presumably does not perturb the structure and function of the enzyme significantly. It is evident from these results that the translated region of *MAOA* is highly conserved. Given the linkage disequilibrium data which indicate that the *MAOA* gene itself is the primary determinant of MAO-A activity levels in fibroblasts (Hotamisligil and Breakefield, 1991), it seems likely that sequence variations which determine these MAO-A activity levels lie in the noncoding regions of the gene, presumably in the 5′-regulatory region that controls the rate of transcription. This would be consistent with the idea

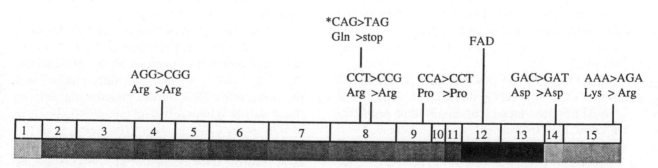

Fig. 1. Known variations in translated region of human *MAOA* gene. The numbers indicate the exons as represented by the empty bars. The density of shading underneath each bar represents the relative degree of homology between human MAO-A and MAO-B amino acid sequences in that exon, with the percent homologies from exon 1 to exon 15 as follows: 41% (exon 1), 71%(2), 74%(3), 77%(4), 70%(5), 77%(6), 74%(7), 68%(8), 66%(9), 67%(10), 79%(11), 94%(12), 89%(13), 52%(14), 58%(15). The covalent binding site for FAD in exon 12 is also indicated. Basepair substitutions described in Tivol et al. (in press) and (*) Brunner et al. (1993b) are indicated.

that a "quantitative" change rather than a "qualitative" change in MAO-A molecules accounts for the variations in activity levels observed in fibroblasts from normal humans (Costa et al., 1980). In contrast, analysis of the coding region of the *MAOA* gene showed a disruptive mutation causing a premature termination signal which correlated with complete loss of enzyme activity in the MAO-A deficient patients (Brunner et al., 1993a).

Although it seems that humans with very high or very low levels of MAO-A activity can lead a normal life, it is possible that certain disease phenotypes can develop in these individuals over time through interaction with other genetic or environmental factors. In other words, abnormal levels of MAO could be risk factors for some disease states. Recent results on Parkinson's disease lend strong support to this hypothesis (Hotamisligil et al., 1994; Kurth et al., 1993). Allele association studies revealed a marked differences in the frequencies of different polymorphic alleles of *MAO* genes in patient populations as compared to control populations. This difference in the frequency of certain alleles suggests that these normal polymorphisms may serve to mark functionally significant mutations in these alleles. Albeit other possible interpretations exist, such as epistasis and ethnic stratification, this approach serves as a first approximation for assessing the role of a candidate gene. The utility of this approach is illustrated by the finding that the E4 allele of the apolipoprotein gene is associated with early-onset Alzheimer's disease (van Duijn et al., 1994).

MAOA alleles can now be typed by the use of two RFLPs and a $(GT)_n$ dinucleotide repeat. The two RFLPs are detected by *EcoRV* and *MspI* cuts in exon 14 (Hotamisligil and Breakefield, 1991) and the noncoding regions (Ozelius et al., 1989), respectively. Combinations of the two RFLPs give rise to four haplotypes: A ($-$ $-$), B ($-$ $+$), C ($+$ $+$), and D ($+$ $-$), by the presence ($+$) or absence ($-$) of *EcoRV* and *MspI* sites, respectively. The $(GT)_n$ repeat element is in intron 1 (Black et al.,

1991). It reveals nine alleles (112, 114, 116, 118, 120, 122, 124, 126 and 130 bp in length). *MAOB* can be typed by a $(GT)_n$ repeat element in intron 2 of the gene (Konradi et al., 1992), which reveals six alleles (174, 176, 178, 180, 182, and 184 bp in length), as well as a single-strand conformational polymorphism in or around exon 13 (Kurth and Kurth, 1992).

Table 1 shows genotyping results for *MAOA* (Hotamisligil and Breakefield, 1991) among 40 human skin fibroblast strains (Costa et al., 1980) which have a wide range of MAO-A activities (from 0.1 to 179 pmol/min per mg protein). There appears to be a higher frequency of the C haplotype, as well as the 122 allele, among cell lines with "high" ($>$ 12 pmol/min per mg protein) MAO-A activities. This suggests that the structural gene is the primary determinant of enzyme activity in these cells. Since kinetic analysis of enzyme activities among a subset of these fibroblast lines has shown different V_{max}, rather than K_m values, and a number of active molecules proportional to activity levels, it is likely that the amount of the enzyme accounts for most of the differences in activity levels (Costa et al., 1980). The fact that no variations in cDNA coding sequences from several of these fibroblast lines have been found (Hotamisligil et al., 1994; Tivol et al., in press) suggests that sequence variations underlying the difference in activities probably reside in the noncoding regions controlling transcription, RNA processing or stability.

Similar genotyping of patients with Parkinson's disease (PD) and normal controls (Table 2) shows that the frequencies of certain alleles, particularly the "C 122" allele are markedly different between the two groups: 22% for the patients and 7% for the controls (Hotamisligil et al., 1994). For the *MAOB* gene, Table 3 shows that allele 180 of the $(GT)_n$ repeat was twice as common in PD patients as in controls (Hotamisligil et al., 1994). Since, as described above, the "C 122" allele appears to be associated with "high" enzyme activity (Table 1), and since the "C 122" allele occurs less frequently among patients with PD than among con-

TABLE 1

MAOA haplotypes and activities in male skin fibroblasts

Cell line[a]	Age (yr)	Activity[b] (pmol/min/mg protein)	Haplotype
HF56	17	0.1 ± 0.1	A 114
GM537	12	0.2 ± 0.1	A 114
GM409	7	0.9 ± 0.2	A —
GM497	4	0.9 ± 0.7	A —
On Ser	7	1.0 ± 0.2	A 114
GM2037	13	1.2 ± 0.6	A 114
A2	11	1.2 ± 0.6	A 114
Gm500	10	1.4 ± 0.3	A 116
Sal Mat	14	1.6 ± 0.4	A 118
To Ser	9	2.2 ± 0.7	C 126
GM498	3	2.7 ± 0.7	A 116
GM152	9	3.5 ± 0.9	A 114
115	13	3.6 ± 0.3	A 114
GM323	11	5.4 ± 0.6	A 114
GM1906	15	6.0 ± 3.1	A 114
GM1662	1	6.2 ± 1.0	C 122
87	12	6.7 ± 0.7	A 114
Al	15	7.4 ± 1.1	A 114
Rid Mor	15	9.2 ± 0.8	A 114
HF17	33	10.6 ± 2.7	A 114
HF9	25	12.1 ± 4.2	B 122
GM2227	12	15.0 ± 3.2	B 122
S3	3	16.1 ± 2.2	C 114
HF46	36	16.5 ± 1.7	C 126
HF8	26	17.7 ± 4.2	C 122
HF45	25	20.0 ± 4.9	C 126
R-E11	9	23.8 ± 3.3	B 122
GM316	12	24.5 ± 2.1	A 114
HF20	19	25.2 ± 3.2	C 122
HF53	36	26.7 ± 3.9	A 114
GM1653	37	27.1 ± 2.4	A 116
Ro Bel	14	31.7 ± 0.3	A 116
El San	8	31.9 ± 9.1	C 122
HF26	38	38.2 ± 2.1	C 122
HF10	23	41.8 ± 16.2	A 116
HF51	57	42.1 ± 10.4	A 114
HF39	54	52.3 ± 10.0	A 114
HF27	38	82.5 ± 16.0	C 122
HF52	47	84.5 ± 8.0	A 114
LN Bur	20	179.2 ± 30.9	A 114

[a]All skin fibroblast lines (except 115, GM537, On Ser, To Ser, Sal Mat, MG152, GM1906, S3, GM1662, GM2227, and LN Bur) are from control human males.
[b] Measured by a modification of the toluene extration procedure of Wurtman and Exelrod.
From Breakefield et al., 1994; with permission from Marcel Dekker, Inc.

TABLE 2

Distribution of *MAOA* haplotypes in controls and Parkinson patients

Haplotype	Controls (n = 129) (#)	Controls (if n = 91) (#)	Controls (%)	Patients (n = 91) (#)	Patients (%)
A 112	3	2.1	2.3	5	5.5
D 112	0	0	0	3	3.3
A 114	49	34.6	38.0	30	33.0
B 114	0	0	0	3	3.3
C 114	6	4.2	4.7	7	7.7
D 114	2	1.4	1.6	2	2.2
A 116	16	11.3	12.4	11	12.1
B 116	0	0	0	3	3.3
C 116	0	0	0	1	1.1
D 116	4	2.8	3.1	2	2.2
B 118	1	0.7	0.8	4	4.4
C 120	2	1.4	1.6	1	1.1
A 122	1	0.7	0.8	4	4.4
B 122	5	3.5	3.9	0	0
C[a] 122	28	19.8	21.7	7	7.7
D 122	0	0	0	4	4.4
C 124	1	0/7	0.8	1	1.1
C 126	10	7.1	7.8	5	5.5
D 126	0	0	0	2	2.2
C 130	1	0.7	0.8	0	0

[a]The frequency of this allele is significantly different in two populations (Fisher's Exact Test, $P = 0.005$).
From Hotamisligik et al, 1994; with permission of the Movement Disorder Society.

TABLE 3

Distribution of *MAOB* alleles in controls and Parkinson patients

Allele	Controls (n = 129)	Controls (if n = 91)	Controls (%)	Patients (n = 91)	Patients (%)	P values from Fisher's Exact Test
174	9	6.3	7.0	2	2.2	0.13
176	24	16.9	18.6	9	9.9	0.44
178	27	19.0	20.9	16	17.6	0.61
180	15	10.6	11.6	19	20.9	0.09
182	47	33.2	36.4	43	47.3	0.13
184	7	4.9	5.4	2	2.2	0.31

$\chi^2(5) = 11.3$, $P = 0.046$. From Hotamisligik et al, 1994; with permission of the Movement Disorder Society.

trols, it is possible that low levels of MAO A may contribute to susceptibility to PD, at least in some patients. This would be consistent with the "environmental toxin" hypothesis (Barbeau et al., 1987; Tanner, 1989), in which MAO-A plays the role of a detoxifying enzyme. However, other data suggest that high MAO activity may be toxic to dopaminergic neurons (Andersen et al., 1994), possibly by formation of free radicals (Cohen, 1987). A similar role for debrisoquine hydroxylase, which is a member of the cytochrome P-450 monooxygenase family, has also been suggested by the finding of an association of certain defective alleles with PD (Armstrong et al., 1992; Smith et al., 1992). Scanning the "C 122" alleles from control and PD patient groups, for sequence differences between groups, particularly in the regulatory regions, may bring insight to the factors that contribute to susceptibility to PD, as well as critical regulatory elements in the *MAO* genes.

In conclusion, advances in the molecular genetics of MAO have ushered in a new era for studying its role in human disease. We can foresee that, in the long run, correlations of sequence variations with disease phenotypes, as in the MAO-A-deficient patients (Brunner et al., 1993a), may begin to emerge by the use of methods based on PCR and SSCP. In addition, the allelic-association approach will continue to provide an efficient means for evaluating the role of *MAO* genes in different disease states. In the short run, detailed mutational analysis of those alleles associated with particular diseases, such as Parkinson's disease, may lead to further understanding of the role of MAO in susceptibility to the disease.

References

Andersen, J.K., Frim, D.M., Isacson, O. and Breakefield, X.O. (1994) Catecholaminergic cell atrophy in a transgenic mouse aberrantly overexpressing MAO-B in neurons. *Neurodegeneration*, 3: 97–109.

Armstrong, M., Daly, A.K., Cholerton, S., Bateman, D.N. and Idle, J.R (1992) Mutant debrisoquine hydroxylation genes in Parkinson's disease. *Lancet*, 339: 1017–1018.

Bach, A.W.J., Lan, N.C., Johnson, D.L., Abell, C.W., Bembenek, M.E., Kwan, S.-W., Seeburg, P.H. and Shih, J.C. (1988) cDNA cloning of human liver monoamine oxidase A and B: molecular basis of differences in enzymatic properties. *Proc. Natl. Acad. Sci. USA*, 85: 4934–4938.

Barbeau, A., Roy, M., Cloutier, T., Plasse, L. and Paris, S. (1987) Environmental and genetic factors in the etiology of Parkinson's disease. *Adv. Neurol.*, 45: 299–306.

Berger, W., Meindl, A. and van de Pol, T.R.J. (1992) Isolation of a candidate gene for Norrie disease by positional cloning. *Nature Genet.*, 1: 199–203.

Black, G.C.M., Chen, Z.-Y., Craig, I.W. and Powell, J.F. (1991) Dinucleotide repeat polymorphism at the MAOA locus. *Nucleic Acids Res.*, 19: 689.

Bond, P.A. and Bond, C.R.L. (1977) Properties of monoamine oxidase(MAO) in human blood platelets, plasma, lymphocytes and granulocytes. *Clin. Chim. Acta*, 80: 317–326.

Breakefield, X.O., Chen, Z.Y., Tivol, E., Shalish, C. and Craig, I. (1994) Molecular genetics and inheritance of human monoamine oxidases A and B. *Monoamine Oxidase Inhibitors in Neurological Diseases*, Marcel Dekker, New York, pp. 95–112.

Breakefield, X.O., Giller, E.L.J., Nurnberger, J.I., Castiglione, C.M., Buchsbaum, M.S. and Gershon, E.S. (1980) Monoamine oxidase type A in fibroblasts from patients with bipolar depressive illness. *Psychiatr. Res.*, 2: 307–314.

Brunner, H.G., Nelen, M., Breakefield, X.O., Ropers, H.H. and van Oost, B. (1993a) Abnormal behavior associated with a point mutation in the structural gene for monoamine oxidase A. *Science*, 262: 578–580.

Brunner, H.G., Nelen, M.R., van Zandvoort, P., Abeling, N.G.G.M., van Gennip, A.H., Wolters, E.C., Kuiper, M.A., Ropers, H.H. and B.A. van Oost (1993b) X-linked borderlne mental retardation with prominent behavioral disturbance: phenotype, genetic localization, and evidence for disturbed monoamine metabolism. *Am. J. Hum. Genet.*, 52: 1032–1039.

Chen, Z.-Y., Powell, J.F., Hsu, Y.-P.P., Breakefield, X.O. and Craig, I.W. (1992a) Organization of the human monoamine oxidase genes and long-range physical mapping around them. *Genomics*, 14: 75–82.

Chen, Z.-Y., Hendriks, R.W., Jobling, M.A., Powell, J.F., Monaco, A., Sims, K.B., Breakefield, X.O. and Craig, I.W. (1992b) Isolation and characterization of a gene implicated in Norrie disease. *Nature Genetics*, 1: 204–208.

Chen, Z.-Y., Hotamisligil, G.S., Huang, J.-K., Wen, L., Ezzeddine, D., Aydin-Muderrisoglu, N., Powell, J.F., Huang, R.H., Breakefield, X.O., Craig, I. and Hsu, Y.-P.P. (1991) Structure of the human gene for monoamine oxidase type A. *Nucleic Acids Res.*, 19: 4537–4541.

Cohen, G. (1987) Monoamine oxidase, hydrogen peroxide, and Parkinson's disease. *Adv. Neurol.*, 45: 119–125.

Costa, M.R.C., Edelstein, S.B., Castiglione, C.M., Chao, H. and Breakefield, X.O. (1980) Properties of monoamine oxidase in control and Lesch-Nyhan fibroblasts. *Biochem. Genet.*, 18: 577–590.

Crabb, D.W., Edenberg, H.J., Bosron, W.F. and Li, T.K. (1989) Genotypes for aldehyde dehydrogenase deficiency and alcohol sensitivity. The inactive ALDH2(2) allele is dominant. *J. Clin. Invest.*, 83: 314–316.

de la Chapelle, A., Sankila, E.-M., Lindlof, M., Aula, P. and Norio, R. (1985) Norrie disease caused by a gene deletion allowing carrier detection and prenatal diagnosis. *Clin. Genet.*, 28: 317–320.

Deguchi, T., Mashimo, M. and Suzuki, T. (1990) Correlation between acetylator phenotypes and genotypes of polymorphic arylamine *N*-acetyltransferase in human liver. *J. Biol. Chem.*, 265: 12757–12760.

Donnai, D., Mountford, R.C. and Read, A.P. (1988) Norrie disease resulting from a gene deletion: clinical features and DNA studies. *J. Med. Genet.*, 25: 73–78.

Edelstein, S.B., Castiglione, C.M. and Breakefield, X.O. (1978) Monoamine oxidase activity in normal and Lesch-Nyhan fibroblasts. *J. Neurochem.*, 31: 1247–1254.

Fowler, C.J., Tipton, K.F., MacKay, A.V.P. and Youdim, M.B.H (1982) Human platelet monoamine oxidase—a useful enzyme in the study of psychiatric disorders. *Neuroscience*, 7: 1577–1594.

Gal, A., Wieringa, B., Smeets, D.F., Bleeker-Wagemakers, L.M. and Ropers, H.H. (1986) Submicroscopic interstitial deletion of the X chromosome explains a complex genetic syndrome dominated by Norrie disease. *Cytogenet. Cell. Genet.*, 42: 219–24.

Gibbs, R.A., Nguyen, P.N. and Caskey, C.T. (1989) Detection of single DNA base differences by competitive oligonucleotide priming. *Nucleic Acids Res.*, 17: 2437–2448.

Giller, E.L.J., Castiglione, C.M., Wojciechowski, J. and Breakefield, X.O. (1982) Molecular properties of platelet MAO in psychiatric patients and controls. *Biological Markers in Psychiatry and Neurology*, Pergamon Press, New York.

Giller, E.L.J., Young, J.G., Breakefield, X.O., Carbonari, C., Braverman, M. and Cohen, D.J. (1980) Monoamine oxidase and catechol-*O*-methyltransferase activities in cultured fibroblasts and blood cells from children with autism and the Gilles de la Tourette Syndrome. *Psychiatry Res.*, 2: 307–314.

Grimsby, J., Chen, K., Wang, L.-J., Lan, N.C. and Shih, J.C. (1991) Human monoamine oxidase A and B genes exhibit identical exon-intron organization. *Proc. Natl. Acad. Sci. USA*, 88: 3637–3641.

Hotamisligil, G.S. and Breakefield, X.O. (1991) Human monoamine oxidase A gene determines levels of enzyme activity. *Am. J. Human Genet.*, 49: 383–392.

Hotamisligil, G.S., Girmen, A.S., Fink, J.S., Tivol, E., Shalish, C., Trofatter, J., Baenziger, J., Diamond, S., Markham, C., Sullivan, J., Growdon, J. and Breakefield, X.O. (1994)

Hereditary variations in monoamine oxidase as a risk factor for Parkinson's disease. *Movement Disorders*, 9: 305–310.

Hsu, Y.-P.P., Weyler, W., Chen, S., Sims, K.B., Rinehart, W.B., Utterback, M.C., Powell, J.F. and Breakefield, X.O. (1988) Structural features of human monoamine oxidase A elucidated from cDNA and peptide sequences. *J. Neurochem.*, 51: 1321–1324.

Hsu, Y.P., Powell, J.F., Sims, K.B. and Breakefield, X.O. (1989) Molecular genetics of the monoamine oxidases. *J. Neurochem.*, 53: 12–18.

Konradi, C., Ozelius, L. and Breakefield, X.O. (1992) Highly polymorphic $(GT)_n$ repeat sequence in intron II of the human MAOB gene. *Genomics*, 12: 176–177.

Kurth, J.H. and Kurth, M.C. (1992) A study of monoamine oxidase alleles as possible predictors of increased risk for developing Parkinson's disease. *Movement Disorder* (Suppl.) 1: 25.

Kurth, J.H., Kurth, M.C., Poduslo, S.E. and Schwankhaus, J.D (1993) Association of a monoamine oxidase B allele with Parkinson's disease. *Ann. Neurol.*, 33: 368–372.

Kwan, S.W., Bergeron, J.M. and Abell, C.W. (1992) Molecular properties of monoamine oxidases A and B. *Psychopharmacology*, (Suppl.) 106: S1–5.

Lan, N.C., Heinzmann, C., Gal, A., Klisak, I., Orth, U., Lai, E., Grimsby, J., Sparkes, R.S., Mohandas, T. and Shih, J.C. (1989) Human monoamine oxidase A and B genes map to Xp11.23 and are deleted in a patient with Norrie disease. *Genomics*, 4: 552–559.

Lauder, M.J. (1985) Roles for neurotransmitters in development; possible interaction with drugs during the fetal and neonatal periods. *Prog. Clin. Biol. Res.*, 163: 375–380.

Levy, E.R., Powell, J.F., Buckle, V.J., Hsu, Y.P., Breakefield, X.O. and Craig, I.W. (1989) Localization of human monoamine oxidase-A gene to Xp11.23–11.4 by in situ hybridization: implications for Norrie disease. *Genomics*, 5: 368–370.

Murphy, D.L., Sims, K.B., Karoum, F., de la Chapelle, A., Norio, R., Sankila, E.M. and Breakefield, X.O. (1990) Marked amine and amine metabolite changes in Norrie disease patients with an X-chromosomal deletion affecting monoamine oxidase. *J. Neurochem.*, 54: 242–247.

Murphy, D.L., Wright, C., Buchsbaum, M., Nicols, A., Costa, J.L. and Wyatt, R.J. (1976) Platelet and plasma amine oxidase activity in 680 normals: sex and age differences and stability over time. *Biochem. Med.*, 16: 254–265.

Orita, M., Iwahana, H., Kanazawa, H., Hayashi, K. and Sekiya, T. (1989a) Detection of polymorphisms of human DNA by gel electrophoresis as single-strand conformation polymorphisms. *Proc. Natl. Acad. Sci. USA*, 86: 2766–2770.

Orita, M., Suzuki, Y., Sekiya, T. and Hayashi, K. (1989b) Rapid and sensitive detection of point mutations and DNA polymorphisms using the polymerase chain reaction. *Genomics*, 5: 874–879.

Ozelius, L., Gusella, J.F. and Breakefield, X.O. (1989) *MspI* RFLP for human MAOA gene. *Nucleic Acids Res.*, 17: 10516.

Powell, J.F., Hsu, Y.P., Weyler, W., Chen, S.A., Salach, J., Andrikopoulos, K., Mallet, J. and Breakefield, X.O. (1989) The primary structure of bovine monoamine oxidase type A. Comparison with peptide sequences of bovine monoamine oxidase type B and other flavoenzymes. *Biochem. J.*, 259: 407–413.

Sandler, M., Reveley, M.A. and Glover, V. (1981) Human platelet monoamine oxidase activity in health and disease: a review. *J. Clin. Pathol.*, 34: 292–302.

Shih, C.J. (1991) Molecular basis of human MAO A and B. *Neuropsychopharmacology*, 4: 1–7.

Sims, K.B., de la Chapelle, A., Norio, R., Sankila, E.-M., Hsu, Y.-P.P.,Rinehart, W.B., Corey, T.J., Ozelius, L., Powell, J.F., Bruns, G., Gusella, J.F., Murphy, D.L. and Breakefield, X.O. (1989) Monoamine oxidase deficiency in males with an X chromosome deletion. *Neuron*, 2: 1069–1076.

Sims, K.B., Lebo, R.V., Benson, G., Shalish, C., Golbus, M.S. and Breakefield, X.O. (1992) The Norrie disease gene maps to a 150 kb region on chromosome Xp11.3. *Hum. Mol. Genet.*, 1: 83–89.

Smith, C.A.D., Gough, A.C., Leigh, P.N., Summers, B.A., Harding, A.E., Maranganore, D.M., Sturman, S.G., Schapira, A.H.V., Williams, A.C., Spurr, N.K. and Wolf, C.R. (1992) Debrisoquine hydroxylase gene polymorphism and susceptibility to Parkinson's disease. *Lancet*, 339: 1375–1377.

Tabakoff, B., Hoffman, P.L., Lee, J.M., Saito, T., Willard, B., L. De and Jones, F. (1988) Differences in platelet enzyme activity between alcoholics and nonalcoholics. *N. Engl. J. Med.*, 318: 134–139.

Tanner, M.C. (1989) The role of environmental toxins in the etiology of Parkinson's disease. *TINS*, 12: 49–54.

Tivol, E.A., Shalish, C., Schuback, D.E., Hsu, Y.-P. and X.O. Breakefield Mutational analysis of the human MAOA gene. *Neuropsych. Genetics*, in press.

van Duijn, C.M., de Kniff, P., Cruts, M., Wehnert, A., Havekes, L.M., Hofman, A. and Broeckhoven, C.V. (1994) Apolipoprotein E4 allele in a population-based study of early-onset Alzheimer's disease. *Nature Genetics*, 7: 74.

von Knorring, A.L., Bohman, M., von Knorring, L. and Oreland, L. (1985) Platelet MAO activity as a biological marker in subgroups of alcoholism. *Acta Psychiatr. Scand.*, 72: 51–58.

Warburg, M. (1966) Norrie's disease: a congenital progressive oculo-acousticocerebral degeneration. *Acta Ophthalmol.* (Suppl.), 89: 1–47.

Weyler, W., Hsu, Y.-P.P. and Breakefield, X.O. (1990) Biochemistry and genetics of monoamine oxidase. *Pharmacol. Ther.*, 47: 391–417.

Wurtman, R.J. and Axelrod, J. (1963) A sensitive and specific assay for the estimation of monoamine oxidase. *Biochem. Pharmacol.*, 12: 1439–1441.

Zhu, D., Antonarakis, S.E., Schmeckpeper, B.J., Biergaarde, P.J., Greb, A. E. and Maumenee, I.H. (1989) Microdeletion in the X-chromosome and prenatal diagnosis in a family with Norrie disease. *Am. J. Hum. Genet.*, 33: 485–488.

Zureick, J.L. and Meltzer, H.Y. (1988) Platelet MAO activity in hallucinating and paranoid schizophrenics: a review and meta-analysis. *Biol. Psychiatry*, 24: 63–78.

Peter M. Yu, Keith F. Tipton and Alan A. Boulton (Eds.)
Progress in Brain Research, Vol 106
© 1995 Elsevier Science BV. All rights reserved.

CHAPTER 8

The correlation between platelet MAO activity and personality: short review of findings and a discussion on possible mechanisms

Lars Oreland[1] and Jarmila Hallman[2]

[1]*Department of Medical Pharmacology, POB 593, BMC, University of Uppsala, 751 24 Uppsala, Sweden, and* [2]*Department of Psychiatry, University Hospital, 7551 85 Uppsala, Sweden*

The literature on platelet monoamine oxidase (MAO; E.C. 1.4.3.4) activity has been reviewed several times (Fowler et al., 1982; Oreland and Hallman, 1989; Oreland, 1993); the present communication is an attempt to update this information and to speculate further on possible mechanisms behind the correlation between this enzyme activity and personality.

Platelet MAO is of the B-type and has the same amino acid sequence as that in the brain (Chen et al., 1993), confirming a previous explanation that the minor kinetic differences between the two were due to a modest influence of membrane microenvironment (Fowler et al., 1989). The enzyme is stable during one's lifetime, however, with a possible increase after the age of 40 (Murphy et al., 1976; Bridge et al., 1985; Bagdy and Rihmer, 1986). Several twin studies have shown a high degree of heritability and in the recent study by Pedersen et al. (1993) a heritability factor of 0.75 was found.

Buchsbaum et al. (1976) presented, approximately 20 years ago, their so-called "vulnerability hypothesis" for platelet MAO. The implication was that low activities of platelet MAO are associated with personality traits which increase the vulnerability of an individual to, for example, drug-abuse and social maladaptation. The hypothesis received strong support when it was simultaneously reported that alcoholics had low levels of platelet MAO and that this low activity was a constitutional trait rather than an effect of alcohol consumption (Wiberg et al., 1977). In a great number of studies, the relationship between low levels of platelet MAO and personality characteristics such as sensation-seeking, impulsiveness, monotony avoidance and, to some degree, aggression has been confirmed (Schalling et al., 1987; see Oreland, 1993). In studies of monkeys, strong correlations between platelet MAO and behaviour have been revealed which, in essence, parallel the findings with humans (Redmond et al., 1979). Other support stems from the report by Sostek et al. (1981) that platelet MAO activity is related to the behaviour in newborn babies such as screaming and motor activity as well as their consolability.

Further confirmation was obtained in our study investigating the correlation between platelet MAO activity and neuropsychological measures (af Klinteberg et al., 1990). Response time and variations (SD) in response to left-sided stimuli were found to be significantly correlated to platelet MAO activity and this was interpreted as a higher degree of activation for the contralateral (right) hemisphere in individuals with low platelet

MAO activity. In a perceptual maze test, there was a significant relationship between low platelet MAO activity and short check times after completing the problem. Of perhaps the greatest interest was the strong correlation with failed inhibition, a measure of how many mistakes the individuals made when a visual sign indicated "press the button" and a simultaneous auditory signal cancelled this order. These results could be interpreted in many ways depending on the conceptual framework. The simplest is to conclude that low MAO probands prefer speed over accuracy. It may also, in line with Luria (1980), indicate a low frontal inhibitory activity, which was associated with low planning and checking capacity. It may also be regarded as an index of motor disinhibition, comparable to the reduced capacity for refraining from making a previously punished spontaneous response, which according to Soubrié (1986) and others is associated with serotonergic depletion.

The associations between platelet MAO activity and personality most probably provide the basis for the associations between platelet MAO activity and various psychiatric disorders. In some cases, such as drug abuse and psychopathy, basic personality could be expected to play a vital role in the development of the disorder, while in other cases, such as schizophrenia, depression or panic disorder, platelet MAO, reflecting premorbid personality, might correlate to symptoms or subclasses of the disorder (see Oreland, 1993).

As already mentioned, low platelet MAO activity has been demonstrated in alcoholics (see Oreland, 1993). The subclassification of alcoholism into types 1 and 2, based on heritable and environmental factors in a series of adopted children (Cloninger et al., 1981), has provided valuable information on the relation between platelet MAO activity and alcoholism. Thus, it could be shown that mainly type 2 alcoholics (with a strongly inherited disposition) and to a lesser degree type 1 alcoholics (environmentally conditioned), have low platelet MAO and the sensation seeking-related personality traits associated with this biochemical marker (von Knorring et al.,

1985). These results have been confirmed by a large number of independent groups and, most recently, in an excellent series of papers by Devor et al. (1994). Several previous results supporting the genetic aspects of alcoholism by showing low platelet MAO activity in first-order relatives of alcoholics has also been confirmed and extended by Devor et al. (1993) showing a significant overrepresentation of alcoholism in those relatives of alcoholics who themselves had low MAO-B activity.

Another interesting area in relation to platelet MAO activity is psychopathy, criminality and aggressive behaviour. Very early, Yu and colleagues contributed to this, although the results were not entirely conclusive (Yu, 1984). Their indications of a connection between criminality and low platelet MAO activity could be verified by the findings of considerably lower platelet MAO activity in consecutive patients undergoing forensic psychiatric examination in comparison with construction builders (Lidberg et al., 1985). It is noticeable that in this study the mean MAO activity among the staff at the clinic was in between that of the patients and the workers. In a more recent study, violence and aggressiveness in crime were associated with low platelet MAO activity (Belfrage et al., 1992). The result with regard to the staff at the clinic of forensic psychiatry has later been extended to show that there are differences between various groups of students, those studying medicine and psychology being at the lower end (Schalling and Oreland, unpublished results). Also among physicians there seem to be differences. In a recent study on specialists in internal medicine, surgeons and psychiatrists, the two former groups had medium mean activities, while the latter group had lower activities (Hallman and Oreland, unpublished).

A question of interest is whether the associations between platelet MAO and personality might be of any clinical use. In a recent study, platelet MAO activity was analysed in men who had committed crime before the age of 15, and associations of MAO activity with continuing criminal activity were determined over the next

15 years (Alm et al., 1994). Those who had continued with such criminal activity were found to have highly significantly lower platelet MAO activity, and it seems as though platelet MAO has a high predictive value. In another recent study, in order to understand this predictive value of platelet MAO activity, the childhood behaviour in 84 male subjects, dichotomized with regard to hyperactivity and aggressiveness, and their platelet MAO at adulthood were analysed. Low platelet MAO activity was found to be specifically associated neither with hyperactive behaviour nor with aggressiveness, but with the combination of the two (af Klinteberg et al., unpublished observations). A possible clinical use of platelet MAO, other than in forensic psychiatry, might be in differentiating between type 1 and type 2 alcoholics so as to choose type-specific treatment programmes.

From the above, it may seem as if low platelet MAO activity is mainly associated with negative factors. However, it is essential to emphasize that low platelet MAO activity need not be negative for the individual; leadership, creativity, and boldness are personality traits which tend to also be characteristic of an individual with low platelet MAO (von Knorring et al., 1984).

At the high end, with regard to platelet MAO activity, panic disorder and agoraphobia have been candidates (e.g. Yu et al., 1983). Results are, however, again conflicting (see Oreland, 1993), possibly reflecting different diagnostic routines. Recently, a series of patients with social phobia diagnosed according to the DSM III-R were investigated and their activities were found to be very high in comparison with controls (Fahlén et al., unpublished results).

With regard to the question which mechanism lies behind those associations, there are some obvious possibilities:

Hypothesis 1: platelet MAO is correlated to brain MAO-B, which then would cause the personality traits of interest as a result of the rate of neurotransmitter degradation.

Hypothesis 2: platelet MAO directly influences the level of some trace amine, e.g. β-phenylethyl-amine, which might be of importance for behaviour.

Hypothesis 3: platelet MAO is regulated together with other mitochondrial enzymes, and low platelet MAO might indicate generally low mitochondrial function (or number), which might result in more marked effects on some transmitter systems than on others.

Hypothesis 4: platelet MAO is a genetic marker, e.g. for the "capacity" of some central transmitter system. Such a common genetic control could occur via common gene promoter activating or inhibiting compounds.

With regard to hypothesis No. 1, there are two studies in which no correlation between platelet and brain MAO activities was found (Winblad et al., 1979; Young et al., 1986). It may, however, be argued that only MAO in some specific compartment, brain region or cell type might correlate. Even if one presupposes that thrombocyte and CNS MAO-B activities are determined by a common genetic pathway, several factors must be taken into consideration which may undermine the possibility that low brain MAO-B activity, in effect, causes those personality traits characteristic for respective individuals. Most of the traits linked to platelet MAO activity seem to indicate that central serotonergic activity should be involved (see below). Serotonin is a poor substrate for MAO-B in comparison with MAO-A and, along the same line, drugs which act as MAO-A inhibitors have a substantially higher effect on serotonergic activity than MAO-B inhibitors (see Murphy et al., 1987). The difference regarding brain MAO-B activity between different individuals within a specific age category is, in retrospect, so small that it is difficult to imagine that it could have any physiological significance (Fowler et al., 1980). In contrast to the case with platelets, brain MAO-B activity increases with age. This increase (approx. 20–30% per decade in some regions) has its basis in an increase in the proportion of glial cells in the brain expressing high MAO-B activity (Ekblom et al., 1993). On a relative basis, this increase is more significant than the difference between different individuals regarding age-corrected MAO-B activities. It has not yet been shown that there are any significant changes in the personality traits in question, even when brain MAO-B is completely inhibited with selegeline, a specific MAO-B inhibitor currently used in the treatment of Parkinson's disease. Further evidence which detracts from the possibility that there exists a causal relationship between low brain MAO-B activity and a low metabolic turnover of serotonin comes from findings that aggression (Eichelman, 1987) and high sexual activity in animals (Meyerson et al., 1985) are characteristic of the opposite, i.e. low serotonergic activity. Indeed, low serotonergic activity should be a direct result of a higher catabolic activity by MAO.

With regard to hypothesis No. 2, that platelet MAO directly influences the level of some trace amine, e.g. β-phenylethylamine, which might be of importance for behaviour, this possibility has been explored in the past with results of possible interest, but further exploration is needed (Yu et al., 1983, 1984). In a recent paper, however, a striking correlation between platelet MAO activity and plasma levels of β-phenylethylamine was reported (Yamada et al., 1994) and the plasma levels of this compound have, indeed been linked to behaviour, although not exactly those behaviors linked to platelet MAO activity (Moises et al., 1985; Yamada et al., 1994). Clear evidence has been published, by using single cell recording, that low doses of β-phenylethylamine given systemically induces marked effects on both central dopaminergic and noradrenergic neurons (Lundberg et al., 1985; Oreland et al., 1985). In summary, the possibility that some trace amine might play a role in this context still deserves some attention.

Hypothesis No. 3, that platelet MAO is regulated together with other mitochondrial enzymes, and that low platelet MAO might indicate generally low mitochondrial function (or number), stems from recent results showing significant correlations between MAO, cytochrome oxidase and isocitrate dehydrogenase activities in platelets

from a series of controls (Prince et al., 1994). Furthermore, these enzyme activities were reduced to approximately the same extent (30%) in patients with Down's syndrome (Prince et al., 1994). In this study, however, the activity of a fourth mitochondrial enzyme, glutamate dehydrogenase, was neither correlated to the other mitochondrial enzymes in controls nor reduced in Down's syndrome patients. If this correlation between MAO and several mitochondrial enzymes also prevails in brain tissue, individuals with low platelet MAO activity might also have a low energy supply in neurons. It could be further speculated that different types of neurons might have a different response towards such a shortage and that serotonergic neurons especially might function at a lower level of transmitter release or with a lower rate of axonal growth.

With regard to hypothesis No. 4, that platelet MAO is a genetic marker which is regulated by mechanisms also regulating some brain function of importance, it has been found with healthy individuals that there is a significant correlation between cerebrospinal fluid levels of the serotonin metabolite 5-HIAA and platelet MAO (Oreland et al., 1981). This is in good agreement with the finding that both adult men with a tendency for aggressive behaviour and aggressive children and youths have low levels of 5-HIAA in cerebral spinal fluid (Brown et al., 1979; Krusei et al., 1990), that is, individuals who also have low levels of trbc-MAO. Recently, low levels of CSF 5-HIAA have also been linked to another category of patients, type 2 alcoholics (Virkkunen and Linnoila, 1993). Furthermore, "failed inhibitions", which is inversely correlated with platelet MAO activity, is considered to be mainly a serotonergic measure (see above). In lieu of this, as well as the fact that the serotonergic neuron, in contrast to other monoaminergic neurons, but similar to the thrombocyte, contains the "wrong type" of the enzyme, i.e. MAO-B (Levitt et al., 1982), we have, since the middle of the seventies, cultivated the hypothesis that platelet MAO is a genetic marker for the size or functional capacity of the central serotonergic system (Oreland, 1979, 1993; Oreland and Shaskan, 1983).

The cloning of both MAO-A and -B was reported for the first time in 1988 by Jean Shih and her group (Bach et al., 1988). Both of these genes reside on the short arm of the X-chromosome (Lan et al., 1989). Despite the rapid increase in knowledge pertaining to the molecular genetic characteristics of MAO, there exists still very little definitive information which could serve as a basis with which to tie together variations in MAO activity between individuals, with respect to either the A- or B-type, to established alleles of the respective gene (Hotamisligil and Breakefield, 1991; Girmen et al., 1992). It seems more reasonable that the regulation of MAO-A and -B is determined to the greatest degree by what level their promoter sequences, i.e. the region which activates and controls the speed with which a gene is expressed, are activated or inhibited (Zhu et al., 1992). The gene's promoter sequences are thus affected by various factors which bind to specific sequences of the promoter region. In other words, much of the regulation behind the activity of the MAO enzymes should rest on the level of transcription, i.e. the speed of synthesis of respective mRNA. This hypothesis is substantiated by the findings of a correlation between mRNA levels of MAO-A and -B and the respective catalytic activity of each enzyme in different tissues (Grimsby et al., 1990). In addition, it has never been possible to validate, despite many studies, qualitative differences in the MAO-A and -B proteins between individuals with different activities (see Oreland, 1993). A genetic control, functioning to the greatest degree through the promoter sequence, opens the possibility of explaining apparently contradictory results. First, the correlation between brain MAO-A and -B which exists in different individuals can be explained by the possibility that both genes have promoter regions with similar binding regions (Zhu et al., 1992). Thus, an individual with low MAO-A activity in one brain region should, in essence, have not only low MAO-A activity in the brain in general, but also low MAO-B activity.

More important, however, is the fact that with the knowledge of the make-up of the promoter region, it should be possible to see whether certain factors are decisive in the regulation of serotonergic neuron growth as well. If this is the case, then it would explain the connection between low or disturbed MAO transcription, resulting in low MAO activities, and low or disturbed development of the brain's serotonergic system with characteristic personality traits and resulting behavioural disturbances.

Brunner et al. recently reported a relationship between familial behavioural disturbances and a defect in the gene which codes for MAO-A (Morell, 1993; Brunner et al., 1993). This Dutch report describes how eight male members of a family of 24 demonstrated moderate mental retardation and repeated episodes of aggressive behaviour including, among other things, attempted murder, arson with intent to murder, and sexual assault. With the help of linkage analysis, it was possible to connect these disturbances to a defect in the gene encoding MAO-A, which is localised close to the gene encoding MAO-B on the short arm of the X chromosome. Further in support of the possibility that these individuals had a defect in the monoamine-metabolising capacity of MAO-A, Brunner found that monoamines and their metabolites in urine were at levels which could be expected if there was a selective reduction in MAO-A activity. It was also directly shown that individuals with excessive aggression and a defect in the MAO-A gene had normal platelet MAO activities. One must therefore infer that the reported syndrome does not imply any molecular explanation for the earlier, well-described associations between MAO-B and aggression. Inhibition of MAO-A produces an anti-depressive effect, a fact which has been demonstrated in clinical trials leading to the registration of, for example, the selective MAO-A inhibitor moclobemide in Sweden. The mechanism behind the effects of MAO-A inhibitors is likely to be an increase in the levels of serotonin in serotonergic synapses, even though the inhibition of the enzyme should occur at another localisation than within serotonergic neurons (which contains MAO-B; see above). A decrease in the activity of MAO-A, as a result of a defect in the gene itself, should similarly produce an increase in serotonin concentration in the synapses. The symptoms observed by Brunner et al. were, however, in direct opposition to those expected, i.e psychological disturbances, with aggression being among the most prominent, instead of the predicted anti-depressive/anti-aggression effect. We can merely state that the cause of this discrepancy between observed and expected effects is not explainable with existing knowledge.

References

af Klinteberg, B., Oreland, L., Hallman, J. Wirsén and Schalling, D. (1990) Exploring the connections between platelet monoamine oxidase (MAO) activity and behavior: Relationships with performance in neuropsychological tasks. *Neuropsychobiology*, 23: 188–196.

Alm, P.O., Alm, M., Humble, K., Leppert, J., Sörensen, S., Lidberg, L. and Oreland, L. (1994) Criminality and platelet monoamine oxidase (MAO) activity in juvenile delinquents grown up. *Acta Psychiatr. Scand.*, 89: 41–45.

Bach, A.W. J., Lan, N.C., Johnson, D.L., Abell, C.W., Bembenek, M.E., Kwan, S-W., Seeburg, P.H. and Shih, J.C. (1988) cDNA cloning of human liver monoamine oxidase A and B: Molecular basis of differences in enzymatic properties. *Proc. Natl. Acad. Sci. USA*, 85: 4934–4938.

Bagdy, G. and Rihmer, Z. (1986) Measurement of platelet monoamine oxidase activity in healthy human volunteers. *Acta Physiol. Hung.*, 68: 19–24.

Belfrage, H., Oreland, L. and Lidberg, L. (1992) Platelet monoamine oxidase activity – a diagnostic tool for mentally disordered non-psychotic violent offenders. *Acta Psychiatr. Scand.*, 85: 218–221.

Bridge, T.P., Soldo, B.J., Phelps, B.H., Wise, C.D., Franacak, M. J. and Wyatt, R.J. (1985) Platelet monoamine oxidase activity: demographic characteristics contribute to enzyme activity variability. *J. Gerontol.*, 40: 23–28.

Brown, G.L., Goodwin, F.K., Ballenger, J.C., Goyer, P.F. and Major, L.F. (1979) Aggression in humans correlates with cerebrospinal fluid amine metabolites. *Psychiatr. Res.*, 1: 131–139.

Brunner, H.G., Nelen, M.R., van Zandvoort, P., Abeling, N.G. G. M., van Gennip, A.H., Wolters, E.C., et al. (1993) X-linked borderline mental retardation with prominent behavioral disturbance: phenotype, genetic localization, and evidence for disturbed monoamine metabolism. *Am. J. Hum. Genet.*, 52: 1032–1039.

Buchsbaum, M.S., Coursey, R.D. and Murphy, D.L. (1976) The biochemical high-risk paradigm: behavioral and familial correlates of low platelet monoamine oxidase activity. *Science*, 194: 339–341.

Chen, K., Wu, H-F. and Shih J.C. (1993) The deduced amino acid sequences of human platelet and frontal cortex monoamine oxidase B are identical. *J. Neurochem.*, 61:187–190.

Cloninger, C.R., Bohman, M. and Sigvardsson, S. (1981) Inheritance of alcohol abuse. *Arch. Gen. Psychiatry*, 38 :861–68.

Devor, E.J., Cloninger, R., Hoffman, P.L. and Tabakoff, B. (1993) Association of monoamine oxidase (MAO) activity with alcoholism and alcoholic subtypes. *Am. J. Med Genet.*, 48: 209–213.

Devor, E.J., Abell, C.W., Hoffman, P.L., Tabakoff, B. and Cloninger, R. (1994) Platelet MAO Activity in Type I and Type II Alcoholism. *Ann. N.Y. Acad. Sci.*, 708: 119–128.

Eichelman, B. (1987) Neurochemical and psychopharmacologic aspects of aggressive behavior. In: H.Y. Meltzer (Ed.), *Psychopharmacology. The Third Generation of Progress*, Raven Press, New York, pp. 697–704.

Ekblom, J., Jossan, S.S., Oreland, L., Walum, E. and Aquilonius, S-M. (1993) Reactive gliosis and monoamine oxidase-B. *Glia*, 8:122–132.

Fowler, C.J., Ekstedt, B., Egashira, T., Kinemuchi, H. and Oreland, L. (1979) The interaction between human platelet monoamine oxidase, its monoamine substrates and oxygen. *Biochem. Pharmacol.*, 28: 3063–3068.

Fowler, C.J., Wiberg, Å., Oreland, L., Marcusson, J. and Winblad, B. (1980) The effect of age on the activity and molecular properties of human brain monoamine oxidase. *J. Neural Transmiss.*, 49: 1–20.

Fowler, C.J., Tipton, K.F., MacKay, A.V. P. and Youdim, M.B. H. (1982) Human platelet monoamine oxidase – A useful enzyme in the study of psychiatric disorders? *Neuroscience*, 7: 1577–1594.

Girmen, A.S., Baenziger, J., Hotamisligil, G.S., Konradi, C., Shalish, C., Sullivan, J.L. and Breakefield, X.O. (1992) Relationship between platelet monoamine oxidase B activity and alleles at the MAO-B locus. *J. Neurochem.*, 59: 2063–2066.

Grimsby, J., Lan, N.C., Neve, R., Chen, K. and Shih, J.C. (1989) Tissue distribution of human monoamine oxidase A and B m RNA. *J. Neurochem.*, 55: 1166–1169.

Hotamisligil, G.S. and Breakefield, X.O. (1991) Human monoamine oxidase a gene determines levels of enzyme activity. *Am. J. Hum. Genet.*, 49: 383–392.

Kruesi, M.J. P., Rapoport, J.L., Hamburger, S., Hibbs, E., Potter, W.Z., Lenane, M., et al. (1990) Cerebrospinal fluid monoamine metabolites, aggression and impulsivity in disruptive behavior disorders of children and adolescents. *Arch. Gen. Psychiatry*, 47: 419–426.

Lan, N.C., Heinzmann, C., Gal, A., Klisak, I., Orth, U., Lai, E., Grimsby, J., Sparkes, R.S., Mohandas, T. and Shih, J.S. (1989) Human monoamine oxidase A and B genes map to Xp11.23 and are deleted in a patient with Norrie disease. *Genomics*, 4: 552–559.

Levitt, P., Pintar, J.E. and Breakefield, X.O. (1982) Immuno-cytochemical demonstration of monoamine oxidase B in brain astrocytes and serotonergic neurons. *Proc. Natl. Acad. Sci. USA*, 79: 6385–6389.

Lidberg, L., Modin, I., Oreland, L., Tuck, J.R. and Kristian-son, M. (1985) Platelet monoamine oxidase activity and psychopathy. *Psychiatr. Res.*, 16:4: 339–343.

Lundberg, P.-Å., Oreland, L. and Engberg, G. (1985) Inhibi-tion of locus coeruleus neuronal activity by beta-phenyleth-ylamine. *Life Sci.*, 36: 1889–1896.

Luria, A.R. (1980) *Higher Cortical Functions in Man*, 2nd edn., Basic Books, New York.

Meyerson, B.J., Malmnäs, C.O. and Everitt, B.J. (1985) Neu-ropharmacology, neurotransmitters and sexual behavior in mammals. In: N. Adler, D. Pfaff and R.W. Goy (Eds.), *Handbook of Behavioral Neurobiology*, Plenum Press, New York, pp. 495–536.

Moises, H.W., Waldmeier, P. and Beckmann, H. (1985) Phenylethylamine and personality. In: A.A. Boulton, L. Maitre, P.R. Bieck and P. Riederer (Eds.), *Neuropsy-chopharmacology of the Trace Amines. Experimental and Clinical Aspects*, Humana Press, Clifton, NJ, pp. 387–394.

Morell, V. (1993) Evidence found for possible "aggression gene". *Science*, 260: 1722–1723.

Murphy, D.L., Wright, C., Buchsbaum, M., Nichols, A., Costa, J.L. and Wyatt, R.J. (1976) Platelet and plasma amine oxidase activity in 680 normals: Sex and age differences and stability over time. *Biochem. Med.*, 16: 254–256.

Murphy, D.L., Aulakh, C.S., Garrick, N.A. and Sunderland, T. (1987) Monoamine oxidase inhibitors as antidepressants: Implications for the mechanism of action of antidepressant and the psychobiology of the affective disorders and some related disorders. In: H.Y. Meltzer (Ed.), *Psychopharma-cology, The Third Generation of Progress*, Raven Press, New York, pp. 546–551.

Oreland, L. (1979) The activity of human brain and thrombo-cyte monoamine oxidase (MAO) in relation to various psychiatric disorders. I. MAO Activity in some disease states. In: T. Singer, R. von Korff, and D. Murphy (Eds.), *Monoamine Oxidase; Structure, Function and Altered Func-tions*, Academic Press, New York, pp. 379–387.

Oreland, L. (1993) Monoamine oxidase in neuropsychiatric disorders. In: H. Yasuhara, S.H. Parvez, M. Sandler, K. Oguchi and T. Nagatsu (Eds.), *Monoamine Oxidase: Basic and Clinical Aspects*, VSP Press, Utrecht, pp. 219–247.

Oreland, L. and Hallman, J. (1988) Monoamine oxidase activi-ties in relation to psychiatric disorders: The state of the art. *Nord. J. Psychiatry*, 42: 95–105.

Oreland, L. and Shaskan, E.G. (1983) Monoamine oxidase activity as a biological marker. *Trends Pharmacol. Sci.*, 4: 339–341.

Oreland, L., Wiberg, Å., Åsberg, M., Träskman, L., Sjöstrand, L., Thorén, P., Bertilsson, L. and Tybring, G. (1981) Platelet MAO activity and monoamine metabolites in cerebrospinal fluid in depressed and suicidal patients and in healthy controls. *Psychiatr. Res.*, 4: 21–29.

Oreland, L., Lundberg, P.-Å. and Engberg, G. (1985) Effects of 2-phenylethylamine and tyramine on central nora-drenaline and dopamine systems: an electrophysiological study. In: A.A. Boulton, L. Maitre, P.R. Bieck and P. Riederer (Eds.), *Neuropsychopharmacology of the Trace Amines. Experimental and Clinical Aspects*, Humana Press, Clifton, NJ, pp. 201–213.

Pedersen, N.L., Oreland, L., Reynolds, C. and McClearn G.E. (1993) Importance of genetic influence on thrombocyte MAO activity in twins reared together. *Psychiat. Res.*, 6: 239–251.

Prince, J., Shia, J., Båve, U., Annerén, G. and Oreland, L. (1994) Mitochondrial enzyme deficiences in Down's syn-drome. *J. Neural Transmiss. Park. Dis. Dement. Sect.*, 8: 171–181.

Redmond, Jr, D.E., Murphy, D.L. and Baulu, J. (1979) Platelet monoamine oxidase activity correlates with social affiliative and agonistic behaviors in normal Rhesus monkeys. *Psy-chosomatic Medicine*, 41: 87–100.

Schalling, D., Åsberg, M., Oreland L. and Edman, G. (1987) Markers for vulnerability to psycho-pathology. Tempera-ment traits associated with platelet MAO activity. *Acta Psychiatr. Scand.*, 76: 172–182.

Soubrié, P.H. (1986) Reconciling the role of central serotonin neurons in human and animal behavior. *Behav. Brain Sci.*, 9: 319–363.

Sostek, A.J., Miller Sostek, A., Murphy, D.L., Bond Martin, E. and Smith Born, W. (1981) Cord blood amine oxidase activities relate to arousal and motor functioning in human newborns. *Life Sci.*, 28: 2561–2568.

Virkkunen M. and Linnoila, M. (1993) Brain serotonin, type 2 alcoholism and impulsive violence. *J. Stud. Alc.* Suppl. 11: 163–69.

von Knorring, A-L., Bohman, M., von Knorring, L. and Ore-land, L. (1985) Platelet oxidase activity as a biological marker in subgroups of alcoholism. *Acta Psychiatr. Scand.*, 72: 51–58.

von Knorring, L., Oreland, L. and Winblad, B. (1984) Person-ality traits related to monoamine oxidase activity in platelets. *Psychiatry Res.*, 12: 11–26.

Wiberg, Å., Gottfries, C-G. and Oreland, L. (1977) Low platelet monoamine oxidase activity in human alcoholics. *Med. Biol.*, 55: 181–186.

Winblad, B., Gottfries, C-G., Oreland, L. and Wiberg, Å. (1979) Monoamine oxidase in human platelets and brains of non-neurological geriatric patients. *Med. Biol.*, 57:129–132.

Yamada, S., Hirano, M., Nishi, S., Inokuchi, T. and Uchimura, H. (1994) Temperament traits associated with platelet monoamine oxidase activity and plasma 2-phenylethylamine in healthy volunteers. *Biogenic Amines*, 10: 295–302

Young, W.F., Laws, E.R., Sharbrough, F.W. and Weinshilboum, R.M. (1986) Human monoamine oxidase. Lack of brain and platelet correlation. *Arch. Gen. Psychiatry*, 43: 604–609.

Yu, P.H., Bowen, R.C., Davis, B.A. and Boulton, A.A. (1983) Platelet monoamine oxidase activity and trace acid levels in plasma of agoraphobic patients. *Acta Psychiatr. Scand.*, 67: 188–194.

Yu, P.H., Davis, B.A., Bowen, R.D., Wormith, S., Addington, D. and Boulton A.A. (1984) The catabolism of trace amines in some psychiatric disorders. In: A. Boulton, W. Baker, W.G. Dewhurst and M. Sandler (Eds.), *Neurobiology of the Trace Amines*, The Humana Press, Clifton, NJ, pp. 475–486.

Zhu, Q.-S., Grimsby, J., Chen, K. and Shih, J.C. (1992) Promoter organization and activity of human monoamine oxidase (MAO) A and B genes. *J. Neurosci.*, 12:11:4437–4446.

Peter M. Yu, Keith F. Tipton and Alan A. Boulton (Eds.)
Progress in Brain Research, Vol 106
© 1995 Elsevier Science BV. All rights reserved.

CHAPTER 9

Platelet MAO activities and MAO-B protein concentrations in Parkinson's disease and controls

C.C. Finch[1], S.L. Ho[2], A.C. Williams[2] and E.E. Billett[1]

[1]*Department of Life Sciences, The Nottingham Trent University, Clifton Lane, Nottingham, NG11 8NS, UK, and*
[2]*Department of Clinical Neurology, Birmingham University, Birmingham B15 2TH, UK*

Introduction

Monoamine oxidase (amine:oxygen oxidoreductase (deaminating) (flavin containing), EC 1.4.3.4) (MAO) is a membrane-bound mitochondrial enzyme responsible for the metabolism of both endogenous and exogenous biogenic amines.

MAO exists in two functionally different forms, A and B, the A form sensitive to the irreversible inhibitor clorgyline and the B form sensitive to L-deprenyl (Knoll and Magyar, 1972). Differences in substrate specificity and immunological properties (Denney et al., 1982) are also indicators of the two forms. The nucleotide and amino acid sequences of the human and bovine subtypes indicate that the two proteins are encoded by separate but related genes (approx. 70% homology) closely linked on the X chromosome (Bach et al., 1988). Various analyses of MAO activity in human tissues, including brain, indicate that both forms are present, but placenta has been reported to contain only MAO-A and blood platelets only MAO-B (Youdim, 1988). Platelet MAO-B has traditionally been used as a model for brain MAO-B (Youdim, 1988), and it is now known that the deduced amino acid sequences of MAO-B derived from human platelets and brain frontal cortex are identical (Chen et al., 1993).

Platelets are also able to accumulate, store and release the neurotransmitter 5-hydroxytrypta-mine. This knowledge has further fuelled the idea that platelets can serve as models for serotonergic neurones. In the human brain dopamine is a substrate for MAO-B, the form predominantly found in this tissue (Stahl, 1977). The expression of MAO in the brain has been a focus of interest in Parkinson's disease (PD) firstly because selective inhibition of MAO-B with L-deprenyl, particularly as an adjunct to L-DOPA, is successfully used therapeutically (Youdim and Finberg, 1986), and secondly because MAO-B oxidises N-methyl-4-phenyl-1,2,3,6-tetrahydropyridine (MPTP) into the 1-methyl-4-phenylpyridium cation, MPP^+, a potent neurotoxin (Maret et al., 1990). Thus MAO-B could reasonably be considered as an activating enzyme for other pro-neurotoxins, possibly of environmental origin, and increased MAO-B activities may therefore be expected in PD patients.

Whether or not platelet MAO-B has a role in predictive testing of PD is still an open question because results obtained to date are conflicting. Some studies have indeed shown relative enzyme excesses compared to controls (Danielczyk et al., 1988; Bonuccelli et al., 1990) and others indicate either relative deficits (Zeller et al., 1976) or no discernible differences (Mann et al., 1983; Yong and Perry, 1986).

More recently, data have suggested that measurements of platelet MAO activity are dependent on the substrate used, the activity being slightly higher in untreated PD patients than controls when using phenylethylamine and significantly lower using dopamine (Humfrey et al., 1990). One recent brief study (Jarman et al., 1993) has disputed the results with dopamine and another study (Checkoway et al., 1992) has suggested that the results with PEA are slightly lower in male PD patients compared to controls but slightly higher in female patients compared to controls. Thus it appears that when using non-hydroxylated monoamines as substrates MAO activity in PD patients is greater than in controls, while using mono- and di-hydroxylated monoamines as substrates leads to a reduction in activity compared to controls. This may imply that in PD a different MAO-B isoenzyme is being expressed. Indeed isoenzymes of MAO-B have been shown to exist in monkey platelets (Obata et al., 1990).

It is possible that conflicting results have arisen because the measurement of MAO activity is unreliable, being influenced by a number of factors, including interfering enzymes, inhibitors and the lipid environment in addition to the variable relative numbers of males and females (often in the menopausal stages) used in the studies, knowing that MAO activity is affected by hormonal status (Poirier et al., 1985). As no attempt has been made to date to monitor the platelet MAO-B protein content of these patients, it is not known whether the effects seen are due to altered rate of expression, altered MAO protein or the presence of modulators. Recently, we have prepared and used a MAO-B specific murine monoclonal in a sensitive enzyme-linked assay which can monitor MAO-B in human tissues and blood platelets (Yeomanson and Billett, 1992). The assay measures total MAO-B protein (both active and inactive) and is based on the competition between a soluble form of MAO (either test or standard) and MAO bound to a solid phase for binding to a limited amount of the MAO-B-specific monoclonal. The aims of the present study were to reassess the status of platelet MAO in recently diagnosed, drug-untreated male patients with clinically defined idiopathic PD compared with age-matched controls (healthy volunteers).

To overcome the problems with MAO activity measurements we have used the sensitive ELISA for the specific measurement of MAO-B protein concentrations. MAO activity assays with dopamine and phenlyethylamine were performed concomitantly to allow an estimation of the molecular activity of MAO-B.

Materials and methods

Patient selection

Parkinson's disease was diagnosed by the presence of three of the following features: tremor, rigidity, bradykinesia, postural instability, gait disturbances, response to L-DOPA. Patients with atypical features including abnormal eye movements, dementia and autonomic dysfunction were excluded, as was parkinsonism due to any other neurological diseases, chemicals or toxins. None of the subjects used in this study were on medication for PD or drugs known to influence MAO-B activity. All sample collection was performed at the Department of Clinical Neurology, Queen Elizabeth Hospital, Birmingham, UK, under the supervision of Professor A.C. Williams and Dr. S.L Ho.

Preparation of platelet rich plasma (PRP)

This is a modification of Corash's method, (1980).

Collection of PRP: whole blood (20 ml) was collected into 0.2 ml 10% (w/v) ethylene diaminetetraacetic acid (EDTA), pH 7.4 and PRP isolated by centrifugation at $600 \times g$ for 5 min. Platelet number was determined and PRP was frozen in aliquots at $-70°C$ overnight or until required.

Platelet washing: PRP was thawed and aliquots (3 ml and 2 ml) centrifuged at $28000 \times g$, 20 min. The resultant pellets were washed by resuspension in washing buffer (5 mM EDTA, 0.154 M NaCl, pH 7.2), and centrifuged at $28000 \times g$, 20 mins before resuspension in 0.3mls potassium phosphate buffer (0.05 M, pH 7.4) containing

0.5% Triton X-100 (w/v) for ELISA or 0.2 ml potassium phosphate buffer (0.05 M, pH 7.4, no Triton X-100) for the activity measurements.

MAO activity studies

Measurement of MAO activity is based on the radiochemical method of Russell and Mayer (1983) using 10 μl concentrated PRP for the dopamine assay (final dopamine concentration of 50 μM) and 30 μl concentrated PRP for the PEA assay (final PEA concentration 20 μM) in a final volume of 200 μl. Time course assays for both substrates were linear for at least 60 min, the incubation time used in the assays.

Determination of MAO-B protein content via ELISA

Principles of the competitive ELISA. Microtitre wells were coated with antigen which competes with free antigen, either standard MAO or MAO in the samples for a limiting amount of murine MAO-B specific antibody. Antibody binding was revealed by an anti-mouse horseradish peroxidase-conjugated secondary antibody. The amount of bound enzyme-conjugated antibody is inversely proportional to the amount of free antigen present. Mitochondrial membranes were used as a source of antigen for coating the wells, (a) to conserve standard MAO and (b) because membranes bind more avidly to ELISA plates than solubilised proteins.

Preparation of antigens

Preparation of mitochondrial membranes for ELISA coating. Mitochondrial membranes were prepared from normal human liver at post mortem i.e. < 24 h after death. The method was as described by Billett et al. (1984).

Solubilisation of mitochondrial membranes. MAO was solubilised from mitochondrial membranes using Triton X-100 (final concentration 1%, w/v) containing phenylmethylsulphonyl fluoride (PMSF) (final concentration, 10 mM) by incubating for 60 min at 4°C, stirring slowly before cen-

trifugation at $100,000 \times g$ for 60 min. The pellet was discarded and the supernatant was used immediately in the ELISA.

Solubilisation of platelet MAO for ELISA. Platelet pellets resuspended in buffer (see above) were incubated (4°C, 60 min) stirring gently. Solubilised platelet protein was collected by centrifugation at $28,000 \times g$, 60 min. (This procedure has been shown to solubilise over 98% of MAO activity in platelet samples.)

Preparation of 'standard' MAO for the ELISA assay. MAO was 'purified' from human liver mitochondrial membranes as described by Billett and Mayer (1986) using a combination of gel filtration, ion-exchange chromatography and ammonium sulphate precipitation. The MAO-A and -B content of 'purified' MAO was monitored by SDS polyacrylamide gel electrophoresis coupled with antibody probing to confirm the identity of the MAO bands. The percentages of MAO-A and -B in the purified MAO extract were estimated by gel densitometer scanning.

Source of antibody and antibody concentration. Antibody secreted by the hybridoma cell line 3F12/G10 (specific for MAO-B) (Billett and Mayer, 1986) was used in these assays.

Results

Preliminary work

Triton X-100 was found to have an adverse effect on the binding of the 3F12/G10 antibody to MAO at concentrations above 0.1% (w/v). Hence for standardisation purposes solubilised MAO, irrespective of source, was incubated at a final concentration of 0.1% Triton X-100. 3F12/G10 was titrated in the presence of 0.1% Triton X-100 against mitochondrial membranes bound to the solid phase. Titre was defined as the reciprocal of the dilution required for 50% saturation of solid phase antigen and was estimated to be 900 (Fig. 1). No difference in sensitivity and range of the assay was detected when using the

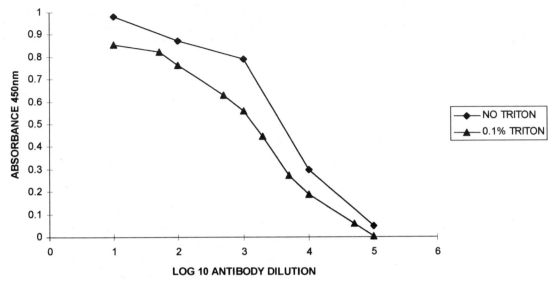

Fig. 1. Titration of 3F12/G10 in the presence and absence of Triton X-100. Wells were coated with mitochondrial membranes and incubated with serial dilutions of the mouse monoclonal antibody, 3F12/G10. Binding of the monoclonal antibody was revealed using an anti-mouse horseradish peroxidase-conjugated secondary antibody.

antibody at 50%, 60% and 75% saturations. Fig. 1 also shows that the titre was greater (3900) in the absence of Triton X-100.

The MAO-B content of patient platelet sam-

ples was determined in the competitive ELISA by comparing the linearised displacement plot of platelet MAO with that of purified MAO. Fig. 2 shows the displacement of 3F12/G10 binding to

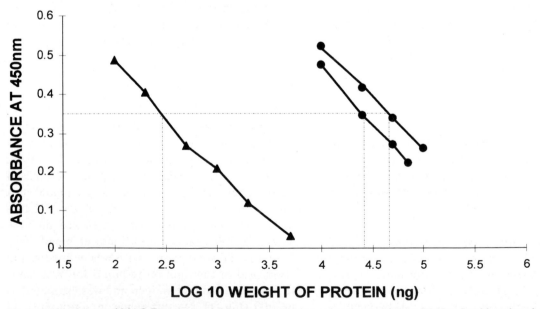

Fig. 2. Measurement of MAO-B concentration in human platelets using the competitive ELISA. Semi-log plot of competitive data for standard MAO (▲) and two platelet samples (●) as examples; $n = 3$. In the absence of competing antigen the mean absorbance value was 0.54 ± 0.03.

the solid phase antigen in the presence of varying concentrations of 'standard' MAO and serial dilutions of solubilised platelet samples. The semi-log plots of the sample data are parallel with the 'standard' MAO data, indicating that 3F12/G10 recognises the same epitope in the extracts and in the 'standard'.

Platelet MAO activities and MAO-B protein concentration in male PD patients and controls

In this small sample the mean concentration of MAO-B protein/mg platelet protein was approx. 40% greater in the PD patients than in the control population. However, this difference was not significant and was very variable within the PD group (Table 1). Indeed MAO activity per mg platelet protein and MAO molecular activity (nmol/h per mg MAO) were similar in the two groups with both PEA and dopamine as substrates. Thus our study shows that the status of MAO in platelets is not altered in PD.

It is worth noting that this study was undertaken as part of a larger study involving both

TABLE 1

Platelet MAO activities and MAO-B protein concentrations in male Parkinson's disease patients and controls

	Controls	Parkinson's disease
Number	7	11
Age ± S.D	56 ± 13	61 ± 12
μg MAO-B per mg total protein	2.33 ± 0.55	3.36 ± 2.01
PEA deamination		
a) nmol/h per mg total protein	3.02 ± 1.53	2.16 ± 0.71
b) nmol/h per mg MAO protein	1291.2 ± 637.2	1092.4 ± 997.1
Dopamine deamination		
a) nmol/h per mg total protein	0.96 ± 0.42	0.82 ± 0.30
b) nmol/h per mg MAO protein	409.5 ± 171.6	410.6 ± 433.6

None of the above differences is significant using the Mann-Whitney U-test, chosen because the sample size is small and unmatched.

TABLE 2

MAO activities in a mixed population

	Controls	Parkinson's disease
Number (M/F)	17 (10/7)	21 (15/6)
Age ± S.D.	58 ± 11	62 ± 11
PEA deamination nmol/h per mg total protein	2.91 ± 1.2	2.67 ± 0.99
Dopamine deamination nmol/h per mg total protein	0.98 ± 0.39	1.00 ± 0.42

None of the above differences is significant using the Mann-Whitney U-test, chosen because the sample size is small and unmatched.

males and females and included PRP samples of small volume which could not be analysed in the ELISA. Platelet MAO activity for this mixed population using both dopamine and PEA as substrates is represented in Table 2. This larger study again shows that PD does not alter platelet MAO activity.

Conclusions

MAO-B protein concentration, monitored using ELISA, is the same in male PD patients as in male age-matched controls. Using both dopamine and PEA as substrates MAO molecular activity (nmol/h per mg MAO) is not altered in PD (males only assayed). Platelet MAO activity per mg total protein is also similar in PD patients (males and females) and controls using both dopamine and PEA as substrates.

As the sample numbers are small, it is unwise to conclude the these observations are necessarily final.

References

Bach, A.W.J., Lan, N.C., Johnson, D.L., Abell, C.W., Bembenek, M.E., Kwan, S.W., Seeburg, P.H. and Shih, J.C. (1988) cDNA cloning of human liver monoamine oxidase A and B: Molecular basis of differences in enzymatic properties. *Proc. Natl. Acad. Sci.*, 85: 4934–4938.
Billett, E.E., Gunn, B. and Mayer, R.J. (1984) Characterisation of two monoclonal antibodies obtained after immuni-

sation with human liver mitochondrial membrane preparations. *Biochem. J.*, 221: 765–776.

Billett, E.E. and Mayer, R.J. (1986) Monoclonal antibodies to monoamine oxidase B and another mitochondrial protein from human liver. *Biochem. J.*, 235: 257–263.

Bonuccelli, U., Piccini, P., Del-dotto, P., Pacifici, G.M., Corsini, G.U. and Muratorio, A. (1990) Platelet monoamine oxidase B activity in Parkinsonian patients. *J. Neurol. Neurosurg. Psychiat.*, 53: 854–855.

Checkoway, H., Costa, L.G., Woods, J.S., Castoldi, A.F., Lund, B.O. and Swanson, P.D. (1992) Peripheral blood cell activities of monoamine oxidase B and superoxide dismutase in Parkinson's Disease. *J. Neural Transm. (P.D. section)*, 4: 283–290.

Chen, K., Wu, H-F. and Shih, J.C. (1993) The deduced amino acid sequences of human platelet and frontal cortex monoamine oxidase B are identical. *J. Neurochem.*, 61: 187–190.

Corash, L. (1980) Platelet Heterogeneity: Relevance to the use of platelets to study psychiatric disorders. *Schizophrenia Bull.*, 6: 254–258.

Danielczyk, W., Streifler, M., Konradi, C., Riederer, P. and Moll, G. (1988) Platelet MAO-B activity and the psychopathology of Parkinson's Disease, senile dementia and multi-infarct dementia. *Acta Psychiatr. Scand.*, 78: 730–736.

Denney, R.M., Fritz, R.R., Patel, N.T. and Abell, C.W. (1982) Human liver MAO-A and MAO-B separated by immunoaffinity chromatogrraphy with MAO-B specific monoclonal antibody. *Science*, 215: 1400–1403.

Humfrey, C.D.N., Steventon, G.B., Sturman, S.G., Waring, R.H., Griffiths, B. and Williams, A.C. (1990) Monoamine oxidase substrates in Parkinson's Disease. *Biochem. Pharmacol.*, 40: 2562–2564.

Jarman, J., Glover, V., Sandler, M., Turjanski, N. and Stern, G. (1993) Platelet monoamine oxidase B activity in Parkinson's Disease: a re-evaluation. *J. Neural Transm. (P.D. Section)*, 5: 1–4.

Knoll, J. and Magyar, K. (1972) Some puzzling pharmacological effects of monoamine oxidase inhibitors. *Adv. Biochem. Psychopharmacol.*, 5: 393–408.

Mann, V.M., Cooper, J.M., Krige, D., Daniel, S.E., Schapira, A.H.V. and Marsden, C.D. (1992) Brain, skeletal muscle and platelet homogenate mitochondrial function in Parkinson's Disease. *Brain*, 115: 333–342.

Maret, G., Testa, B., Jenner, P., El-Tayer, N. and Carrupt, P.A. (1990) The MPTP story: MAO activates tetrahydropyridine derivatives to toxins causing Parkinsonism. *Drug Metab. Rev.*, 22: 291–332.

Obata, T., Egashira, T. and Yamanaka, Y. (1990) Isoelectric focusing of isoenzymes of monkey platelet monoamine oxidase. *Biochem. Pharmacol.*, 40: 1689–1693.

Poirier, M-F., LUo, H., Dennis, T., Le Fur, G. and Scatton B. (1985) Platelet monoamine oxidase activity and plasma 3,4-dihydroxyphenylethylene glycol levels during the menstrual cycle. *Neuropsychobiol.*, 14: 165–169.

Russell, S.M. and Mayer, R.J. (1983) Degradation of transplanted rat liver mitochondrial outer membrane proteins in hepatoma cells. *Biochem. J.*, 216: 163–175.

Stahl, S.M. (1977) The human platelet. *Arch. Gen. Psychiatr.*, 34: 509–516.

Yeomanson, K.B. and Billett, E.E. (1992) An enzyme immunoassay for the measurement of human monoamine oxidase B protein. *Biochim. Biophys. Acta*, 1116: 261–268.

Yong, V.W. and Perry, T.L. (1986) Monoamine oxidase B, smoking and Parkinson's Disease. *J. Neurol. Sci.*, 72: 265–272.

Youdim, M.B.H. (1988) Platelet monoamine oxidase B: Use and misuse. *Experientia*, 44: 137–142.

Youdim, M.B.H. and Finberg, J.P.M. (1986) MAO Type B Inhibitors as adjunct to L-DOPA therapy. *Adv. Neurol.*, 45: 127–136.

Zeller, E.A., Boshes, B., Arbit, J., Bieber, M., Blonsky, E.R., Dolkart, M. and Huprikar, S.V. (1976) Molecular biology of neurological and psychiatric disorders. I. Effect of Parkinsonism, age, sex and L-DOPA on platelet monoamine oxidase. *J. Neural Transm.*, 39: 63–77.

Peter M. Yu, Keith F. Tipton and Alan A. Boulton (Eds.)
Progress in Brain Research, Vol 106
© 1995 Elsevier Science BV. All rights reserved.

CHAPTER 10

Aromatic L-amino acid decarboxylase modulation and Parkinson's disease

N.H. Neff and M. Hadjiconstantinou

Departments of Pharmacology and Psychiatry, The Ohio State University College of Medicine, Columbus, OH 43210, USA

Aromatic L-amino acid decarboxylase (AAAD): general characteristics

AAAD is a relatively non-selective enzyme found in both neuronal and non-neuronal tissues (see Bowsher and Henry, 1986). From enzyme isolation studies its molecular mass is about 50 kDa, depending on the species, and it is thought to exist as a dimer in nature. From cloning studies, including our own, the molecular mass is about 50 kDa (Bowsher and Henry, 1986; Lovenberg et al., 1962; Bouchard et al., 1981; Siow and Dakshinamurti, 1990). Krieger et al. (1991) reported that different mRNAs code for AAAD in tissues of neuronal and non-neuronal origin. In neuronal tissue AAAD is required for the synthesis of catecholamines, serotonin, melatonin and trace amines (Blaschko, 1959; Paterson et al., 1990). AAAD is not considered to be the rate-limiting enzyme for catecholamine synthesis (Levitt et al., 1965). There is evidence, however, that it might be rate-limiting for the synthesis of the trace amines (Paterson et al., 1990). Moreover, it has generally been assumed that AAAD is not modulated by neuronal activity. Studies, primarily from our laboratory, with retina and striatum have provided evidence that this assumption is no longer tenable (Rossetti et al., 1989, 1990; Hadjiconstantinou et al., 1988, 1993; Zhu et al., 1992, 1993).

AAAD and retina

Our original studies focused on the rat retina because DA is the principal biogenic amine neu-

rotransmitter and dopaminergic neurons are activated when rats are placed in a lighted environment (Kramer, 1971). There are no identified serotonergic neurons in retina, although melatonin is present in some photoreceptive cells (Pang et al., 1980; Wiechmann, 1986). The rat retina, therefore, is an ideal model tissue for studying the neurochemical changes that follow activation of dopaminergic neurons (Iuvone and Neff, 1981). AAAD of retina, found primarily in dopaminergic amacrine cells and some interplexiform cells (Park et al., 1986), is regulated by both physiological stimuli and pharmacological agents. For example, exposure of dark-adapted rats to room light increases retinal AAAD activity to twice the values found in the dark (Hadjiconstantinou et al., 1988) when studied over 3 h. This increase appears to result from an increase of enzyme protein and it can be inhibited by cycloheximide. Light-adapted animals form more DA from exogenous administered L-DOPA compared to dark-adapted animals, suggesting that the light-induced increase of AAAD activity is functional (Xu et al., 1985).

Retinal AAAD activity is modulated via specific neurotransmitter receptors. For example, administration of α_2-adrenoceptor antagonists (Rossetti et al., 1989) or DA D_1 receptor antagonists (Rossetti et al., 1990) to dark-adapted animals results in a two-fold increase of AAAD activity in dark. For both treatments, kinetic analysis indicates changes of V_{max} rather than a change of K_m for the substrate L-DOPA or the cofactor pyridoxal-5'-phosphate. Administration of an α_2-adrenoceptor agonist suppresses both the light-induced rise of AAAD and the rise of the enzyme induced by α_2-adrenoceptor antagonists in the dark (Rossetti et al., 1989). The light-induced increase of AAAD activity can also be prevented by administering a DA D_1 agonist (Rossetti et al., 1990). Furthermore, DA D_1 agonists can reduce enzyme activity when given after it increases following exposure to light. This response can be prevented by prior administration of DA D_1 receptor antagonists. Apparently occupation of both DA D_1 and α_2-adrenergic receptors is necessary to suppress AAAD activity. Derepressing either receptor results in a rise of AAAD.

AAAD and striatum

The modulation of AAAD activity is not unique to the retina. Both DA D_1 and DA D_2 receptor antagonists can increase AAAD activity in the striatum of the mouse (Hadjiconstantinou et al., 1993). We have not been able to modulate activity with α-adrenergic drugs, however. AAAD activity in striatum is enhanced after administering the DA antagonists haloperidol, sulpiride or SCH 23390. Treatment with MPTP decreases AAAD activity and administration of DA receptor antagonists doubles enzyme activity in striatum. Striatal denervation with the neurotoxin MPTP results in animals that are more sensitive to the DA antagonists, i.e., responding earlier and to lower doses of the antagonists than control mice. There might be two phases associated with enhanced AAAD activity. There is an early transient increase, about 15 min after the administration of the drugs, followed by a second increase several hours later (Fig. 1). The late occurring increase is associated with a change in V_{max} for AAAD (Hadjiconstantinou et al., 1993) and can be prevented by treatment with cycloheximide. Zhu et al. (1992, 1993) corroborated our work in another species, the rat. They observed an increase of rat striatal AAAD after administering DA antagonists, which occurred within 30 min and lasted about 2 h. Interestingly, the increase of AAAD at 30 min was not inhibited by cycloheximide. AAAD enhancement

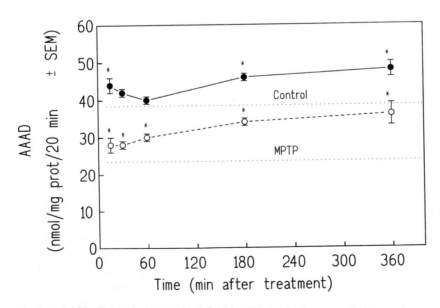

Fig. 1. Sulpiride time-response study. Sulpiride, 120 mg/kg i.p., was administered to control and MPTP-treated mice. Data are presented as the mean ± SEM for eight or more animals per group. From Hadjiconstantinou et al., 1993. $*P < 0.05$ when compared with basal value for the respective group.

induced by the D_2 antagonists was reported for the nucleus accumbens and the olfactory tubercle as well (Zhu et al., 1992, 1993).

Subchronic administration of L-DOPA or D_1 or D_2 receptor agonists lowers striatal AAAD (Hadjiconstantinou et al., 1993), while subchronic treatment with haloperidol, sulpiride and SCH 23390 or treatment with reserpine increases AAAD (Hadjiconstantinou et al., 1993). Reserpine has been reported to increase tyrosine hydroxylase (TH) and AAAD mRNA in locus coeruleus but not midbrain of rat (Wessel and Joh, 1992). Buckland et al. (1992) found that chronic treatment with haloperidol or loxapine increased AAAD mRNA but not TH mRNA in the rat brain. They speculated that AAAD may be more important than TH for long-term regulation of DA production. This concept is not new. Most studies of the enzyme have been performed in animals. Yet studies with human brain have consistently shown lower activities than in animals (Rahman and Nagatsu, 1982). For example, it has been reported that AAAD activity in the rat caudate is 6402 nmol · g wet weight while for the human caudate it is 14 nmol · g wet weight (Bowsher and Henry, 1986). Indeed, early assays of AAAD in human brain were problematic and led to a meeting, "Is there DOPA decarboxylase in the human brain", where low activity and variability were discussed (Sacks et al., 1979). These early observations led Sacks et al. (1979) to speculate that AAAD activity may be rate-limiting for monoamine synthesis in human brain.

The ability to regulate AAAD is not limited to the CNS and retina. Recent reports provided evidence that AAAD mRNA in adrenal medulla is increased following reserpine treatment (Wessel and Joh, 1992) and dexamethasone increases AAAD mRNA in PC12 cells (Kim et al., 1993). Furthermore, deprenyl, a MAO B, inhibitor increases AAAD mRNA in PC12 cells (Li et al., 1992), as do inhibitors of AAAD (Li et al., 1993). DA-containing elements in the rat nephron proximal convoluted tubules contain AAAD (Ferguson and Bell, 1991). DA modulates the tubule secretion of Na^+. Low salt intake results in a significant decrease of the V_{max} for AAAD without changing the apparent K_m for L-DOPA (Hayashi et al., 1990).

Modulation of AAAD

More than one mechanism may modulate AAAD activity. In retina when the room lights are turned off, AAAD activity drops rapidly at first (half-life about 3 min) and then more slowly (half-life about 73 min) (Hadjiconstantinou et al., 1988). It takes about 3 h of exposure to room light for AAAD to reach full activity in animals kept in the dark for 12 h. In contrast, it only takes about 15 min to reach full activity after 30 min in the dark (Hadjiconstantinou et al., 1988). In addition, the observation that DA receptor antagonists increase AAAD activity of the striatum in a biphasic manner, with the early increase insensitive and a late increase sensitive to protein synthesis inhibition, implies that at least two mechanisms are implicated (Hadjiconstantinou et al., 1993; Zhu et al., 1992). The early increase may represent activation while the late phase may represent induction of AAAD. Phosphorylation of the enzyme is a possible mechanism for activation. Indeed, the deduced amino acid sequence of bovine adrenal AAAD (Gudehithlu et al., 1992) has several potential phosphorylation sites for cAMP-dependent protein kinase (PKA), Ca^{2+}-calmodulin-dependent protein kinase II (CAM kin II), protein kinase C (PKC) and proline-directed protein kinase (Kemp and Pearson, 1990). Two charged isoforms of AAAD have been identified which may be the consequences of post-translational modification, perhaps phosphorylation (Park et al., 1992; Li et al., 1992; Juorio et al., 1993).

Intracerebroventricular (ICV) administration of forskolin (Fig. 2) induces a rapid transient rise of AAAD in both the striatum and midbrain of mice (Young et al., 1993). The increase is not inhibited by pretreatment with the protein synthesis inhibitor cycloheximide. A similar increase of AAAD was observed when 8-Br-cyclic AMP was injected i.c.v. (Young et al., 1993). The PKC activator PMA also increases AAAD activity (Table 1) in

TABLE 1

PMA and okadaic acid increase AAAD activity in the mouse striatum: the response to PMA is blocked by chelerythrine

Treatment	AAAD (nmol/mg protein/20 min ± SEM)
Vehicle	34 ± 1
PMA	52 ± 4*
Chelerythrine	38 ± 3
PMA + chelerythrine	37 ± 2
Vehicle	33 ± 1
Okadaic acid	39 ± 1*

Two nmol PMA in DMSO or chelerythrine 0.132 nmol and okadaic acid 0.2 nmol in 2 μl of artificial CSF was injected i.c.v. into ether-anesthetized mice. The mice were killed 30 min later. * $P < 0.5$ compared with appropriate control group. $n = 5$–10. From Young et al., 1994.

the striatum and midbrain of mice (Young et al., 1994). Chelerythrine, a selective inhibitor of PKC,

blocks the response to PMA when administered together, while protein synthesis inhibition with cycloheximide had no effect. Kinetic analysis revealed that both forskolin and PMA increased the apparent V_{max} for the enzyme without affecting the K_m for the cofactor or the substrate. Support for phosphorylation also comes from studies with okadaic acid (Table 1), a protein phosphatase inhibitor. Okadaic acid administered alone increased AAAD activity (Young et al., 1994). The studies cited, especially with okadaic acid, suggest that there is basal phosphorylation-dephosphorylation of AAAD that normally modulates AAAD activity.

The physiological reason for enzyme modulation remains to be investigated. It is doubtful, however, that there would be active modulation without a physiological meaning. Our postulated mechanisms for modulating AAAD activity are similar to those previously reported for modulating TH in retina and brain, short-term modula-

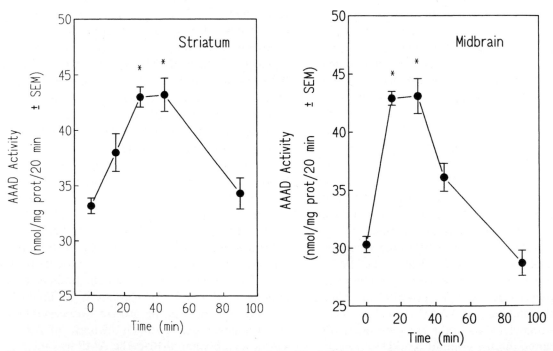

Fig. 2. The rise of AAAD activity in the mouse striatum and midbrain following an i.c.v. injection of forskolin. Forskolin, 20 nmol in 2 μl, was injected i.c.v. in mice under diethyl ether anesthesia. The animals were killed at the intervals indicated and AAAD was assayed. Data are presented as the mean ± SEM for groups of five or more animals. From Young et al., 1993. * $P < 0.05$ compared with zero time.

tion by phosphorylation activation and long-term modulation by induction (Iuvone et al., 1982, 1978). Hahn et al. (1993) reported that the sequence of each promoter region of the AAAD gene shows putative binding sites for octamer factors and AP-2, suggesting ability for transcriptional modification.

The trace amines, *p*-tyramine, *o*-tyramine, 2-phenylethylamine and tryptamine, are normal constituents of brain and AAAD is thought to be rate-limiting for their synthesis (Paterson et al., 1990). Kang et al. (1992) showed that the decarboxylation of administered L-DOPA in striata of rats with a unilateral substantia nigra lesion is mediated by AAAD located in dopaminergic terminals as demonstrated by immunohistochemistry and in situ hybridization. Glia cells which have been reported to express AAAD mRNA (Marks et al., 1992; Li et al., 1992), however, are not capable of decarboxylating L-DOPA (Juorio et al., 1987). There are neurons in hypothalamus, brain stem, striatum and spinal cord that contain immunoreactive AAAD but not TH (Jaeger et al., 1983, 1984). Interestingly, the trace amine content of the striatum increases after treatment with neuroleptics (Paterson et al., 1990), the same treatment that we and Zhu et al. (1992, 1993) have shown to increase AAAD activity in the striatum. This may represent indirect physiological evidence for enhanced AAAD activity following blockade of DA receptors.

Conclusions

Our finding that AAAD activity can be modulated has both theoretical and practical implications. The belief that AAAD is not modulated is erroneous and therefore it is important to carefully document the pharmacology and neurochemistry for enhancing AAAD activity. An understanding of the mechanism(s) underlying enzyme modulation may provide valuable clues for resolving the biological significance of the phenomenon.

In Parkinson's disease there is progressive loss of nigrostriatal dopaminergic neurons. Current therapy for the disease is to administer L-DOPA which in the striatum is converted to DA by AAAD in the surviving neurons. With time, however, the ability to decarboxylate L-DOPA diminishes and clinical symptomatology intensifies as neurons degenerate. If AAAD activity could be enhanced the productive life of parkinsonian patients might be extended. The finding that AAAD can be enhanced pharmacologically provides a new therapeutic approach for treating this disease. In the late stages of Parkinson's disease the symptoms of the "on-off phenomenon" are expressed where there are fluctuations between off-periods of marked akinesia over several hours with on-periods of improved motility which may be related to oscillating or poorly modulated AAAD activity and conversion of L-DOPA to DA. We postulate that AAAD activity might be stabilized by drugs that enhance AAAD. Clearly, the study of AAAD has provided insight into neuronal mechanisms and furnished new therapeutic possibilities for treating Parkinson's disease.

Summary

Aromatic L-amino acid decarboxylase (AAAD) is the second enzyme in the sequence leading to the synthesis of the catecholamines and serotonin, and it is the rate-limiting enzyme for the synthesis of the trace amines. In the striatum AAAD activity is increased by neuronal firing and diminished or enhanced by activation or blocking dopamine (DA) D_1 or D_2 receptors, respectively. At least two biochemical mechanisms appear responsible for modulation, short-term involving second messengers and possible phosphorylation, and long-term involving protein synthesis. In Parkinson's disease AAAD is the rate-controlling enzyme for the synthesis of DA when L-DOPA is administered and any change of AAAD activity could have clinical consequences. Indeed, the "on-off phenomenon" where there are fluctuations between off-periods of marked akinesia over several hours with on-periods of improved motility may be related to oscillating or poorly modulated AAAD activity and conversion of L-DOPA to DA. Studies are presented demonstrating how

AAAD activity can be enhanced in an animal model of Parkinson's disease and how rapid fluctuations of AAAD can be provoked via second messenger system activation.

References

Blaschko, H. (1959) The development of current concepts of catecholamine formation. *Pharmacol. Rev.*, 11: 307–316.

Bouchard, S., Bousquet, C. and Roberge, A.G. (1981) Characteristics of dihydroxy-phenylalanine/5-hydroxytryptophan decarboxylase activity in brain and liver of cat. *J. Neurochem.*, 37: 781–787.

Bowsher, R.R. and Henry, D.P. (1986) Aromatic L-amino acid decarboxylase: biochemistry and functional significance.In: A.A. Boulton, G.B. Baker and P.H. Yu (Eds.), *Neuromethods: Series 1: Neurochemistry, Neurotransmitter Enzymes,* Humana Press, NJ, pp. 33–77.

Buckland, P.R., O'Donovan, M.C. and McGuffin, P. (1992) Changes in dopa decarboxylase mRNA but not tyrosine hydroxylase mRNA levels in rat brain following antipsychotic treatment. *Psychopharmacology*, 108: 98–102.

Ferguson, M. and Bell, C. (1991) Two patterns of dopa decarboxylase immunoreactivity in sympathetic axons supplying rat renal cortex. *Renal Physiol. Biochem.*, 14: 55–62.

Gudehithlu, K.P., Duchemin, A.-M., Silvia, C.P., Neff, N.H. and Hadjiconstantinou, M. (1992) Expression of cloned aromatic L-amino acid decarboxylase in Xenopus laevis oocytes. *Neurochem. Int.*, 21: 275–279.

Hadjiconstantinou, M., Rossetti, Z.L., Silvia, C., Krajnc, D. and Neff, N.H. (1988) Aromatic L-amino acid decarboxylase activity of the rat retina is modulated in vivo by environmental light. *J. Neurochem.*, 51 : 1560–1564.

Hadjiconstantinou, M., Wemlinger, T.A., Silvia, C.P., Hubble, J. and Neff, N.H. (1993) Aromatic L-amino acid decarboxylase activity of mouse striatum is modulated via dopaminergic receptors. *J. Neurochem.*, 60: 2175–2180.

Hahn, S.L., Hahn, M., Kang, U.J. and Joh, T.H. (1993) Structure of the rat aromatic L-amino acid decarboxylase gene: Evidence for an alternative promoter usage. *J. Neurochem.*, 60: 1058–1064.

Hayashi, M., Yamaji, Y., Kitajima, W. and Saruta, T. (1990) Aromatic L-amino acid decarboxylase activity along the rat nephron. *Am. J. Physiol.*, 258: F28-F33.

Iuvone, P.M., Galli, C.L. and Neff, N.H. (1978) Retinal tyrosine hydroxylase: comparison of short-term and long-term stimulation by light. *Mol. Pharmacol.*, 14: 1212–1219.

Iuvone, P.M. and Neff, N.H. (1981) Dopamine neurons of the retina: a simple method system for studying synaptic regulatory mechanisms. Essays. *Neurochem. Neuropharmacol.*, 5: 75–94.

Iuvone, P.M., Rauch, A.L., Marshburn, P.B., Glass, D.B. and Neff, N.H. (1982) Activation of retinal tyrosine hydroxylase in vitro by cyclic AMP-dependent protein kinase: characterization and comparison to activation in vivo by photic stimulation. *J. Neurochem.*, 39: 1632–1640.

Jaeger, C.B., Ruggiero, D.A., Albert, V.R., Park, D.H., Joh, T.H. and Reis, D.J. (1984) AADC in the rat brain: Immunocytochemical location in neurons of the brain stem. *Neuroscience*, 11: 691–713.

Jaeger, C.B., Teitelman, G., Joh, T.H., Albert, V.R., Park, D.H. and Reis, D.J. (1983) Some neurons of the rat central nervous system contain AADC but not monoamines. *Science*, 219: 1233–1235.

Juorio, A.V., Walz, W. and Sloley, B.D. (1987) Absence of decarboxylation of some aromatic-l-amino acids by cultured astrocytes. *Brain Res.*, 426: 183–186.

Juorio, A. V., Li, X.-M., Walz, W. and Paterson, I. A. (1993) Decarboxylation of L-Dopa by cultured mouse astrocytes. *Brain Res.* 626: 306–309

Kang, U.J., Park, D.H., Wessel, T., Baker, H. and Joh, T.H. (1992) DOPA-decarboxylation in the striata of rats with unilateral substantia nigra lesions. *Neurosci. Lett.*, 147: 53–57.

Kemp, B.E. and Pearson, R.B. (1990) Protein kinase recognition sequence motifs. *Trends Biochem. Sci.*, 15: 342–346.

Kim, K.-T., Park, D.H. and Joh, T.H. (1993) Parallel up-regulation of catecholamine biosynthetic enzymes by dexamethasone in PC12 cells. *J. Neurochem.*, 60: 946–951.

Kramer, S.G. (1971) Dopamine: A retinal neurotransmitter. I Retinal uptake, storage, and light stimulated release of ^{3}H-dopamine in vivo. *Invest. Ophthalmol. Vis. Sci.*, 10: 438–452.

Krieger, M., Coge, F., Gros, F. and Thibault, T. (1991) Different mRNAs code for dopa decarboxylase in tissues of neuronal and nonneuronal origin. *Proc. Natl. Acad. Sci USA*, 88: 2161–2165.

Levitt, M., Spector, S., Sjoerdsma, A. and Udenfriend, S. (1965) Elucidation of the rate-limiting step in norepinephrine biosynthesis in the perfused guinea pig heart. *J. Pharmacol. Exp. Ther.*, 148: 1–8.

Li, X.-M., Juorio, A.V. and Boulton, A.A. (1993) NSD-1015 alters the gene expression of aromatic L-amino acid decarboxylase in rat PC12 pheochromocytoma cells. *Neurochem. Res.*, 18 : 915–919.

Li, X.-M., Juorio, A.V., Paterson, I.A. and Zhu, M.Y. (1992) Specific irreversible monoamine oxidase B inhibitors stimulate gene expression of aromatic L-amino acid decarboxylae in PC12 cells. *J. Neurochem.*, 59: 2324–2327.

Li, X.-M., Juorio, A. V., Paterson, I. A., Walz, W., Zhu M-Y. and Boulton, A. A. (1992) Gene expression of aromatic L-amino acid decarbosylase in cultured rat glial cells. *J. Neurochem.*, 59: 1172–1175.

Lovenberg, W., Weissbach, H. and Udenfriend, S. (1962) Aromatic L-amino acid decarboxylase. *J. Biol. Chem.*, 237: 89–93.

Marks, M.J., Pauly, J.R., Gross, S.D., Deneris, E.S., Hermans-Borgmeyer, I., Heinemann, S.F. and Collins, A.C. (1992) Nicotine binding and nicotinic receptor subunit RNA after chronic nicotine treatment. *J. Neurosci.*, 12: 2765–2784.

Pang, S.F., Yu, H.S., Suen, H.C. and Brown, G.M. (1980) Melatonin in the retina of rats: A diurnal rhythm. *J. Endocrin.*, 87: 89–93.

Park, D.H., Kim K-T., Choi, M.-U., Samanta, H. and Joh, T.H. (1992) Characterization of bovine aromatic L-amino acid decarboxylase expressed in a mouse cell line: comparison with native enzyme. *Mol. Brain Res.*, 16: 232–238.

Park, D.H., Teitelman, G., Evinger, M.J., Woo, J.I., Ruggiero, D.A., Albert, V.R., Baetge, E.E., Pickel, V.M., Reis, D.J. and Joh, T.H. (1986) Phenylethanolamine *N*-methyltransferase-containing neurons in rat retina: immunohistochemistry, immunochemistry, and molecular biology. *J. Neurosci.*, 6: 1108–1113.

Paterson, I.A., Juorio, A.V. and Boulton, A.A. (1990) 2-Phenylethylamine: A modulaor of catecholamine transmission in the mammalian central nervous system. *J. Neurochem.*, 55: 1827–1837.

Rahman, M.K. and Nagatsu, T. (1982) Demonstration of AADC activity in human brain with L-DOPA an Int. d 5HTP as substrates by high performance liquid chromatography with electrochemical detection. *Neurochem.*, 4: 1–6.

Rossetti, Z., Krajnc, D., Neff, N.H. and Hadjiconstantinou, M. (1989) Modulation of retinal aromatic L-amino acid decarboxylase via alpha 2 adrenoceptors. *J. Neurochem.*, 52: 647–652.

Rossetti, Z.L., Silvia, C.P., Krajnc, D., Neff, N.H. and Hadjiconstantinou, M. (1990) Aromatic L-amino acid decarboxylase is modulated by D_1 dopamine receptors in rat retina. *J. Neurochem.*, 54: 787–791.

Sacks, W., Vogel, W.H., Nagatsu, T., Lloyd, K.G. and Sandler, M. (1979) Round table on: Is there DOPA decarboxylase in human brain? In: E. Usdin, I.J. Kopin and J. Barchas (Eds.), *Catecholamines: Basic and Clinical Frontiers*, Pergamon, New York, pp. 127–131.

Siow, Y.L. and Dakshinamurti, K. (1990) Neuronal dopa decarboxylase. *Ann. N.Y. Acad. Sci.*, 585: 173–188.

Wessel, C.W. and Joh, T.H. (1992) Parallel upregulation of catecholamine-synthesizing enzymes in rat brain and adrenal gland: effects of reserpine and correlation with immediate early gene expression. *Mol. Brain Res.*, 15: 349–360.

Wiechmann, A.F. (1986) Melatonin: parallels in pineal gland and retina. *Exp. Eye Res.*, 42: 507–527.

Xu, J., Hadjiconstantinou, M. and Neff, N.H. (1985) Exposure to light accelerates the formation of dopamine from exogenous L-DOPA in the rat retina. *J. Ocul. Pharmacol.*, 1: 177–181.

Young, E.A., Neff, N.H. and Hadjiconstantinou, M. (1993) Evidence for a cyclic AMP-mediated increase of aromatic L-amino acid decarboxylase activity in the striatum and midbrain. *J. Neurochem.*, 60: 2331–2333.

Young, E.A., Neff, N.H. and Hadjiconstantinou, M. (1994) Phorbol ester administration transiently increases aromatic L-amino acid decarboxylase activity of the mouse striatum and midbrain. *J. Neurochem.*, 63: 694–697.

Zhu, M.-Y., Juorio, A.V., Paterson, I.A. and Boulton, A.A. (1993) Regulation of striatal aromatic L-amino acid decarboxylase: effects of blockade or activation of dopaminergic receptors. *Eur. J.Pharmacol.*, 238: 157–164.

Zhu, M.Y., Juorio, A.V., Paterson, I.A. and Boulton, A.A. (1992) Regulation of aromatic L-amino acid decarboxylase by dopamine receptors in the rat brain. *J. Neurochem.*, 58: 637–641.

Peter M. Yu, Keith F. Tipton and Alan A. Boulton (Eds.)
Progress in Brain Research, Vol 106

CHAPTER 11

Some new mechanisms underlying the actions of (−)-deprenyl: possible relevance to neurodegeneration

Xin-Min Li, Augusto V. Juorio and Alan A. Boulton

*Neuropsychiatry Research Unit, Department of Psychiatry, University of Saskatchewan, Saskatoon, Saskatchewan,
S7N 0W0 Canada*

Introduction

Neuroprotective effect of (−)-deprenyl

(−)-Deprenyl is a selective MAO B inhibitor; it blocks the oxidative deamination of biogenic amines such as dopamine (DA) and phenylethylamine (Johnston, 1968; Knoll and Magyar, 1972; Philips and Boulton, 1979). MAO is located on the outer membrane of the mitochondrion where it catalyzes the deamination of monoamine neurotransmitters and other monoamines (Schnaitman et al., 1967; Tipton, 1973). MAO exists in two forms (A and B), differentiated according to the sensitivity of the enzyme to inhibitors. The A-form is highly sensitive to clorgyline, while the B-form is highly sensitive to (−)-deprenyl (Johnston, 1968; Neff and Yang, 1974). (−)-Deprenyl acts as a "suicide inhibitor", binding rapidly and irreversibly to the flavine moiety of the enzyme (Youdim, 1978). Both the A and B forms of MAO have been detected in human brain tissue (Konradi et al., 1989).

Many clinical studies have shown that the treatment of parkinsonian patients with a combination of L-Dopa and (−)-deprenyl therapy leads to an optimal drug regimen (Birkmayer et al., 1977; Riederer et al., 1978; Rinne, 1983; Tetrud and Langston, 1989; The Parkinson Study Group, 1989; 1993). Long-term administration of (−)-de-

prenyl can delay the introduction of L-Dopa therapy; it has also been claimed to delay the degeneration of the nigrostriatal dopamine system and prolong life expectancy (The Parkinson Study Group, 1989; Birkmayer et al., 1983).

More recent clinical trials have shown that the administration of (−)-deprenyl is useful in the treatment of Alzheimer's disease. It improves performance on episodic memory and learning tasks requiring complex information-processing and sustained conscious effort, it slows the progression of cognitive loss, and it delays clinical deterioration (Tariot et al., 1987; Sunderland et al., 1987; Mangoni et al., 1991; Goad et al., 1991; Cooper, 1991; Palmer and De Kosky, 1993; Davis and Haroutunian, 1993). A multi-center large-scale investigation into the efficacy of (−)-deprenyl in Alzheimer's disease patients has recently been launched (Gottlieb and Kumar, 1993).

(−)-Deprenyl has also been shown to possess neuro-protective/rescue properties. It is capable of protecting and rescuing dying neurons in an MPTP neurotoxin model (Tatton and Greenwood, 1991; Nomoto and Fukuda, 1993, Yu et al., 1994), protecting hippocampal neurons from damage by a cholinergic toxin (Ricci et al., 1992), and kainate (Gelowiz and Paterson, 1994), preventing the DSP-4 (*N*-(2-chloroethyl)-2-bromobenzylamine hydrochloride) induced loss of noradrenaline (NA) in the hippocampus (Gibson, 1987; Bertocci et al., 1988; Finnegan et al., 1990, Yu et al., 1994), reducing the death of motoneurons caused by axotomy (Salo and Tatton, 1992; Ansari et al., 1993), preventing striatal neuronal death induced by transient forebrain ischemia (Matsui and Kumagae, 1991, Barber et al., 1993), as well as prolonging life-span and enhancing sexual activity in rats (Knoll et al., 1989; Milgram et al., 1990; Kitani et al., 1992). Although there are several hypotheses to explain these actions, such as blockade of DA metabolism (Knoll, 1978), blockade of DA uptake (Zsilla et al., 1986), conversion to $(-)$-amphetamine (Karoum et al., 1982), induction of superoxidase dismutase and catalase (Carrillo et al., 1991), potentiation of NA and DA transmission by 2-phenylethylamine (Paterson et al., 1991), the detailed mechanism(s) of $[-)$-deprenyl's action are not yet clear. It is clear, however, that mechanisms of action other than MAO B inhibition are involved. An in vitro study has demonstrated that some newly synthesized proteins may be involved in the inhibitory effects of $(-)$-deprenyl against apoptosis (Tatton et al., 1994). A recent report on increased mRNA expression of trkC in the rat brain after treatment with $(-)$-deprenyl has now introduced the notion that neurotrophins and their receptors may be involved (Ekblom et al., 1994).

We will discuss here some of our recent findings in the regulation of gene expression, which may suggest some new mechanisms of actions for $(-)$-deprenyl in neurodegenerative disorders.

Methodology

Cell cultures. PC12 cells and C6 cells were cultured as described in protocols provided by the supplier (American Type Culture Collection, Rockville, MD). PC12 cells were grown in RPMI 1640 tissue culture medium (Gibco) supplemented with 10% heat-inactivated horse serum and 5% fetal calf serum and C6 cells in Ham's F-10 medium with 15% horse serum and 2.5% fetal calf serum. All cultures were maintained in 5% CO_2 at 37 °C. The cells were collected for detecting mRNA, protein contents and activities of AADC. Primary cultures of mouse and rat astrocytes were obtained by disruption and sieving in modified Eagle's minimum essential medium containing 20% horse serum. The studies were done with monolayer cultures grown for 3 weeks (Li et al., 1992a; Juorio et al., 1993a).

cDNA probes. AADC cDNA was obtained from rat adrenal total RNA by reverse transcription and polymerase chain reaction (RT/PCR) and was verified according to the published rat AADC cDNA sequence (Tanaka et al., 1989; Li et al., 1993a). The full length rat GFAP cDNA (2.7 kb) cloned in a vector Blue Script SK minus (rGFA15) clone, which is expressed in astrocytes and in Schwann cells, was kindly provided by Dr. Feinstein (Cornell University, NY; Feinstein et al., 1992). The cDNA probes were labelled with $[\alpha$-$^{32}P]dCTP$ (New England Nuclear) (Fainberg and Vogelstein, 1983).

Extraction of RNA. Cultured cells were lysed in 4 M guanidium thiocyanate solution and total cellular RNA was collected by centrifugation through 5.7 M CsCl. RNA was quantitated by absorbance at 260 nm, and purity checked by the 260 nm/280 nm ratio (Maniatis et al., 1982).

Slot blot and filter hybridization. mRNA were assayed by Northern blots from cultured cells and rat neural tissues as previously described (Li et al., 1993a). For better quantification some assays were performed by slot blot. Total RNA was denatured and aliquots were blotted to nylon membranes using slot-blot manifold apparatus (Bio-Rad). RNA was cross-linked to the membranes by a UV Stratalinker 2400 (Stratagene). Membranes were hybridized with cDNA or cRNA probes, washed and then exposed to X-Omat AR film (Eastman Kodak) with intensifying screens at -70 °C to obtain autoradiograms, which were then scanned with a densitometer (Du 640, Beckman). Membranes were then washed and rehybridized with a γ-actin probe. The data are expressed as ratios of areas under the scanning curves for blots hybridized with the AADC, GFAP cDNA probes and corresponding values for the γ-actin probe, in which the control ratios were normalized to 100%.

Immunoblot for AADC. The soluble cell extract from tissues and cultured cells was obtained by homogenization, sonication and centrifugation. We have previously determined, by Western blots, that the specific rabbit anti-AADC serum interacts with a single band of AADC protein (Li et al., 1992a). For better quantitation, aliquots of protein for each sample were blotted onto nitrocellulose filters using a dot-blot manifold apparatus (Bio-Rad). The filters were blocked with milk, incubated with specific rabbit anti-AADC antibody (1:2000), washed and reincubated with a second antibody (^{125}I-labelled donkey anti-rabbit IgG, New England Nuclear) as previously described (Maniatis et al., 1982). After three washes with TBS, filters were exposed to X-Omat AR film (Eastman Kodak). Relative changes in protein content were quantitated using a densitometer.

AADC assay. AADC activity was assayed by the method previously described (Nagatsu et al, 1979, Zhu et al. 1992) based on the enzymatic conversion of L-Dopa to DA with measurement of DA by HPLC with electro-chemical detection (HPLC-EC). The samples from cultured cells or brain tissues were homogenized in 0.25 M ice cold sucrose, centrifuged at $12\,000 \times g$ for 10 min and the supernatant was used for incubation. The incubation mixture contained 50 mM sodium phosphate buffer (pH 7.2), 0.04 mM L-Dopa (D-Dopa for blank), 0.17 mM ascorbic acid, 0.01 mM pyridoxal 5-phosphate, 0.1 mM pargyline, 1 mM 2-mercaptoethanol, 0.1 mM EDTA and 50 μl enzyme in a total volume of 400 μl. After incubation (20 min, at 37 ° C), the reaction was stopped by addition of 0.1 M perchloric acid, containing isoproterenol as internal standard. The mixture was centrifuged again and the supernatant (50 μl) was used for HPLC assay. Protein concentration was determined by the Lowry method and the enzyme activity was expressed as nmol/20 min/mg protein at 37 ° C. The K_m and V_{max} values obtained from an Eadie-Hofstee plot.

Detection of DA and DOPAC. The detection of dopamine and 3,4-dihydroxyphenylacetic acid (DOPAC) was carried out by high-performance liquid chromatography with electrochemical detection as previously described (Kwok and Juorio, 1986).

Statistical analyses. Results were analyzed by one- or two-way analysis of variance. In the presence of significant F values, individual comparisons between means were made using Duncan's New Multiple Range Test.

Results and discussion

Stimulation of gene expression of AADC

Aromatic amino acid decarboxylase (AADC, EC4.1.1.28) is directly involved in the synthesis of the neurotransmitters, DA and serotonin (5HT), since it decarboxylates their respective amino acids precursers 3,4-dihydroxy-phenylalanine (L-Dopa) and 5-hydroxytryptophan. It is also directly involved in the synthesis of other biogenic amines, particularly so-called trace amines which have been shown to possess neuromodulatory properties (Christenson et al., 1972; Lovenberg et al., 1962; Boulton and Juorio, 1982; Juorio and Boulton 1982). Since AADC is quite abundant in brain tissues, it has not been considered to be rate-limiting in the synthesis of DA and 5HT (Brodie et al., 1962; Bowsher and Henry, 1983). AADC can be found throughout the central and peripheral nervous systems, where it is localized in catecholamine- and serotonin-containing neurons, as well as in chromaffin cells of the adrenal medulla. AADC activity is also present in some neurons (D cells) that neither produce nor contain DA or 5HT (Jaeger et al., 1983; Komori et al., 1991) as well as astrocytes (Juorio et al., 1993a). AADC activity, however, is also distributed widely in peripheral tissues where monoamine neurotransmitters are not produced

(Albert et al., 1987), suggesting that this enzyme may possess some other functional significance. It has been shown that a single gene encodes the sequence of AADC in both neuronal and non-neuronal tissues (Albert et al., 1987; Coge et al., 1990). The cDNA of AADC from rat (Tanaka et al., 1989), human (Ichinose et al., 1989) and bovine tissues (Kang and Joh, 1990) has been cloned and characterized. The isolated clones have proved to be useful tools in the investigation of the molecular aspects of AADC (Beall and Hirsh, 1987; Li et al., 1992a; Sumi-Ichinose et al., 1992; Eaton et al., 1993).

Some early reports showed that the chronic administration of some non-selective MAO inhibitors (MAOIs) could stimulate AADC activity in rat brain (Robinson et al., 1979; Campbell et al., 1980). It has been shown recently that AADC activity in rat retina is modulated in vivo by environmental light (Hadjiconstantinou et al., 1988) and is up-regulated by both haloperidol and the D_1 antagonist SCH23390 (Rossetti et al., 1990). This increase in activity appears to be the result of an increase in the enzyme protein. In our laboratory, we have also been able to show that the acute D_1 antagonist SCH23390 and the D_2 antagonist pimozide increase striatal AADC activity (Zhu et al., 1992, 1994) and that this short-term effect is not due to de novo protein synthesis. This suggests the involvement of second-messenger systems (Young et al., 1993). Chronic treatment with neuroleptics such as haloperidol and loxapine has been shown to increase AADC gene expression while tyrosine hydroxylase (TH) gene expression was not affected (Buckland, 1992). In another study chronic (−)-deprenyl administration transiently decreases TH activity and its mRNA in the rat nigrostriatal pathway (Vrana et al., 1992). Such results suggest that change in DA receptor activity is one of the mechanisms involved in AADC regulation and this in turn suggests that AADC possesses a dynamic role in the control of the synthesis of monoamines. This regulation is complicated and exists at different levels in in vivo models (Gjedde et al., 1993).

In Parkinson's disease, degeneration of the nigrostriatal system is accompanied by depletion of DA and marked reductions in striatal tyrosine hydroxylase and AADC activities (Lloyd and Hornykiewicz, 1970). AADC is rate-limiting for patients on L-Dopa therapy and its therapeutic efficacy is attributed to its enzymatic decarboxylation of L-Dopa and the replenishment of DA levels in the striatum (Hornykiewicz, 1974). AADC activity is also reduced in aging animals (David et al., 1989). Post mortem studies carried out on the brains of Alzheimer's disease patients have shown a reduction in NA and 5-HT levels (Reisberg, 1983; Chan-Palay and Asan, 1989), again perhaps indicating some involvement of AADC in these conditions as well. L-Dopa is thought to be converted to DA predominantly within DA terminals (Langelier et al., 1973) as well as in 5HT terminals (Ng et al., 1972). We have demonstrated, however, the presence of AADC gene expression in cultured glial cells (Li et al., 1992a; Juorio et al., 1993a). AADC is present in human brain tissue at a much lower level than in other species and this suggests that AADC might be rate-limiting in monoamine synthesis in human brain, especially in parkinsonian patients (Robins et al., 1967; Gjedde et al., 1993).

We have shown that (−)-deprenyl stimulates AADC gene expression in PC12 cells (Li et al., 1992b), suggesting that (−)-deprenyl could exerting its anti-parkinsonian effects and potentiation of L-Dopa, therapy by producing more DA, a mechanism additional to straightforward MAO B inhibition, thus increasing DA levels (Birkmayer et al., 1975). Since MAO B activity has not been detected in PC12 cells (Youdim et al., 1986; Li, unpublished results), this stimulation suggests the presence of a novel site of action for (−)-deprenyl.

We have shown that (−)-deprenyl (0.1–10 μM) and other irreversible MAO B inhibitors stimulate AADC gene expression iin PC12 cells (see Table 1; Li et al., 1992b). The specificity of this effect was examined by comparing (−)-deprenyl with other MAOIs. PC12 cells were treated with

10 μM of each of the following drugs for 72 h; (−)-deprenyl, MDL 72,974A ((E)-2-(4-fluoro-phenethyl)-3-fluoroallylamine, an irreversible MAO B inhibitor) and pargyline (a less selective irreversible MAO B inhibitor). They all produced a dose- and time-related stimulation of AADC gene expression whilst clorgyline (a selective irreversible MAO A inhibitor) and Ro 19-6327 (N-(2-aminoethyl)-5-chloro-2-pyridine carboxamide, a reversible MAO B inhibitor) had no effect (Table 1).

These effects, of the irreversible MAO B inhibitors on AADC gene expression, were strikingly similar to their claimed neuroprotective efficacy. DSP-4-induced NA depletion in the hippocampus is prevented by (−)-deprenyl, pargyline, and some aliphatic propargylamines (Yu et al., 1992, 1994), but not by clorgyline or Ro 19-6327 (Gibson, 1987; Bertocci et al., 1988). (−)-Deprenyl and other MAO B inhibitors can block MPTP-induced parkinsonism by preventing the activation of MPTP to its toxic metabolite MPP^+ by MAO B (Heikkila et al., 1984). Delayed (−)-deprenyl administration can rescue dying neurons in an MPTP murine parkinsonian model, indicating that the effects are mediated by an unidentified mechanism of action not related to the conversion of MPTP to MPP^+ (Tatton and Greenwood, 1991; Ansari et al., 1993). Similarly a wash-out study whereby MPTP is removed before (−)-deprenyl is added also indicated neuroprotection (Finnegan et al., 1990). Low levels of (−)-deprenyl can reduce the death of motor neurons caused by axotomy (Salo and Tatton, 1992). In this model, no neurotoxin is involved, suggesting that (−)-deprenyl may in some way compensate for the loss of target-derived trophic support. An increase in AADC gene expression may be one of several parallel events in the neuroprotective effects of (−)-deprenyl that are mediated at a novel site of action.

AADC is present in glial cells and is stimulated by MAO B inhibitors

AADC is present not only in neurons but also in glial cells. Using Northern blot and Western immunoblot analyses we have shown a single species of mRNA for AADC and a single protein band at 52 kDa for AADC enzyme protein in cultured rat astrocytes and in C6 glioma cells (Figs. 1 and 2) (Li et al., 1992a). Recently we have also demonstrated the presence of AADC activity (Table 2) (Juorio et al., 1993a). These results demonstrate, for the first time, the existence of AADC gene expression in glial cells at both the transcriptional and the translational levels. In addition, C6 glioma cell cultures have retained the gene expression for AADC and preliminary data show that (−)-deprenyl stimulates AADC gene expression in cultured C6 cells (Li, unpublished data).

In healthy striatum, the AADC in glial cells is unlikely to contribute to catecholamine production since glia have not been reported to contain tyrosine hydroxylase (TH) (Jaeger et al., 1983). It is likely, however, that some trace amines which do not require prior hydroxylation such as p- and m-tyramine, 2-phenylethylamine and tryptamine are produced by AADC in glial cells; these trace amines could then modulate (i.e. amplify) monoaminergic neurotransmission (Boulton, 1976; Paterson et al., 1990; Juorio and Paterson, 1990). Because of the substantial loss of DA terminals in Parkinson's disease, however, the

TABLE 1

Effect of some MAO inhibitors on AADC mRNA levels in PC12 cells

Treatment	Mean ± S.E.
Deprenyl	146 ± 3.7[a]
MDL 72,974A	154 ± 7.0[a]
Ro 19–6327	101 ± 3.5
Clorgyline	111 ± 4.1
Pargyline	144 ± 4.5[a]

[a] $P < 0.01$. $n = 3$. Values are expressed as percentage of the control. MAO inhibitor concentrations were 10 μM and incubation times 72 h. Data taken from Li et al., 1992b.

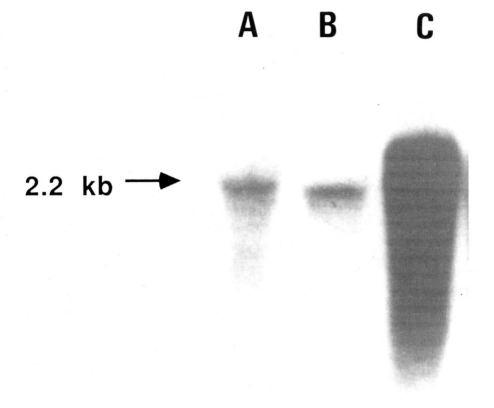

A   B   C

2.2 kb →

Fig. 1. Northern blot analysis of AADC mRNA. Poly(A)RNA from cultured astrocytes (20 μg, lane A), C6 glioma cells (20 μg, lane B) and rat kidney (10 μg, lane C). Taken with permission from Li et al., 1992a.

activity of AADC in glia may become very important in the decarboxylation of exogenously administered L-Dopa. It has been shown in both rat and primates that treatment with MAO inhibitors significantly affects L-Dopa and DA metabolism in the brain (Juorio et al., 1993b). The effects of MAO inhibitors also occur outside catecholaminergic neurons, since in animals pretreated with 6-hydroxydopamine DA accumulation following L-Dopa administration remains considerable (Buu

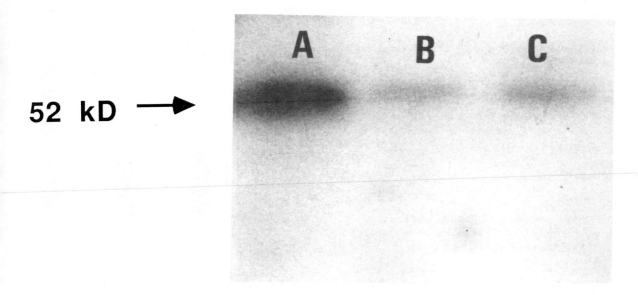

52 kD →

Fig. 2. Western blot analysis of AADC protein. Cell lysate protein from rat kidney (10 μg, lane A), C6 glioma cells (50 μg, lane B) and cultured astrocytes (50 μg, lane C). Taken with permission from Li et al., 1992a.

and Angers, 1987). Further studies are needed to characterize in vivo AADC regulation after drug treatment.

Inhibition of gene expression of GFAP

It is interesting to compare the pattern of the effect of various MAOIs on AADC mRNA with their effects on GFAP gene expression in C6 glioma cells since in the former stimulation occurs whilst in the latter there is inhibition. (−)-

TABLE 2

The synthesis of DA in primary glial cultures

L-Dopa concentration (M)	DA (ng/mg protein) DA DOPAC
0	< 0.5
10^{-6}	2.2 ± 0.2
10^{-5}	6.7 ± 0.5
10^{-4}	20 ± 1.3
10^{-3}	64 ± 4.5

Mean $\pm$ SE ($n = 5$). Data taken from Juorio et al., 1993a.

Deprenyl decreases the abundance of GFAP mRNA in a time- and dose-dependent manner. The effect again seems to be specific to irreversible MAO B inhibitors, since (−)-deprenyl, MDL72974A and pargyline exhibited similar effects while (+)-deprenyl and clorgyline (an MAO A inhibitor) had no effect (Table 3; Li et al., 1993b). Recent data (Li, unpublished results) also indicate that (−)-deprenyl can moderately inhibit C6 cell proliferation as measured by [^{3}H]thymidine incorporation.

GFAP accumulation is a prominent feature of astrocytic gliosis, which commonly occurs in the CNS following neural tissue damage. GFAP also accumulates in aging and neurodegenerative diseases, as in Alzheimer's disease (Norton et al., 1992; Tardy et al., 1989) and Parkinson's disease (Damier et al., 1993). An inhibition or delay in GFAP synthesis (i.e. glial cell proliferation) might reduce or eliminate scar formation and thus reduce the formation of a physical barrier. The consequence of this would be to allow neurons and oligodendrocytes to reestablish a functional environment, which might be beneficial (Aschner

TABLE 3

Effect of some MAO inhibitors on GFAP mRNA levels in C6 glioma cells

Treatment	GFAP mRNA (% of controls)
(−)-Deprenyl	68 ± 6.3[a]
MDL 72,974A	74 ± 6.1[a]
Pargyline	75 ± 3.6[a]
Clorgyline	96 ± 2.6
(+)-Deprenyl	92 ± 2.6

Mean ± SE values ($n = 4$). MAO inhibitor and (−)-deprenyl analogue concentrations are 1 μM and incubation times 24 h. [a]$P < 0.01$ by Newman-Keuls test with respect to controls. Data taken from Li et al., 1993b.

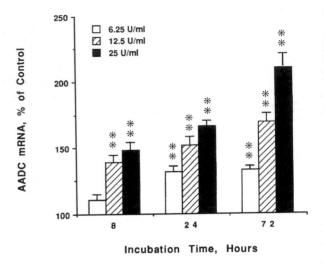

Fig. 3. Effect of IL-1β on AADC mRNA levels in cultured PC12 cells. Data are means ± SE, $n = 6$. **$P < 0.01$ with respect to the control values by Newman-Keuls test. Data from Li et al., 1993c.

and Kimelberg, 1991). It has recently been demonstrated that in the frontal cortex of rats treated chronically with (−)-deprenyl, GFAP-immunoreactive astrocyte profiles are decreased in comparison with age-matched untreated controls (Amenta et al., 1994). Our findings also suggest that (−)-deprenyl might be useful for regulating astrogliosis (Aschner and Kimelberg, 1991). A recent in vivo study, however, showed treatment of rats with (−)-deprenyl following a striatal lesion produced an increase in GFAP immunoreactivity (Biagini et al. 1993): clearly more investigations will be required to unravel these somewhat conflicting findings.

Neurotrophic factors may be involved in the apparent neuroprotective efficacy of some irreversible MAO B inhibitors

Recently we have demonstrated that AADC gene expression can also be regulated by IL 1-β and PG E$_2$ in PC12 cells (Figs. 3 and 4; Li et al., 1993c). IL 1-β and PGE$_2$ produce a dose- and time-dependent up-regulation in AADC mRNA levels (up to 200% of control values) which is followed by a stable increase in AADC protein. Because IL-1 is synthesized and acts locally within the brain to influence neuronal and glial function, it has been proposed to be a mediator with both beneficial and detrimental responses to inflam-

mation and injury. The regulation of AADC by IL-1 may indicate the possible involvement of AADC in neuronal injury and recovery. IL-1 (Carman-Krzan et al., 1991; Olson et al., 1990) and PGE$_2$ (Toso et al., 1988) also stimulate neurotrophic factor (including NGF) gene expression in cultured neurons and astrocytes, suggesting that the regulation of AADC gene expression by these cytokine treatments is similar to the effects on NGF gene expression. AADC activity is reduced in aging animals (David et al., 1989) while NGF and BDNF mRNAs are decreased in the hippocampus of individuals with Alzheimer's disease (Phillips et al., 1991). Catecholamines have been reported to increase the NGF mRNA content in cultured astroglial cells and fibroblasts (Furukawa et al., 1992). NGF synthesis in cultured cells is growth-dependent, suggesting that the expression of some genes related to cell growth is associated with up-regulation of NGF synthesis. It is interesting to note that AADC activity in many kinds of cultured cells is also growth-dependent. In fact the specific activity of AADC in culture is about 2-fold higher during the exponential phases of growth than during the

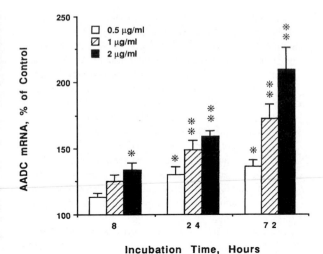

Fig. 4. Effect of PGE$_2$ on AADC mRNA levels in cultured PC12 cells. Data are means ± SE, $n = 6$. *$P < 0.05$ and **$P < 0.01$ with respect to the control values by Newman-Keuls test. Taken with permission from Li et al., 1993c.

(Fusco et al., 1991). A trophic deficiency could represent an important pathogenic mechanism in aging and neurodegenerative conditions; in principle, therefore, administration of trophic factors might reverse symptoms related to this deficiency. Pathophysiological observations and complementary animal experiments suggest the possible use of neurotrophins as a therapeutic tool for degenerative neuronal disorders such as Parkinson's disease and Alzheimer's disease (Levi-Montalcini, 1987; Sendtner et al., 1992). Applications for therapeutic purposes, however, are limited because neurotrophins, as macromolecules, cannot pass through the blood–brain barrier (Friden et al., 1993). In view of this, enhancement or regulation of neurotrophic factors or their receptors by a drug(s) that can pass through the blood–brain barrier is a promising chemotherapeutic approach (Furukawa and Furukawa, 1990; Furukawa et al., 1992; Shinoda et al., 1990; Takeuchi et al., 1990).

Acknowledgements

We thank Saskatchewan Health and the Health Services Utilization and Research Commission (HSURC) for financial support.

References

Albert, V.R., Allen, J.M. and Joh, T. (1987) A single gene codes for aromatic L-amino acid decarboxylase in both neuronal and non-neuronal tissues. *J. Biol. Chem.*, 262: 9404–9411.

Altar, C.A., Boylan, C.B., Jackson, C., Hershenson, S., Miller, J., Wiegand, S.J., Lindsy, M. and Hyman, C. (1992) Brain-derived neurotrophic factor augments rotational behavior and nigrostriatal dopamine turnover in vivo. *Proc. Natl. Acad. Sci. USA*, 89: 11347–11351.

Amenta, F., Bograni, S., Cadel, S., Ferrante, F., Valsecchi, B. and Vega, J. (1994) Microanatomical changes in the frontal cortex of aged rats: effect of l-deprenyl treatment. *Brain Res. Bull.*, 34: 125–131.

Ansari, K.S., Tatton, W.G., Yu, P.H. and Kruck, T.P. A. (1993) Death of axotomized immature rat facial motoneurons: stereospecific rescue by R(−)-deprenyl independently of MAO inhibition. *Neuroscience*, 13: 4042–4053.

Arakawa, Y., Sendtner, M. and Thoenen, H. (1990) Survival effect of ciliary neurotrophic factor (CNTF) on chick em-

plateau phases and 3–5-fold higher during the increase in cells in the G$_2$-M phase (Francis et al., 1983). (−)-Deprenyl seems to possess the trophic capacity to activate cultured astrocytes at their arrest phase of growth (G$_0$ phase) back into active cell cycles (Skibo et al., 1992).

The neurotrophic factors NGF, BDNF, and CNTF are involved in neuronal growth, differentiation and survival (Easter et al., 1985; Thoenen and Barde, 1980; Varon and Bunge, 1978; Levi-Montalcini, 1987; Leibrock et al., 1989; Altar et al., 1992; Arakawa et al., 1990). NGF is predominantly synthesized in the target areas of NGF-responsive neurons (Whittemore and Seiger, 1987) while BDNF is synthesized in neurons as well as glial cells (Leibrock et al., 1989). Astroglial cells, fibroblast cells, and Schwann cells all synthesize and secrete NGF and CNTF in culture (Assouline et al., 1987). NGF and other neurotrophic factors bind to specific cell surface receptors and are retrogradely transported to the cell bodies of neurons, where various gene programmes are regulated in response to receptor activation. They are synthesized and their receptors (LNGFR, Trk A, Trk B and Trk C) are expressed in the CNS

108

bryonic motoneurons in culture: comparison with other neurotrophic factors and cytokines. *J. Neurosci.*, 10: 3507–3515.

Aschner, M. and Kimelberg, H.K. (1991) The use of astrocytes in culture as model systems for evaluating neurotoxic-induced-injury. *Neurotoxicology*, 12: 505–517.

Assouline, J.G., Bosch, P., Lim, R., Kim, I.S., Jensen, R. and Pantazis, N.J. (1987) Rat astrocytes and Schwann cells in cultures synthesize nerve growth factor-like neurite-promoting factors. *Dev. Brain Res.*, 31: 103–18.

Barber, A.J., Paterson, I.A., Gelowitz, D.L. and Voll, C.L. (1993) Deprenyl protects rat hippocampal pyramidal cells from ischaemic insult. *Soc. Neurosci. Abstr.*, 19: 674.6.

Beall, C.J. and Hirsh, J. (1987) Regulation of the *Drosophila* dopa decarboxylase gene in neuronal and glial cells. *Gene Dev.*, 1: 510–520.

Bertocci, B., Gill, G. and DaPrada, M. (1988) Prevention of the DSP4-induced noradrenergic neurotoxicity by irreversible, not by reversible MAO-B inhibitors. *Pharmacol. Res. Commun.*, 20 (Suppl 5), 131–132.

Biagini, G., Zoli, M.,Fuxe, K. Agnati, L.F. (1993) L-Deprenyl increases GFAP immunoreactivity selectively in activated astrocytes in rat brain. *Neuroreport*, 4,955–958.

Birkmayer, W., Knoll, J., Riederer, P. (1983) (−)-Deprenyl leads to prolongation of l-Dopa efficacy in Parkinson's disease. In: H. Beckmann, and P. Riederer (Eds.), *Monoamine Oxidase and its Selective Inhibitors*, Karger, Basel, pp. 170–176.

Birkmayer, W., Riederer, P., Youdim, M.B. and Linauer, W. (1975) The potentiation of the anti-akinetic effect of l-dopa treatment by an inhibitor of MAO-B, l-deprenyl. *J. Neural Transm.*, 36: 303–336.

Birkmayer W, Riederer P, Ambrozi, L. and Youdim, M.B. (1977) Implications of combined treatment with 'Madopar' and L-deprenyl in Parkinson's disease, a long term study. *Lancet*, 1: 439–443.

Boulton, A.A. (1976) Cerebral aryl alkyl aminergic mechanisms. In: E. Usdin and M. Sandler (Eds.), *Trace Amines and the Brain. Vol. I: Psychopharmacology Series*, M. Dekker, New York, pp 22–39.

Boulton, A.A. and Juorio, A.V. (1982) Brain trace amines. In: A. Lajtha (Ed.), *Handbook of Neurochemistry*, Vol. I, Plenum Press, New York, pp. 189–222.

Bowsher, R.R. and Henry, D.P. (1983) Decarboxylation of *p*-tyrosine: a potential source of *p*-tyramine in mammalian tissues. *J. Neurochem.*, 40: 992–1002.

Brodie, B.B., Kuntzman, R., Hirch, C.W. and Costa, E. (1962) Effects of decarboxylase inhibition on the biosynthesis of brain monoamines. *Life Sci.*, 1: 81–84.

Buckland, P.R., O'Donovan, M.C. and McGuffin, P. (1992) Changes in dopa decarboxylase mRNA but not tyrosine hydroxylase mRNA levels in rat brain following antipsychotic treatment. *Psychopharmacology*, 108: 98–102.

Buu, N.T. and Angers, M. (1987) Effects of different monoamine oxidase inhibitors on the metabolism of L-Dopa in the rat brain. *Biochem. Pharmacol.*, 36: 1731–1735.

Campbell, I.C., Murphy, D.L., Walker, M.N. and Lovenberg, W. (1980) Monoamine oxidase inhibitors (MAOI) increase rat brain aromatic amino acid decarboxylase activity. *Br. J. Clin. Pharmacol.*, . 9: 431–432.

Carman-Krzan, M., Vige, X. and Wise, B.C. (1991) Regulation by interleukin-1 of nerve growth factor secretion and nerve growth factor mRNA expression in rat primary astroglial cultures. *J. Neurochem.*, 56: 636–643.

Carrillo, M.C., Kanai, S., Nokubo, M. and Kitani, K. (1991) (−)Deprenyl induces activities of both superoxide dismutase and catalase but not of glutathione peroxidase in the striatum of young male rats. *Life Sci.*, 4 8: 517–521.

Chan-Palay, V. and Asan, E. (1989) Alteration in catecholamine neurons of the locus coeruleus in senile dementia of the Alzheimer type and in Parkinson's disease with and without dementia and depression. *J. Comp. Neurol.*, 287: 373–392.

Christenson, J.W., Dairman, W. and Udenfriend, S. (1972) On the identity of DOPA decarboxylase and 5-hydroxytryptophan decarboxylase. *Proc. Natl. Acad. Sci. USA*, 69: 343–347.

Coge, F., Krieger-Poullet, M., Gros, F. and Thibault, J. (1990) Comparative and quantitative study of L-DOPA decarboxylase mRNA in rat neuronal and non-neuronal tissues. *Biochem. Biophys. Res. Commun.*, 170: 1006–1012.

Cooper, J. (1991) Drug treatment of Alzheimer's disease. *Arch. Intern. Med.*, 151: 245–249.

Damier, P., Hirsch, E.C., Zhang, P., Agid, Y. and Javoy-Agid, F. (1993) Glutathione peroxidase, glial cells and Parkinson's disease. *Neuroscience*, 52: 1–6.

David, J.C., Coulon, J.F., Cavoy, A. and Delacour, J. (1989) Effects of aging on *p*- and *m*-octopamine, catecholamines, and their metabolizing enzymes in the rat. *J. Neurochem.*, 53: 149–154.

Davis, K.L. and Haroutunian, V. (1993) Strategies for the treatment of Alzheimer's disease. *Neurology*, 43 (suppl. 4): 52–55.

Easter, W., Purves, D., Rakee, P. and Spitzer, N.C. (1985) The changing view of neural specificity. *Science*, 230: 507–511.

Eaton, M.J., Gudehithlu, K.P., Quach, T., Silvia, C.P., Hadjiconstantinou, M. and Neff, N.H. (1993) Distribution of aromatic l-amino acid decarboxylase mRNA in mouse brain by in situ hybridization histology. *J. Comp. Neurol.*, 337: 640–654.

Ekblom, J., Jossan, S.S., Ebendal, T., Soderstrom, S., Oreland, L. and Aquilonius, S.-M. (1994) mRNA expression of neurotrophins and members of the trk family in the rat brain after treatment with l-deprenyl. *Acta Neurol. Scand.*, 89: 147–148.

Fainberg, A. P. and Vogelstein, B. (1983) A technique for radiolabelling DNA restriction endonuclease fragments to high specific activity. *Anal. Biochem.*, 132: 6–13

Feinstein, D.L., Weinmaster, G.A., and Milner, R.J. (1992) Isolation of cDNA clones encoding rat glial fibrillary acidic protein: expression in astrocytes and in Schwann cells. *J. Neurosci. Res.*, 32: 1–14.

Finnegan, K.T., Skratt, J.J., Irwin, I., DeLanney, L.E. and Langston, J.W. (1990) Protection against DSP-4-induced neurotoxicity by deprenyl is not related to its inhibition of MAO B. *Eur. J. Pharmacol.*, 184: 119–126.

Francis, J., Thompson, R., Bernal, S.D., Luk, G.D. and Baylin, S.B. (1983) Effects of dibutyryl cyclic adenosine 3':5'-monophosphate on the growth cultured human small-cell lung carcinoma and the specific cellular activity of L-Dopa decarboxylase. *Cancer Res.*, 43: 639–645.

Friden, P.M., Walus, L.R., Watson, P., Doctrw, S.R., Kozarich, J.W., Backman, C., Bergman, H., Hoffer, B., Bloom, F. and Granholm, A.-C. (1993) Blood-brain barrier penetration and in vivo activity of an NGF conjugate. *Science*, 259: 373–377.

Furukawa, S. and Furukawa, Y. (1990) Nerve growth factor synthesis and its regulatory mechanisms: an approach to therapeutic induction of nerve growth factor synthesis. *Cerebrovasc. Brain Metab. Rev.*, 2: 328–44.

Furukawa, Y., Tomioka, N., Sato, W., Satoyoshi, E., HayashiK. and Furukawa, S. (1992) Catecholamines increase nerve growth factor mRNA content in both mouse astroglial cells and fibroblast cells. *FEBS Lett.*, 247: 463–467.

Fusco, M., Polato, P., Vantini, G., Cavicchioli, L., Bentivoglio, M. and Leon, A. (1991) Nerve growth factor differentially modulates the expression of its receptor within the CNS. *J. Comp. Neurol.*, 312: 477–491.

Gelowitz, D.L. and Paterson, I.A. (1994) L-deprenyl reduces kainic acid-induced neuronal death in the hippocampus. *Soc. Neurosci. Abstr.*, 20: 113.2.

Gibson, C.J. (1987) Inhibition of MAO B, but not MAO A, blocks DSP-4 toxicity on central NE neurons. *Eur. J. Pharmacol.*, 141: 135–138.

Gjedde, A., Leger, G.C., Cumming, P., Yasuhara, Y., Evans, A.C., Guttman, M. and Kuwabara, H. (1993) Striatal l-dopa decarboxylase activity in Parkinson's disease in vivo: implications for the regulation of dopamine synthesis. *J. Neurochem.*, 61: 1538–1541.

Gottlieb, G.L. and Kumar, A. (1933) Conventional pharmacologic treatment for patients with Alzheimer's disease. *Neurology*, 43(suppl 4), 56–63.

Goad, D.L., Davis, C.M., Liem, P., Fuselier, C.C., McCormack, J.R. and Olsen, K.M. (1991) The use of selegiline in Alzheimer's patients with behavior problems. *J. Clin. Psychiat.*, 52: 342–345.

Hadjiconstantinou, M., Rossetti, Z., Silvia C, Krajnc, D. and Neff, N.H. (1988) Aromatic l-amino acid decarboxylase activity of the rat retina is modulated in vivo by environmental light. *J. Neurochem.*, 51: 1560–1564.

Heikkila, R.E., Manzino, L., Cabbat, F.S. and Duvoisin, R. C (1984). Protection against the dopaminergic neurotoxicity of 1-methyl-4-phenyl-1,2,3,6-tetraydropyridine by monoamine oxidase inhibitors. *Nature*, 311: 467–469.

Hornykiewicz, O. (1974) The mechanisms of action of L-dopa in Parkinson's disease. *Life Sci.*, 15: 1249–1259.

Hörtnagl, H., Berger, M.L., Havelec, L. and Hornykiewicz, O. (1993) Role of glucocorticoids in the cholinergic degeneration in rat hippocampus induced by ethylcholine aziridinium (AF64A). *J. Neurosci.*, 13: 2939–2945.

Ichinose, H., Kurosawa, Y., Titani, K., Fujita, K. and Nagatsu, T. (1989) Isolation and characterization of a cDNA clone encoding human aromatic L-amino acid decarboxylase. *Biochem. Biophys. Res. Commun.*, 164: 1024–1030.

Jaeger, C.B., Teitelman, G., Joh, T.H., Albert, V.R., Park, D.H. and Reis, D.J. (1983) Some neurons of the rat central nervous system contain aromatic l-amino acid decarboxylase but not monoamine. *Science*, 219: 1233–1235.

Johnston, J.P. (1968) Some observations upon a new inhibitor of monoamine oxidase in brain tissue. *Biochem. Pharmacol.*, 17: 1285–1297.

Juorio, A.V. and Boulton, A.A. (1982) The effect of some precursor amino acids and enzyme inhibitors on the mouse striatal concentration of tyramines and homovanillic acid. *J. Neurochem.*, 39: 859–863.

Juorio, A.V. and Paterson, I.A. (1990) Tryptamine may couple dopaminergic and serotonergic transmission in the brain. *Gen. Pharmacol.*, 21 , 759–762.

Juorio, A.V., Li, X.-M., Walz, W. and Paterson, I.A. (1993a) Decarboxylation of L-Dopa by cultured mouse astrocytes. *Brain Res*, 626: 306–309.

Juorio, A.V., Li, X.-M., Paterson, I.A. and Boulton, A.A. (1993b) Effects of monoamine oxidase B inhibitors on dopaminergic function: role of 2-phenylethylamine and aromatic L-amino acid decarboxylase. In: C.W. Olanow and A. Lieberman (Eds.), *MAO Inhibitors in Neurological Disease*, Budapest, pp. 181–200.

Kang, U.J. and Joh, T.H. (1990) Deduced amino acid sequence of bovine aromatic L-amino acid decarboxylase: homology to other decarboxylase. *Mol. Brain Res.*, 8: 83–87.

Karoum, F., Chuang, L.W., Eisler, T., Calne, D.B., Liebowitz, M.R., Quitkin, F.M., Klein, D.F. and Wyatt, R.J. (1982) Metabolism of (−)deprenyl to amphetamine and methamphetamine may be responsible for deprenyl's therapeutic benefit: A biochemical assessment. *Neurology*, 32: 503–509.

Kitani, K., Kanai, S., Sato, Y., Ohta, M., Ivy, G.O. and Carrillo M-C. (1992) Chronic treatment of (−)deprenyl prolongs the life span of male fischer 344 rats: further evidence. *Life Sci.*, 52: 281–288.

Knoll, J. and Magyar, K. (1972) Some puzzling pharmacological effects of monoamine oxidase inhibitors. *Adv. Biochem. Psychopharmacol.*, 5: 393–408.

Knoll, J. (1978) The possible mechanisms of action of (−)deprenyl in Parkinson's disease. *J. Neural. Transm.*, 43: 117–198.

Knoll, J., Dallo, J. and Yen, T.T. (1989) Striatal dopamine, sexual activity and lifespan, longevity of rats treated with (−)deprenyl. *Life Sci.*, 45: 525–531.

Komori, D., Fujii, T., Karasawa, N., Yamada, K. and Nagatsu, I. (1991) Some neurons of the nouse cortex and caudoputamen contain aromatic L-amino acid decarboxylase but not monoamines. *Acta Histochem. Cytochem.*, 24: 571–577.

Konradi, C., Kornhuber, J., Froelich, L., Fritze, J., Heinsen, H., Beckmann, H., Schulz, E. and Riederer, P. (1989) Demonstration of MAO A and B in the hyman brainstem by a histochemical technique. *Neuroscience*, 33: 383–400.

Kwok, R.P.S. and Juorio, A.V (1986) The concentration of striatal tyramine and dopamine metabolism in diabetic rats and effect of insulin administration. *Neuroendocrinology*, 43: 590–596.

Langelier, P., Roberge, A.G., Boucher, R. and Poirier, L. (1973) Effects of chronically administered L-DOPA in normal and lesioned cats. *J. Pharmacol. Exp. Ther.*, 187: 15–22.

Leibrock, J., Lottspeich, F., Hohn, A., Hofer, M., Hengerer, B., Masiakowski, P., Thoenen, H. and Barde, Y.A. (1989) Molecular cloning and expression of brain-derived neurotrophic factor. *Nature*, 351: 149–152.

Levi-Montalcini, R. (1987) The nerve growth factors 35 years later. *Science*, 237: 1154–1162.

Li, X-M., Juorio, A.V., Paterson, I.A., Walz, W., Zhu, M.Y. and Boulton, A.A. (1992a) Gene expression of aromatic L-amino acid decarboxylase in rat cultured glial cells. *J. Neurochem.*, 59: 1172–1175.

Li, X-M., Juorio, A.V., Paterson, I.A., Zhu, M.Y. and Boulton, A.A. (1992b) Specific irreversible MAO B inhibitors stimulate gene expression of aromatic l-amino acid decarboxylase in PC12 cells. *J. Neurochem.*, 59: 2324–2327.

Li, X.-M., Juorio, A.V., Boulton, A.A. (1993a) Gene regulation of aromatic l-amino acid decarboxylase (AADC) by NSD-1015 in rat PC12 pheochromocytoma cells. *Neurochem. Res.*, 18: 915–919.

Li, X.-M., Qi, J., Juorio, A.V. and Boulton, A.A. (1993b) Reduction in GFAP mRNA abundance induced by (−)-Deprenyl and other MAO B inhibitors in C6 Glioma Cells. *J. Neurochem.*, 61: 1573–1576.

Li, X.-M., Juorio, A.V. and Boulton, A.A. (1993c) Induction of aromatic l-amino acid decarboxylase mRNA by interleukin-1 β and prostaglandin E2. *Neurochem. Res*, 19: 593–597.

Lloyd, K.G. and Hornykiewicz, O. (1970) Parkinson's disease, activity of L-dopa decarboxylase in discrete brain regions. *Science*, 170: 1212–1213.

Lovenberg, W., Weissbach, W. and Udenfriend, S. (1962) Aromatic L-amino acid decarboxylase. *J. Biol. Chem.*, 237: 89–93.

Maniatis, T., Fritsch, E.F. and Sambrook, J. (1982) *Molecular Cloning, a Laboratory Manual*, Cold Spring Harbor, New York.

Mangoni, A., Grassi, M.P., Frattola, L., Piolti, R., Bassi, S.,

Motta, A., Marcone, A. and Smirne, S. (1991) Effects of a MAO-B inhibitor in the treatment of Alzheimer disease. *Eur. Neurol.*, 31: 100–107.

Matsui, Y. and Kumagae, K. (1991) Monoamine oxidase inhibitors prevent striatal neuronal necrosis induced by transient forebrain ischemia. *Neurosci. Lett.*, 126: 175–178.

Milgram, N.W., Racine, R.J., Nellis, P., Mendonca, A. and Ivy, G.O. (1990) Maintenance on l-deprenyl prolongs life in aged male rats. *Life Sci.*, 47: 415–420.

Nagatsu, Y., Yamamoto, T. and Kato, T. (1979) A new and highly sensitive voltammetric assay for AADC activity by high-performance liquid chromatography. *Anal. Biochem.*, 100: 160–165.

Neff, N.H. and Yang, H.-Y.T. (1974) Another look at the monoamine oxidases and the monoamine oxidase inhibitor drugs. *Life Sci.*, 14: 2061–2074.

Ng, L.K. Y., Chase, T.N., Colburn, R.W. and Kopin, I.J. (1972) L-dopa in parkinsonism: a possible mechanism of action. *Neurology*, 22: 688–696.

Nomoto, M. and Fukuda, T. (1993) A selective MAO B inhibitor Ro19-6327 potentiates the effects of levodopa on parkinsonism induced by MPTP in the common marmoset. *Neuropharmacology*, 32: 473–477.

Norton, W.T., Aquino, D.A., Hozumi, I., Chiu, F.C., and Brosnan, C.F (1992) Quantitative aspects of reactive gliosis: a review. *Neurochem. Res.*, 17: 877–885.

Olson, L., Henschen, A., Eriksdotter-Nilsson, M., Stromberg, E. Wetmore, C., Ernfors, P., Friedman, W., Persson, H. and Ebendal, T. (1990) The expanding role of nerve growth factor in the central nervous system. In: V. Sara (ed.), *Growth Factors: From Genes to Clinical Application*, Raven Press, New York, pp. 167–177.

Palmer, A.M. and DeKosly, S.T. (1993) Monoamine neurons in aging and Alzheimer's disease. *J. Neural. Transm.*, 91: 135–139.

Paterson, I.A., Juorio, A.V., Berry, M.D. and Zhu, M.Y. (1991) Inhibition of monoamine oxidase-B by (−)-deprenyl potentiates neuronal responses to dopamine agonists but not inhibit dopamine catabolism in the rat striatum. *J. Pharmacol. Exp. Ther.*, 258: 1019–1026.

Paterson, I.A., Juorio, A.V. and Boulton, A.A. (1990) 2-Phenylethylamine: a modulator of catecholamine transmission in the central nervous system? *J. Neurochem.*, 55: 1827–1837.

Philips, S.R. and Boulton, A.A. (1979) The effect of monoamine oxidases on some arylalkylamines in rat striatum. *J. Neurochem.*, 33: 159–167.

Phillips, H.S., Hains, J.M., Armanini, M., Laramee, G.R., Johnson, S. A. and Winslow, J.W. (1991) BDNF mRNA is decreased in the hippocampus of individuals with Alzheimer's disease. *Neuron*, 7: 695–702.

Reisberg, B. (1983) An overview of current concepts of Alzheimer's disease, senile dementia, and age-associated cognitive decline. In: B. Reisberg (Ed.), *Alzheimer's Dis-*

ease, The Standard Reference, Free Press, New York, pp. 6–9.

Ricci, A., Mancini, M., Strocchi, P., Bongrani, S. and Bronzetti, E. (1992) Deficits in cholinergic neurotransmission markers induced by ethylcholine mustard aziridinium (AF64A) in the rat hippocampus: sensitivity to treatment with the monoamine oxidase-B inhibitor l-deprenyl. *Drugs Exp. Clin. Res.*, 18: 163–171.

Riederer P, Youdim, M.B. and Rausch, W.D. (1978) On the mode of action of L-deprenyl in the human central nervous system. *J. Neural Transm.*, 43: 217–226.

Rinne, U.K. (1983) Deprenyl (selegiline) in the treatment of Parkinson's disease. *Acta Neurol. Scand.*, 95 (suppl.): 107–111.

Robins, E., Robins, J.M., Croninger, A.B., Moses, S.G., Spencer, J. and Hudgens, R.W. (1967) The low level of 5-HTP decarboxylase in human brain. *Biochem. Med.*, 1: 240–251.

Robinson, D.S., Campbell, I.C., Walker, M., Statham, N., Lovenberg, W. and Murphy, D.L. (1979) Effect of chronic monoamine oxidase inhibitor treatment on biogenic amine metabolism in rat brain. *Neuropharmacology*, 18: 771–776.

Rossetti, Z.L., Silvia, C.P., Krajnc, D., Neff, N.H. and Hadji-constantinou, M. (1990) Aromatic l-amino acid decarboxylase is modulated by D1 dopamine receptors in rat retina. *J. Neurochem.*, 54: 787–791.

Salo, P.T. and Tatton, W.G. (1992) Deprenyl reduces the death of motoneurons caused by axotomy *J. Neurosci. Res.*, 31: 394–400.

Schnaitman, C., Erwin, V.G. and Greenawalt, J.W. (1967). The submitocondrial localization of monoamine oxidase: an enzymatic marker for the outer membrane of rat liver mitocondria. *J. Cell Biol.*, 32: 719–735.

Sendtner, M., Schmalbruch, H., Stockli, K.A., Carroll, P., Kreutzberg, G. W. and Thoenen, H. (1992) Ciliary neurotrophic factor prevents degeneration of moter neurons in mouse mutant progressive motor neuronopathy. *Nature*, 358: 502–504.

Shinoda, I., Furukawa, Y. and Furukawa, S. (1990) Stimulation of nerve growth factor synthesis/secretion by propento-fylline in cultured mouse astroglial cells. *Biochem. Pharmacol.*, 39: 1813–1816.

Skibo G, Ahmed, I., Yu, P., Boulton, A.A. and Fedoroff, S. (1992) l-Deprenyl, a monoamine oxidase-B inhibitor acts on the astroglia cell cycle at the G1/G0 boundary. *Abstr. Annu. Meet. Am. Soc. Cell Biol.*

Sumi-Ichinose, C., Ichinose, H., Takahashi, E., Hori, T. and Nagatsu, T. (1992) Molecular cloning of genomic DNA and chromosomal assignment of the gene for human aromatic L-amino acid decarboxylase, the enzyme for catecholamine and serotonin synthesis. *Biochemistry*, 31: 2229–2238.

Sunderland, T., Tariot, P.N., Cohen, R.M., Newhouse, P.A., Mellow, A. M., Mueller, E.A. and Murphy, D.L. (1987)

Dose-dependent effects of deprenyl on CSF monoamine metabolites in patients with Alzheimer's disease. *Psychopharmacology*, 91: 293–296.

Takeuchi, R., Murase, K., Furukawa, Y., Furukawa, S. and Hayashi, K. (1990) Stimulation of nerve growth factor synthesis/secretion by 1,4-benzoquinone and its derivatives in cultured mouse astroglial cells. *FEBS. Lett.*, 12: 63–66.

Tanaka, T., Horio, Y., Taketoshi, M., Imamura, I., Ando-Yamamoto, M., Kangawa, K., Matsuo, H., Kuroda, M. and Waka, H. (1989) Molecular cloning and sequencing of a cDNA of rat dopa decarboxylase, partial amino acid homologies with other enzymes synthesizing catecholamines. *Proc. Natl. Acad. Sci. USA*, 86: 8142–8146.

Tardy, M., Fages, C., Riol, H., LePrince, G., Rataboul, P., Charriere-Bertrand, C. and Nunez, J. (1989) Developmental expression of the glial fibrillary acidic protein mRNA in the central nervous system and in cultured astrocytes. *J. Neurochem.*, 52: 162–167.

Tariot, P.N., Sunderland, T., Weingartner, H., Murphy, D.L., Welkowitz, J.A., Thompson, K. and Cohen, R.M. (1987) Cognitive effects of l-deprenyl in Alzheimer's disease. *Psychopharmacology*, 91: 489–495.

Tatton, W.G. and Greenwood, C.E. (1991) Rescue of dying neurons, a new action for deprenyl in MPTP parkinsonism. *J. Neurosci. Res.*, 30: 666–672.

Tatton, W.G., Ju, W.Y.L., Holland, D.P., Tai, C. and Kwan, M. (1994) (−)-Deprenyl Reduceds PC12 cell apoptosis by inducing new protein synthesis. *J Neurochem*, 63: 1572–1575.

Tetrud, J.W. and Langston, J.W. (1989) The effect of deprenyl (selegiline) on the natural history of Parkinson's disease. *Science*, 245: 519–522.

The Parkinson Study Group (1989) Effect of deprenyl on the progression of disability in early Parkinson's disease. *N. Engl. J. Med.*, 321: 1364–1371.

The Parkinson Study Group (1993) Effect of tocopherol and deprenyl on the progression of disability in early Parkinson's disease. *N. Engl. J. Med.*, 328: 176–183.

Thoenen, H. and Barde Y.-A. (1980) Physiology of nerve growth factor. *Physiol. Rev.*, 60: 1285–1335.

Tipton, K. (1973) Biochemical aspects of monoamine oxidase. *Br. Med. Bull.*, 29: 116–119.

Toso, R., De Bernardi, M., Brooker, G., Costa, E. and Mocchetti, (1988) Beta adrenergic and prostaglandin receptor activation increases nerve growth factor mRNA content in C6–2B rat astrocytoma cells. *J. Pharmacol. Exp. Ther.*, 246: 1190–1193.

Vrana, S.L., Azzaro, A.J. and Vrana, R.E. (1992) Chronic selegiline trasiently decreases tyrosine hydroxylase activity and mRNA in the rat nigrostriatal pathway. *Mol. Pharmacol.*, 41: 839–844.

Varon, S. and Bunge, R.P. (1978) Trophic mechanisms in the peripheral nervous system. *Annu. Rev. Neurosci.*, 1: 327–361.

Whittemore, S.W. and Seiger, A. (1987) The expression, localization and functional significance of b-nerve growth factor in the central nervous system. *Brain Res. Rev.*, 12: 439–464.

Youdim, B.M. H. (1978) The active centres of monoamine oxidase types 'A' and 'B': binding with (14C)-clorgyline and (14C)-deprenyl. *J. Neural Transm.*, 43: 199–208.

Youdim, B.M. H., Heldman, E., Pollard, H.B., Fleming, P. and McHugh, E. (1986) Contrasting monoamine oxidase activity and tyramine induced catecholamine release in PC 12 and chromaffin cells. *Neuroscience*, 19: 1311–1318.

Young, E.A., Neff, N.H. and Hadjiconstantinou, M. (1993) Evidence for cyclic AMP-mediated increase of aromatic L-amino acid activity in the striatum and midbrain. *J. Neurochem.*, 60: 2331–2333.

Yu, P.H., Davis, B.A. and Boulton, A.A. (1992) Aliphatic propargylamines: potent, selective irreversible monoamine oxidase B inhibitors. *J. Med. Chem.*, 35: 3705–3713.

Yu, P.H., Davis, B.A. Fang, J. and Boulton, A.A. (1994a) Neuroprotective effects of some MAOIs against DSP-4 induced NA depletion iin the mouse hioppocampus. *J. Neurochem.*, 63: 1820–1828.

Yu, P.H., Davis, B.A. Durden, D.A., Barber, A., Terleckyj, I., Nicklas, W.G. and Boulton, A.A. (1994b) Neurochemical and neuroprotective effects of some aliphatic propargylamines: new selective non-amphetamine-like MAO B inhibitors. *J. Neurochem.*, 62: 697–704.

Zhu, M.Y., Juorio, A.V., Paterson, I.A. and Boulton, A.A. (1992) Regulation of aromatic l-amino acid decarboxylase by dopamine receptors in the rat brain. *J. Neurochem.*, 58: 636–641.

Zhu, M.-Y., Juorio, A.V., Paterson, I.A. & Boulton, A.A. (1994) Regulation of aromatic L-amino acid decarboxylase in rat striatal synaptosomes: Effects of dopamine receptor agonists and antagonists. *Br. J. Pharmacol.*, 112: 23–30.

Zsilla, G., Földi, P., Held, G., Székely, A.M. and Knoll, J. (1986) The effect of repeated doses of repeated doses of (−) deprenyl on the dynamics of monoaminergic transmission. Comparison with clorgyline. *Pol. J. Pharmacol. Pharm.*, 38: 57–67.

Peter M. Yu, Keith F. Tipton and Alan A. Boulton (Eds.)
Progress in Brain Research, Vol 106
© 1995 Elsevier Science BV. All rights reserved.

CHAPTER 12

Neurochemical, neuroprotective and neurorescue effects of aliphatic *N*-methylpropargylamines; new MAO-B inhibitors without amphetamine-like properties

P.H. Yu, B.A. Davis, X. Zhang, D.M. Zuo, J. Fang, C.T. Lai, X.M. Li, I.A. Paterson and A.A. Boulton

Neuropsychiatry Research Unit, Department of Psychiatry, University of Saskatchewan, Saskatoon, Saskatchewan,
S7N 5E4 Canada

Introduction

$R(-)$-Deprenyl (selegiline, Eldepryl), the archetypical MAO-B inhibitor, has been shown to be useful in the treatment of Parkinson's and Alzheimer's diseases (PD and AD, respectively). It was first used as an adjunct drug to potentiate L-DOPA in the treatment of PD (i.e. to reduce the oxidation of dopamine) (Birkmayer et al., 1983). The drug reduces the requirement for L-DOPA and thus decreases related side effects. The problem with L-DOPA chemotherapy, however, is that its efficacy lasts for only a limited period and its side-effects gradually become intolerable. $R(-)$-Deprenyl has been shown to be capable of prolonging the efficacy of L-DOPA in the more advanced stages of treatment (i.e. it eases the "on-off" effect) (Lieberman and Fazzini, 1991). The treatment of PD with L-DOPA seems to be mostly symptomatic; it does not appear to cure or prevent the progression of the illness. Dopamine neurons continue to die.

$R(-)$-Deprenyl can, by itself, significantly delay the onset of disability associated with early, otherwise untreated, cases of PD (The Parkinson Study Group, 1989, 1993). These findings have been confirmed in several centres around the world (Tetrud and Langston, 1989; Allain et al., 1991). $R(-)$-Deprenyl has also been claimed to improve the clinical condition of some Alzheimer's patients (Mangoni et al., 1991; Tariot et al., 1987). In addition $R(-)$-deprenyl has been claimed to prolong the life span and improve the sexual activity of rodents (Knoll et al., 1989) and perhaps humans (Birkmayer et al., 1985). Unlike MAO-A inhibitors, MAO-B inhibitors do not usually cause hypertensive crises, and thus they possess the potential to become useful neuropsychiatric and geriatric drugs. $R(-)$-Deprenyl probably possesses other effects in addition to its ability to potentiate dopamine function. It has been shown that $R(-)$-deprenyl can protect against neurotoxins, such as MPTP (Heikkila et al., 1984) and DSP-4 (Finnegan et al., 1990; Yu et al., 1994a,b), when the drug is administered before the insult. It can even rescue nerve cells that have been damaged by neurotoxins or axotomy, when administered after the insult (Tatton and Greenwood 1991; Salo and Tatton, 1991). The mechanism(s) of this neurorescue effect is, however, not yet established.

MPTP is a neurotoxin that can damage the nigro-striatal nerve pathway and induce PD symptoms in humans (Langston et al., 1983) and primates (Langston et al., 1984; Burn et al., 1984). The neuronal damage is responsive to L-DOPA treatment (Davis et al., 1979). $R(-)$-Deprenyl, as well as other MAO inhibitors, has been shown to be capable of preventing MPTP-induced Parkinson-like neurotoxicity in animals (Heikkila et al., 1984). MPTP itself is not directly involved in the toxic action; in the brain, MPTP is converted to the distal toxin MPP^+ by MAO-B in glial cells (Chiba et al., 1984), wwhere it is taken up by neurons with subsequent interference in the respiratory chain in mitochondria resulting in cell death (Ramsay et al., 1991). It has been suggested that PD might be caused by MPTP-like substances existing in the environment which might be ingested or absorbed by PD patients (Snyder and D'Amato, 1986); alternatively, it has been suggested that such neurotoxins might be formed endogenously. Several compounds, such as N-methylated tetrahydroisoquinolines, have been proposed as candidates (Ohta et al., 1987; Naoi et al., 1993). Blocking MAO-B activity therefore prevents such neurotoxic action. Recently it has been shown that some of the metabolites of $R(-)$-deprenyl are themselves capable of protecting against the neuronal damage induced by MPP^+, 6-hydroxydopamine and DSP-4 (Sziráki et al., 1994; Ahoda et al., 1994).

$R(-)$-Deprenyl also exhibits neuroprotective effects against another neurotoxin, namely DSP-4, which causes the depletion of noradrenaline in the nerve terminals of the hippocampus (Finnegan et al., 1990). Unlike MPTP, DSP-4 is not metabolized by MAO-B. It has been claimed that $R(-)$-deprenyl competes with DSP-4 for noradrenergic uptake sites and that this could be the mechanism of protection against the neurotoxic damage caused by this particular neurotoxin.

It has also been proposed that MAO-catalyzed deamination reactions can enhance oxidative stress and that the resultant free radicals may cause damage to nerve cells (Cohn and Spina, 1989). Such oxidations lead to the production of hydrogen peroxide, and this in turn can be converted into the hazardous hydroxyl free radical in the presence of ferrous ions. Inhibition of MAO activity would thus reduce this oxidative stress and slow down any associated damage. It is also possible that $R(-)$-deprenyl may reduce oxidative stress via other, yet to be identified, mechanisms (Chiueh et al., 1994).

It has been proposed that neurotrophic factors may be stimulated by $R(-)$-deprenyl. Recent evidence shows that $R(-)$-deprenyl may be involved in the regulation of the cell cycle where it might prevent the senescence of astroglial cells; these cells may provide trophic support to nerve cells (Skibo et al., 1992). It has also been shown that MAO-B inhibitors stimulate the gene expression of L-aromatic amino acid decarboxylase, an important enzyme involved in the synthesis of biogenic amines (Li et al., 1992); they also inhibit the expression of glial fibrillary acidic protein (GFAP) in C6 cells (Li et al., 1993).

Although $R(-)$-deprenyl "rescues" nerve cells under "stress", it only restores some of these cells. Is this action of $R(-)$-deprenyl unique? Are other MAO-B inhibitors also capable of regulating neuronal survival? Since these neuroprotective and rescue effects are unrelated to the inhibition of MAO-B activity, what mechanisms might be involved? In order to answer these questions, it seems useful to investigate other MAO-B inhibitors along with $R(-)$-deprenyl in neuroprotection and neurorescue paradigms. We have recently synthesized a series of aliphatic N-propargylamine compounds, e.g. N-(2-heptyl)-N-methylpropargylamine (2-HMP), N-(2-hexyl)-N-methylpropargylamine (2-HxMP) and N-methyl-N-(2-pentyl)-propargylamine (M-2-PP). Some of these compounds are highly potent and selective MAO-B inhibitors (Yu et al., 1993). They also protect nerve cells against MPTP- and DSP-4-induced damage, as well as exhibiting neuroprotective and neurorescue effects in several in vitro and in vivo paradigms.

Deamination of aliphatic amines by MAO-B

MAO-B has been shown to be involved in the metabolism of the anti-epileptic prodrug, 2-(n-pentyl)-aminoacetamide (Milacemide) (De Varebeke et al., 1988). Milacemide can cross the blood–brain barrier, where it is oxidized by MAO-B to form glycinamide, which is subsequently cleaved to glycine. We have recently shown that 2-propylpentylamine (2-propyl-1-aminopentane) and 2-propylpentylglycinamide can similarly be deaminated by rat liver MAO-B, where they are then converted to 2-propylpentaldehyde and valproic acid (VPA) (Yu and Davis, 1991a,b) both in vitro and in vivo. It is interesting that MAO-B can catalyze these atypical aliphatic substrates. Aliphatic monoamines are metabolized by MAO-B (Yu, 1989) and the straight-chain aliphatic amines with carbon numbers between 5 and 10 exhibit very high affinity for MAO-B. We have taken advantage of this high affinity to design and synthesize the aliphatic propargyl MAO-B inhibitors.

Aliphatic propargylamines as MAO-B inhibitors

$R(-)$-Deprenyl, a structural analogue of amphetamine, is catabolized to produce $R(-)$-desmethyldeprenyl, $R(-)$-methamphetamine and $R(-)$-amphetamine (Heinonen et al., 1989); this has caused some concern, since its amphetamine-like properties might be associated with its clinical efficacy, although it is a fact that the $R(-)$-enantiomer of deprenyl and its corresponding metabolites are behaviorally much less active than the the $S(+)$-enantiomers. In order to understand the action(s) of $R(-)$-deprenyl, other types of MAO-B inhibitor, i.e. those not possessing an amphetamine moiety or amphetamine-like properties, should be assessed (Langston, 1990). The structural and functional relationships of a number of racemic aliphatic N-methylpropargylamines have been elucidated (Yu et al., 1993). $(\pm)$-N-2-Hexyl-N-methylpropargylamine (2-HxMP) and $(\pm)$-N-2-pentyl-N-methylpropargylamine (M-2-PP), for example, are highly potent, selective and irreversible MAO-B inhibitors. MAO-inhibitory activity appears to be correlated with the lipophilicity of the compounds. The length of the carbon chain of the N-alkyl group is not only related to the inhibitory potency, but it also affects the relative selectivity towards MAO-A and MAO-B. The MAO-B inhibitory activity of these compounds is stereospecific; for example, the $R(-)$ stereoisomers of N-2-butyl-N-methylpropargylamine (2-BuMP), M-2-PP, 2-HxMP and N-2-butyl-N-methylpropargylamine (2-HMP) are estimated to be 20–100-fold more potent than their corresponding $S(+)$ enantiomers. Such a finding of differential enantiomer potency is consistent with the stereospecific effects exhibited by $R(-)$- and $S(+)$-deprenyl (Robinson, 1985).

Aliphatic propargylamines with intermediate carbon chain lengths appear to be more potent than their longer-chain analogs in the inhibition of brain MAO-B activity (i.e. as assessed from their ED_{50} values) following intraperitoneal administration. These shorter-chain-length molecules are more easily absorbed and/or more readily transported into the brain. Members of the series with longer carbon chain lengths are more lipophillic and very potent in vitro, but less effective in inhibiting brain MAO-B activity in vivo; this is probably related to their lipophillic interactions before entering or within the brain. $(\pm)$-2-HxMP and $(\pm)$-M-2-PP following oral administration were found to be 5-fold more potent than $R(-)$-deprenyl at blocking brain MAO-B activity. It is also interesting to note that the aliphatic propargylamines, such as M-2-PP, are considerably more stable in aqueous solution than is $R(-)$-deprenyl.

A series of substituted N-alkylpropargylamines, using N-2-butyl-N-methylpropargylamine (2-BuMP) as the model compound, have been synthesized and the relationship of structural modification on effectiveness and selectivity in the inhibition towards MAO activities investigated. When the N-methyl group was replaced by a hydrogen atom, an ethyl group or a propargyl group, MAO inhibitory activity was reduced. Modification of the propargyl group, e.g. to 3-butynyl, N-cyanomethyl or to allyl, destroyed the inhibitory activity. The potency of the inhibitors was related to the carbon chain length of the alkyl group as well as to the substitution of the alpha or terminal carbon atoms of the aliphatic group. Substitution with hydroxyl, carboxyl or carboethoxyl groups on the terminal carbon of the alkyl chain also considerably reduced the inhibitory activity. An increase in MAO-inhibitory activity was observed for those molecules posssessing a single methyl group substitution on the alpha carbon in comparison to those substituted with two hydrogens or two methyl groups. Other branched alkyl N-methylpropargylamines, e.g. N-methyl-N-(3-pentyl)propargylamine, appear to be slightly less selective in their MAO-B inhibitory activity (Yu et al., 1993).

At a dose of 2 mg/kg, M-2-PP selectively inhibited MAO-B activity in mice. After daily treatments for 10 or 21 days an increased inhibition of MAO-B was observed, but by these times MAO-A had also become slightly inhibited. Treatment with 2-HxMP or M-2-PP at a lower dose (0.25 mg/kg, i.p.) was without obvious effect on either MAO-A or MAO-B in the brain 24 h following a single i.p. injection; after 13 days of daily treatments, however, the MAO-B activity was inhibited. At lower oral doses (i.e. 1 and 10 μg/ml in drinking water), selective inhibition of MAO-B activity was also achieved, but at higher doses (i.e. 100 μg/ml), MAO-A also became inhibited following 3 weeks of treatment. This chronic treatment could clearly be the result of an accumulative inhibitory effect on MAOs. A prolonged inhibition in MAO-B activity following a single higher acute dose (2 mg/kg, i.p.) of several aliphatic propargylamines was observed, and this confirms that the inhibition of MAO-B by aliphatic propargylamines is, as with $R(-)$-deprenyl, also irreversible in vivo.

Neurochemical effects

($\pm$)-2-HxMP was without significant effect on levels of DA, NE or 5-HT in the caudate nucleus following an acute i.p. dose of up to 20 mg/kg. At doses above 10 mg/kg, however, some amine metabolites, such as DOPAC and HVA, became significantly reduced. There was little effect on 5-HIAA levels. Similar results have been obtained with respect to ($\pm$)-M-2-PP and ($\pm$)-N-(2-butyl)-N-methylpropargylamine.

The effects of ($\pm$)-M-2-PP, ($\pm$)-2-HxMP and $R(-)$-deprenyl on trace amines in the mouse caudate have also been assessed. β-Phenylethylamine (a typical MAO-B substrate) levels were increased substantially by these MAO-B inhibitors even at doses as low as 0.5 mg/kg. Both the above compounds were more potent than $R(-)$-deprenyl in causing an increase of β-phenylethylamine levels. Levels of p-tyramine, which is a mixed-type substrate for MAO, were only slightly increased when higher doses (i.e. 20 mg/kg) of the inhibitors were used. Similar results were observed with respect to the effects on m-tyramine. Chronic treatment with ($\pm$)-M-2-PP and $R(-)$-deprenyl (i.e. daily p.o. administration) caused a selective inhibition of mouse brain MAO-B activity and a significant increase in DA and 3-MT levels in the mouse striatum. The aliphatic N-propargylamines were without any effect on the uptake of dopamine and noradrenaline (Fang and Yu, 1994; Yu et al., 1994b).

Neuroprotective and neurorescue effects

Several aliphatic N-methylpropargylamines, when given before the toxin, have been shown to be capable of preventing the depletion of striatal dopamine indduced by MPTP (Yu et al., 1994a) as well as the depletion of noradrenaline in the hippocampus of CD1 Swiss white mice as caused by DSP-4 (Yu et al., 1994b). The observed neuroprotective effect against MPTP is not surprising, since these compounds are quite potent MAO-B inhibitors (Yu et al., 1992). The neuroprotective effect of aliphatic N-propargylamines against DSP-4 neurotoxin, however, is quite interesting, since its action is unrelated to the inhibition of MAO activity or to the uptake of the toxin into the hippocampus (Yu et al., 1994b).

These neuroprotective effects of ($\pm$)-2-HxMP in the DSP-4 model have been confirmed by morphological examinations (Zhang et al., unpublished observation). NA fibres have been visualized immunohistochemically using an antibody to dopamine-β-hydroxylase (DBH) followed by the

TABLE 1

The effects of $R(-)$-deprenyl and $(\pm)$2-HxMP on DSP-4-induced depletion of DBH-positive axons in rat hippocampus and cortex

	Relative survival of DBH-positive axons	
	Cortex	Hippocampus
Saline	100 ± 5	100 ± 3
DSP-4	$12 \pm 2*$	$8 \pm 1*$
$(\pm)$2-HxMP + DSP-4	85 ± 5	85 ± 3
$R(-)$-Deprenyl + DSP-4	66 ± 8	95 ± 7

$* P < 0.01$ compared to controls.

assessment of stain density using a computer-assisted image analysis method (see Table 1).

Noradrenergic neurons in the locus coeruleus die slowly following destruction of hippocampal noradrenergic nerve terminals by a single administration of DSP-4. About 90% of the axon and nerve terminals were depleted within a short period (i.e. within 7 days) but only approx, 30 % of the DβH-positive neurons (cell bodies of noradrenergic neurons) were dead 3 months later (Table 2). A single dose of both $(\pm)$-2-HxMP and $R(-)$-deprenyl (administered 1 h before DSP-4) (i.e. a neuroprotective effect) is capable of pro-

TABLE 2

Effects of $R(-)$-deprenyl and $(\pm)$-2-HxMP on DSP-4-induced loss of locus coeruleus neurons

	LC cell numbers 3 months after DSP-4 treatment
Saline	2230 ± 89
DSP-4 (50 mg/kg)	$1482 \pm 39*$
$(\pm)$2-HxMP (10 mg/kg) + DSP-4	2011 ± 91
$R(-)$-Deprenyl (10 mg/kg) + DSP-4	1981 ± 95

$*P < 0.05$ compared to controls; drugs administered 1 h before toxin and three additional daily doses thereafter.

tecting against the death of noradrenergic neurons in the rat locus coeruleus (Zhang et al., 1995b).

In addition to neuroprotection several aliphatic propargylamines also exhibit a neurorescue effect against DSP-4-induced damage to the noradrenergic system. We have previously shown that $(\pm)$-2-HxMP given 1 h before DSP-4 protects noradrenergic nerve terminals and axons from depletion of NA. Three additional daily doses of the drugs, administered after the toxin (i.e a maximal neuroprotective/rescue effect) significantly increased the survival of hippocampal noradrenergic axons. When $(\pm)$-N-(2-heptyl)-N-methylpropargylamine $((\pm)$-2-HMP) was administered 30 min after DSP-4 treatment followed by three further additional daily treatments (i.e. a "neurorescue" effect), a further sparing of hippocampal NE was observed. Interestingly the "rescue" effect seems to be stereospecific; i.e. $R(-)$ form is more potent than $S(-)$ form), while the "protective" effect is clearly stereo-nonspecific (Table 3).

We have also shown that DSP-4 treatment depletes nitric oxide synthase (NOS) containing neurons in the dentate gyrus. $(\pm)$-2-HxMP (10 mg/kg, i.p.) given 1 h before DSP-4 protects these neurons as shown in Table 4.

$(-)$-2-HMP, $(\pm)$-2-HxMP and $(\pm)$-M-2-PP at low dose (0.25 mg/kg, s.c.) have been shown to be capable of rescuing damaged neurons in the hippocampal CA1 region following transient global ischemia (Davis et al., 1995). $R(-)$-2-HxMP (0.25 mg/kg, s.c.) has also been shown to be capable of rescuing mouse hippocampal neurons following damage caused by a single peripheral injection of the neurotoxin kainic acid (10 mg/kg) in the mouse (Davis et al., 1995). Zhang et al. (1995a) have also shown rescue of hippocampal neurons following a single injection of kainic acid in rats. Kainic acid induces the production of heat-shock protein 70 kDa (HSP70), which is known to be a marker for cells responding to stress caused by a chemical or physical insult. Interestingly, $R(-)$-2-HxMP and, to a lesser extent, $S(+)$-2-HxMP effectively block the kainate-induced expression

118

TABLE 3

Stereospecific neuroprotective and neurorescue effects of aliphatic ($\pm$)-2-HMP against DSP-4 (50 mg/kg, i.p.)

	Neurorescue (%)	Neuroprotection (%)
$R(-)$-2-HMP	48 ± 13	79 ± 5
$S(+)$-2-HMP	23 ± 2	86 ± 10

The percent of rescue or protection is based on the restoration of hippocampal NE levels; for details of method see Yu et al. (1994b).

of HSP70 in rat hippocampal and other tissues (Zhang et al., 1995a).

$R(-)$-Deprenyl has been shown to rescue motoneurons in 14-day-old mice following axotomy of their facial nerve (Ansari et al., 1993a). ($\pm$)-2-HxMP exhibited a similar effect in this model (Ansari et al., 1993b). $R(-)$-Deprenyl, several aliphatic propargylamines and some other irreversible MAO-B inhibitors, but not MAO-A or reversible inhibitors, have been shown to enhance gene expression of AADC (aromatic L-amino acid decarboxylase) mRNA in PC12 cells and to reduce of GFAP mRNA expression in C6 glioma cells (Li et al., 1993 and personal communication). Such an enhancement of the expression of mRNA of AADC has been proposed to provide an alter-

TABLE 4

Effects of DSP-4, $R(-)$-deprenyl and ($\pm$)-2-HxMP on NOS-positive neurons in the rat dentate gyrus

	Cell numbers of NOS-positive neurons in dentate gyrus
Saline	360 ± 7
DSP-4 (50 mg/kg)	4 ± 3*
($\pm$)2-HxMP (10 mg/kg) + DSP-4	321 ± 16
$R(-)$-Deprenyl (10 mg/kg) + DSP-4	317 ± 16

* $P < 0.01$ compared to controls.

native mechanism with respect to $R(-)$-deprenyl's action in the treatment of Parkinson's disease (Li et al., 1992).

Miscellaneous effects

Aliphatic propargylamines do not exhibit any apparent toxicity. The LD_{50} for ($\pm$)-2-HxMP towards adult mice, for example, is estimated to be about 800 mg/kg, p.o., which is somewhat better than $R(-)$-deprenyl. The doses applied in many of the above-described neuroprotection or neurorescue models were considerably lower, i.e. 0.25 mg/kg. We have administered $R(-)$-deprenyl and ($\pm$)-M-2-PP chronically to old mice in their drinking water (10 μg/ml) for 37 weeks and shown a selective inhibition of brain MAO-B activity. In this experiment $R(-)$-deprenyl, but not ($\pm$)-M-2-PP, reduced the body weight of the animals (Barber et al., 1993). ($\pm$)-M-2-PP exhibited no apparent toxicity in this chronic study.

We have also observed that $R(-)$-deprenyl can potentiate dopamine-induced neurotoxic effects towards neuroblastoma cells (SH-SY5Y), while the aliphatic propargylamines do not (Lai and Yu, 1994). This seems to be consistent with a recent report that $R(-)$-deprenyl can potentiate p-chloroamphetamine-induced neurotoxicity (Benmansour and Brunswick, 1994), although the mechanism for this is unclear.

Conclusion

The $R(-)$-enantiomers of aliphatic N-propargylamines, such as 2-HMP, 2-HxMP and M-2-PP, are highly potent, irreversible and selective MAO-B inhibitors both in vitro and in vivo. The corresponding $S(+)$-enantiomers are approx. 20–100-fold less potent. Although these compounds exhibit properties similar to those of $R(-)$-deprenyl with respect to the inhibition of MAO-B activity, neuroprotection and neurorescue, they do not possess any amphetamine moiety within their structure, nor do they exhibit any amphetaminergic behavioural properties. They are able to protect nigrostriatal dopamine neurons and hippocampal noradrenaline nerve terminals against MPTP- and DSP-4-induced depletions of DA and NE, respectively. They exert a neurorescue effect toward motoneurons following facial axotomy and are capable of rescuing neurons damaged by an ischaemia insult or by the neurotoxin kainic acid. They may become useful in the treatment of some neurodegenerative disorders.

Summary

A series of aliphatic N-methylpropargylamine MAO-B inhibitors have been synthesized and their structural and functional relationships have been investigated. 2-Hexyl-N-methylpropargylamine (2-HxMP), for example, has been found to be a highly potent, irreversible, selective, MAO-B inhibitor both in vitro and *in vivo*. The R-($-$)-enantiomers are much more active than the S-($+$)-enantiomers at inhibiting MAO-B activity. Some of these compounds protect mouse nigrostriatal dopamine neurons against the neurotoxin MPTP and the mouse hippocampal noradrenergic system against the neurotoxin N-(2-chloroethyl)-N-ethyl-2-bromobenzylamine (DSP-4). They rescue hippocampal neurons after damage induced by ischemia and kainic acid treatment, as well as motoneurons in young mice following facial nerve axotomy. Such rescue effects are, interestingly, unrelated to inhibition of MAO-B activity. Some of the aliphatic propargylamines enhance the survival of neuroblastoma cells co-cultured with astrocytes following serum depletion. They stimulate the expression of AADC mRNA and inhibit GFAP mRNA expression. They do not possess amphetamine-like properties and exhibit no effect on noradrenaline or dopamine uptake nor do they increase hypertensive effects in the tyramine pressor test. Unlike R($-$)-deprenyl, 2-HxMP does not potentiate dopamine toxicity in vitro. These new MAO-B inhibitors may possess significant chemotherapeutic implications for certain psychiatric and neurodegenerative disorders.

References

Ahoda, T., Haapalinna, A., Heinonen, E., Suhonen, J. and Hervonen, A. (1994) 6-OHDA neurotoxicity is prevented by selegiline and its metabolites. *24th Am. Soc. Neurosci. Meet. Abstr.*, 20: 674.2.

Allain, H., Cougnard, J., Neukirch, H.C., the FMST members. (1991) Selegiline in de novo Parkinsonian patients: The French selegiline multicenter trial (FSMT). *Acta Neurol. Scand. 84 (Suppl.)*, 136: 73–78.

Ansari, K.S., Tatton, W.G., Yu, P.H. and Kruck, T.X. (1993a) Death of axotomized immature rat facial motoneurons: Stereospecificity of deprenyl-induced rescue. *J. Neurosci.*, 13: 4042–4053.

Ansari, K.S., Zhang, F., Holland, D.P., Yu, P.H. and Tatton, W.G. (1993b) R($-$)-Deprenyl, not its major metabolites, rescues axotomized immature rat facial motoneurons. 23rd Am. Soc. Neurosci. Meeting, Washington, USA.

Barber, A.J., Yu, P.H. and Boulton, A.A. (1993) Chronic monoamine oxidase-B inhibition in aged mice: a behavioral and biochemical assessment. *Life Sci.*, 53: 739–747.

Benmansour, S. and Brunswick, D.J. (1994) The MAO-B inhibitor deprenyl, but not the MAO-A inhibitor clorgyline, potentiates the neurotoxicity of p-chloroamphetamine. *Brain Res.*, 650: 305–312.

Birkmayer, W., Knoll, J., Riederer, P., Hars, V. and Marton, J. (1985) Increased life expectancy resulting from addition of R($-$)-deprenyl to Madopar treatment in Parkinson's disease: A long term study. *J. Neural Transm.*, 64: 113–127.

Birkmayer, W., Knoll, J., Riederer, P. and Youdim, M.B.H. (1983) (-)-Deprenyl leads to prolongation of l-Dopa efficacy in Parkinson's disease. *Mod. Pbl. Pharmacopsychiatr.*, 19: 170–176.

Burn, R.S., Chiueh, C.C., Markey, S.P., Ebert, M.H., Jacobowitz, D.M. and Kopin, I.J. (1983) A primate model of Parkinsonism: selective destruction of dopaminergic neurons in the pars compacta of the substantia nigra by N-methyl-4-phenyl-1,2,3,6-tetrahydropyridine. *Proc. Natl. Acad. Sci. USA*, 80: 4546–4550.

Chiba, K., Trevor, A. and Castagnoli, N. Jr. (1984) Metabolism of the neurotoxic tertiary amine, MPTP, by brain monoamine oxidase. *Biochem. Biophys. Res. Commun.*, 120: 574–578.

Chiueh, C.C., Huang, S.J. and Murphy, D.L. (1994) Suppression of hydroxyl radical formation by MAO inhibitors: a novel possible neruoprotective mechanism in dopaminergic neurotoxicity. *J. Neural Transm.* 41(Suppl.): 189–196.

Cohn, G. and Spina, M.B. (1989) Deprenyl suppresses the oxidant stress associated with increased dopamine turnover. *Am. Neurol.*, 26: 689–690.

Davis, G.C., Williams, A.C., Markey, S.P., Evert, M.H., Caine, E.D., Reichert, C.M. and Kopin, I.J. (1979) Chronic Parkinsonism secondary to intravenous injection of meperidine analogues. *Psychiat. Res.*, 1: 249–254.

Davis, B.A., Yu, P.H., Paterson, I.A., Li, X.M., Durden, D.A., Tatton, W.G. and Boulton, A.A. (1995) Neurorescue by the optically active enantiomers of some aliphatic methylpropargylamines. *Abstr, Proc. 26th Am. Neurochem. Soc. Meet.*

De Varebeke, P.J., Cavalier, R., David-Remacle, M. and Youdim, M.B.H. (1988) Formation of the neurotransmitter glycine from the anticonvulsant milacemide is mediated by brain monoamine oxidase-B. *J. Neurochem.*, 50: 1011–1016.

Fang, J. and Yu, P.H. (1994) Effect of l-deprenyl, its structural analogues and some monoamine oxidase inhibitors on dopamine uptake. *Neuropharmacology*, 33: 763–768.

Finnegan, K.T., Skratt, J.S., Irwin, I., DeLanney, L.E. and Langston, J.W. (1990) Protection against DSP-4-induced neurotoxicity by deprenyl is not related to its inhibition of MAO-B. *Eur. J. Pharmacol.*, 184: 119–126.

Heikkila, R.E., Hess, A. and Duvoisin, R.C. (1984) Dopaminergic neurotoxicity of l-methyl-4-phenyl-1,2,3,6-tetrahydropyridine in mice. *Science*, 224: 1451–1453.

Heinonen, E.H., Myllyla, V., Sotaniemi, K., Lammintausta, R., Salonen, J.S., Anttila, M., Savijarvi, M. and Rinne, U.K. (1989) Pharmacokinetics and metabolism of selegiline. *Acta Neurol. Scand.*, 126: 93–99.

Knoll, J., Dallo, J. and Yen, T.T. (1989) Striatal dopamine, sexual activity and life span longevity of rats treated with (−)-deprenyl. *Life Sci.*, 45: 525–531.

Lai, C.T. and Yu, P.H. (1994) Effect of antioxidants and L-deprenyl on cytotoxicities of dopamine and L-dopa in cultured dopamine neuroblastoma cells. *Abstr. 16th Annu. Meet. Canad. Coll. Neuro-Psychopharmacol.*, Quebec City, Canada.

Langston, J.W. (1990) Selegiline as neuroprotective therapy in Parkinson's disease: concepts and controversies. *Neurology*, 40(Suppl.): 61–66.

Langston, J.W., Ballard, P.A., Tetrud, J.W. and Irwin, I. (1983) Chronic parkinsonism in humans due to product of meperidine-analog synthesis. *Science*, 219: 979–980.

Langston, J.W., Forno, L.S., Rebert, C.S. and Irwin, I (1984) Selective nigral toxicity after systemic administration of 1-methyl-4-phenyl-1,2,3,6-tetrahydropyridine in the squirrel monkey. *Brain Res.*, 292: 390–394.

Li, X.M., Juorio, A.V., Paterson, I.A., Zhu, M.Y. and Boulton, A.A. (1992) Specific irreversible monoamine oxidase B inhibitors stimulate gene expression of aromatic l-amino acid decarboxylase in PC12 cells. *J. Neurochem.*, 59: 2324–2327.

Li, X.M., Qi, J., Juorio, A.V., and Boulton, A.A. (1993) Reduction in glial fibrillary acidic protein mRNA abundance induced by (−)-deprenyl and other monoamine oxidase B inhibitors in C6 glioma cells. *J. Neurochem.*, 61: 1573–1576.

Lieberman, A. and Fazzini, E. (1991): Experience with selegiline and levodopa in advanced Parkinson's disease. *Acta Neurol. Scand.* 84(Suppl.) 136: 66–69.

Mangoni, A., Grassi, M.P., Frattola, L., Piolti, R., Brassi, S., Motta, A., Marcone, A. and Smirne, S. (1991) Effects of a

MAO-B inhibitor in the treatment of Alzheimer disease. *Eur. Neurol.*, 31: 100–107.

Naoi, M., Dostert, P., Yoshida, M. and Nagatsu T. (1993) *N*-Methylated tetrahydroisoquinolines as dopaminergic neurotoxins. *Adv. Neurol.*, 60: 212–217.

Ohta, S., Kohno, M., Makino, Y., Tachikawa, O. and Hirobe, M. (1987) Tetrahydroisoquinoline and 1-methyltetrahydroisoquinoline are present in the human brain: relation to parkinson's disease. *Biomed. Res.*, 8: 453–456.

The Parkinson Study Group (1989) Effect of deprenyl on the progression of disability in early Parkinson's disease. *New Engl. J. Med.* 321: 1364–1371.

The Parkinson Study Group (1993) Effects of tocopherol and deprenyl on the progression of disability in early Parkinson's disease. *New Engl. J. Med.*, 328: 176–183.

Ramsay, R.R., Krueger, M.J., Youngster, S.K., and Singer, T.P. (1991) Evidence that the inhibition sites of the neurotoxic amine, 1-methyl-4-phenylpyridinium (MPP$^+$) and of the respiratory chain inhibitor, piericidin A, are the same. *Biochem. J.*, 273: 481–484.

Robinson, B.J. (1985) Stereo-selectivity and isozyme selectivity of monoamine oxidase inhibitors: enantiomers of amphetamine, *N*-methylamphetamine and deprenyl. *Biochem. Pharmacol.*, 34: 4105–4108.

Salo, P.T. and Tatton, W.G. (1991) Deprenyl reduces the death of motoneurons caused by axotomy. *J. Neurosci. Res.*, 31: 394–400.

Skibo, G., Ahmed, I., Yu, P.H., Boulton, A.A. and Fedoroff, S. (1992) l-Deprenyl, a monoamine oxidase-B (MAO-B) inhibitor, acts on the astroglia cell cycle at the G1/G0 boundary. *Am. Soc. Cell Biol.*, A13.

Snyder, S.H. and D'Amato, R.J. (1986) MPTP: a neurotoxin relevant to the pathophysiology of Parkinson's disease. *Neurology*, 36: 250–258.

Sziráki, I., Kardos, V., Patthy, M., Pátfalusi, M., Gáal, J., Solti, M. and Tömösközi, Z.S. (1993) Metabolites of deprenyl are involved in protection against the neurotoxicity of MPTP and its analogs in mice. *J. Neurochem.*, 61: S64.

Tariot, P.N., Cohen, R.M., Sunderland, T., Newhouse, P.A., Yount, D., Mellow, A.M., Weingartner, H., Mueller, E.A. and Murphy, D.L. (1987) L-Deprenyl in Alzheimer's disease-preliminary evidence for behavioral change with monoamine oxidase B inhibition. *Arch. Gen. Psychiatry,* 44: 427–433.

Tatton, W.G. and Greenwood, C.E. (1991) Rescue of dying neurons: a new action for deprenyl in MPTP Parkinsonism. *J. Neurosci. Res.*, 30: 666–672.

Tetrud, J.W. and Langston, J.W. (1989) The effect of deprenyl (selegiline) on the natural history of Parkinson's disease. *Science*, 245: 519–522.

Yu, P.H. (1989) Deamination of aliphatic amines of different chain lengths by rat liver monoamine oxidase A and B. *J. Pharm. Pharmacol.*, 41: 205–208.

Yu, P.H. and Davis, B.A. (1991a) 2-Propyl-1-aminopentane, its deamination by monoamine oxidase and semicarbazide-sensitive amine oxidase, conversion to valproic acid and behavioral effects. *Neuropharmacology*, 30: 507–515.

Yu, P.H. and Davis, B.A. (1991b) Simultaneous delivery of valproic acid and glycine to the brain; deamination of 2-propylpentylglycinamide by monoamine oxidase B. *Mol. Chem. Neuropathol.*, 15: 37–49.

Yu, P.H., Davis, B.A. and Boulton, A.A. (1992) Aliphatic propargylamines: potent selective irreversible monoamine oxidase B inhibitors. *J. Med. Chem.*, 35: 3705–3713.

Yu, P.H., Davis, B.A and Boulton, A.A. (1993) Effect of structural modification of alkyl *N*-propargylamines on the selective inhibition of monoamine oxidase B activity. *Biochem. Pharmacol.*, 46: 753–757.

Yu, P.H., Davis, B.A. and Boulton, A.A. (1994a) Neurochemical and neuroprotective effects of some aliphatic propargylamine MAO-B inhibitors. *J. Neurochem.*, 62: 697–704.

Yu, P.H. Davis, B.A., Fang J. and Boulton, A.A. (1994b) Neuroprotective effect of some monoamine oxidase-B inhibitors against DSP-4 induced noradrenaline depletion in the mouse hippocampus. *J. Neurochem.*, 63: 1820–1828.

Zhang, X., Yu, P.H., Davis, B.A., Zuo, D.M. and Boulton, A.A. (1995a) Neuroprotective effects of *N*-methylpargylamines againsty kainic acid induced neruonal damage in the rat brain. *Abstr. Proc. 26th Am. Soc. Neurochem. Meet.*

Zhang, X., Zuo, D.-M. and Yu, P.H. (1995b) Neuroprotection of *R*(−)-deprenyl and *N*-2-hexyl-*N*-methylpropargylamine on DSP-4 induced degeneration of noradrenergic neurons in tbe rat locus coeruleus. *Neurosci. Lett.*, 186: 45–48.

Peter M. Yu, Keith F. Tipton and Alan A. Boulton (Eds.)
Progress in Brain Research, Vol 106
© 1995 Elsevier Science BV. All rights reserved.

CHAPTER 13

Enantioselective recognition of two anticonvulsants, FCE 26743 and FCE 28073, by MAO, and relationship between MAO-B inhibition and FCE 26743 concentrations in rat brain

M. Strolin Benedetti, P. Tocchetti, M. Rocchetti, M. Martignoni, P. Marrari, I. Poggesi and P. Dostert

Pharmacia, Via per Pogliano, 20014 Nerviano, Milan, Italy

Introduction

The two alanine derivatives FCE 26743 ((S)-2-(4-(3-fluorobenzyloxy)-benzylamino)propionamide) and its enantiomeric counterpart FCE 28073 (Fig. 1) have been found to display similar, potent anticonvulsant activities in animal models of epilepsy (Dostert et al., 1991; Maj et al., 1993; Bonsignori, personal communication). These molecules belong to a series (Dostert et al., 1990) of analogues of milacemide (2-(n-pent-yl amino) acetamide), a glycine derivative with atypical anti-epileptic and potential psychotropic properties (Houtkooper et al., 1986; Saletu et al., 1986). Both FCE 26743 and FCE 28073 differ from milacemide in that an alaninamide residue replaces the glycinamide residue, and in the presence of a polyaromatic moiety instead of the pentyl group in milacemide.

FCE 26743 has been shown to be also a potent and selective inhibitor of monoamine oxidase (EC 1.4.3.4, MAO) type B (Strolin Benedetti et al., 1994). It has been suggested that molecules that, in addition to their anticonvulsant properties, possess potent MAO-inhibitory activities might decrease oxidative stress associated with epilepsy as a consequence of hydrogen peroxide formation impairment (Dostert et al., 1991; Strolin Benedetti et al., 1994). In this respect, it is worth noting that a significantly higher MAO-B activity was found in hippocampi from epileptic patients as compared with non-epileptic control subjects after correction for age-related changes (Kumlien et al., 1995).

In this paper we report on the in vitro and ex vivo MAO inhibitory properties of FCE 26743 and FCE 28073 in the rat, and on the in vitro MAO inhibitory properties of the aldehyde (4-(3-fluorobenzyloxy)benzaldehyde), which would be produced by MAO should FCE 26743 and/or FCE 28073 be substrates of that enzyme. In addition, to examine whether products formed by MAO-independent oxidative metabolism of FCE 26743 could contribute to its MAO-B inhibitory properties, experiments were carried out in rats pretreated with SKF-525A, an inhibitor of oxidative drug metabolism (Rossi et al., 1987; Murray and Reidy, 1990; Robertson and Bland, 1993; Lewis et al.; 1994). Finally, the relationship between ex vivo MAO-B inhibition and FCE

FCE 26743

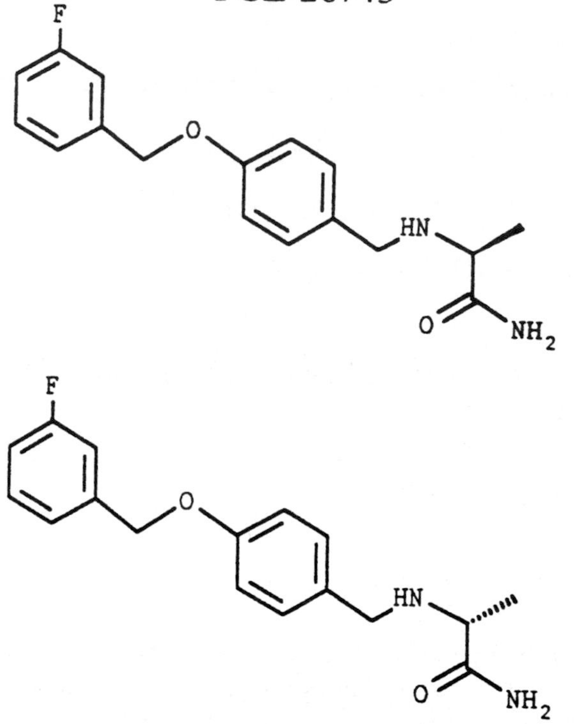

FCE 28073

Fig. 1. Chemical structure of FCE 26743 and FCE 28073.

26743 concentrations in the rat brain was investigated by developing a pharmacokinetic-pharmacodynamic model.

Materials and methods

Chemicals

FCE 26743, FCE 28073 (as methanesulphonate salts) and the corresponding aldehyde (4-(3-fluorobenzyloxy)benzaldehyde) were synthesized by Dr. P. Pevarello at Pharmacia-Farmitalia Carlo Erba. 5-Hydroxytryptamine (5-HT) creatinine sulphate and phenylethylamine (PEA) hydrochloride were from Sigma, USA. ^{14}C-5-HT (57 mCi/mmol) and ^{14}C-PEA (55 mCi/mmol) were purchased from Amersham, UK. SKF-525A hydrochloride was purchased from RBI, USA. All other chemi-

cals were of the highest reagent grade commercially available.

Animals and treatment

Sprague-Dawley male rats (Charles River, Italy), 200–230 g body weight, were used. For the ex vivo determinations of MAO activity and for the pharmacokinetic experiments single, oral doses ranging from 1 to 60 mg/kg were administered to animals fasted overnight. The doses of FCE 26743 and FCE 28073 were calculated as free base, and both compounds were administered as the methanesulphonate salt in aqueous solution (2 ml/kg body weight).

For the experiments in rats pretreated with SKF-525A hydrochloride, this compound was given i.p. in aqueous solution (2 ml/kg body weight) at a dose of 50 mg/kg (as free base) 1 h before FCE 26743 according to Yoshida et al. (1987).

For the in vitro MAO activity determinations brains from Sprague-Dawley male rats fasted overnight were also used.

MAO activity

Rats were killed by decapitation and the whole brain was rapidly removed, weighed, frozen in liquid nitrogen and stored at −20°C until assayed. After thawing, brains were homogenized in 0.1 M phosphate buffer, pH 7.4 (1 g tissue/16 ml buffer). In some in vitro and ex vivo experiments higher dilutions were used, up to 1 g tissue/512 ml buffer.

Brain MAO-A and MAO-B activities were assayed essentially as described by Cao Dahn et al. (1984). Aliquots (0.1 ml) of brain homogenate were added with [14]C 5-HT or ^{14}C-PEA so as to obtain a final volume of 0.5 ml containing 160 μM 5-HT or 4 μM PEA.

In vitro experiments were carried out after different times (0 to 60 min) of preincubation with the inhibitors prior to residual MAO activity determination. Concentrations of the inhibitors were expressed as free base and the inhibitors were used as methanesulphonate salts in aqueous solution.

Plasma and brain concentrations of FCE 26743

FCE 26743 was extracted from plasma with diethyl ether, then back-extracted with a 25 mM solution of phosphoric acid.

Brain was homogenized with acetone and the acetone phase was evaporated to dryness. Then, phosphoric acid was added to the residue and the aqueous phosphoric acid solution was repeatedly washed with hexane. After neutralization of the phosphoric acid solution with 1 M NaOH, FCE 26743 was extracted with diethyl ether, then back-extracted with phosphoric acid solution as described for plasma.

The HPLC system used for the determination of FCE 26743 concentrations in brain homogenates and plasma consisted of a SP 8700 XR pump equipped with a Rheodyne Model 7125 sampling valve with a 200 μl loop, a Chromjet Computing Integrator connected to a Labnet Data Capture Module, and a Jasco model 821-FP fluorescence detector. The chromatographic separation was performed using a 250×4 mm C18 column (particle size 3 μm). The mobile phase was acetonitrile:50 mM KH_2PO_4 (adjusted to pH 2 with 85% phosphoric acid) (32:68, v/v) and the flow rate 0.5 ml/min. The excitation and emission wavelengths were 224 and 302 nm, respectively. The limit of quantitation was 10 ng/ml plasma and 20 ng/g brain.

Pharmacokinetic-pharmacodynamic data analysis

Estimation of pharmacokinetic parameters was performed by non-linear least-squares regression (PCNONLIN software, Metzler and Weiner, 1992) using a weighting function of $1/y^2$. The goodness of fit was assessed by evaluating the residuals and the accuracy of parameters estimation (Boxenbaum et al., 1974). Analogous procedures were used for the estimation of the pharmacodynamic parameters. Model discrimination was performed using the *F*-test (Boxenbaum et al., 1974) and

Akaike's Information Criterion (Yamaoka et al., 1978).

Results and discussion

In the in vitro studies with rat brain homogenates FCE 26743 was found to be a potent inhibitor of MAO-B ($IC_{50} = 1.7 \pm 0.1 \times 10^{-7}$ M, mean $\pm$ SD, 2 min of preincubation) and to weakly inhibit MAO-A ($IC_{50} = 3.7 \pm 0.35 \times 10^{-4}$ M), while FCE 28073 was approx. 10-times less potent as a MAO-B inhibitor ($IC_{50} = 17.7 \pm 1.4 \times 10^{-7}$ M) and 7-times more potent as a MAO-A inhibitor ($IC_{50} = 0.5 \pm 0.03 \times 10^{-4}$ M).

The inhibition of brain MAO-A and -B by the two enantiomers was also determined ex vivo 1 h after oral administration of 1, 5, 10 and 60 mg/kg doses (Table 1). From the 5 mg/kg dose up, FCE 26743 inhibited strongly and selectively the B form of MAO (86% inhibition after 5 mg/kg dosing), whereas its enantiomeric counterpart FCE 28073 inhibited MAO-B by 50% at the highest dose of 60 mg/kg only. No notable inhibition of MAO-A was observed for both compounds up to the highest administered dose.

The time-course of the inhibition of brain MAO-B by the two compounds was determined ex vivo after oral administration of a 10 mg/kg dose, for which both molecules were shown to elicit a similar, marked anticonvulsant effect. As shown in Fig. 2, the inhibition of rat brain MAO-B was much higher after FCE 26743 than after FCE 28073. The large difference in MAO inhibitory potency between the two enantiomers is consistent with the influence of the absolute configuration on the selective recognition of the enantiomers of *N*-α-alkyl-substituted derivatives by the MAO forms (Strolin Benedetti and Dostert, 1985; Dostert and Strolin Benedetti, 1991; Dostert et al.,1992). It is interesting to observe that another glycine derivative, (2-(4-(3-chlorobenzoxy) phenethylamino)acetamide), very similar to the compounds discussed in this paper but without the *N*-α-methyl group, has been shown to display

TABLE 1

Ex vivo inhibition of rat brain MAO 1 h after oral administration of FCE 26743 and FCE 28073

| MAO type | % inhibtion (mean ± SD, $n = 5$) | | | | | | | |
| | FCE 26743 | | | | FCE 28073 | | | |
	1 mg/kg	5 mg/kg	10 mg/kg	60 mg/kg	1 mg/kg	5 mg/kg	10 mg/kg	60 mg/kg
MAO-A	0	0	2 ± 3	7 ± 7	0	0	0	0
MAO-B	38 ± 9	86 ± 3	84 ± 6	94 ± 1	2 ± 2	11 ± 6	33 ± 3	50 ± 4

Brain homogenate: 1 g tissue/16 ml buffer. Data are expressed as means ± SD of the ratio of individual values of treated rats vs. mean control value.

similar inhibitory potency towards MAO-A and -B (O'Brien et al., 1994).

When FCE 26743 (10^{-7} M concentration) was preincubated in rat brain homogenates for different times from 0 up to 60 min, the percent inhibition of MAO-B was found to reach a maximum in about 10–15 min and to slightly decrease thereafter (Table 2). It is worthy of note that no changes in the percentage of inhibition have been shown to occur with reversible inhibitors whatever the time of incubation (Mazouz et al., 1988); conversely, increased percent inhibition with time is found with irreversible inhibitors and competitive, slow and tight-binding reversible inhibitors (Strolin Benedetti, 1984; Mazouz et al., 1993). When brain homogenates were diluted prior to FCE 26743 addition, the IC_{50} value decreased (or the percent inhibition of MAO-B for a given concentration increased) with dilution (Table 3),

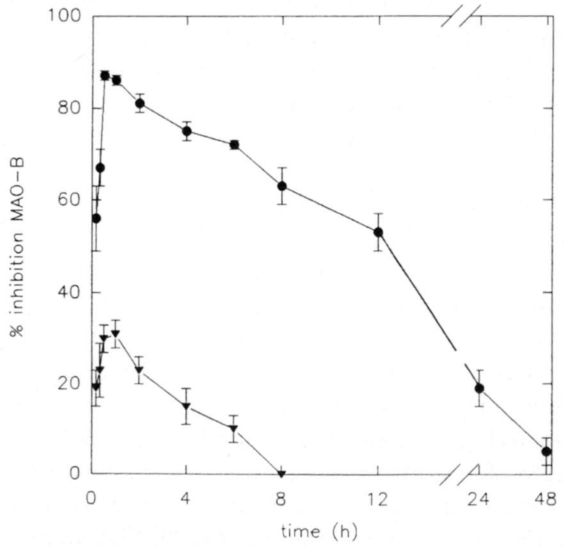

Fig. 2. Ex vivo inhibition of rat brain MAO-B by FCE 26743 (●) and FCE 28073 (▼) after oral administration (10 mg/kg). Data are expressed as mean ± standard error of the ratio. Brain homogenates were prepared using 1 g tissue/16 ml of buffer; MAO-B was assayed using ^{14}C-PEA (4 μM) as substrate.

TABLE 2

Effect of the preincubation time on the in vitro inhibition of rat brain MAO-B by FCE 26743

Time of preincubation (37 °C, 10^{-7} M)	% inhibition (mean ± SD)
0 min	10
1 min	20 ± 4
2 min	33 ± 5
3 min	41 ± 5
5 min	51 ± 2
7 min	50 ± 3
10 min	55 ± 3
15 min	53 ± 2
30 min	50 ± 2
60 min	47 ± 2

Rat brain homogenate: 1 g tissue/16 ml buffer. Each value is the mean of three experiments, made in triplicate, in which three different brains were used.

TABLE 3

Effect of dilution of rat brain homogenates on the in vitro inhibition of MAO-B by FCE 26743

Time of preincubation (37°C, 10^{-7} M)	% inhibition MAO-B (mean ± SD)			
	1 g/16 ml	1 g/128 ml	1 g/256 ml	1 g/512 ml
2 min	30 ± 2	54 ± 3	59 ± 1	63 ± 2
60 min	45 ± 2	74 ± 6	70 ± 8	82 ($n = 2$)

Time of preincubation (37°C, concentrations range: 10^{-9}–10^{-3} M)	IC_{50} (10^{-7} M) (mean ± SD)			
	1 g/16 ml	1 g/128 ml	1 g/256 ml	1 g/512 ml
2 min	1.79 ± 0.04	0.77 ± 0.10	0.51 ± 0.09	0.4 ± 0.07
60 min	1.06 ± 0.20	0.25 ± 0.01	0.23 ± 0.04	0.18 ($n = 2$)

% inhibition and IC_{50} values are the mean of three experiments, each performed in triplicate.

TABLE 4

Effect of dilution of rat brain homogenates on the ex vivo inhibition of MAO-B at different times after oral administration of FCE 26743 (10 mg/kg)

Dilution	% inhibition (mean ± s.e.r.)		
	30 min	4 h	16 h
1 g/16 ml	86 ± 1	85 ± 1	24 ± 2
1 g/256 ml	83 ± 1	88 ± 2	29 ± 3
1 g/512 ml	87 ± 2	90 ± 2	37 ± 2

MAO-B was assayed immediately after dilution; s.e.r: standard error of the ratio.

suggesting that FCE 26743 behaves as an irreversible inhibitor of MAO-B (Strolin Benedetti et al., 1982, 1983).

The effect of dilution of the brain homogenates was also studied ex vivo after oral administration of a 10 mg/kg dose of FCE 26743. The percentage of MAO-B inhibition was found to remain virtually unaffected by dilution (Table 4), as could be expected for an irreversible inhibitor of the enzyme (Strolin Benedetti et al., 1982, 1983; Strolin Benedetti, 1984).

Although the in vitro preincubation experiments and the in vitro and ex vivo dilution experiments are in favour of FCE 26743 acting as an irreversible MAO-B inhibitor, the time-curve of the ex vivo inhibition of rat brain MAO-B after a 10 mg/kg oral dose of FCE 26743 is typical of a short-acting inhibitor. A possible mechanism that may account for the apparently contrasting results is presented in Fig. 3. After a first step where the enzyme (E) and the inhibitor (I) are rapidly in equilibrium with the enzyme-inhibitor complex EI, as for a classical reversible inhibition, a second step occurring through initial single-electron transfer from the nitrogen-nonbonding electrons to the oxidized FAD followed by α-proton abstraction, as suggested by Silverman's studies (Silverman and Zieske, 1985; Silverman and Zelechonok, 1992), or through direct hydrogen atom abstraction by an enzyme-bound radical (FAD·) according to Yue et al. (1993), would lead to the formation of an intermediate imine. In the case of classical substrates the imine is subsequently hydrolysed to yield the corresponding aldehyde. In the present case, one may assume that the imine reacts with a SH group present in the MAO protein, with production of an enzyme-

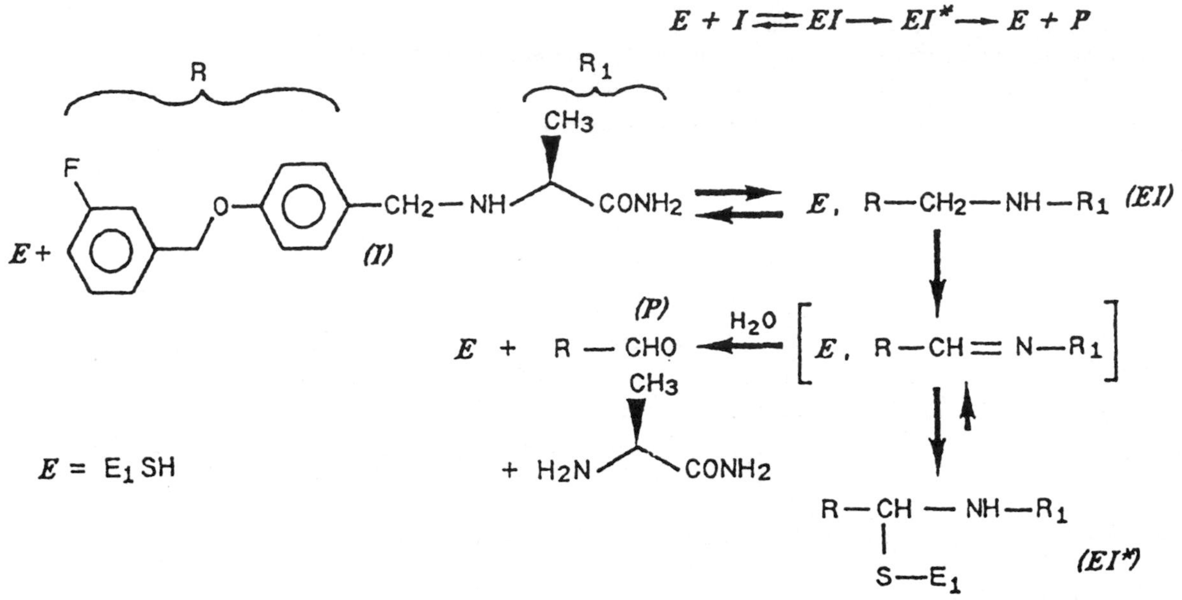

128

Fig. 3. Proposed mechanism for the interaction of FCE 26743 with MAO-B.

inhibitor adduct (termed EI∗) and subsequent MAO inhibition as a result. This adduct might slowly dissociate to regenerate the imine, which would be then hydrolysed. In an in vitro system, the equilibrium would be strongly displaced towards the formation of the enzyme-inhibitor adduct EI∗, so that the compound behaves as an irreversible inhibitor. In contrast, under in vivo conditions, the aldehyde formed by hydrolysis could be cleared, favouring the reversibility of the reaction from EI∗ back to the imine, with FCE 26743 behaving as a short-acting ex vivo inhibitor as a result.

Compared to FCE 26743, the corresponding aldehyde was found to be a weaker inhibitor of MAO-B (IC$_{50}$ = 2.3 × 10^{-6} M, 2 min preincubation, rat brain homogenate 1 g/16 ml), suggesting that the formation of this aldehyde, if any, by the action of MAO should not contribute, at least to a significant extent, to the inhibition of MAO by FCE 26743. SKF-525A has been shown to be an inhibitor of some cytochrome P-450 isoenzymes (Rossi et al., 1987; Murray and Reidy, 1990; Lewis et al., 1994) as well as of aldehyde oxidase (Ro-

bertson and Bland,1993). Pretreatment of rats with SKF-525A given at a dose (50 mg/kg, i.p.) which was shown not to affect MAO-B activity in a separate experiment, increased the percentage inhibition of brain MAO-B by FCE 26743 (Table 5). This result suggests that products formed by MAO-independent oxidative metabolism should not contribute, at least to a significant degree, to the inhibitory effect of FCE 26743 towards brain MAO-B in vivo.

The concentrations of FCE 26743 were measured, both in plasma and brain, after oral administration of a 10 mg/kg dose. Brain levels were found to be much higher than plasma levels, with the ratio brain concentrations/plasma concentrations being about 20 at 1 h post-dosing (Fig. 4). The peak level in plasma appears to occur slightly earlier (20–30 min) than in brain (30–60 min). However, the shape of the two curves was very similar, at least until 6 h, after which time the plasma levels were no longer detectable. When the plasma levels vs. time points are presented as a semi-log plot, a monoexponential decay characterized by a half-life of about 0.9 h is observed.

TABLE 5

Effect of SKF-525A (50 mg/kg, i.p.) on the ex vivo inhibition of rat brain MAO-B by FCE 26743 (2.5 or 10 mg/kg, p.o.)

Treatment	% inhibition (mean ± s.e.r)						
	1 h	2 h	4 h	8 h	24 h	30 h	48 h
FCE 26743 (10 mg/kg)	ND	81 ± 2	ND	63 ± 4	19 ± 4	ND	ND
SKF-525A + FCE 26743	ND	90 ± 1	ND	91 ± 1	44 ± 2	ND	ND
FCE 26743 (2.5 mg/kg)	48 ± 8	53 ± 2	53 ± 1	31 ± 2	6 ± 1	3 ± 1	0
SKF-525A + FCE 26743	43 ± 2	75 ± 2	78 ± 1	66 ± 1	14 ± 3	15 ± 7	0

SKF-525A was administered 1 h before FCE 26743; ND = not determined.

When the brain levels vs. time points are also presented as a semi-log plot (Fig. 5), a biexponential decay characterized by a first half-life of about 0.9 h is noted, followed by a second half-life for the terminal phase of about 9.6 h. It is interesting to observe that the only half-life measurable in plasma has the same value as the first half-life in brain, suggesting that both brain and plasma belong to the central compartment. A similar conclusion can be drawn by interpreting brain and plasma kinetics in terms of compartmental analysis (Fig. 6, Table 6). The fact that the peripheral compartment could not be observed from plasma data is probably due to the low concentrations of FCE 26743 in plasma compared to brain.

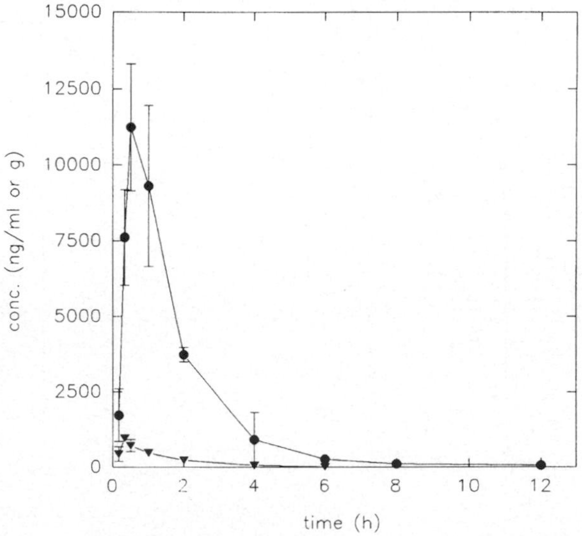

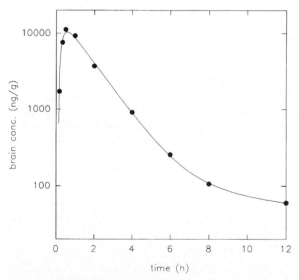

Fig. 5. Mean brain concentrations ($n = 3$) vs. time plot for FCE 26743 following oral administration of a 10 mg/kg dose to rats. The solid curve represents the best fitting of the equation:

$$Y(t) = A \cdot e^{-\alpha \cdot (t - t_{\text{lag}})} + B \cdot e^{-\beta \cdot (t - t_{\text{lag}})} - C \cdot e^{-k01 \cdot (t - t_{\text{lag}})}$$

to the data (where A and B are the pre-exponential terms, $C = A + B$, α, β, k_{01} are the rate macroconstants and t_{lag} is the lag time). Parameters ± standard error of the estimates: $A = 17722 \pm 2514$ ng/g; $\alpha = 0.805 \pm 0.062$ h^{-1}; $B = 137 \pm 101$ ng/g; $\beta = 0.072 \pm 0.065$ h^{-1}; $k_{01} = 4.73 \pm 1.04$ h^{-1}; $t_{lag} = 0.140 \pm 0.005$ h ($r^2 = 0.99$).

Fig. 4. Plasma (ϑ) and brain (●) concentrations of FCE 26743 after oral administration of 10 mg/kg to rats. Data are expressed as mean ± SD ($n = 3$).

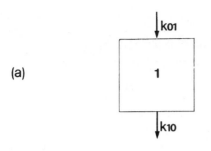

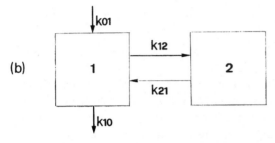

Fig. 6. Scheme of the models used for the interpretation of plasma (a) and brain (b) pharmacokinetics. Equations of the models:

(a) Plasma

$$Y(t) = C_{plasma}(t) = \frac{k_{01} \cdot F \cdot \text{Dose}}{V_1 \cdot (k_{01} - k_{10})}$$

$$\cdot (e^{-k_{10} \cdot (t - t_{lag})} - e^{-k_{01} \cdot (t - t_{lag})})$$

(where k_{01} and k_{10} are the absorption and elimination rate constants, respectively, F is the bioavailability of the drug (assumed to be 1), V_1 is the volume of distribution of the compartment 1, and t_{lag} is the lag time).

(b) Brain

$$Y(t) = C_{brain}(t) = \frac{k_{01} \cdot F \cdot \text{Dose}}{V_1}$$

$$\cdot \left\{ \frac{(k_{21} - \alpha) \cdot e^{-\alpha \cdot (t - t_{lag})}}{(k_{01} - \alpha)(\beta - \alpha)} + \frac{(k_{21} - \beta) \cdot e^{-\beta \cdot (t - t_{lag})}}{(k_{01} - \beta)(\alpha - \beta)} \right.$$

$$\left. + \frac{(k_{21} - k_{01}) \cdot e^{-k_{01} \cdot (t - t_{lag})}}{(\alpha - k_{01})(\beta - k_{01})} \right\}$$

(where k_{12} and k_{21} are the transfer rate microconstants between compartment 1 and 2, α and β are the rate macroconstants (see Fig. 5) and the other parameters are defined above).

When the percent inhibition of brain MAO-B is plotted against the brain concentrations of FCE 26743, an anticlockwise hysteresis loop is obtained (Fig. 7), i.e. for the same brain concentration a higher inhibition is observed at later times,

TABLE 6

Plasma and brain pharmacokinetic parameters: rate microconstants from compartmental analysis

	k_{01} (h^{-1})	k_{10} (h^{-1})	k_{12} (h^{-1})	k_{21} (h^{-1})
Plasma	58.15 ± *	0.732 ± 0.020	na	na
Brain	4.73 ± 1.04	0.737 ± 0.070	0.062 ± 0.018	0.079 ± 0.069

Data are expressed as estimate ± standard error of the estimate. *CV% > 100%; na: not applicable.

indicating equilibration delay between the brain concentrations and the concentrations at the effect site. Such a hysteresis behaviour has already been reported for several drugs (Holford and Sheiner, 1981). For example, an anticlockwise hysteresis loop was found when consecutive neuromuscular blockade measurements were plotted against the concentration of metocurine in plasma (Shafer et al., 1989), whereas a clockwise hysteresis loop was noted when plasma levels of cocaine

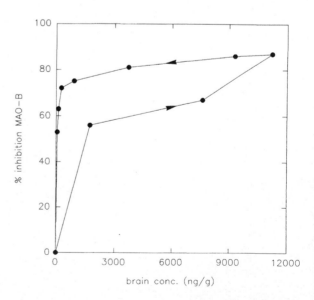

Fig. 7. Ex vivo inhibition of rat brain MAO-B vs. FCE 26743 brain concentrations following oral administration of a 10 mg/kg dose of FCE 26743 to rats.

were related to the degree of euphoria after intranasal administration of the compound (Van Dyke et al., 1977; Holford and Sheiner, 1981). Recently, the relationship between the time-course of MAO-A inhibition, indirectly estimated by the plasma concentrations of monoamine metabolites, and the plasma concentrations of unchanged drug in humans has been reported for moclobemide, another MAO inhibitor (Holford et al., 1994). However, from the data reported in this paper no estimate as to whether hysteresis occurs can be made. In another recent work on lazabemide, a reversible MAO-B inhibitor, no time delay between plasma drug concentrations and resulting inhibition of platelet MAO-B in humans was found to occur (Guentert et al., 1994). The anticlockwise hysteresis observed in the present study indicates that the effect, the inhibition of MAO-B, is not directly related to FCE 26743 brain concentrations. Therefore, it was deemed necessary to develop a model aiming to evaluate the concentrations of the drug at the effect site, which would account for the effect observed without being affected by equilibration delay. The central compartment (compartment 1, Fig. 8), which, as discussed above, includes brain, was assumed to be related to the effect compartment (compartment E) by a first-order process through an entry rate constant k_{1e}. An elimination rate constant k_{e0} controls the disappearance of the drug from this compartment. The equation describing the effect site concentrations (CE(t)) for the proposed pharmacokinetic model was adapted from the equations developed by Sheiner et al. (1979) and Holford and Sheiner (1981). Then, the concentrations of the drug in the effect compartment (CE(t)) are related to the effect (E, % MAO-B inhibition) by the relationship:

$$E = E_{max} \cdot CE(t)/CE_{50} + CE(t)$$

used in enzyme kinetics for the reaction enzyme-substrate (Michaelis–Menten equation/E_{max} model), where E_{max} is the maximal effect and CE_{50} is the concentration of the drug in the effect compartment producing 50% of the maximal effect.

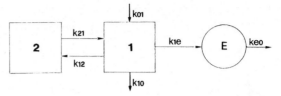

Fig. 8. Scheme of the pharmacokinetic-pharmacodynamic model. Equations of the model:

$$(t) = \frac{k_{e0} \cdot k_{01} \cdot F \cdot \text{Dose}}{V_1}$$

$$\cdot \left\{ \frac{(k_{21} - k_{01}) \cdot e^{k_{01} \cdot (t - t_{lag})}}{(\alpha - k_{01})(\beta - k_{01})(k_{e0} - k_{01})} \right.$$

$$+ \frac{(k_{21} - \alpha) \cdot e^{-\alpha \cdot (t - t_{lag})}}{(k_{01} - \alpha)(\beta - \alpha)(k_{e0} - \alpha)}$$

$$+ \frac{(k_{21} - \beta) \cdot e^{-\beta \cdot (t - t_{lag})}}{(k_{01} - \beta)(\alpha - \beta)(k_{e0} - \beta)}$$

$$\left. + \frac{(k_{21} - k_{e0}) \cdot e^{-k_{e0}(t - t_{lag})}}{(k_{01} - k_{e0})(\alpha - k_{e0})(\beta - k_{e0})} \right\}$$

(where CE(t) is the FCE 26743 effect site concentration and the other parameters were previously defined).

$$E = \frac{E_{max} \cdot CE(t)}{CE_{50} + CE(t)}$$

(where E is the % of MAO-B inhibition and the other parameters are defined in the text).

By substituting the equation CE(t) in the E_{max} model, it is possible to obtain the equation (E) describing the time course of the effect. This equation depends on the pharmacokinetic parameters, which, in the present case, were previously estimated by non-linear fitting of the brain levels vs. time curve, on the elimination rate constant from the effect compartment (k_{e0}) and on the parameters of the E_{max} model (E_{max}, CE_{50}). By non-linear regression analysis, the values of k_{e0}, E_{max} and CE_{50} which allow the best fitting of the experimental effect values vs. time (Fig. 9) can be estimated. For k_{e0} a value of 6.02 h^{-1}, which corresponds to an equilibration half-time of about 7 min, was obtained. This means that about 20 min are necessary for an equilibrium between the concentrations in the brain and the effect compartment to be reached. This value

132

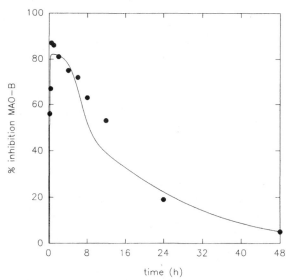

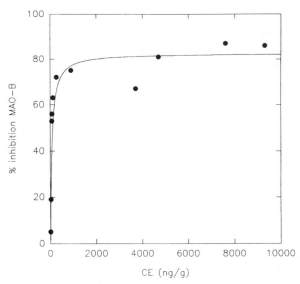

Fig. 9. Ex vivo inhibition of rat brain MAO-B by FCE 26743 vs. time plot following oral administration of 10 mg/kg to rats. The solid line represents the best fitting of the equations of the pharmacokinetic-pharmacodynamic model. Parameters ± standard error of the estimates: $k_{e0} = 6.02 \pm 3.01$ h^{-1}; $E_{max} = 82.7 \pm 5.2$ %; CE$_{50} = 67.3 \pm 9.7$ ng/g ($r^2 = 0.92$).

Fig. 10. Ex vivo inhibition of rat brain MAO-B by FCE 26743 vs. estimated FCE 26743 concentrations in the effect compartment.

is not very different from the time necessary in the in vitro experiment (10–15 min, Table 2) to obtain a stable MAO-B inhibition. An E_{max} value of 82.7% was found, while a value of 67.3 ng/g for CE$_{50}$ (2.2×10^{-7} M) was obtained, in good agreement with the IC$_{50}$ value (1.8×10^{-7} M) previously found in the in vitro experiments.

The pharmacodynamic model used (E_{max} model) was tested against a more general model (Sigmoid E_{max} model: $E = E_{max} \cdot CE(t)^N / CE_{50}^N + CE(t)^N$). However, the sigmoidicity factor ($N = 1.10 \pm 0.11$, mean ± SE) was not significantly different from 1. F-test and AIC confirmed that the restricted E_{max} model was sufficient to describe the data.

The curve Effect–CE (Fig. 10) is in reasonable agreement with the experimental values of the effect plotted vs. the concentrations in the effect compartment calculated considering the time at which the effect has been measured and using the estimated value of k_{e0}. As compared with Fig. 7, it can be observed that, in Fig. 10, only a single

point shows a substantial deviation from the sigmoidal curve, indicating that the hysteresis is reduced. Therefore, the adopted pharmacokinetic-pharmacodynamic model appears to be acceptable.

Conclusion

MAO-B was found to selectively recognize the two enantiomers of 2-(4-(3-fluorobenzyloxy)benzylamino)propionamide, with the S enantiomer (FCE 26743) being a more potent inhibitor of that enzyme form than its enantiomeric counterpart (FCE 28073). After oral administration of FCE 26743 to rats, the brain concentrations of unchanged drug were much higher than the plasma concentrations. At the time corresponding to 50% inhibition of brain MAO-B (about 13 h, Fig. 2), FCE 26743 brain concentration can be estimated as being 55.6 ng/g, i.e. about 1.8×10^{-7} M, in good agreement with the IC$_{50}$ values (1.8 and 1.1×10^{-7} M after 2 and 60 min of preincubation, respectively, Table 3) determined in the in vitro experiments. Thus, the inhibition of brain MAO-B by FCE 26743 appears to be due to the molecule itself rather than to metabolites. The aldehyde that would correspond to the oxidative metabolism of FCE 26743 by MAO was found to inhibit brain MAO-B. However, its potency as MAO-B inhibitor is roughly 10-times lower than that of FCE 26743. Therefore, a significant participation of this aldehyde in the inhibition of brain MAO-B in vivo appears to be unlikely. The inhibition of brain MAO-B was enhanced by pretreatment of rats with SKF-525A. Various hypotheses could account for this effect. The most likely hypothesis is that SKF-525A inhibits the FCE 26743-metabolizing enzymes, with formation of higher brain levels of FCE 26743 as a result. However, the brain concentrations of FCE 26743 in rats pretreated with SKF-525A were not determined. The inhibition of SKF-525A-dependent metabolic pathway(s) might also favour the formation of otherwise minor metabolites, with MAO-B inhibitory properties, at the expense of the metabolites formed in the absence of the inhibitor. SKF-525A is an inhibitor of aldehyde oxidase (Robertson and Bland, 1993), and a variety of aldehydes have been shown to be substrates of brain aldehyde oxidase (Peet et al., 1993). Therefore, one can ask whether the aldehyde which would result from the action of MAO on FCE 26743 might contribute to the enhancement of brain MAO-B inhibition observed in SKF-525A-pretreated rats, once its catabolism by aldehyde oxidase is inhibited. Although direct evidence is still missing, the anticlockwise hysteresis observed when the MAO-B inhibitory potency of FCE 26743 is plotted against the brain concentrations of the compound is probably due to the suggested mechanism of interaction of FCE 26743 with MAO-B, rather than to the action of metabolites.

References

Boxenbaum, H.G., Riegelmann, S. and Elashoff, R.M. (1974) Statistical estimation in pharmacokinetics. *J. Pharmacokinet. Biopharm.*, 2: 123–148.

Cao Dahn, H., Strolin Benedetti, M. and Dostert, P. (1984) Differential changes in monoamine oxidase A and B activity in aging rat tissues. In: K.F. Tipton, P. Dostert and M. Strolin Benedetti (Eds.), *Monoamine Oxidase and Disease. Prospects for Therapy with Reversible Inhibitors*, Academic Press, London, pp. 301–317.

Dostert, P. and Strolin Benedetti, M. (1991) Structure-modulated recognition of substrates and inhibitors by monoamine oxidases A and B. *Biochem. Soc. Trans.*, 19: 207–212.

Dostert, P., Pevarello, P., Heidempergher, F., Varasi, M., Bonsignori, A. and Roncucci, R. (1990) Preparation of α-(phenylalkylamino)carboxamides as drugs. *Eur. Pat. Appl.*, EP 400, 495.

Dostert, P., Strolin Benedetti, M. and Tipton K.F. (1991) New anticonvulsants with selective MAO-B inhibitory activity. *Eur. Neuropsychopharmacol.*, 1: 317–319.

Dostert, P., O'Brien, E.M., Tipton, K.F., Meroni, M., Melloni, P. and Strolin Benedetti, M. (1992) Inhibition of monoamine oxidase by the *R* and *S* enantiomers of *N*[3-(2,4-dichlorophenoxy)propyl]-*N*-methyl-3-butyn-2-amine. *Eur. J. Med. Chem.*, 27: 45–52.

Guentert, T.W., Holford, N.H.G., Pfefen, J.P. and Dingemanse, J. (1994) Mixed linear and non-linear disposition of lazabemide, a reversible and selective inhibitor of monoamine oxidase B. *Br. J. Clin. Pharmacol.*, 37: 545–551.

Holford, N.H.G. and Sheiner, L.B. (1981) Understanding the dose-effect relationship: clinical application of pharmacokinetic-pharmacodynamic models. *Clin. Pharmacokinet.*, 6: 429–453.

Holford, N.H.G., Guentert, T.W., Dingemanse, J. and Banken, L. (1994) Monoamine oxidase-A: pharmacodynamics in humans of moclobemide, a reversible and selective inhibitor. *Br. J. Clin. Pharmac.*, 37: 433–439.

Houtkooper, M., van Oorschot, C.A.E.H., Rentmeester, T.W., Höppener, P.J.E.A. and Onkelinx, C. (1986) Double-blind study of milacemide in hospitalized therapy-resistant patients with epilepsy. *Epilepsia*, 27: 255–262.

Kumlien, E., Sherif, F, Ge, L. and Oreland, L. (1995) Platelet and brain GABA-transaminase and monoamine oxidase activities in complex partial epilepsy. *Epilepsy Res.*, 20: 161–170.

Lewis, D.F.V., Moereels, H., Lake, B.G., Ioannides, C. and Parke, D.V. (1994) Molecular modeling of enzymes and receptors involved in carcinogenesis: QSARs and COMPACT-3D *. *Drug. Metab. Rev.*, 26: 261–285.

Maj, R., Antongiovanni, V., Bonsignori, A., Breda, M., Dostert, P., Fariello, R.G., McArthur, R.A., Varasi, M. and Bianchetti, A. (1993) Anticonvulsant profile of benzylaminopropanamide derivatives in mice and rats. Abstract presented at the Focus on Epilepsy II, International Conference, Whistler (Canada) 11–14.

Mazouz, F., Lebreton, L., Milcent, R. and Burstein, C. (1988) Inhibition of monoamine oxidase types A and B by 2-aryl-

4H-1,3,4-oxadiazin-5(6H)-one derivatives. *Eur. J. Med. Chem.*, 23: 441–451.

Mazouz, F., Gueddari, S., Burstein, C., Mansuy, D. and Milcent, R. (1993) 5-[4-(benzyloxy)phenyl]-1,3,4-oxadiazol-2(3H)-one derivatives and related analogues: new reversible, highly potent, and selective monoamine oxidase type B inhibitors. *J. Med. Chem.*, 36: 1157–1167.

Metzler, C.M. and Weiner, D.L. (1992) PCNONLIN User Guide, version 4.0. Statistical Consultant Inc., Lexington.

Murray, M. and Reidy, G.F. (1990) Selectivity in the inhibition of mammalian cytochromes *P*-450 by chemical agents. *Am. Soc. Pharmacol. Exp. Ther.*, 42: 85–101.

O'Brien, E.M., Dostert, P., Pevarello, P. and Tipton, K.F. (1994) Interactions of some analogues of the anticonvulsant milacemide with monoamine oxidase. *Biochem. Pharmacol.*, 48: 905–914.

Peet, C.F., Smith, J.A. and Beedham, C. (1993) Aldehyde oxidase catalysed formation of 5-hydroxyindoleacetic acid in guinea pig liver and brain. *Br. J. Pharmacol.*, 110 (Proc. Suppl. Oct.), 171P.

Robertson, I.G.C. and Bland, T.J. (1993) Inhibition by SKF-525A of the aldehyde oxidase-mediated metabolism of the experimental antitumour agent acridine carboxamide. *Biochem. Pharmacol.*, 45: 2159–2162.

Rossi, M., Markovitz, S. and Callahan, T. (1987) Defining the active site of cytochrome *P*-450: the crystal and molecular structure of an inhibitor, SKF-525A. *Carcinogenesis*, 8: 881–887.

Saletu, B., Grünberger, J. and Linzmayer, L. (1986) Acute and subacute CNS effects of milacemide in elderly people: double-blind, placebo-controlled quantitative EEG and psychometric investigations. *Arch. Gerontol. Geriatr.*, 5: 165–181.

Shafer, S.L., Varvel, J.R. and Gronert, G.A. (1989) A comparison of parametric with semiparametric analysis of the concentration versus effect relationship of metocurine in dogs and pigs. *J. Pharmacokinet. Biopharmacol.*, 17: 291–304.

Sheiner, L.B., Stanski, D.R., Vozeh, S., Miller, R.D. and Ham, J. (1979). Simultaneous modeling of pharmacokinetics and pharmacodynamics: application to d-tubocurarine. *Clin. Pharmacol. Ther.*, 25: 358–371.

Silverman, R.B. and Zelechonok, Y. (1992) Evidence for a hydrogen atom transfer mechanism or a proton/fast electron transfer mechanism for amine oxidase. *J. Org. Chem.*, 57: 6373–6374.

Silverman, R.B. and Zieske, P.A. (1985) Mechanism of inactivation of monoamine oxidase by 1-phenylcyclopropylamine. *Biochemistry*, 24: 2128–2138.

Strolin Benedetti, M. (1984) Some pharmacological and clinical aspects of reversible MAO inhibitors. In: W. Paton, J. Mitchell and T. Turner (Eds.), *Proceedings of IUPHAR 9th International Congress of Pharmacology*, Vol. 2, MacMillan, London, pp. 219–230.

Strolin Benedetti, M. and Dostert, P. (1985) Stereochemical aspects of MAO interactions: reversible and selective inhibitors of monoamine oxidase. *Trends Pharmacol. Sci.*, 6: 246–251.

Strolin Benedetti, M., Dostert, P., Boucher, T. and Guffroy, C. (1982) A new reversible selective type B monoamine oxidase inhibitor: MD 780236. In: K. Kamijo, E. Usdin and T. Nagatsu (Eds.), *Monoamine Oxidase. Basic and Clinical Frontiers*, International Congress Series 564, Excerpta Medica, Amsterdam, pp. 209–220.

Strolin Benedetti, M., Dostert, P., Guffroy, C. and Tipton, K.F. (1983) Partial or total protection of long-acting monoamine oxidase inhibitors (MAOIs) by new short-acting MAOIs of type A MD 780515 and type B MD 780236. *Mod. Probl. Pharmacopsychiat.*,19: 82–104.

Strolin Benedetti, M., Marrari, P., Colombo, M., Castelli, M.G., Arand, M., Oesch, F. and Dostert, P. (1994) The new anticonvulsant FCE 26743 is a selective and short-acting MAO-B inhibitor devoid of inducing properties towards cytochrome *P*-450-dependent testosterone hydroxylation. *J. Pharm. Pharmacol.*, 46: 814–819.

Van Dyke, C., Jatlow, P., Ungerer, J., Barash, P.G. and Byck, R. (1977) Oral cocaine: plasma concentrations and central effects. *Science*, 200: 211–213.

Yoshida, T., Oguro, T. and Kuroiwa, Y. (1987) Hepatic and extrahepatic metabolism of deprenyl, a selective monoamine oxidase (MAO) B inhibitor, of amphetamines in rats: sex and strain differences. *Xenobiotica*, 17: 957–963.

Yamaoka, K., Nakagawa, T. and Uno, T. (1978) Application of Akaike's Information Criterion (AIC) in the evaluation of linear pharmacokinetic equations. *J. Pharmacokinet. Biopharmacol.*, 6: 165–175.

Yue, K.T., Bhattacharyya, A.K., Zhelyaskov, V.R. and Edmondson, D.E. (1993) Resonance Raman spectroscopic evidence for an anionic flavin semiquinone in bovine liver monoamine oxidase. *Arch. Biochem. Biophys.*, 300: 178–185.

Peter M. Yu, Keith F. Tipton and Alan A. Boulton (Eds.)
Progress in Brain Research, Vol 106
© 1995 Elsevier Science BV. All rights reserved.

CHAPTER 14

Selectivity of MDL 72,974A for MAO-B inhibition based on substrate and metabolite concentrations in plasma

N.D. Huebert, V. Schwach, C. Hinze and K.D. Haegele

Marion Merrell Dow Research Centre, 16, rue d'Ankara, 67080 Strasbourg Cédex, France

Introduction

In vitro and in vivo studies in animals have shown that MDL 72,974A ((E)-4-fluoro-β-fluoromethylene benzene butaneamine hydrochloride) is a potent, selective, enzyme-activated, irreversible inhibitor of the B form of monoamine oxidase (MAO-B). It inhibits MAO activity in rat brain, heart, liver and duodenum with a selectivity ratio of between 40 and 100 for the B-form as opposed to the A-form of the enzyme (Zreika et al., 1989).

In man, a dose-dependent inhibition of platelet MAO-B activity was demonstrated for single, daily oral doses of 0.1 to 12 mg MDL 72,974A (Duléry et al., 1993). Inhibition at doses of 0.5 mg and above was greater than 95 % within 1 h of drug administration. Sub-chronic administration at doses of 0.1, 1, 12 and 24 mg given as single, daily, oral doses over a 10-day period resulted in a sustained inhibition of platelet MAO-B which returned to predrug levels within 7 to 15 days. After 10 days treatment, inhibition of MAO-B was $84.8 \pm 4.4\%$ at the 0.1 mg dose and $97.7 \pm 0.4\%$ at the 24 mg dose. Thus, complete or nearly complete inhibition of platelet MAO-B can be demonstrated over a wide dose range.

While the inhibition of MAO-B can be assessed readily by the measurement of platelet enzyme activity, no easily accessible source of MAO-A exists for the evaluation of its inhibition in human. The neurotransmitter NA is a preferred substrate of MAO-A (Fowler and Ross, 1984) and plasma concentrations of two of its metabolites, DOPEG and 3-methoxy-4-hydroxy-phenylethylglycol (MHPG), have been used as indirect indicators of effects on NA metabolism (Pickar et al., 1981; Goldstein et al., 1988; Koulu et al., 1989). Similarly, PEA is a preferred substrate of MAO-B (Boulton, 1991) and plasma PEA concentrations could be indicative of MAO-B inhibition. The present report describes the results of the analysis of plasma catechol DOPEG, NA, A, DOPA, DOPAC, DA and PEA concentrations before, during and after the subchronic, oral administration of single, daily doses of MDL 72,974A over a 10-day period to healthy, male volunteers.

Methods

Study design

The study was carried out as an open trial in two groups of six subjects who were administered 12 or 24 mg/day MDL 72,974A over a 10-day period. Subjects were between the ages of 19 and 43 years (height 177 ± 7 cm; weight 72 ± 9 kg) and all had given informed consent. The study was approved by the local Ethics Committee.

Plasma samples for biochemical measurements were taken on three occasions before the beginning of drug treatment (Day −2, Day −1 and on Day 1 before the initial dose of MDL 72,974A), during drug treatment (Days 3, 4, 5, 6, 7, 8, 9 and 10) and during the follow-up period (Days 17 and 21). All plasma samples for biochemical marker analysis were taken between 07:30 h and 08:00 h. On each day, 10 ml blood were drawn into chilled heparin tubes and the plasma was separated immediately in a refrigerated centrifuge. Following separation, the plasma was removed, frozen immediately and stored at −20°C until analyzed.

Materials and chemicals

All chemicals and solvents were of the purest analytical grade available and water with a resistance greater than 10 MΩ cm^{-1} was obtained from a MilliQ apparatus (Millipore, St Quentin-Yvelines, France). All reference standards were purchased from Sigma (Saint Quentin Fallavier, France).

Catechol analysis

Plasma catechol analysis was carried out according to the method of Eisenhofer et al. (1986) with minor modifications. Plasma catechols were adsorbed onto 20 mg alumina from 1 ml plasma (made basic with 0.5 ml 0.1 M Tris-HCl buffer (pH 8.0)) in the presence of 2 ng of the internal standard, 3,4-dihydroxybenzylamine (DHBA)). After two succesive washes with 1.5 ml water, the catechols were desorbed in 250 μl 0.2 N HClO$_4$ of which 100 μl were injected by a WISP automatic injector (Waters, Saint Quentin, Yvelines, France). Separation of the catechols was achieved on a reverse-phase HPLC Spherisorb ODS2 column (25 cm × 4.6 mm i.d., 5 μm particle size) (SFCC, Neuilly-Plaisance, France) at a flow rate of 1 ml/min using a mobile phase composed of NaH$_2$PO$_4$ · H$_2$O (13.80 g/l), sodium octanesulphonic acid (200 mg/l) and disodium EDTA (90 mg/l) adjusted to pH 2.80 with 85% o-phosphoric acid and a linear gradient of 0 to 8% acetonitrile over 15 min. Quantification was by reductive electrochemical detection using an ESA coulometric detector (Eurosep, Cergy-Pontoise, France) with the conditioning cell potential set at +0.30 V, the

first working cell at +0.15 V and the second working cell at −0.35 V. The method was calibrated over the concentration range 50 pg/ml to 2000 pg/ml with calibration curves run in duplicate with each daily analysis. Identification, integration and calculations were carried out using a Maxima 820 Chromatography Manager (Waters).

PEA analysis

PEA analysis was carried out using a previously described method (Huebert et al. (1994a). A brief description is given here. PEA was extracted with cyclohexane (2 × 2 ml) from 1 ml plasma, which had been adjusted to basic pH with 50 μl 10 N NaOH and which contained 11 ng phenylpropylamine (PPA) as internal standard. The organic phase was separated, acidified with 20 μl ethylacetate containing 2 M acetic acid and evaporated to dryness under N$_2$. The residue was reconstituted in 200 μl water.

The amine groups of PEA and PPA were derivatized with o-phthalaldehyde (OPA) and 2-mercaptoethanol to yield their isoindole adducts by an automated precolumn derivatization method using a Waters WISP 715 automatic injector in the auto-transfer mode (Waters). Ten μl of the OPA reagent were added to the 200 μl sample and mixed three times with a mixing volume of 100 μl. The derivatized sample was injected immediately with an injection volume of 100 μl.

Reverse-phase HPLC (Spherisorb C8 column : 7.5 × 100 mm; 5 mm) (SFCC) separated the adducts from unreacted reagent and other amines. The mobile phase (0.0375 N acetate buffer (pH 5.4)/acetonitrile (44/56)) was delivered at a flow rate of 1.5 ml/min and the amines were separated with retention times of 7.5 and 9.5 min for PEA and PPA, respectively.

Amperometric detection (Waters) on a glassy carbon electrode, maintained at a potential of +0.75 V versus a Ag/AgCl reference electrode, provided the sensitive and specific quantification of PEA. The method was calibrated over the concentration range from 60 pg/ml to 2 ng/ml with calibration curves run in duplicate with each daily analysis. Identification, integration and calculations were carried out using a Maxima 820 Chromatography Manager (Waters).

Statistical analysis

The plasma concentrations of the biochemical parameters were analyzed by repeated measures analysis of variance (ANOVA) in order to determine changes over time. When statistically significant changes were seen the results were analysed using Dunnett's multiple comparisons test to determine differences from the baseline measure which was represented by the arithmetic mean of the three predose values (Days −2, −1 and 1).

Results

No statistically significant changes in A, DOPA, DOPAC or DA concentrations were seen at either dose (data not shown). Analysis of variance indicated a statistically significant change in NA concentrations from baseline at the 12 mg dose ($P = 0.003$) but not at the 24 mg dose. Dunnett's multiple comparison test showed no statistically

significant changes during the drug administration period but indicated a significant difference between the concentrations on follow-up Day 17 compared with control ($P < 0.05$) (Fig. 1). No statistically significant change in DOPEG concentration was seen with the administration of 12 mg MDL 72,974A (Fig. 2) but statistically significant differences were seen with the 24 mg dose (Fig. 3). The plasma concentrations on days 4, 5, 6, 8, and 9 were significantly lower compared to baseline values ($P < 0.05$).

No statistically significant change in PEA concentration was seen with the administration of 12 mg MDL 72,974A but a statistically significant change over time was seen with the 24 mg dose (Fig. 4). The plasma PEA concentration was significantly elevated only on day 9 compared to baseline values ($P < 0.05$).

Discussion

MDL 72,974A has been shown to be a very specific inhibitor of MAO-B in vitro and in vivo in rats

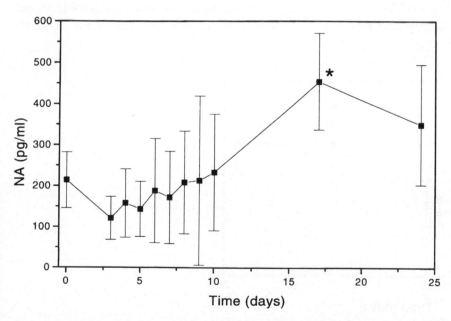

Fig. 1. Plasma NA concentrations before, during and after the administration of single, daily doses of 12 mg MDL 72,974A over a 10-day period. *$P < 0.05$ (Dunnett's multiple comparison test).

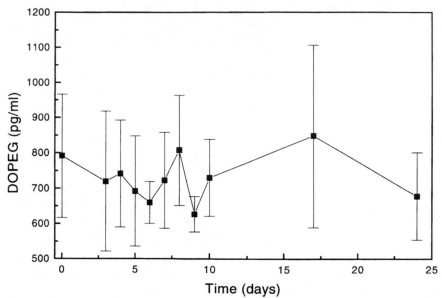

Fig. 2. Plasma DOPEG concentrations before, during and after the administration of single, daily doses of 12 mg MDL 72,974A over a 10-day period.

(Zreika et al., 1989). This drug has also been shown to be a very potent inhibitor of platelet MAO-B in man with > 95% inhibition achieved with single doses as low as 0.5 mg (Duléry et al., 1993). In order to verify the selectivity of inhibi- tion, a measure of MAO-A activity equivalent to that of platelet MAO-B activity would be prefer- able; however, there is no appreciable MAO-A activity in plasma and no readily accessible source of the enzyme in man. The specificity of MAO

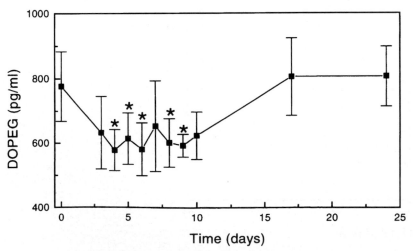

Fig. 3. Plasma DOPEG concentrations before, during and after the administration of single, daily doses of 24 mg MDL 72,974A over a 10-day period. *$P < 0.05$ (Dunnett's multiple comparison test).

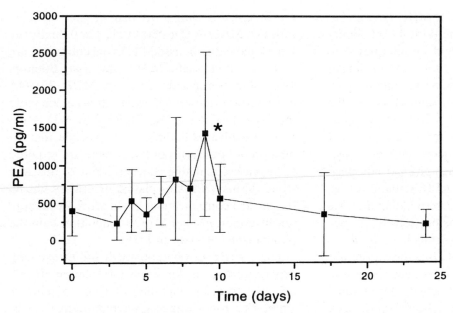

Fig. 4. Plasma PEA concentrations before, during and after the administration of single, daily doses of 24 mg MDL 72,974A over a 10-day period. *$P <$ 0.05 (Dunnett's multiple comparison test).

inhibition was therefore investigated using indirect measures of MAO-A and MAO-B activity.

Amines have been classified as substrates of MAO-A or MAO-B based on their relative affinities for the two forms of the enzyme (Fowler and Ross, 1984). Consequently, NA, A and serotonin have been classed as substrates of MAO-A because their affinities, as determined by relative K_m values, are greater than for MAO-B, whereas DA has been classed as a nonspecific substrate since it is metabolized equally well by both forms of the enzyme. On the other hand, PEA is oxidized by MAO-B at much lower concentrations than by MAO-A and is the best known endogenous substrate for MAO-B (Boulton, 1991). Since MAO represents the major catabolic pathway for the biogenic amines, its inhibition would be expected to result in increases in the concentration of substrates and decreases in the concentration of the corresponding metabolites.

The effect of pharmacological manipulations on the noradrenergic system have been studied extensively by a number of groups (Pickar et al., 1981; Goldstein et al., 1983, 1985, 1986, 1988;

Howes et al., 1986; Kallio et al., 1988; Scheinin et al., 1988; Koulu et al., 1989). Howes et al. (1986) have shown that NA is a better indicator of sympathetic activity than its metabolite, DOPEG. On the other hand, the results of other studies seem to indicate that DOPEG is a better indicator of intraneuronal NA metabolism (Goldstein et al., 1983, 1985, 1988). Both plasma DOPEG (Eisenhofer et al., 1986; Howes et al., 1986; Koulu et al., 1989) and plasma MHPG (Pickar et al., 1981) have been used as indicators of MAO-A inhibition in human but DOPEG would seem to be a better choice for two reasons. Firstly, while DOPEG concentrations are lower than MHPG concentrations, plasma DOPEG appears to constitute a small metabolic pool with a fast turnover rate and, thus, is more sensitive to inhibition of its formation. Secondly, plasma DOPEG concentrations do not exhibit the diurnal variations seen with plasma MHPG (DeMet et al,. 1985; Dennis et al., 1986; Gwirtsman et al., 1989) and thus changes are more easily interpreted.

In the present study, plasma DOPEG concentrations remained unchanged during the administration of 12 mg daily doses of MDL 72,974A but decreased significantly by the third day of administration of 24 mg. This might be interpreted to indicate that the 24 mg dose is no longer biochemically specific and some inhibition of intraneuronal MAO-A is occurring. However, the magnitude of the change in DOPEG concentrations, while significant, was much less that that seen with other MAO inhibitors such as tranylcypromine and deprenyl (when given at nonspecific doses of 30 to 60 mg/day) (Eisenhofer et al., 1986). Thus the lack of a corresponding increase in NA or A concentrations is not surprising since these amines can also be metabolized by other enzymes such as catechol-O-methyltransferase and would suggest that there is nevertheless no change in sympatho-adrenal activity. In addition, changes in plasma DOPA concentrations seen with the previous MAO inhibitors indicating feedback inhibition of the catecholamine metabolic pathways were not seen in the present study.

Unlike the catechols, PEA is metabolized almost exclusively by MAO and its affinity for MAO-B is much greater than its affinity for MAO-A ($K_m^A/K_m^B = 35$) (Dostert et al., 1989). Since the inhibition of MAO-B is known to increase tissue concentrations of this substrate significantly (Boulton, 1991), it was decided to investigate whether an increase in the plasma concentrations of this substrate would be associated with doses of MDL 72,974A capable of inhibiting completely the platelet enzyme and thus provide a more functional measure of MAO-B inhibition. MDL 72,974A did not increase PEA concentrations at the 12 mg dose but a significant increase was seen at the 24 mg dose. Since platelet MAO-B is completely inhibited at these two doses and since, at the higher dose, effects on MAO-A inhibition were also evident, it would seem likely that MAO-B inhibition alone is not sufficient to result in increases in the circulating concentrations of this substrate. Although PEA is considered a specific substrate for MAO-B its affinity

for MAO-A is similar to that of specific substrates of MAO-A (Dostert et al., 1989). Since the largest increases in tissue PEA concentrations are seen with nonspecific MAO inhibitors (Boulton, 1991) and nonspecific doses of MDL 72,974A increase rat brain PEA concentrations much more than selective doses (M. Zreika and N.D. Huebert, unpublished findings), it is possible that inhibition of both forms of the enzyme are required to increase circulating concentrations of this substrate. Urinary PEA or plasma or urinary phenylacetic acid concentrations could prove to be more sensitive indicators of MAO-B inhibition than the plasma concentration of PEA.

The occurrence of a potentially life-threatening hypertensive crisis, known as the "cheese effect", resulting from the ingestion of sympathomimetic amine-rich foods (especially tyramine-rich foods) during MAO inhibitor treatment has hindered the widespread use of these inhibitors as therapeutic agents. Intestinal MAO plays an important role in the breakdown of orally ingested p-tyramine that is present in foodstuffs (Marley and Blackwell, 1970; DaPrada et al., 1988) and the inhibition of intestinal and hepatic MAO results in enhanced bioavailability of p-tyramine. The potentiation of the hypertensive effect of p-tyramine has been demonstrated with selective inhibitors of the A form, with nonspecific inhibitors which inhibit both forms of the enzyme and with nonselective doses of MAO-B inhibitors, that is doses of MAO-B-selective inhibitors that are sufficiently high to inhibit also MAO-A, but not with MAO-B selective doses (Zimmer, 1990). In a previously published study (Huebert et al., 1994b), we showed that the sub-chronic administration of 1, 12 or 24 mg MDL 72974A did not potentiate the effects of orally administered p-tyramine or enhance its oral bioavailability. In addition, there were no changes in any of the pharmacokinetic parameters of p-tyramine or its major metabolite, p-hydroxyphenylacetic acid, indicating no changes in the systemic metabolism of p-tyramine. The potentiation of a p-tyramine pressor response has three possible components: decreased presystemic clearance of *p*-tyramine in the gastrointestinal tract and liver, decreased systemic metabolism of *p*-tyramine and increased systemic sensitivity to circulating *p*-tyramine concentrations due to the inhibition of NA metabolism by MAO-A. The present study combined with that published previously (Huebert et al., 1994b) would suggest that at daily doses up to and including 24 mg, there should be no risk of hypertensive crises being provoked by dietary *p*-tyramine. However, the small but significant decreases in plasma DOPEG seen with 24 mg MDL 72974A would suggest that further studies would be required if dosing were to be extended beyond the current dose range.

Summary

Plasma concentrations of 3,4-dihydroxyphenylethylglycol (DOPEG), noradrenaline (NA), adrenaline (A), 3,4-dihydroxyphenylalanine (DOPA), 3,4-dihydroxyphenylacetic acid (DOPAC), dopamine (DA) and phenylethylamine (PEA) were analyzed in samples taken prior to, during and following the administration of single, daily doses of 12 or 24 mg MDL 72,974A to healthy male volunteers. No effects on the concentrations of DOPA, A, DA or DOPAC were seen during the administration of either dose over 10 days. No treatment-related changes in the concentration of NA were evident at either dose. No changes in DOPEG or PEA concentrations were seen with the 12 mg dose; however, small but significant decreases in plasma DOPEG concentrations and a significant increase in PEA were seen during the administration of the 24 mg dose. This would suggest that at the 24 mg dose some intraneuronal inhibition of MAO-A may be occurring although the lack of increases in NA and A concentrations indicates no accompanying change in sympatho-adrenal activity. Plasma PEA concentrations do not provide a more sensitive or functional indication of MAO-B inhibition. The increase in PEA concentrations at the higher dose may suggest that the inhibition of both forms of the enzyme is necessary to increase its plasma concentration.

References

Boulton, A.A. (1991) Phenylethylaminergic modulation of catecholaminergic neurotransmission. *Prog. Neuropsychopharmacol. Biol. Psychiatry*, 15: 139–156.

Da Prada, M., Zurcher, G., Wuthrich, I. and Haefely, W.E. (1988) On tyramine, food, beverages and the reversible MAO inhibitor moclobemide. *J. Neural Transm. 26(Suppl): 31–56.*

DeMet, E.M. Halaris, A.E., Gwirtsman, H.E. and Reno, R.M. *(1985) Diurnal rhythm of 3-methoxy-4-hydroxyphenylglycol (MHPG): relationship between plasma and urinary levels. Life Sci., 37: 1731–1741.*

Dennis, T., Benkelfat, C., Touitou, Y., Auzeby, A., Poirier, M-F., Scatton, B. and Loo, H. (1986) Lack of circadian rhythm in plasma levels of 3,4-dihydroxyphenylethyleneglycol in healthy human subjects. *Psychopharmacology*, 90: 471–474.

Dostert, P.L., Stroloine Benedetti, M.S. and Tipton, K.F. (1989) Interactions of monoamine oxidase with substrates and inhibitors. *Med. Res. Rev.*, 9: 45–89.

Duléry, B.D., Schoun, J., Zreika, M., Dow, J., Huebert, N., Hinze, C. and Haegele, K.D. (1993) Pharmacokinetics of and monoamine oxidase B inhibition by (*E*)-4-fluoro-β-fluoromethylene benzene butaneamine in man. *Arzneim-Forsch./Drug Res.*, 43: 297–302.

Eisenhofer, G., Goldstein, D.S., Stull, R., Keiser, H.R., Sunderland, T., Murphy, D.L. and Kopin, IJ. (1986) Simultaneous liquid-chromatrographic determination of 3,4-dihydroxyphenylglycol, catecholamines and 3,4-dihydroxyphenylalanine in plasma and their responses to inhibition of monoamine oxidase. *Clin. Chem.*, 32: 2030–2033.

Fowler, C.J. and Ross, S.B. (1984) Selective inhibitors of monoamine oxidase A and B: Biochemical, pharmacological and clinical properties. Med. Res. Rev., 4: 323–358.

Goldstein, D.S., Eisenhofer, G., Stull, R., Fodio, C.J., Keiser, H.R.and Kopin, I.J. (1988) Plasma dihydroxyphenylglycol and the intraneuronal disposition of norepinephrine in humans. *J. Clin. Invest.*, 81: 213–220.

Goldstein, D.S., McCarty, R., Polinsky, R.J. and Kopin, I.J. (1983) Relationship between plasma norepinephrine and sympathetic neural activity. *Hypertension*, 5: 552–559.

Goldstein, D.S., Zimlichman, R., Stull, R., Folio, J., Levinson, P.D. and Keiser, H.R. (1985) Measurement of regional neuronal removal of norepinephrine in man. *J. Clin. Invest.*, 76: 15–21.

Goldstein, D.S., Zimlichman, R., Stull, R., Keiser, H.R. and Kopin, I.J. (1986) Estimation of intrasynaptic norepinephrine concentrations in humans. *Hypertension*, 8: 471–475.

Gwirtsman, H.E., Halaris, A.E., Wolf, A.W., DeMet, E,. Piletz, J.E. and Marler, M. (1989) Apparent phase advance in diurnal MHPG rhythm in depression. *Am. J. Psychiat*, 146: 1427–1433.

Howes, L.G., Hawksby, C.C., Reid, J.L. (1986) Comparison of plasma 3,4-dihydroxyphenyl-ethyleneglycol (DHPG) and norepinephrine levels as indices of sympathetic activity in man. *Eur. J. Clin. Invest.*, 16: 18–21.

Huebert, N.D., Schwach, V., Richter, G., Zreika, M., Hinze, C. and Haegele, K.D. (1994a) Analytical method for the bio-analysis of β-phenylethylamine. *Anal. Biochem.*, 221: 42–47.

Huebert, N.D., Schwach, V., Hinze, C. and Haegele, K.D. (1994b) Kinetics and metabolism of *p*-tyramine during monoamine oxidase inhibition by mofegiline. *Clin. Pharmacol. Ther.* (in press).

Kallio, A., Koulu, M., Ponkilainen, R., Scheinin, H. and Scheinin, M. (1988) Plasma DHPG does not reflect reduction of noradrenaline release after alpha2-adrenoceptor agonist administration in man. *Psychopharmacology (Berlin)*, 96(Suppl): 375.

Koulu, M., Scheinin, M., Kaarttinen, A., Kallio, J., Pyykko, K., Vuorinen, J., and Zimmer, R.H. (1989) Inhibition of monoamine oxidase by moclobemide: effects on monoamine metabolism and secretion of anterior pituitary hormones and cortisol in healthy volunteers. *Br. J. Clin. Pharmacol.*, 27: 243–255.

Marley, E. and Blackwell, B. (1970) Interactions of monoamine oxidase inhibitors, amines and foodstuffs. *Adv. Pharmacol. Chemother.*, 8: 185–239.

Pickar, D., Cohen, R.M., Jimerson, D.C., Lake, C.R. and Murphy, D.L. (1981) Tyramine infusions and selective monoamine oxidase inhibitor treatment: II Interrelationships among pressor sensitivity changes, platelet MAO inhibition, and plasma MHPG reduction. *Psychopharmacology*, 74: 8–12.

Scheinin, M., Koulu, M., Zimmer, R., Kaartinen, A., Kallio, and J. Pyykkoe, K. (1988) *Psychopharmacology (Berlin)* 96(Suppl.): 228.

Zimmer, R. (1990) Relationship between tyramine potentiation and monoamine oxidase (MAO) inhibition: comparison between moclobemide and othe MAO inhibitors. *Acta Psychiatr. Scand.*, 360(Suppl.): 81–83.

Zreika, M., Fozard, J.R., Dudley, M.W., Bey, P.H., McDonald, I.A. and Palfreyman, M.G. (1989) MDL 72974: a potent and selective enzyme-activated irreversible inhibitor of monoamine oxidase type B with potential for use in Parkinson's disease. *J. Neural Transm. [P-D Sect.]*, 1: 283–254.

Peter M. Yu, Keith F. Tipton and Alan A. Boulton (Eds.)
Progress in Brain Research, Vol 106
© 1995 Elsevier Science BV. All rights reserved.

CHAPTER 15

The distribution of orally administered (−)-deprenyl-propynyl-^{14}C and (−)-deprenyl-phenyl-^{3}H in rat brain

K. Magyar[1], J. Lengyel[2], I. Szatmári[3] and J. Gaál[3]

[1]*Department of Pharmacodynamics,* [2]*Central Isotope Laboratory, Semmelweis University of Medicine, and* [3]*CHINOIN Pharmaceutical and Chemical Works Co. Ltd., Budapest, Hungary*

Introduction

It has been confirmed in many laboratories, as in ours, that (−)-deprenyl is metabolized to methylamphetamine and amphetamine (Reynolds et al., 1978; Magyar and Szüts, 1982; Magyar and Tóthfalusi, 1984; Heinonen et al., 1989). In spite of the formation of amphetamines, deprenyl did not prove to be a potent releaser of biogenic amines (Knoll and Magyar, 1972). The lack of releasing effect of (−)-deprenyl could be due firstly to the fact that from (−)-deprenyl only the (−)-isomers of amphetamines can be formed, which have lower releasing potency than the (+)-forms. It was proved earlier in parkinsonian patients that racemase did not convert the (−)-amphetamines to their (+)-forms (Schachter et al., 1980). The second explanation for the poor releasing effect of (−)-deprenyl is that not the amphetamines themselves, but their metabolites (e.g. *p*-hydroxy-norephedrine) are responsible for the release of noradrenaline from the depot granules (Brodie et al., 1970). Only the (+)-*p*-hydroxy-amphetamine is converted to (+)-*p*-hydroxy-norephedrine in vivo (the (−)-*p*-hydroxy-amphetamine is not a substrate for beta-hydroxylase). This can explain the difference between the releasing potency of the different enantiomers (Goldstein and Anagnoste, 1965).

Pretreatment with (−)-deprenyl is able to prevent the toxic effect of MPTP (*N*-methyl-4-phenyl-1,2,3,6-tetrahydropyridine) in the dopaminergic (Langston, 1985), DSP-4 (*N*-(2-chloroethyl)-*N*-ethyl-2-bromobenzylamine, in the noradrenergic (Finnegan et al., 1990; Finnegan, 1993; Magyar, 1991, 1993, 1994) and AF64A (methyl-β-acetoxyethyl-2-chloroethylamine) in the cholinergic (Ricci et al., 1992) neurons. All of the MAO-B inhibitors are effective to prevent MPTP toxicity, but only (−)-deprenyl and not the MDL72974 compound (in spite of being a potent MAO-B inhibitor) was effective against DSP-4 toxicity (Finnegan et al., 1990).

The inhibition of the carrier-mediated uptake process of noradrenaline plays an essential role in the prevention of DSP-4-induced neurotoxicity. We proved rather early that deprenyl and its optical isomers inhibit [^{3}H]noradrenaline uptake into cerebral cortex slices of mice (Knoll and Magyar, 1972; Magyar, 1980). Recent experiments revealed that not only the parent compound but also its metabolites are responsible for inhibition of the synaptosomal uptake of noradrenaline and dopamine (Magyar, 1994). Neither (−)-deprenyl nor its metabolites inhibit the synaptosomal uptake of serotonin.

In inhibiting noradrenaline uptake (−)-methylamphetamine, a metabolite of (−)-deprenyl, is about 10-times as potent as the parent compound. Based upon the preventive role of (−)-deprenyl metabolites in the carrier-mediated selective neurotoxicity induced by DSP-4 (and probably by AF64A), we investigated the in vivo metabolism and pharmacokinetic behaviour of (−)-deprenyl in rats. The usual chromatographic methods (HPLC and GC) were not sensitive enough for this purpose and we therefore chose the isotope technique for these studies.

Experiments were undertaken in rats to investigate the in vivo pharmacokinetics of (−)-deprenyl by using the two alternatively and positionally labelled radioisomers of the compound: (−)-deprenyl-propynyl-^{14}C (^{14}C-deprenyl) and (−)-deprenyl-phenyl-^{3}H (^{3}H-deprenyl).

The animals received 1.5 mg/kg (−)-deprenyl orally. The substance administered contained a mixture of ^{3}H- and ^{14}C-labelled (−)-deprenyl. By measuring the radioactivity of both labels simultaneously the levels of (−)- deprenyl in the plasma and in 15 regions of the brain were determined as a function of time, on the basis of the specific activities of the two radioisomers, separately. The alternate label (^{3}H or ^{14}C) provided an estimation of the metabolic disintegration of the compound.

Materials, animals and methods

Labelled substances

^{3}H-deprenyl: (−)-N-methyl-N-propynyl-2-phenyl-1-methyl-ethylamine · HCl-(phenyl-^{3}H), specific activity: 740 GBq/mmol (dissolved in 96% ethanol; 54.76 MBq/ml).

^{14}C-deprenyl: (−)-N-methyl-N-propynyl-2-phenyl-1-methyl-ethylamine · HCl-(propynyl-^{14}C), specific activity: 715.0 MBq/mmol. The ^{14}C-labelled radioisomer was synthesized in the Drug Research Institute (Budapest, Hungary), while the ^{3}H-deprenyl was labelled in the Biological Research Center of the Hungarian Academy of Sciences (Szeged, Hungary). The unlabelled (−)-de-

prenyl was produced and supplied by CHINOIN (Budapest, Hungary).

Animals and treatment

Male Wistar rats (LATI, Budapest, Hungary) weighing 150–160 g were used in this study. The animals were housed three to a cage at a temperature of $22.0 \pm 2.0°C$. The animals received 1.5 mg/kg of (−)-deprenyl orally from a stock solution, which contained 0.15 mg/ml (−)-deprenyl, with 0.86 MBq ^{3}H and 0.19 MBq ^{14}C radioactivy. Before treatment, the animals were deprived of food for 12 h, but they had free access to water. 1 ml per 100 g body weight of the above stock solution was administered via a gastric probe.

Determination of plasma levels

Blood samples were taken at 15, 30, 45 and 60 min, 2, 4, 6, 8, 12, 24, 48, 72 and 96 h after drug intake. The rats were decapitated, and blood was collected in centrifuge tubes containing 500 IU of heparin. The blood was left undisturbed for 1 h, then centrifuged at $1500 \times g$ for 10 min. From plasma 50 μl samples were taken for radioactivity measurement.

Determination of radioactivity in the cerebral tissues

Decapitation was performed just below the foramen magnum. The skull was opened along the suturae. The cerebral tissues dissected were: corpus pineale, bulbus olfactorius, hypophysis, hypothalamus, tuberculum olfactorium, substantia nigra, corpus mamillare, frontal cortex, corpus striatum, hippocampus, colliculus superior, cerebellum, pons + colliculus inferior, medulla oblongata. After removing the brain, the bulbus olfactorius and hypophysis remained in the cranium, and they were excised following the removal of the brain. Apart from the cortex, of which only a sample was taken, each other part of the brain was treated as a whole. Dissection of the brain was carried out according to the atlas of Paxinos and Watson (1986). The cerebral tissues (irrespective of the mass) were placed in a mixture of 500 μl Soluene-350 and 350 μl isopropyl alcohol, and they were completely dissolved within 72 h. Radioactivity was determined by the liquid scintillation technique.

Liquid scintillation measurements

The radioactivity of plasma and brain tissues was counted using a Beckman LS 1801 apparatus. Quench correction was made by using ^{137}Cs as an external standard. The composition of the scintillation cocktail was: 833 ml dioxane, 137 ml methylcellosolve, 60 g naphthalene, 84 ml liquifluor. The liquifluor was composed of: 100.0 g PPO, 1.25 g POPOP, 1000 ml toluene. 50 μl aliquots of plasma were added to 10 ml scintillation cocktail. For counting the radioactivity of the brain tissues a volume of 15 ml acidic cocktail (dioxane cocktail plus 0.5 N HCl, in a ratio of 10:1) was used.

Checking of the stability of radiolabels

The stability studies were performed as follows. (1) The stock solution of ^{3}H-deprenyl was diluted (100 $\times$) with distilled water. A known quantity of ^{14}C-deprenyl (tracer) was added, and the solution was kept at 37°C for 24 h, then let to flow through a column packed with XAD-2 absorbent resin (Serva). The substance was eluted by methanol, and the radioactivity of the aqueous solution (^{3}H-water exchange) was determined. This was found to be as low as 0.17 or 0.48 percent of the total radioactivity transferred to the column for ^{3}H or ^{14}C, respectively. If (−)-deprenyl had not been adsorbed by XAD-2, both ^{3}H and ^{14}C activity would have been high. Provided that the ^{3}H label, as a result of isotope-exchange, had been incorporated in water, then this activity should have been detected in the aqueous phase. The position of ^{3}H label in the molecule appeared to be stable. (2) The stability of the propargyl residue was checked by adding 0.1 N HCl and keeping the compound at 37°C for 60 min. The ratio of the compound and its decomposed part was also determined using the method described above. In this case, the aqueous eluate contained 2.4 percent of the initial ^{14}C-radioactivity, indicating the stability of the propargyl group. The stability of the labelled radioisomers indicates that any

change in the molar ratio of (−)-deprenyl as calculated either from the specific activity of the ^{14}C or ^{3}H tracer should be due to the metabolic disintegration of the active ingredient.

Results

Based upon the specific activity of ^{3}H measurements in the plasma, the molar concentration of (−)-deprenyl was determined (Table 1, Fig. 2). The peak plasma level was detected as early as 15 min after oral administration of 1.5 mg/kg (−)-deprenyl. The concentrations measured at 30 and 45 min after drug intake were found to be similar to the 15 min level. The ^{3}H-radioactivity in the plasma started to decrease 60 min following the ingestion of the substance. The decrease was going on continuously, then at the 6th h another peak was observed. The further elimination took place at a low speed. It should be noted that when calculating the concentrations from ^{3}H, as late as 96 h after (−)-deprenyl intake, still 25% of the maximum level was measured in the plasma. The plasma levels could not be modelled using the traditional compartment analysis (one or two compartment open model), because of the lack of sufficient sampling during the rapid upward phase of absorption. Therefore, only the AUC_{0-t} values, which amounted to 107.9 nmol/ml per h, were calculated.

When the molar concentrations of deprenyl in the plasma were calculated from the ^{14}C tracer (after giving 1.5 mg/kg deprenyl), the values were higher than those calculated from the ^{3}H label, the ratio being 1.6:1 within 45 min following drug intake (Table 1, Fig. 2). This ratio decreased in the later phase; then, in the 4th h, it was reversed, i.e. the amount of ^{3}H label exceeded the quantity of ^{14}C tracer. ^{14}C radioactivity could not be detected in the plasma 48 h after the administration of the compound. The AUC_{0-t} value in the plasma according to the ^{14}C-label was found to be 33.59 nmol/ml per h.

In the brain regions studied, on the basis of ^{3}H-radioactivity the peak concentrations (C_{max}) were seen 30 to 45 min (t_{max}) after drug adminis-

TABLE 1

Time-related changes in the concentrations of orally given $(-)$-deprenyl detected in the plasma and brain tissues

Time (h)	Plasma (nmol/ml)		Frontal cortex (pmol/mg)		Parietal cortex (pmol/mg)		Hypothalamus (pmol/mg)	
	^{3}H	^{14}C	^{3}H	^{14}C	^{3}H	^{14}C	^{3}H	^{14}C
0.25	1.60 ± 0.11	2.47 ± 0.25	2.76 ± 0.22	1.27 ± 0.08	2.75 ± 0.24	1.15 ± 0.19	2.38 ± 0.67	1.06 ± 0.33
0.5	1.69 ± 0.19	2.61 ± 0.11	3.31 ± 0.44	1.02 ± 0.10	3.45 ± 0.77	0.97 ± 0.09	1.92 ± 0.16	1.17 ± 0.59
0.75	1.60 ± 0.33	2.54 ± 0.25	3.54 ± 0.40	1.20 ± 0.24	3.41 ± 1.56	1.12 ± 0.20	2.55 ± 0.23	1.38 ± 0.43
1	1.15 ± 0.33	1.66 ± 0.44	2.62 ± 0.14	0.60 ± 0.37	2.19 ± 0.32	0.82 ± 0.15	1.78 ± 0.74	0.67 ± 0.18
2	1.14 ± 0.22	1.25 ± 0.23	1.11 ± 0.20	0.73 ± 0.17	1.19 ± 0.14	0.84 ± 0.24	1.45 ± 0.62	0.94 ± 0.35
4	0.93 ± 0.21	0.71 ± 0.02	1.12 ± 0.20	0.57 ± 0.10	0.81 ± 0.22	0.60 ± 0.05	0.50 ± 0.12	0.64 ± 0.50
6	1.26 ± 0.18	0.75 ± 0.20	2.81 ± 2.20	0.75 ± 0.05	0.93 ± 0.31	0.91 ± 0.23	0.67 ± 0.17	0.52 ± 0.18
8	1.17 ± 0.06	0.52 ± 0.08	0.81 ± 0.56	0.67 ± 0.05	1.17 ± 0.06	0.58 ± 0.05	1.02 ± 0.38	0.55 ± 0.21
12	0.89 ± 0.23	0.30 ± 0.08	1.34 ± 0.16	0.40 ± 0.15	1.13 ± 0.24	0.38 ± 0.08	0.91 ± 0.10	0.45 ± 0.21
24	0.79 ± 0.66	0.16 ± 0.00	1.25 ± 0.21	0.41 ± 0.08	1.09 ± 0.36	0.35 ± 0.06	0.82 ± 0.02	0.38 ± 0.
48	0.59 ± 0.08	0	1.02 ± 0.28	0.36 ± 0.11	0.80 ± 0.20	0.31 ± 0.19	0.73 ± 0.47	0.43 ± 0.13
72	0.48 ± 0.09	0	0.60 ± 0.09	0.16 ± 0.04	0.54 ± 0.13	0.29 ± 0.03	0.77 ± 0.42	0.32 ± 0.10
96	0.38 ± 0.04	0	0.58 ± 0.09	0.26 ± 0.09	0.53 ± 0.04	0.23 ± 0.05	0.67 ± 0.19	0.28 ± 0.07

Treatment and calculations as in Fig. 1. (mean ± S.D.; $n = 3$)

tration. Based upon the 45 min values, the cerebral tissues can be divided into three groups (Fig. 1): (1) the level in corpus striatum was similar to that found in the plasma; (2) concentrations exceeding those of the plasma (but less than double the latter) were detected in several brain tissues, such as corpus pineale, bulbus olfactorius, hypothalamus, tuberculum olfactorium, corpus mamillare, frontal and parietal cortex, hippocampus, cerebellum, pons + colliculus inf. and medulla oblongata; (3) more than double the level of plasma was found in the hypophysis, substantia nigra and colliculus inferior.

Between 6 and 12 h following drug intake, just as in the plasma, another rise of radioactivity was seen in some of the cerebral tissues (Figs. 2 and 3). This was especially marked in tissues weighing around 1 mg (substantia nigra, corpus pineale, nucleus mamillaris). In these tissues, the ^{3}H activity was reduced below the detection limit between the 2 and 6 h period, but thereafter the detectability returned. In the early phase of the experiments, the brain tissues contained twice as

much ^{3}H-radioactivity as did the plasma (Tables 1–4). This difference, however, disappeared by 4 to 6 h following drug ingestion, and in the small tissues weighing about 1 mg there was no detectable radioactivity. The highest level was found in the substantia nigra, though the values in this region showed the largest variability. As in the plasma, the elimination from the cerebral tissues was quite slow: 96 h after the administration of $(-)$-deprenyl, the ^{3}H-related activity in the brain exceeded that found in the plasma (Figs. 2 and 3). The numerical data demonstrating the ^{3}H-radioactivities in the tissues studied are summarized in Tables 1–4.

The data calculated from the ^{14}C label obtained 45 min after deprenyl administration are presented in Fig. 1. At this time the ^{14}C-related radioactivy in the plasma exceeded that detected in any cerebral tissues studied (Tables 1–4). The levels in the small tissues, weighing about 1 mg (substantia nigra, corpus pineale, nucleus mamillaris), were below the detection limit. Low values were measured in the corpus striatum; hypophysis

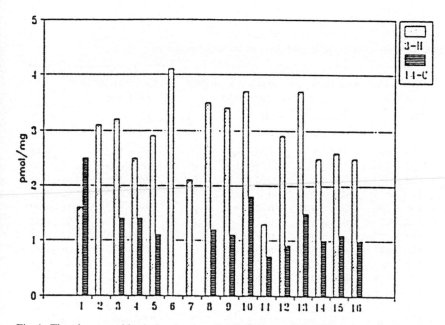

Fig. 1. The plasma and brain levels of orally administered alternatively and positionally labelled (−)-deprenyl (1.5 mg/kg) to rats 45 min after treatment. The radioactive doses from ^{3}H and ^{14}C labels were 0.86 and 0.19 MBq/100 g, respectively. The tissue levels were calculated on the basis of the specific activities of the ^{3}H and ^{14}C labelled radioisomers. 1 plasma, 2 corpus pineale, 3 bulbus olfactorius, 4 hypothalamus, 5 tuberculum olfactorium, 6 substantia nigra, 7 nucleus mamillaris, 8 frontal cortex, 9 parietal cortex, 10 hypophysis, 11 corpus striatum, 12 hippocampus, 13 colliculus superior, 14 medulla oblongata, 15 cerebellum, 16 pons + colliculus inferior.

TABLE 2

Time-related changes in the concentrations of orally given (−)-deprenyl detected in the brain tissues

Time (h)	Hypophysis (pmol/mg)		Hippocampus (pmol/mg)		Corpus striatum (pmol/mg)		Substantia nigra (pmol/mg)	
	^{3}H	^{14}C	^{3}H	^{14}C	^{3}H	^{14}C	^{3}H	^{14}C
0.25	1.87 ± 0.20	1.25 ± 0.21	1.63 ± 0.26	0.81 ± 0.16	1.04 ± 0.31	0.60 ± 0.17	4.54 ± 1.85	0
0.5	3.50 ± 0.95	1.58 ± 0.29	3.17 ± 0.05	0.76 ± 0.15	2.57 ± 0.71	0.69 ± 0.23	6.03 ± 1.30	0
0.75	3.67 ± 0.48	1.82 ± 0.24	3.00 ± 0.34	0.94 ± 0.22	1.82 ± 0.61	0.71 ± 0.30	4.34 ± 1.75	0
1	2.39 ± 0.46	1.42 ± 0.15	1.31 ± 0.22	0.52 ± 0.19	1.00 ± 0.28	0.42 ± 0.22	1.71 ± 0.81	0
2	1.32 ± 0.29	1.43 ± 0.21	1.10 ± 0.28	0.46 ± 0.28	0.71 ± 0.40	0.37 ± 0.12	0	0
4	0.51 ± 0.20	0.62 ± 0.10	1.17 ± 0.16	0.54 ± 0.12	0.75 ± 0.18	0.32 ± 0.05	0	0
6	0.53 ± 0.80	2.11 ± 1.74	1.13 ± 2.35	0.69 ± 0.24	0.61 ± 0.11	0.38 ± 0.06	0	0
8	0.64 ± 0.20	0.47 ± 0.10	0.91 ± 0.24	0.50 ± 0.11	0.73 ± 0.12	0.34 ± 0.09	2.14 ± 0.69	0
12	0.53 ± 0.15	0.71 ± 0.15	1.00 ± 0.17	0.27 ± 0.10	0.66 ± 0.23	0.20 ± 0.07	1.55 ± 0.51	0
24	0.55 ± 0.08	0.51 ± 0.17	0.86 ± 0.15	0.27 ± 0.05	0.51 ± 0.21	0.22 ± 0.09	1.64 ± 0.40	0
48	0.44 ± 0.13	0.46 ± 0.12	0.82 ± 0.32	0.30 ± 0.13	0.39 ± 0.07	0.21 ± 0.09	1.13 ± 0.37	0
72	0.44 ± 0.14	0	0.56 ± 0.19	0.21 ± 0.06	0.41 ± 0.14	0.17 ± 0.08	1.06 ± 0.34	0
96	0.50 ± 0.08	0	0.51 ± 0.12	0.18 ± 0.06	0.41 ± 0.10	0.14 ± 0.05	0.54 ± 0.30	0

Treatment and calculations as in Fig. 1. (mean ± S.D.; $n = 3$)

TABLE 3

Time-related changes in the concentrations of orally given (−)-deprenyl detected in the brain tissues

Time (h)	Bulbus olfactorius (pmol/mg) ^{3}H	^{14}C	Tuberculum olfactorium (pmol/mg) ^{3}H	^{14}C	Nucleus mamillaris (pmol/mg) ^{3}H	^{14}C	Colliculus superior (pmol/mg) ^{3}H	^{14}C
0.25	2.02 ± 1.11	1.20 ± 0.49	2.53 ± 0.88	1.07 ± 0.35	2.38 ± 0.72	0	3.01 ± 1.02	1.52 ± 0.44
0.5	2.57 ± 0.36	1.08 ± 0.18	3.46 ± 0.80	1.10 ± 0.25	2.28 ± 0.46	0	4.29 ± 0.95	1.49 ± 0.39
0.75	2.98 ± 0.81	1.33 ± 0.41	3.05 ± 0.33	1.17 ± 0.16	2.06 ± 0.19	0	3.92 ± 1.26	1.53 ± 0.43
1	2.15 ± 0.43	0.87 ± 0.17	2.49 ± 0.79	0.97 ± 0.29	0	0	2.38 ± 1.43	1.10 ± 0.32
2	1.42 ± 0.44	0.90 ± 0.33	1.36 ± 0.60	0.81 ± 0.41	0	0	1.96 ± 0.82	1.35 ± 0.49
4	1.15 ± 0.22	0.58 ± 0.15	1.44 ± 0.29	0.71 ± 0.12	0	0	2.11 ± 0.30	1.00 ± 0.44
6	1.07 ± 0.32	0.71 ± 0.19	1.01 ± 2.07	0.65 ± 0.28	0	0	1.29 ± 0.51	0.97 ± 0.29
8	0.92 ± 0.12	0.52 ± 0.07	1.16 ± 0.42	0.63 ± 0.19	0.82 ± 0.17	0	1.79 ± 0.62	1.04 ± 0.27
12	1.38 ± 0.50	0.46 ± 0.10	1.74 ± 0.40	0.80 ± 0.43	1.12 ± 0.16	0	1.72 ± 0.40	0.62 ± 0.14
24	1.09 ± 0.17	0.27 ± 0.05	1.42 ± 0.38	0.43 ± 0.08	0.98 ± 0.06	0	1.97 ± 0.44	0.62 ± 0.19
48	0.72 ± 0.33	0.34 ± 0.14	1.06 ± 0.56	0.41 ± 0.18	1.11 ± 0.07	0	1.44 ± 0.35	0.46 ± 0.04
72	0.57 ± 0.08	0.23 ± 0.05	0.76 ± 0.14	0.31 ± 0.08	0.66 ± 0.12	0	1.15 ± 0.45	0.41 ± 0.15
96	0.54 ± 0.13	0.23 ± 0.09	0.58 ± 0.21	0.28 ± 0.05	1.00 ± 0.23	0	0.84 ± 0.38	0.30 ± 0.17

Treatment and calculations as in Fig. 1. (mean ± S.D.; $n = 3$)

TABLE 4

Time-related changes in the concentrations of orally given (−)-deprenyl detected in the brain tissues

Time (h)	Corpus pineale (pmol/mg) ^{3}H	^{14}C	Cerebellum (pmol/mg) ^{3}H	^{14}C	Medulla oblongata (pmol/mg) ^{3}H	^{14}C	Pons + colliculus inferior (pmol/mg) ^{3}H	^{14}C
0.25	3.18 ± 0.97	0	2.09 ± 0.41	1.07 ± 0.16	1.82 ± 0.49	0.90 ± 0.18	2.28 ± 0.23	1.52 ± 0.09
0.5	5.71 ± 0.60	0	2044 ± 0.27	1.96 ± 0.08	2.43 ± 0.46	0.91 ± 0.18	2.28 ± 0.43	1.49 ± 0.12
0.75	3.09 ± 1.35	0	2.52 ± 0.42	0.95 ± 0.21	2.46 ± 0.40	0.96 ± 0.25	2.51 ± 1.38	1.53 ± 0.11
1	1.12 ± 0.20	0	1.89 ± 0.37	0.74 ± 0.16	1.99 ± 0.31	0.71 ± 0.09	1.68 ± 1.24	1.10 ± 0.07
2	0.37 ± 0.03	0	1.22 ± 0.28	0.82 ± 0.19	1.11 ± 0.33	0.67 ± 0.19	1.30 ± 0.26	1.35 ± 0.18
4	0	0	1.13 ± 0.27	0.59 ± 0.08	0.95 ± 0.15	0.44 ± 0.11	1.00 ± 0.08	1.00 ± 0.05
6	0	0	1.14 ± 0.24	0.83 ± 0.21	1.07 ± 0.28	0.68 ± 0.20	1.03 ± 0.25	0.97 ± 0.21
8	0.99 ± 0.30	0	1.12 ± 0.13	0.60 ± 0.05	1.09 ± 0.27	0.58 ± 0.18	1.01 ± 0.16	1.04 ± 0.09
12	0.93 ± 0.01	0	1.21 ± 0.23	0.37 ± 0.07	1.13 ± 0.31	0.35 ± 0.07	1.17 ± 0.19	0.62 ± 0.05
24	1.86 ± 0.21	0	1.16 ± 0.19	0.38 ± 0.07	0.85 ± 0.09	0.27 ± 0.04	0.95 ± 0.13	0.62 ± 0.04
48	0.75 ± 0.12	0	0.98 ± 0.33	0.34 ± 0.16	0.78 ± 0.14	0.29 ± 0.09	0.86 ± 0.23	0.46 ± 0.09
72	0.65 ± 0.37	0	0.66 ± 0.12	0.26 ± 0.04	0.55 ± 0.21	0.22 ± 0.04	0.59 ± 0.15	0.41 ± 0.07
96	0.60 ± 0.26	0	0.57 ± 0.05	0.23 ± 0.05	0.47 ± 0.09	0.19 ± 0.06	0.51 ± 0.03	0.30 ± 0.08

Treatment and calculations as in Fig. 1. (mean ± S.D.; $n = 3$)

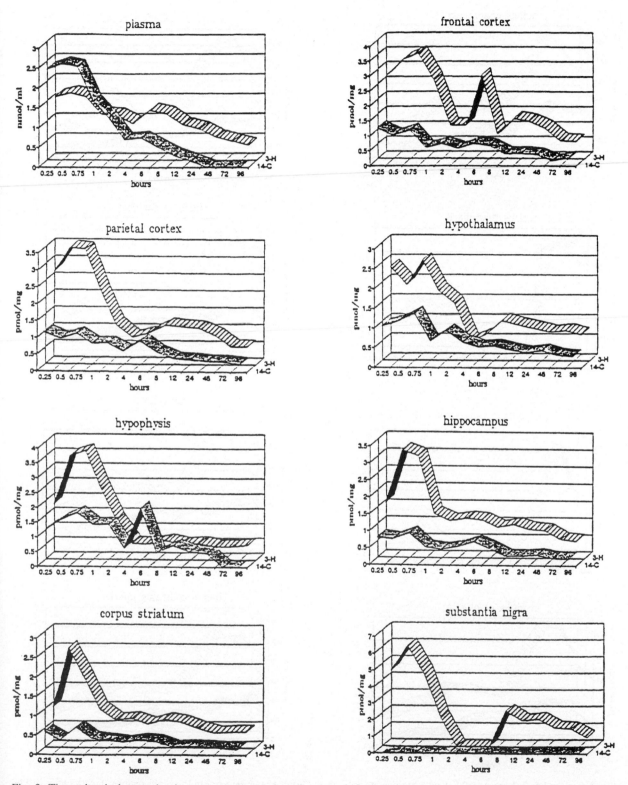

Fig. 2. Time-related changes in the concentrations of orally given (−)-deprenyl detected in the plasma and brain regions. Treatment as in Fig. 1. Time scale is not linear.

150

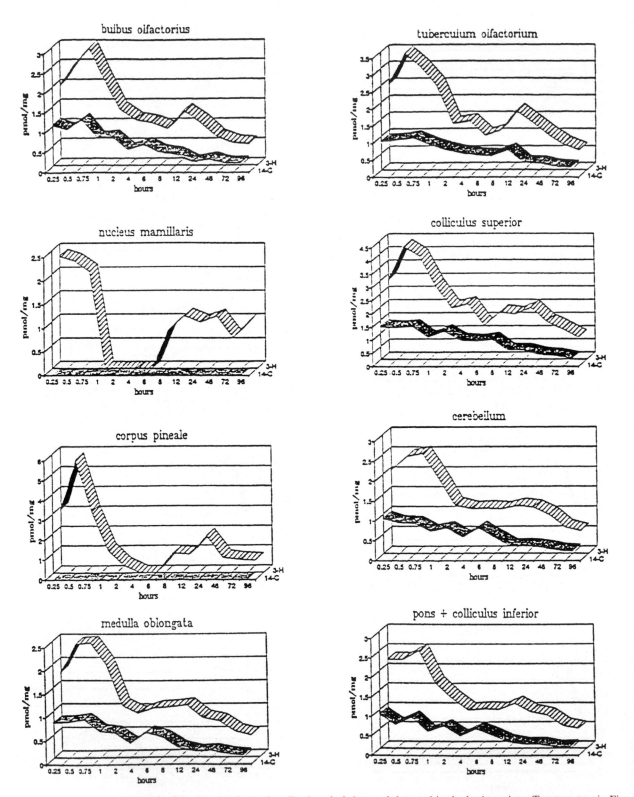

Fig. 3. Time-related changes in the concentrations of orally given (−)-deprenyl detected in the brain regions. Treatment as in Fig. 1. Time scale is not linear.

TABLE 5

AUC_{0-t} values (pmol/mg per h) of cerebral tissues from rats treated orally with (−)-deprenyl (1.5 mg/kg)

Tissues	^{3}H-(−)-deprenyl	^{14}C-(−)-deprenyl
Plasma	107.89	33.59
Corpus pineale	133.70	0
Bulbus olfactorius	100.70	45.10
Hypophysis	55.25	33.27
Hypothalamus	166.31	48.92
Hub. olfactorium	137.32	55.13
Substantia nigra	152.56	0
Nucl. mamillaris	116.56	0
Frontal cortex	159.89	34.26
Parietal cortex	122.64	37.45
Corpus striatum	70.34	23.41
Hippocampus	118.62	32.18
Colliculus sup.	189.71	56.31
Cerebellum	183.90	50.46
Pons + colliculus inf.	147.08	38.92
L medulla obl.	143.92	37.63

AUC_{0-t} values ($t = 96$ h) were determined from the concentration–time curves.

contained the highest concentration. In the other cerebral tissues, the values amounted to nearly half of that seen in the plasma.

The ^{14}C tracer in the cerebral tissues of higher mass could be detected up to 96 h after deprenyl administration. As with ^{3}H, there was a minor increase in ^{14}C label in the period of 6 to 8 h (Figs. 2 and 3). Since this increase was seen with both of the tracers, it may be due to the presence of a substance which still carries both radiolabels. The increase could result from the entero-hepatic cycle of the intact deprenyl molecule. From the concentration–time curves determined on the basis of the specific activities of both labels the AUC_{0-t} values were calculated and presented in Table 5.

Discussion

The (−)-deprenyl labelled by ^{3}H and ^{14}C made it

possible to obtain information on the fate of the molecule in the body. (a) By detecting the ^{3}H label (phenyl-^{3}H) as a function of time we were able to follow the fate of some moieties, such as the parent molecule, and all the metabolites both with (methylamphetamine, amphetamine, desmethyl-deprenyl) and without an amino group; (b) using ^{14}C label (propargyl-^{14}C) we could follow the fate of the parent compound, desmethyl-deprenyl, para- or β-hydroxylated deprenyl, the propargyl group as well as of the metabolite(s) of this last residue.

The molar concentration–time curve of (−)-deprenyl in the plasma, as calculated from the two kinds of label, indicated that in the first 4 h the activity carried by ^{14}C exceeded that related to the ^{3}H tracer. This may be due to the smaller distribution volume of the propargyl residue, or to its strong binding to plasma proteins. The rapid change in the ^{3}H/^{14}C radioactivity ratio indicates a "first pass" metabolic transformation of (−)-deprenyl.

In the cerebral tissues, the presence of ^{3}H label predominates: its level was found to be 2–3-times higher than that of ^{14}C. The maximum plasma radioactivity was detected 15–30 min after deprenyl ingestion, whereas the peak concentration in brain tissues was seen in the 45th min.

The time-related changes of the molar concentrations (calculated from ^{14}C and ^{3}H labels) in the plasma and brain after the oral administration of (−)-deprenyl are presented in Figs. 2 and 3. These data show that over the 96 h period, the tissue levels of ^{3}H were higher than those of ^{14}C. It is also clear that the concentrations of the parent compound, and especially its metabolite(s), vary greatly in the cerebral tissues. Since the surplus of ^{3}H label in the brain regions studied could not stem from the parent compound, the findings indicate that considerable amounts of metabolites, such as methylamphetamine and amphetamine, have been formed and were present in the central nervous system.

Based upon the calculated AUC_{0-t} values (Table 5) obtained from the plasma and brain tissues of rats that have ingested 1.5 mg/kg (−)-deprenyl, three groups of cerebral regions can be distinguished. AUC_{0-t} values are: (1) below 80 pmol/mg per h, hypophysis, corpus striatum; (2) 80–140 pmol/mg per h, corpus pineale, bulbus olfactorius, nucleus mamillaris, parietal cortex, hippocampus, pons + colliculus inferior, medulla oblongata; (3) above 140 pmol/mg per h, hypothalamus, substantia nigra, frontal cortex, colliculus superior, cerebellum.

The relatively low amounts of ^{14}C-related radioactivity in the central nervous system after oral administration of radiolabelled deprenyl indicates that a minor fraction of the compound is responsible for the selective MAO-blocking action, because the selective inhibition of MAO-B definitely requires the integrity of the molecule.

From the data obtained, the concentration of (−)-methylamphetamine could be estimated: it was quite high (around $1–2 \times 10^{-6}$ M) in brain tissue after the oral intake of 1.5 mg/kg (−)-deprenyl. This concentration of (−)-methylamphetamine can significantly inhibit amine uptake, especially if we consider that the inhibitory potency of (−)-methylamphetamine on noradrenaline uptake is about 10-times higher than that of the parent compound. The inhibitory action of (−)-deprenyl metabolites could be responsible for the prevention of the carrier-mediated neurotoxicity induced by DSP-4 on noradrenergic neurons.

The MAO-B inhibition of (−)-deprenyl is an irreversible "hit and run" effect, which after an initial phase is independent of the presence of the substance which caused it. In contrast to this, the inhibition of uptake induced by (−)-deprenyl or its metabolites is reversible in its nature and strictly proportional to the actual concentration of the substance responsible for the effect. MAO inhibition is caused by the parent compound, but the inhibition of uptake in addition to the parent compound is coupled to the effect of its metabolites. Our recent studies, by using the alternatively and positionally label radioisomers of (−)-deprenyl, presented evidence in vivo on the pharmacokinetic profile of the formation of (−)-deprenyl metabolites in rats.

Summary

Using alternatively labelled (−)-deprenyl (^{3}H label in the ring and ^{14}C in the propargyl group) the distribution of the compound was studied in 15 brain regions and the plasma of rats over a period of 96 h, after oral administration of 1.5 mg/kg of (−)-deprenyl. The compound is rapidly absorbed (within 15–30 min) from the gastrointestinal tract, as indicated by its high plasma level. It penetrates to the central nervous system, where it reaches a peak level within 45–60 min. During the first 2 h in the plasma the ^{14}C label, whilst in cerebral tissues during the whole period of the experiment the ^{3}H tracer dominates. The difference in the ratio of ^{3}H to ^{14}C radioactivity (compared to the 0 time relation) develops as early as in the first 15 min, which indicates the operation of a rapid "first pass" biotransformation of the compound.

Our data represent the tissue molar concentration-time curves of (−)-deprenyl calculated from both the ^{3}H and ^{14}C radiolabels. A ratio of 1 of the concentrations of the two tracers would indicate that the molecule remained unchanged. The changes in the ratio, therefore, suggest the formation of considerable quantities of metabolites (methylamphetamine and amphetamine) and their presence in the brain. The difference between the area under the curves (AUC_{0-t} for ^{3}H and AUC_{0-t} for ^{14}C) represents the amount of metabolites expected to be formed during the experiment. The concentration of the metabolites should be taken into account while evaluating the pharmacological effect of (−)-deprenyl. We proved earlier that a dose of 1.5 mg/kg of (−)-deprenyl completely blocks MAO-B activity in the central nervous system. The fast metabolism of the inhibitor indicates that a minor part of the orally administered (−)-deprenyl is sufficient to produce a high level of selective MAO-B inhibition in the brain.

References

Brodie, B.B., Cho, A.K. and Gessa, G.L. (1970) Possible role of *p*-hydroxynorephedrine in the depletion of norepinephrine induced by d-amphetamine and in tolerance to this drug. In: E. Costa and S. Garattini (Eds.), *Amphetamines and Related Compounds*, Raven Press, New York, pp. 217–230.

Finnegan, K.T., Skratt, J.J., Irwin, l., DeLanney, L.E. and Langston, J.W. (1990) Protection against DSP-4-induced neurotoxicity by deprenyl is not related to its inhibition of MA0-B. *Eur. J. Pharmacol.*, 184: 119–126.

Finnegan, K.T. (1993) Neurotoxins and monoamine oxidase inhibition: new aspects. *Movement Disorders*, 8 Suppl. 1: S14–S19.

Goldstein, M. and Anagnoste, B. (1965) The conversion in vivo of d-amphetamine to (+)-*p*-hydroxy-norephedrine. *Biochim. Biophys. Acta*, 107: 166–168.

Heinonen, E.H., Myllyla, V., Sotaniemi, K., Lammitausta, R., Salonen, J.S., Anttila, M., Savijarvi, M., Kotila, M. and Rinne, U.K. (1989) Pharmacokinetics and metabolism of selegiline. *Acta Neurol. Scand.*, 126: 93–99.

Knoll, J. and Magyar, K. (1972) Some puzzling pharmacological effects of monoamine oxidase inhibitors. In: E. Costa and M. Sandler (Eds.) *Monoamine Oxidases. New Vistas*, Raven Press, New York, pp 393–408.

Langston, J.W. (1985) I. MPTP Neurotoxicity an overview and characterization of phases of toxicity. *Life Sci.*, 36: 201–206.

Magyar, K. (Ed.) (1980) *Monoamine Oxidases and Their Selective Inhibition*, Pergamon Press, Akadémiai Kiadó, Budapest, pp. 11–21.

Magyar, K. (1991) Neuroprotective effect of deprenyl and *p*-fluor-deprenyl. *Paneuropean Society of Neurology, Second Congress*, Vienna, 26.

Magyar, K. (1993) Pharmacology of monoamine oxidase type B inhibitors. In: I. Szelenyi (Ed.), *Inhibitors of Monoamine Oxidase B*, Birkhauser Verlag, Basel, pp. 125–143.

Magyar, K. (1994) Behaviour of (−)-deprenyl and its analogues. *J. Neural Transm. (Suppl.)*, 41: 167–175.

Magyar, K. and Szüts, T. (1982) The fate of (−)-deprenyl in the body. Preclinical studies In: *Proceedings of the International Symposium on (−)-Deprenyl*, Jumex, Szombathely, Hungary, Chinoin, Budapest, pp. 25–31.

Magyar, K. and Tóthfalusi, L. (1984) Pharmacokinetic aspects of deprenyl effects. *Pol. J. Pharmacol. Pharm.*, 36: 373–384.

Paxinos, G. and Watson, C. (1986) *The Rat Brain in Stereotaxic Coordinates*, 2nd edn., Academic Press, Australia.

Reynolds, G.P., Elsworth, J.D., Blau, K., Sandler, M., Lees, A.J. and Stern, G.M. (1978) Deprenyl is metabolized to methylamphetamine and amphetamine in man. *Br. J. Clin. Pharmacol.*, 6: 542–554.

Ricci, A., Mancini, M., Stricchi, P., Bongrani, S. and Bronzetti E. (1992) Deficits in cholinergic neurotransmission markers induced by ethylcholine mustard aziridinium (AF64A) in the rat hippocampus: sensitivity to treatment with the monoamine oxidase-B inhibitor l-deprenyl. *Drugs Exp. Clin. Res.*, 8: 163–171.

Schachter, M., Marsden, C.D., Parkes, J.D., Jenner, P. and Testa B. (1980) Deprenyl in management of response fluctuations in patients with Parkinson's disease on levodopa. *J. Neurol. Neurosurg. Psychiatr.*, 43: 1016–1021.

Peter M. Yu, Keith F. Tipton and Alan A. Boulton (Eds.)
Progress in Brain Research, Vol 106
© 1995 Elsevier Science BV. All rights reserved.

CHAPTER 16

Novel sites of action for deprenyl in MPTP-parkinsonism: metabolite-mediated protection against striatal neurotoxicity and suppression of MPTP-induced increase of dopamine turnover in C57BL mice

I. Sziráki[1], V. Kardos[1], M. Patthy[1], J. Gaál[2], P. Arányi[2], E. Kollár[1], Z. Tömösközi[2] and I. Király[1]

[1]*Institute for Drug Research, and* [2]*CHINOIN Pharmaceutical and Chemical Works, Budapest, Hungary*

Introduction

l-Deprenyl (DEP) was originally used in combination with l-DOPA (Birkmayer et al., 1977; Birkmayer et al., 1985), in the treatment of Parkinson's disease (PD). Recent results suggest that DEP delays the onset of disability associated with early, otherwise untreated PD (Tetrud and Langston, 1989; Parkinson Study Group, 1989, 1993). The mode of action of DEP that accounts for its beneficial effects is not yet clear. DEP is metabolized to l-methamphetamine (l-METH) and l-amphetamine (l-AMPH) in man (Reynolds et al., 1978)and in mice (Philips, 1981). At present, it is a matter of controversy whether metabolites of DEP are involved in the therapeutic action of DEP in the treatment of PD (Parkes et al., 1975; Karoum and Wyatt, 1982).

1-Methyl-4-phenyl-1,2,3,6-tetrahydropyridine

(MPTP) induces parkinsonism in man (Davis et al., 1979; Langston et al., 1983) and injury of nigrostriatal dopaminergic neurons in animals, including mice (Hallman et al., 1984; Heikkila et al., 1984a,b). It is now generally accepted that MPTP is a protoxin and must be activated before it exerts its neurotoxic actions. The first step in the development of neurotoxicity is the oxidation of MPTP by MAO-B in glial cells to 1-methyl-4-phenyl-2,3-dihydropyridinium ($MPDP^+$), which is then further oxidized to 1-methyl-4-phenylpyridinium (MPP^+). After its formation, MPP^+ enters dopaminergic neurons via the dopamine re-uptake system (see Tipton and Singer, 1993, for recent review). In fact, the marked decrease in striatal dopamine level, the most characteristic neurochemical alteration in the brain of MPTP-treated mice, can be prevented by pretreatment with nonselective MAO inhibitors or DEP, a selective MAO-B inhibitor (Heikkila et al., 1984b) and also by pretreatment with dopamine uptake inhibitors (Mayer et al., 1986).

During the last few years three lines of evidence have emerged suggesting that the mode of action of DEP in protection against neurotoxicity

---

Address correspondence to: I. Sziráki, Neurotoxicology and Neuroprotection Unit, Laboratory of Clinical Science, NIMH, NIH, Bldg. 10, Rm. 3D41, 10 Center Dr. MSC 1264, Bethesda, MD 20892-1264, USA.

induced by MPTP and its analogs is more complex: (1) DEP, when administered 3 days after the last MPTP treatment (30 mg/kg daily, 5 days), can increase survival of dopaminergic neurons in the substantia nigra of mice (Tatton and Greenwood, 1991; Tatton, 1993) by a mechanism unrelated to the blockade of formation of MPP$^+$ and of its subsequent uptake by dopaminergic neurons; (2) It has been reported that DEP suppresses hydroxyl radical formation associated with the autooxidation of released dopamine elicited by 2′Me-MPTP and MPP$^+$ (Chiueh et al., 1992; Wu et al., 1993; Chiueh et al., 1994); (3) We have demonstrated that DEP has an additional neuroprotective element associated with the ability of l-METH and l-AMPH generated from DEP to block the uptake of MPP$^+$ into the dopaminergic neurons. Moreover, we have shown that DEP also protects against neurotoxicity induced by 1-methyl-4-(2′-methylphenyl)-1,2,3,6-tetrahydropyridine (2′Me-MPTP) or 1-methyl-4-(2′-ethylphenyl)-1,2,3,6-tetrahydropyridine (2′Et-MPTP), which are bioactivated partly or primarily by MAO-A (Kardos et al., 1992; Sziráki et al., 1992, 1993, 1994b).

The present work was undertaken: (i) to further characterize the metabolite-mediated neuroprotective effect of DEP against neurotoxicity induced by MPTP and its 2′-substituted analogs; and (ii) to investigate whether subacute DEP treatment of mice with severe damage in the terminal field of the nigrostriatal dopaminergic neurons (an animal model of DEP monotherapy in the early phase of PD) affects the MPTP-induced striatal dopamine depletion and the compensatory increase of dopamine turnover.

Materials and methods

Male C57 black mice LATI, Gödöllö, Hungary; 25–32 g body weight were used in the experiments of this study. MPTP-HCl, 2′Me-MPTP-HCl, clorgyline-HCl and SKF 525A-HCl were purchased from Research Biochemicals International. Deprenyl-HCl and 2′Et-MPTP-HCl were synthesized in Chinoin Pharmaceutical and Chemical Co., and in the Institute Research for Drug Research, respectively. Unlabeled mazindol and [^{3}H]mazindol were obtained from Alkaloida Pharmaceuticals (Hungary) and NEN, respectively. Drugs were dissolved in 0.9% NaCl, with the exception of mazindol, which was suspended in 1% Tween 80. Mice were injected intraperitoneally with MPTP-HCl/2′Me-MPTP-HCl/2′Et-MPTP-HCl either alone or in combination with DEP, clorgyline, or mazindol according to the treatment schedules indicated in the legends for figures and tables. Three to 7 days after the last treatment, the mice were killed by cervical dislocation. The brains were removed and the corpora striata were dissected out and kept at −80°C until assayed. The paired striata were weighed and then sonicated in 200 μl distilled water for 15 s. Aliquots of water homogenates were resonicated in HPLC-mobile phase containing α-methyl dopamine as the internal standard. After centrifugation (10 000 × g, 15 min at 4°C) aliquots of supernatants were assayed for dopamine and its metabolites (dihydroxyphenylacetic acid (DOPAC) and homovanillic acid (HVA)) by HPLC-ED (Patthy and Gyenge, 1988). In some experiments, aliquots of water homogenates were assayed for mazindol binding as described by Javitch et al. (1984). Striatal membrane (10–15 μg protein; BioRad protein assay) was incubated for 60 min at 0°C in the presence of [^{3}H]mazindol (12 nM final concentration) and 300 nM NaCl. Specific binding was defined as the difference between total binding and binding in the presence of 50 mM unlabeled mazindol. The values were expressed as pmol/g tissue or pmol/mg protein. For statistical analysis one-way ANOVA was used with Duncan's multiple range test.

Results and discussion

Metabolite-mediated protection by DEP against dopaminergic neurotoxicity induced by MPTP or its analogs

Protection against MPTP toxicity in various experimental animals pretreated with DEP and other selective MAO-B and nonselective MAO inhibitors including pargyline is well documented.

We have recently reported (Sziráki et al., 1992, 1994b) that post-treatment by DEP or its metabolites (l-METH and l-AMPH; Reynolds et al., 1978) protects against striatal dopamine depletion in mice induced by MPTP or 2'Me-MPTP. At the post-MPTP time points when DEP and its metabolites were protective, the level of unconverted MPTP in the striatum of C57BL mice is negligible (Jonsson et al., 1986). However, a 30-min post treatment by pargyline, which is not metabolized to l-METH or l-AMPH, had no effect on the MPTP-induced striatal DA depletion despite producing a 90% inhibition of striatal MAO-B activity at this time point (Sziráki et al., 1994b). Both metabolites of DEP inhibited MPP^+ uptake by striatal synaptosomes with IC_{50} values close to that of the DA uptake by blocker mazindol. Therefore we proposed that the protection by DEP post-treatment is associated with its rapid metabolism to l-methamphetamine and l-amphetamine which, after formation, block the uptake of MPP^+ or $2'Me-MPP^+$ into dopaminergic neurons.

It has been reported that a 1-h pretreatment, but not a 24-h post-treatment, with DEP almost completely prevented the xylamine-induced depletion of norepinephrine in the cerebral cortex of rats (Dudley, 1988) and the DSP-4-induced depletion of norepinephrine in mice (Finnegan et al., 1990). Our evidence that metabolites generated from DEP are involved in its neuroprotective action against MPTP and 2'Me-MPTP toxicity support the speculation of these authors that protection against xylamine and DSP-4 toxicity by DEP is due to the formation of metabolites which block the uptake of the respective noradrenergic toxin.

SKF 525A attenuates metabolite-mediated protection of DEP

If the mechanism of neuroprotection by DEP involves an uptake inhibitory component associated with its metabolites, inhibition of the formation of DEP metabolites would be expected to antagonize the metabolite-mediated protective element of DEP treatment. Inhibition of the metabolism of DEP by pretreatment with the microsomal liver enzyme inhibitor, SKF 525A (50 mg/kg, i.p. 30 min), almost completely prevented the DEP-induced dose-dependent increase of the spontaneous locomotor activity and striatal DOPA accumulation in rats. SKF 525A, however, did not antagonize the l-methamphetamine-induced increase of locomotor activity after treatment. In fact, the duration of increased locomotor activity was prolonged by SKF 525A. This effect of was probably due to the inhibition of the metabolism of l-METH (Engberg et al., 1991).

To further assess the role of metabolite formation in the protection by DEP post-treatment the mice received SKF 525A (25 mg/kg, i.p.) between the MPTP-treatment (40 mg/kg, i.p.) and the DEP treatment (10 mg/kg). In line with our previous findings, a 30-min post-treatment by DEP completely protected against MPTP-induced striatal DA depletion. SKF 525A significantly reduced the protective effect of DEP post-treatment but did not have any effect either on MPTP-induced DA depletion or on striatal DA levels (Table 1). SKF 525A, however, did not antagonize the protective effect of post-treatment with l-METH or l-AMPH (data not shown).

We attempted to evaluate the effect of SKF 525A on the protection related to the metabolization of DEP in higher doses and with various treatment schedules. A 30-min pretreatment or a co-treatment with SKF 525A, even at a dose of 25 mg/kg, and higher doses (30 or 50 mg/kg) at the same time point, resulted in an increase of MPTP lethality. Enhanced MPTP toxicity may be explained by recent results (Shahi et al., 1990; see also for further references) showing that MPTP is a substrate for hepatic microsomal cytochrome *P*-450. They suggest that inactivation of isozymes of cytochrome *P*-450 involved in the detoxification of MPTP could increase the bioactivation of MPTP and the subsequent toxicity.

Deprenyl treatment prevents the dopaminergic neurotoxicity of 2'-substituted analogs of MPTP bioactivated partly by MAO-A

Previous studies on structural requirements for neurotoxicity of MPTP demonstrated that 2'Me-MPTP and 2'Et-MPTP are potent dopaminergic

158

neurotoxins and are bioactivated to a significant extent by MAO-A (Youngster et al., 1986; Heikkila and Sonsalla, 1987; Sonsalla et al., 1987; Heikkila et al., 1988). It has been reported that neurotoxicity induced by repeated treatment with 2'Me-MPTP cannot be prevented by pretreatment with DEP even at a dose of 40 mg/kg. Protection was observed at a nonselective dose of MDL 72145 or by pretreatment with dopamine uptake inhibitors (mazindol or GBR 13069), indicating that the 2'Me-MPTP neurotoxicity is mediated by MAO-A and that it also requires the uptake of the pyridinium species by the dopaminergic neurons (Sonsalla et al., 1987). They also reported that the neurotoxicity of 2'Et-MPTP cannot be prevented by DEP. Pretreatment with a combination of DEP and clorgyline, however, afforded complete protection (Heikkila et al., 1988). Neurotoxicity induced by 2'Et-MPTP (but not by 2'Me-MPTP or MPTP) was significantly attenuated by clorgyline alone, suggesting that the 2'Et-MPTP neurotoxicity is mediated primarily by MAO-A.

We have presented evidence that a 30-min pre- or post-treatment with DEP (10 mg/kg) provides an almost complete protection against striatal DA depletion induced by a single dose (15 mg/kg) of 2'Me-MPTP. Moreover, 2'Me-MPTP neurotoxicity was also prevented by l-METH or l-AMPH (5–5 mg), regardless of whether they were administered 30 min prior to or 30 min after 2'Me-MPTP (Kardos et al., 1992; Sziráki et al., 1994b). In view with our recent findings that d- and l-enantiomers of methamphetamine and amphetamine block the uptake of MPP^+ by striatal synaptosomes of rats and that mazindol posttreatment protects against MPTP and 2'Me-MPTP neurotoxicity (Sziráki et al., 1994a,b), it is concluded that protection by DEP treatment against 2'Me-MPTP neurotoxicity is associated with the blockade of $2'Me-MPP^+$ uptake into dopaminergic neurons (for further discussion see Sziráki et al., 1994b).

To distinguish the two distinct features of the mechanism of action of DEP we contrasted the MAO-B related protection against MPTP neurotoxicity and the MAO-B unrelated, metabolite-mediated protection against 2'Me-MPTP (Fig. 1). Due to the irreversible inhibition of MAO-B (the blockade of the conversion of MPTP to MPP^+), DEP protected against striatal DA depletion induced by two injections of MPTP, as shown on

TABLE 1

Effect of SKF 525A on metabolite-mediated protection by deprenyl against MPTP-induced striatal DA depletion in mice

Treatment-1	Time elapsed (min)	Treatment-2	Time elapsed (min)	Treatment-3	n	DA (μg/g)	% of control
Saline	10	Saline	20	Saline	7	14.0 ± 0.35	100
MPTP	"	Saline	"	Saline	6	3.0 ± 0.26^a	21
Saline	"	SKF 525A	"	Saline	7	14.1 ± 0.42	101
MPTP	"	SKF 525A	"	Saline	9	3.3 ± 0.30^a	24
MPTP	"	SKF 525A	"	DEP	7	$11.1 \pm 0.76^{a,b}$	79
MPTP	"	Saline	"	DEP	5	$14.1 \pm 0.83^{b,c}$	101

Mice received a single dose of MPTP·HCl (40 mg/kg; i.p.) either alone or in combination with SKF 525A (2.5 mg/kg, i.p.) and/or deprenyl (10 mg/kg, i.p.). The animals were killed 3 days after the treatments. Results are the means ± S.E.M.
[a]Statistically different ($P < 0.01$) from saline controls. [b]Statistically different ($P < 0.01$) from MPTP-group. [c]Statistically different ($P < 0.01$) from MPTP + SKF 525A + DEP group.

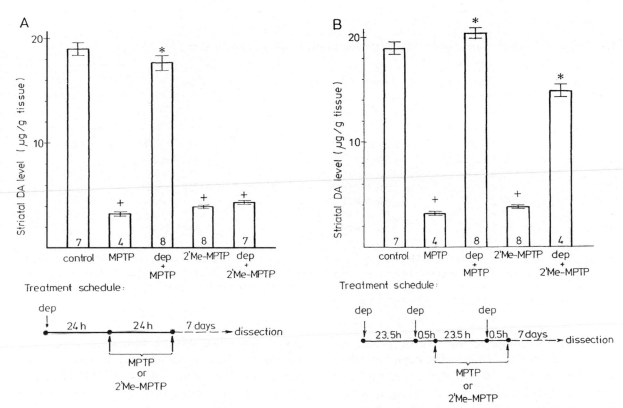

Fig. 1. Long-lasting versus short-lasting protection by deprenyl pretreatment against striatal DA depletion induced by MPTP and 2'Me-MPTP. Mice were i.p. injected with MPTP·HCl (40 mg free base per kg) or 2'Me-MPTP-HCl (15 mg/base per kg) on two consecutive days. Animals received deprenyl HCl (10 mg/kg) 24h before the first injection with 2'Me-MPTP/2'Me-MPTP (A) and two additional DEP treatments 30 min before each injection with MPTP/2'Me-MPTP (B). Numbers in bars indicate the number of animals in each group. Results are the means ± S.E.M. +Statistically different ($P < 0.01$) from saline controls. *Statistically different ($P < 0.01$) from animals treated with MPTP/2'Me-MPTP alone.

the treatment schedule of Fig. 1A. In line with the results of other investigators on the lack of its protective effect against 2'Me-MPTP-toxicity in this treatment schedule, DEP, at a dose of 10 mg/kg, had no effect on striatal DA depletion. When two additional DEP treatments were applied 30 min prior to each 2'Me-MPTP-treatment (15 mg/kg, Fig. 1B), however, it significantly reduced the striatal DA depletion due to the ability of its rapidly generated metabolites to block the 2'Me-MPP$^+$ uptake into dopaminergic neurons.

To determine the length of the period within which pretreatment with DEP can protect against the MAO-A-mediated 2'Me-MPTP toxicity, groups of mice were given a single dose of 2'Me-MPTP (15 mg/kg) at the indicated time points following DEP and killed 4 days after the treatments (Table 2). Deprenyl applied 0.5, 1 and 2 h prior to 2'Me-MPTP significantly reduced the DA depletion. Its protective effect, however, sharply declined, when 4 h or 8 h were allowed to elapse

between DEP and 2'Me-MPTP administration. In fact, treatment with DEP 4 h prior to 2'Me-MPTP potentiated its DA depleting effect. This potentiation may be associated with an interaction of a sustained DA-release induced by DEP metabolites (for further references and discussion see Engberg et al., 1991) and the sustained DA overflow induced by 2'Me-MPTP (Chiueh et al., 1992).

In a post-treatment schedule DEP at 10 mg/kg

TABLE 2

Time course of the effect of deprenyl on 2′Me-MPTP-induced striatal DA depletion in mice

Treatment 1	Time elapsed (h)	Treatment 2	n	DA (μg/g)	% of control
Saline	1	Saline	7	23.2 ± 0.9	100
Saline	1	2′Me-MPTP	6	8.6[a] ± 0.5	37
DEP	0.5	2′Me-MPTP	4	19.8[b] ± 0.4	85
DEP	1	2′Me-MPTP	7	17.5[b] ± 1.2	75
DEP	2	2′Me-MPTP	6	18.0[b] ± 3.0	78
DEP	4	2′Me-MPTP	6	2.5[b] ± 0.3	11
DEP	8	2′Me-MPTP	7	5.5[NS] ± 0.7	24

Mice received a single dose of 2′Me-MPTP-HCl (15 mg per base per kg; i.p.). At various time point prior to 2′Me-MPTP injection groups of mice were treated with l-deprenyl·HCl (10 mg/kg, per oral). The animals were killed 4 days after the treatments. Results are the means ± S.E.M. [a] Statistically different ($P < 0.01$) for saline controls. [b] Statistically different ($P/$ lt$/0.01$) from 2′Me-MPTP group. [NS] Statistically not different from 2′Me-MPTP-only group.

dose provided complete and partial protection against 2′Me-MPTP-induced DA depletion when administered 30 and 60 min after a single dose of 2′Me-MPTP (15 mg/kg). At 20 mg/kg, however, the antagonism of the DA-depleting effect of 2′Me-MPTP was less pronounced at both time points (data not shown). Moreover, DEP at 20 mg/kg resulted in an enhanced mortality compared to treatment with 2′Me-MPTP alone. (However, increased mortality was also observed in our experimentation with mazindol at 10 mg/kg dose, although mazindol at a dose of 5 mg/kg

TABLE 3

Effect of deprenyl on 2′Et-MPTP-induced depletion of striatal DA and its metabolites in mice

Treatment 1	Time elapsed (h)	Treatment 2	DA (μg/g)	% of control	DOPAC (μg/g)	% of control	HVA (μg/g)	% of control
Saline	0.5	Saline	17.07 ± 0.63	100	1.28 ± 0.09	100	1.48 ± 0.05	100
Saline	″	2′Et-MPTP	2.07 ± 0.40[a]	12	0.57 ± 0.09[a]	44	0.70 ± 0.05[a]	47
2′Et-MPTP	″	CLORG	1.33 ± 0.16[a]	8	0.20 ± 0.02[ab]	16	0.41 ± 0.05[ab]	28
2′Et-MPTP	″	DEP	12.23 ± 0.37[ab]	72	0.90 ± 0.05[ab]	70	1.44 ± 0.09[b]	97
2′Et-MPTP	″	MAZ	16.53 ± 0.76[b]	97	1.58 ± 0.08[ab]	123	1.78 ± 0.06[ab]	120
DEP	0.5	2′Et-MPTP	13.75 ± 0.58[ab]	81	1.17 ± 0.08[b]	91	1.29 ± 0.04[b]	87
MAZ	″	2′Et-MPTP	14.78 ± 0.43[dab]	87	1.09 ± 0.1[b]	85	1.34 ± 0.11[b]	91
DEP	4	2′Et-MPTP	4.38 ± 0.71[ac]	26	0.47 ± 0.07[a]	37	0.86 ± 0.06[a]	58
CLORG	″	2′Et-MPTP	6.06 ± 1.09[ab]	35	0.42 ± 0.03[a]	33	0.69 ± 0.05[a]	47
DEP + CLORG	″	2′Et-MPTP	17.90 ± 0.44[b]	105	0.42 ± 0.02[a]	33	0.92 ± 0.03[ac]	62

Mice ($n = 5$–6) received a single dose of 2′Et-MPTP-HCl (30 mg free base per kg; i.p.) and MAO inhibitors (10 mg/kg; i.p.) or mazindol (5 mg/kg) either after (30 min) or before (30 min or 4 h) the 2′Et-MPTP treatment. Results are the mean ± SEM. [a,d] Statistically different ($P < 0.01$; $P < 0.05$) from saline controls. [b,c] Statistically different ($P < 0.01$, $P < 0.05$) from 2′Et-MPTP-only group.

TABLE 4

Effect of deprenyl on striatal dopamine depletion induced by repeated treatments with 2'Et-MPTP in mice

Groups	Deprenyl pretreatments		DA (μg/g)	% of control
	24 h	2 × 30		
Saline	−	−	16.7 ± 0.37	100
2'Et-MPTP	−	−	5.1 ± 0.34[a]	30
DEP + 2'Et-MPTP	+	−	6.8 ± 0.41[a]	40
DEP + 2'Et-MPTP	+	+	11.3 ± 1.48[a,b]	67

Mice received i.p. injections of 2'Et-MPTP·HCL (30 mg free base per kg) on two consecutive days. Two groups of mice were treated with l-deprenyl·HCl (10 mg/kg; i.p.) 24 h prior to the first 2'Et-MPTP treatment. Animals in one of these groups received two additional doses of deprenyl 30 min before each 2'Et-MPTP treatment. The mice were killed 7 days after the last injection. Results are the means ± S.E.M. [a]Statistically different ($P < 0.01$) from saline controls. [b]Statistically different ($P < 0.01$) from 2'Et-MPTP-only group.

provided complete or nearly complete protection against MPTP- or 2'Me-MPTP-induced neurotoxicity without any effect on mortality. Increased mortality in animals treated with MPTP and mazindol (10 mg/kg) was observed also by other investigators (Heikkila, 1990 personal communication).

Depending upon the treatment conditions, d-amphetamine was found to potentiate (Sershen et al., 1986b) or to antagonize (Chiueh et al., 1986a; Sershen et al., 1986a) the toxic effect of MPTP. As with d-amphetamine, d-methamphetamine has also been reported to potentiate (Sershen et al., 1986a) or to antagonize MPTP neurotoxicity (Sziráki et al., 1994a) using a treatment schedule in which d-methamphetamine alone did not alter the striatal DA levels of C57BL mice when measured 4 days later.

To further elucidate the metabolite-mediated effect of DEP treatment on the neurotoxicity of 2'-substituted MPTP analogs, we investigated whether DEP can antagonize the 2'Et-MPTP in-duced striatal DA depletion, using various conditions (Tables 3 and 4). A 30-min pre- or post-

treatment with DEP provided substantial protection against 2'Et-MPTP-induced depletion of DA and its metabolites (Table 3). The DA uptake blocker, mazindol, applied 30 min prior to or after 2'Et-MPTP provided complete protection. A 30-min post-treatment with clorgyline has no effect on 2'Et-MPTP neurotoxicity. A 4-h pre-treatment either with DEP or with clorgyline attenuated the 2'Et-MPTP-induced DA deple-tion. In line with the results of Heikkila et al. (1988) the combination of DEP and clorgyline completely prevented the striatal DA depletion. When the mice received a single injection of DEP 24 h prior to the first 2'Et-MPTP treatment (simi-lar to the treatment schedule as applied in the experiment shown in Fig. 1A) it had no effect on the 2'Et-MPTP neurotoxicity. In contrast with this, when mice received additional DEP injec-tions before each 2'Et-MPTP treatment, DEP produced a substantial protection against 2'Et-MPTP-induced toxicity.

Metabolite-mediated protective element of DEP against decrease of striatal [^{3}H]mazindol binding in mice treated with MPTP or its 2'-substituted analogs

Neurochemical changes in MPTP-treated mice include (in addition to the DA and noradrenaline depletion) reduction of DA uptake (Heikkila et al., 1984), decrease of tyrosine hydroxylase activ-ity in various brain regions (Hallman et al., 1985; Sziráki et al., 1986) and decrease in striatal [^{3}H]mazindol binding (Sershen et al., 1986a,b). The decrease in binding of [^{3}H]mazindol after MPTP treatment correlates with the decrease in striatal DA levels (Sershen et al., 1986a,b). The magnitude of the MPTP-induced DA depletion directly corresponds to density of [^{3}H]mazindol binding to DA transport sites (but not the DA concentration) in intact mouse striatal regions, suggesting that regional differences in susceptibil-ity of DA terminal populations depend upon the local density of uptake sites for MPP$^+$ (Marshall and Navarrete, 1990). Previous research reveals temporal differences between the antagonizing effects of pargyline and nomifensine against MPTP-induced neurotoxicity as monitored by analyzing catecholamine levels in different brain regions and [³H]mazindol binding of striatal homogenates of mice (Sundstrom and Jonsson, 1986). A 30-min post-treatment with nomifensine completely prevented the MPTP-induced striatal DA depletion and decrease in mazindol binding. In contrast, pargyline treatment at this time point had no effect on MPTP neurotoxicity (Sundstrom and Jonsson, 1986).

To further characterize the MAO-B-unrelated protective element of DEP against dopaminergic neurotoxicity we contrasted the 30-min pargyline post-treatment with the 30-min DEP and mazindol post-treatment with respect to their effect on MPTP-induced decreases in striatal DA levels and [³H]mazindol binding (Fig. 2). In line with our previous findings (Sziráki et al., 1994b) the 30-min post-treatment with DEP, but not pargyline, almost completely prevented the MPTP-induced striatal DA depletion and provided substantial protection against the decrease of striatal [³H]mazindol binding. As shown in Fig. 1, the MPTP-induced decrease in striatal [³H]mazindol binding and the protective effect of DEP and mazindol correlate positively with the changes in striatal DA levels. Neither pargyline nor DEP alone had any effect on DA level and [³H]mazindol binding (data not shown). Mazindol treatment alone resulted in a slight decrease (28%) of the [³H]mazindol binding.

In order to get further evidence that supports our finding that DEP treatment (10 mg/kg) protects against dopaminergic neurotoxicity of 2'substituted MPTP-analogs, we investigated the effect of 30-min post-treatment on the decrease of [³H]mazindol binding in striatal homogenates of mice treated with 2'Me-MPTP (15 mg/kg, i.p.) or with 2'Et-MPTP (30 mg/kg, i.p.) (Table 5). Deprenyl at this time point provided complete or nearly complete protection against the decrease of [³H]mazindol binding in mice treated with 2'Me-MPTP and 2'Et-MPTP.

Subacute DEP treatment applied from the 3rd post-MPTP day enhances the recovery of striatal DA levels and suppresses the MPTP-induced increase of striatal DA turnover in mice

It has been shown that DEP in monotherapy may slow the progression of Parkinson's disease (Parkinson Study Group, 1989, 1993; Tetrud and Langston, 1989). Surviving nigrostriatal neurons in Parkinson patients exhibit increased DA turnover as reflected by the elevated ratio of homovanillic acid (HVA) to that of DA at autopsy (see Homykiewicz, 1986). An oxygen free radical mechanism associated with the hydrogen peroxide generating enzymatic oxidation of DA by MAO (Cohen and Spina, 1989, 1989; Cohen, 1990) and/or DA autooxidation (Chiueh et al., 1993; see also for further discussion and references) has been suggested as a prime consideration in the mechanism of the development of PD.

The beneficial effects of DEP either in addition to the standard treatment of PD with L-DOPA plus peripheral DOPA decarboxylase inhibitor

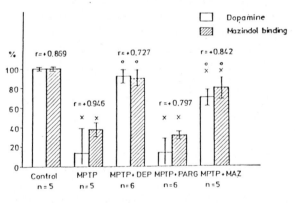

Fig. 2. Comparison of the metabolite-mediated neuroprotective effects of deprenyl as monitored by MPTP-induced decreases in striatal dopamine level and mazindol binding. Mice received a single dose of MPTP·HCl (40 mg/kg i.p.). Deprenyl, pargyline or mazindol were administered 30 min after MPTP treatment and the animals were killed 4 days later. Control values for DA level and [³H]mazindol binding were 27.0 ± 1.12 mg/g and 12.8 ± 8.26 pmol/g, respectively. Note that the DA levels and the mazindol binding were determined from different aliquots of striatal homogenate of each individual animal.

TABLE 5

Protection against 2'Me-MPTP-/2'Et-MPTP-induced reduction of [^{3}H]mazindol binding of striatal homogenate in mice by post-treatment with deprenyl

Experiment-1				Experiment-2			
Treatment-1	Treatment-2	Mazindol binding pmol/mg protein	% of Control	Treatment-1	Treatment-2	Mazindol binding pmol/mg protein	% of Control
Saline	Saline	4.96 ± 0.23	100	Saline	Saline	10.85 ± 0.79	100
2'Me-MPTP	Saline	1.24 ± 0.01[a]	25	2'Et-MPTP	Saline	4.14 ± 0.46[a]	38
2'Me-MPTP	DEP	5.02 ± 0.84[b]	101	2'Et-MPTP	Clorgyline	3.06 ± 0.87[a]	28
				2'Et-MPTP	DEP	9.01 ± 0.84[b]	83
				2'Et-MPTP	Mazindol	9.39 ± 1.59[c]	86

In experiment-1 the mice received a simple dose of 2'Et-MPTP·HCl (15 mg free base per kg i.p.) and 30 min later they were treated with l-deprenyl·HCl (10 mg/kg i.p.). In experiment 2 the mice received 2'Et·MPTP·HCl (30 mg free base per kg i.p.) and 30 min later they were treated either with MAO inhibitors (10 mg/kg) or with mazindol (5 mg/kg). In both experiments the mice (n = 3–5) were killed 3 days after the treatments. Results are the means ± S.E.M. [a]Statistically different (P < 0.01) from saline controls. [b,c]Statistically different (P < 0.01 and P < 0.05) from the groups received only 2'Me-MPTP or 2'Et.MPTP.

(Birkmayer et al., 1977; Birkmayer et al., 1985) or alone (Parkinson Study Group, 1989, 1993; Tetrud and Langston, 1989) is probably related to its inhibitory effect on oxidative stress associated with increased DA turnover and/or DA autooxidation. In fact, inhibition of MAOs with DEP and clorgyline can suppress the peroxidative stress associated with haloperidol-induced (Cohen and Spina, 1989; Cohen, 1990) or reserpine-induced (Spina and Cohen, 1989; Cohen, 1990) increase of DA turnover as monitored by analyzing the striatal level of oxidized glutathione in mice.

Various dopaminergic neurotoxins can also induce an increase of DA turnover in the nigrostriatal dopaminergic system in rodents. Partial lesions of the substantia nigra by injecting different amounts of 6-hydroxydopamine (6-OHDA) resulted in an increase of the conversion of [^{3}H]tyrosine to [^{3}H]DA in the striatum (Agid et al., 1973) and in the formation of metabolites in the dendrites of the dopaminergic neurons (Hefti et al., 1980) in rats. Recent data indicate that unilateral intranigral infusion of Fe^{2+}-citrate (4.2 nmol) resulted in an increase of DA turnover in terminal regions as reflected by an elevated DOPAC to DA ratio in the ipsilateral striatum of rats

(Mohanakumar et al., 1994). Intranigral infusion of high doses of Fe^{3+} (50 μg) was also reported to evoke increased DA turnover in rat striatum as reflected by an elevated (DOPAC + HVA)/DA ratio (Ben-Shachar and Youdim, 1991).

An increase in the striatal DA turnover has been reported in MPTP-treated mice as reflected by an increase in both the relative rates of DA synthesis and the elevated HVA/DA ratio (Reinhard and Nichol, 1986) or by an elevated (DOPAC + HVA)/DA ratio (Sershen et al., 1985; Sziráki, 1989) in different strains of mice.

To further test the hypothesis that DEP exerts its neuroprotective effects against MPTP neurotoxicity at several sites of action in mice, we investigated whether DEP can alter the MPTP-induced changes in the terminal fields of the nigrostriatal DA-ergic system after it has been damaged by MPTP using the treatment schedule described by Tatton and Greenwood (1991). The mice were injected five times with MPTP (30 mg/kg, i.p.) on five consecutive days. Three days later (day-3) one group of MPTP-treated animals was killed and the other groups were injected eight times either with saline (MPTP-2) or with various doses of DEP (as indicated in Tables 6

TABLE 6

Effect of subacute deprenyl post-treatment (from the 3rd post-MPTP day) on MPTP-induced changes in striatal levels of DA and its metabolites in mice (I)

Treatment (MPTP 5×, 30 mg/kg)	Post-treatment (DEP 8×, mg/kg)	DA μg/g	% of control	DOPAC μg/g	% of control	HVA μg/g	% of control	(DOPAC+ HVA)/DA	% of control
Control-1	—	15.8 ± 0.7	100	1.5 ± 0.08	100	2.2 ± 0.2	100	0.23 ± 0.2	100
MPTP-1	—	3.5 ± 0.2^a	22	0.5 ± 0.06^a	33	1.1 ± 0.09^a	50	0.48 ± 0.05^a	209
Control-2	—	17.3 ± 0.8	100	1.1 ± 0.04	100	1.9 ± 0.09	100	0.17 ± 0.01	100
MPTP-2	—	4.9 ± 0.5^a	28	0.5 ± 0.04^a	45	1.3 ± 0.09^a	73	0.42 ± 0.07^a	247
MPTP	0.01	6.3 ± 0.2^b	36	0.6 ± 0.02	55	1.3 ± 0.1	68	0.30 ± 0.02^{bd}	176
MPTP	10	5.7 ± 0.2^c	33	0.4 ± 0.04	36	1.4 ± 0.02	68	0.29 ± 0.02^{bd}	171

Four groups of mice were treated with MPTP·HCl (30 mg free base per kg, i.p.) daily on 5 consecutive days. On the 3rd day after the last MPTP treatment animals in one group (MPTP-1) and in one saline-injected group (Control-1) were killed and their striata were kept at −80°C. Animals in other MPTP-treated groups were given two doses of deprenyl (i.p.) eight times during a period of 18 days beginning on the 3rd post-MPTP day. In one of the MPTP-treated groups mice received saline on the days of deprenyl treatment (MPTP-2). Animals in Control-1 and Control-2 groups received saline injections 5 and 5 + 8. Animals in Control-2, MPTP-2 and in groups with both MPTP and deprenyl treatments were killed 2 days after the last deprenyl treatment and the striata were kept at −80°C until processing for HPLC-determination of levels of DA and its metabolites. The number of animals varied from 5 to 8 per group. Values represent the means ± SEM.
[a] Significantly different ($P < 0.01$) from control groups. [b,c] Significantly different ($P < 0.01$ and $P < 0.05$) from MPTP-1. [d] Significantly different from MPTP-2 group.

and 7) over a period of 18 days and then after a further 2 or 3 days (day-20 and day-21) were killed. The MPTP-1 groups were included in these experiments for two reasons: (1) to verify that the terminal field of nigrostriatal DA-ergic neurons has been damaged by the time when the DEP treatment began, (2) to investigate whether the DA levels in MPTP-treated animals without DEP (MPTP-2) or with DEP change from day-3 to day-20 and -21.

In agreement with previous data (Chiueh et al., 1986), intraperitoneal treatment with five injections of MPTP (24 h apart) resulted in an 80–90% depletion of striatal DA, and a 50–70% depletion of DA metabolites at the 3d post-MPTP day. MPTP treatment caused a 2–4-fold increase in DA turnover, as demonstrated by the elevated (DOPAC + HVA)/DA ratio in line with the results of other workers (Sershen et al., 1985; Reinhard and Nichol, 1986). MPTP-1 animals exhib-

ited a lower DA depletion and also a smaller increase in DA turnover compared to MPTP-1 animals in experiment-2 (Table 7). These results clearly demonstrate that the repeated treatment with MPTP caused neurochemical changes (severe DA depletion and elevated DA turnover) in mice by the 3rd post-MPTP day (the 1st day of DEP treatment) that had taken place in the nigrostriatal neurons. In both experiments, the MPTP-treated animals without DEP treatment which were killed on day-20 or day-21 had somewhat higher levels of DA and DA-metabolites than the MPTP-treated animals killed on day-3. The differences between animals killed on day-3 and day-20, or day-21, although statistically not significant, reveal a spontaneous recovery of striatal DA levels in MPTP-treated mice in agreement with earlier evidence about a slow but complete recovery of MPTP-induced depletion of striatal DA in C57BL mice (Chiueh et al., 1986) and a

TABLE 7

Effect of subacute deprenyl post-treatment (from the 3rd post-MPTP day) on MPTP-induced changes in striatal levels of DA and its metabolites in mice (II)

Treatment (MPTP 5×, 30 mg/kg)	Post-treatment (DEP 8×, mg/kg)	DA µg/g	% of control	DOPAC µg/g	% of control	HVA µg/g	% of control	(DOPAC + HVA)/DA	% of control
Control-1	—	10.9 ± 0.7	100	1.0 ± 0.1	100	1.5 ± 0.1	100	0.22 ± 0.1	100
MPTP-1	—	1.1 ± 0.2[a]	10	0.3 ± 0.1[a]	30	0.6 ± 0.05[a]	40	0.86 ± 0.07[a]	391
Control-2	—	12.1 ± 0.6	100	1.5 ± 0.1	100	1.4 ± 0.05	100	0.24 ± 0.01	100
MPTP-2	—	1.8 ± 0.1[a]	15	0.5 ± 0.1[a]	33	0.8 ± 0.04[a]	57	0.71 ± 0.08[a]	295
MPTP	0.1	3.3 ± 0.5[be]	27	0.7 ± 0.1[be]	47	1.0 ± 0.04[be]	71	0.48 ± 0.05[be]	200
MPTP	1.0	2.7 ± 0.3[c]	22	0.5 ± 0.04	33	0.9 ± 0.04[b]	64	0.54 ± 0.07[be]	225
MPTP	10	1.9 ± 0.2	16	0.3 ± 0.03	20	0.5 ± 0.05[e]	36	0.41 ± 0.03[bd]	171

Five groups of mice were treated with MPTP·HCl (30 mg free base per kg, i.p.) daily on 5 consecutive days. On the 3rd day after the last MPTP treatment animals in one group (MPTP-1) and in one saline-injected group (Control-1) were killed and their striata were kept at −80°C. Animals in other MPTP-treated groups were given various doses of deprenyl (i.p.) eight times during a period of 18 days beginning on the 3rd post-MPTP day. In one of the MPTP-treated groups mice received saline on the days of deprenyl treatment (MPTP-2). Animals in Control-1 and Control-2 groups received saline injections 5 and 5 + 8. Animals in Control-2, MPTP-2 and in groups with both MPTP and deprenyl treatments were killed 3 days after the last deprenyl treatment and the striata were kept at −80°C until processing for HPLC-determination of levels of DA and its metabolites. The number of animals varied from 5 to 8 per group. Values represent the means ± SEM.
[a] Significantly different ($P < 0.01$) from control groups. [b,c] Significantly different from MPTP-2 group ($P < 0.01$ and $P < 0.05$). [d,e] Significantly different from MPTP-2 group ($P < 0.01$ and $P < 0.05$).

partial recovery observed after a shorter period of time in N.M.R.I. mice (Hallman et al., 1985).

In mice that received DEP treatment with a cumulative dose of 0.08 and 80 mg/kg in the first experiment (Table 6) and 0.8 and 8.0 mg/kg in the second experiment (Table 7) the striatal DA levels were significantly higher than in the animals killed on the 3rd post-MPTP day, indicating that DEP may increase the spontaneous recovery of the striatal DA level. In fact, in the second experiment-DEP-treatment with the lowest dose (0.1 mg/kg/injection) significantly increased the striatal levels of DA and its metabolites even compared to the MPTP-2 group which were killed on the same post-MPTP day (day-21). The 0.1 mg/kg/2 days dose of DEP applied in our experiment from the 3rd post-MPTP day is comparable with the dosage used in DATATOP trial (10 mg per day ∼ 0.13–0.2 mg per kg body weight assuming that the patients weighed 50–75 kg). In

animals that received DEP in higher doses, the striatal DA levels were near or practically identical to the striatal levels of animals which received MPTP alone and were killed on day-21. In fact, the striatal levels of DOPAC and HVA in animals treated with 10 mg/kg DEP were lower (in the case of HVA the difference was significant) than in the MPTP-2 group, suggesting that the DEP treatment resulted in nonselective MAO-inhibition. In both experiments the DEP treatment (cumulative dose 0.8–80 mg/kg) significantly decreased the MPTP-induced shift to a higher striatal (DOPAC + HVA)/DA ratio seen in MPTP-1 and MPTP-2 groups. The antagonism of the MPTP-induced shift in (DOPAC + HVA)/DA ratio (Sershen et al., 1985; Sziráki, 1989) indicates that DEP treatment suppresses the MPTP-induced increase of striatal DA turnover and therefore reduces the risk of the oxidative stress associated with higher DA turnover.

The suppression of striatal DA turnover and the enhancement of striatal DA level by subacute DEP treatment in mice with already severe DA depletion and a 2–4-fold increase in DA turnover may be associated with several elements of its complex pharmacological action. It is evident that these effects of DEP can be related neither to its inhibitory effect on the bioactivation of MPTP by MAO-B, nor to the capacity of l-METH and l-AMPH generated from DEP to block the MPP$^+$ uptake by DA-ergic neurons. Suppression of MPTP-induced increase in DA turnover by subacute DEP treatment (1 and 10 mg/kg, eight times) starting from the 3rd post-MPTP day is probably associated with the inhibition of intraneuronal and extraneuronal metabolism of DA by MAOs similar to the reported suppression of the reserpine- and haloperidol-induced increase of striatal DA turnover by clorgyline and DEP (Cohen and Spina, 1989; Spina and Cohen, 1989; Cohen, 1990). (Repeated administration of DEP even at a dose of 1.0 mg/kg results in nonselective inhibition of MAO.) The (apparent) suppression of the MPTP-induced increase of DA turnover at lower doses (0.01 and 0.1 mg/kg, eight times) which are insufficient to cause significant inhibition of MAO-B (0.01 mg/kg, see Tatton, 1993) and MAO-A (Heikkila et al., 1990) may well be a partial prevention of the increase of DA turnover as a result of an enhanced neuronal repair associated with some not fully understood effects of lower-dose DEP treatment. In other words, DEP at low doses may decrease the necessity of compensatory changes in DA-turnover in the terminal field of nigrostriatal DA-ergic neurons, and therefore the risk of an increased oxidative stress associated with enzymatic and/or autooxidation of DA. It has been reported that delayed DEP treatment (0.01, 0.25, 10 mg/kg, i.p., eight times over a period of 18 days) can reduce the loss of tyrosine hydroxylase (TH) immunoreactive neurons in substantia nigra zona compacta (the cell body region of the nigrostriatal dopaminergic system) in C57BL mice after their DA-ergic neurons are damaged by MPTP treatment (Tatton and Greenwood, 1991; Tatton, 1993). These authors argued

that DEP treatment at cumulative doses of 2.0 and 80 mg/kg, which were equipotent in rescuing neurons, may act through MAO-B inhibition (Tatton and Greenwood, 1991). However, DEP treatment at a cumulative doses of 0.08 causing little or no MAO-B inhibition was also effective in reducing the loss of TH immunoreactive neurons, indicating that the mode of action of DEP in rescuing the DA neurons at this dose is unrelated to the inhibition of MAO-B (Tatton, 1993). Using C57BL/6J mice, they demonstrated that DEP (1.0 mg/kg every second day, for 21 days) can increase the number of surviving facial motor neurons after axotomy (Oh et al., 1994). (The separation of motorneurons from their target muscles by axotomy is a model for testing the dependence of motorneuron survival on muscle-derived trophic factor (for discussion see Oh et al., 1994)). In a mutant substrain of C57BL/6J mice, however, DEP at the same dose or its major metabolites, l-METH + l-AMPH (0.5 − 0.5 mg/kg, eight times), decreased the survival of motorneurons after axotomy. (This dose of the major metabolites of DEP is probably too high to mimic the effect of l-METH and l-AMPH generated from DEP at a dose of 1 mg/kg.) The decrease of survival of motorneurons in axotomized mutant mice treated with DEP or l-METH and l-AMPH, which exerted even a more pronounced effect, was related to a possible interaction with the normal mechanisms of programmed cell death (apoptosis) (Oh et al., 1994). In a more recent paper from the same group (Tatton et al., 1994), direct evidence has been provided that DEP can reduce the apoptotic death and internucleosomal DNA degradation in PC12 cells in a concentration-dependent manner at a maximum dose of 10^{-9} M. At high concentration (10^{-3} M), however, DEP significantly increased the PC12 death related to the withdrawal of trophic factors. The d-stereoisomer of DEP did not increase the PC12 cell survival at low concentration, but increased the death of the cells at high concentration. Pargyline was also effective in reducing the apoptotic cell death in PC12 cultures without increasing cell death at high concentrations. Pargyline (10 mg/kg) has been also shown to reduce the neuronal death of motorneurons after axotomy; d-DEP, however, was ineffective (see Tatton, 1993).

In experiment-2, one group of the MPTP-treated animals received eight injections of pargyline (cumulative dose 8 mg/kg). The subacute pargyline treatment, which was at 10-times lower dose than used in axotomized rats (see Tatton, 1993) and was applied from the 3rd post-MPTP day, also increased the striatal DA level and suppressed the increase of striatal DA turnover (data not shown). Unlike the metabolite-mediated neuroprotective effect of DEP, which is manifested in a brief time window, the DA-ergic neuroprotective/neurorescue effect of DEP in mice damaged already by MPTP seems partly to be related to shared pharmacological action(s) of DEP and pargyline. In a separate experiment, subacute DEP treatment starting from the 3rd post-MPTP day was applied at doses of 0.01, 0.1, 1.0, 10 and 20 mg/kg per injection. In that experiment, one group of MPTP-treated mice received d-DEP (10 mg/kg, eight times). Striatal DA levels in each of the groups treated with MPTP and DEP and killed on day-21 were higher than in the MPTP-treated mice killed on day-3. Similarly to the effect of DEP treatment on the survival of TH-immunoreactive somata of nigrostriatal DA-ergic neurons in mice that received DEP in a wide range of doses (0.01; 0.25; 10 mg/kg/2days; Tatton and Greenwood, 1991; Tatton, 1993), the enhancement of striatal DA levels was not proportional to DEP dosage. The lack of definable dose-response curve in the case of the effect of DEP treatment on the recovery of striatal DA level may be explained by the assumption that the measured actual DA levels reflect the net result of several antagonistic pharmacological actions of DEP including potential toxicity of its metabolites. DEP treatment in this experiment suppressed the MPTP-induced increase of DA turnover in a dose dependent manner. Subacute treatment with d-deprenyl (cumulative dose 80 mg/kg) also resulted in an enhanced striatal DA level compared to MPTP-1 group and in the suppression of MPTP-induced DA turnover, suggesting that the effect of DEP treatment on the MPTP-induced compensatory changes in the terminal field of the nigrostriatal DA-ergic neurons at this high dose is not stereoselective (data not shown).

Recently, increasing evidence has accumulated indicating that DEP may decrease the risk of oxidative stress via promotion of the scavenger function of the DA-ergic neurons in addition to the inhibition of oxidative stress associated with the compensatory increase of DA turnover. It has been reported that chronic treatment with DEP (0.25 and 2 mg/kg, daily; 3 weeks) causes an induction of superoxide dismutase (SOD) activity in the striatum of rats (Knoll, 1988). Selective increase of striatal SOD activity was confirmed later by Carrillo et al. (1991), and Clow et al. (1991), although these authors found an increased SOD activity only at a 2 mg/kg dose. Vizuete et al. (1993) demonstrated a protection against MPP^+-toxicity in striatal slices and an increase in both SOD and catalase activity in rats treated with DEP (2 mg/kg per day for 3 weeks), suggesting that the protective effect of DEP was independent of the induction of SOD and catalase activities. A more recent study (Lai et al., 1994) claims that the effect of chronic DEP treatment on striatal SOD activity in rats is uncertain.

Intrastriatal infusion of 2'Me-MPTP and MPP^+ has been found to cause sustained dopamine release and subsequent formation of hydroxyl radical ($\cdot$OH) in rats (Chiueh et al., 1992; Wu et al., 1993). Pretreatment with DEP and clorgyline (each 5 mg, i.p.) completely suppressed the $\cdot$OH formation due to 2'Me-MPTP infusion via the inhibition of the formation of pyridinium ions and the enzymatic and or autooxidation of DA (Chiueh et al., 1992). Recent in vitro studies indicate that DEP, clorgyline, and pargyline suppress non-enzymatic DA autooxidation and associated free radical formation (Chiueh et al., 1994). Intrastriatal perfusion of DEP significantly decreased the $\cdot$OH formation induced by intrastriatal administration of MPP^+, and intranigral infusion of DEP completely prevented the MPP^+-induced mild to moderate striatal DA-depletion and nigral injury probably via its apparent antioxidant properties (Wu et al., 1993). They recently provided evidence (Wu et al., 1994) that supplementary treatment with DEP (0.25 mg/kg twice daily for 4 days) significantly rescued nigrostriatal DA-ergic neurons from partial striatal DA depletion induced by intranigral infusion of MPP$^+$ (8.4 nmol) coadministered with DEP (4.2 nmol).

Taken together, these are the first data to show that DEP, in MPTP-treated animals with already damaged nigrostriatal dopaminergic neurons, can enhance the spontaneous recovery of DA levels and suppress the MPTP-induced increase of striatal DA turnover, an increased risk for oxidative stress for the surviving neurons.

Summary

In the present study we provide further evidence for our recent finding that DEP has neuroprotective effects against dopaminergic toxicity of MPTP and its 2′-substituted analogs in mice, which are associated with the ability of its major metabolites, l-methamphetamine and l-amphetamine to block the neuronal uptake of the toxic pyridinium metabolites of MPTP and its analogs. Here we demonstrated that protection by a 30-min DEP posttreatment (10 mg/kg) against MPTP (40 mg/kg)-induced decrease of striatal dopamine level is reduced when mice received SKF 525A (25 mg/kg), an inhibitor of the metabolism of DEP 10 min prior to DEP treatment. For the first time, we demonstrated that a 30-min pre- or post-treatment with DEP (10 mg/kg) provided substantial protection against striatal dopamine depletion induced by 2′Et-MPTP (30 mg/kg), which is primarily bioactivated by MAO-A. A 30-min posttreatment with DEP (but not by pargyline or clorgyline), in addition to protection against dopamine depletion, also prevents the decrease in striatal mazindol binding (an indicator of the integrity of dopaminergic terminals) induced by MPTP (40 mg/kg), 2′Me-MPTP (15 mg/kg) or 2′Et-MPTP (30 mg/kg).

A subacute DEP treatment of mice with severe injury in the terminal fields of the nigrostriatal dopaminergic system (80–90% loss of dopamine; 2–4-fold increase in dopamine turnover as reflected by higher metabolite/DA ratios) enhanced the recovery of striatal dopamine level and suppressed the MPTP-induced elevation of dopamine turnover. Deprenyl treatment was applied in a wide range of dose (0.01–20 mg/kg, i.p., eight times over 18 days from the 3rd day after the last MPTP injection) to mice that had received MPTP (30 mg/kg; i.p.) for 5 consecutive days. The effect of subacute DEP treatment on the recovery of striatal dopamine level was most pronounced at a cumulative dose of 0.8 mg/kg, indicating that higher dosage of DEP may be less beneficial.

Conclusions

The present study extended our previous findings that the action of DEP treatment on dopaminergic neurotoxicity in the mouse model of MPTP-parkinsonism involves the inhibition of uptake of toxic pyridinium metabolites of MPTP and its 2′-substituted analogs. The uptake inhibitory protective element, which is associated with the rapid metabolism of l-deprenyl to l-methamphetamine and l-amphetamine, is only manifested when DEP is administered within a short period either before or after treatment with MPTP or its 2′-substituted analogs.

The suppression of compensatory increase of DA turnover and the enhancement on striatal DA levels by subacute DEP treatment in mice with already severe damage of the nigrostriatal dopaminergic systems may provide further experimental rationale for a low dose DEP therapy in the treatment of Parkinson's disease and perhaps other neurodegenerative diseases.

Acknowledgments

We thank I. Berekhelyi, I. Sz. Törzsök, J. Vámosi, M. Jobbágy, E. Blazsek and D. Szántó for technical assistance. We also thank Professor Keith F. Tipton, Trinity College, Dublin, for his suggestions related to the experimentation on the metabolite-mediated protection of DEP against MPTP neurotoxicity. The first author is grateful to Wilma Davis and Dr. Dennis L. Murphy, Laboratory of Clinical Science, NIMH, for the excellent manuscript processing and the helpful discussions, respectively.

References

Agid, Y., Javoy, F. and Glowinski, J. (1973) Hyperactivity of remaining dopaminergic neurons after partial destruction of the nigrostriatal dopaminergic system in the rat. *Nature New Biol.*, 245: 150–151.

Ben-Shachar, D. and Youdim, M.B.H. (1991) Intranigral iron injection induces behavioral and biochemical "Parkinsonism" in rats. *J. Neurochem.*, 57: 2133–2135.

Birkmayer, W., Knoll, J., Riederer, P., Youdim, M.B.H., Hars, V. and Marton, J. (1985) Increased life expectancy resulting from addition of L-deprenyl to madopar treatment in Parkinson's disease: A longterm study. *J. Neural Transm.*, 64: 113–127.

Birkmayer, W., Riederer, P., Ambrozi, L. and Youdim, M.B.H. (1977) Implications of combined treatment with Madopar and L-deprenyl in Parkinson's disease. *Lancet*, i: 439–443.

Carrillo, M.C., Kanai, S., Nokubo, M. and Kitani, K. (1991) (-) Deprenyl induces activities of both superoxide dismutase and catalase but not of glutahione peroxidase in the striatum of young male rats. *Life Sci.*, 48: 517–521.

Chiueh, C.C., Huang, S.-J. and Murphy, D.L. (1994) Suppression of hydroxyl radical formation by MAO inhibitors: a novel possible neuroprotective mechanism in dopaminergic neurotoxicity. *J. Neural Transm.*, 41: 189–196.

Chiueh, C.C., Johannessen, J.N., Sun, J.L., Bacon, J.P. and Markey, S.P. (1986) Reversible neurotoxicity of MPTP in the nigrostriatal dopaminergic system of mice. In: S.P. Markey, N.J. Castagnoli, A.J. Trevor and I.J. Kopin (Eds.), *MPTP–A Neurotoxin Producing a Parkinsonian Syndrome*, Academic Press, New York, pp. 473–479.

Chiueh, C.C., Miyake, H. and Peng, M. (1993) Role of dopamine autoxidation, hydroxyl radical generation and calcium overload in underlying mechanism involved in MPTP-induced parkinsonism. *Adv. Neurol.*, 60: 251–257.

Chiueh, C.S., Huang, S.-J. and Murphy, D.L. (1992) Enhanced hydroxyl radical generation by 2′-methyl analog of MPTP: suppression by clorgyline and deprenyl. *Synapse*, 11: 346–348.

Clow, A., Hussain, T., Glover, V., Sandler, M., Dexter, D.T. and Walker, M. (1991) (-)-Deprenyl can induce soluble superoxide dismutase in rat striata. *J. Neural Transm.*, 86: 77–80.

Cohen, G. (1990) Monoamine oxidase and oxidative stress at dopaminergic synapses. *J. Neural Transm.*, 32: 229–238.

Cohen, G. and Spina, M.B. (1989) Deprenyl suppresses the oxidant stress associated with increased dopamine turnover. *Ann. Neurol.*, 26: 689–690.

Davis, G.C., Williams, A.C., Markey, S.P., Ebert, M.H., Caine, E.D., Reichert, C.M. and Kopin, I.J. (1979) Chronic Parkinsonism secondary to intravenous injection of meperidine analogs. *Psychiatry Res.*, 1: 249–254.

Dudley, M.W. (1988) The depletion of rat cortical norepinephrine and the inhibition of [^{3}H]-norepinephrine uptake by xylamine does not require monoamine oxidase activity. *Life Sci.*, 43: 1871–1877.

Engberg, G., Elebring, T. and Nissbrandt, H. (1991) Deprenyl (selegiline), a selective MAO-B inhibitor with active metabolites: Effects on locomotor activity, dopaminergic neurotransmission and firing rate of nigral dopamine neurons. *J. Pharmacol. Exp. Ther.*, 259(2): 841–847.

Finnegan, K.T., Skratt, J.J., Irwin, I., DeLanney, L.E. and Langston, J.W. (1990) Protection against DSP-4-induced neurotoxicity by deprenyl is not related to its inhibition of MAO-B. *Eur. J. Pharmacol.*, 184: 119–126.

Hallman, H., Lange, J., Olson, L., Stromberg, I. and Jonsson, G. (1985) Neurochemical and histochemical characterization of neurotoxic effects of 1-methyl-4-phenyl-1,2,3,6-tetrahydropyridine on brain catecholamine neurones in the mouse. *J. Neurochem.*, 44: 117–127.

Hallman, H., Olsen, L. and Jonsson, G. (1984) Neurotoxicity of the meperidine analogue N-methyl-4-phenyl-1,2,3,6-tetrahydropyridine on brain catecholamine neurons in the mouse. *Eur. J. Pharmacol.*, 97: 133–136.

Hefti, F., Melamed, E. and Wurtman, R.J. (1980) Partial lesions of the dopaminergic nigrostriatal system in rat brain: biochemical characterization. *Brain Res.*, 195: 123–137.

Heikkila, R.A., Terleckyj, I. and Sieber, B.A. (1990) Monoamine oxidase and the bioactivation of MPTP and related neurotoxins: relevance to DATATOP. *J. Neural Transm.*, 32: 217–227.

Heikkila, R.E. and Sonsalla, P.K. (1987) The use of the MPTP-treated mouse as an animal model of parkinsonism. *Can. J. Neurol. Sci.*, 14: 436–440.

Heikkila, R.E., Hess, A. and Duvoisin, R.C. (1984a) Dopaminergic neurotoxicity of 1-methyl-4-phenyl-1,2,3,4-tetrahydropiridine in mice. *Science*, 224: 1451–1453.

Heikkila, R.E., Manzino, L., Cabbat, F.S. and Duvoisin, R.C. (1984b) Protection against the dopaminergic neurotoxicity of l-methyl-4-phenyl-1,2,5,6-tetrahydropyridine by monoamine oxidase inhibitors. *Nature*, 311: 467–469.

Heikkila, R.E., Kindt, M.V., Sonsalla, P.K., Giovanni, A., Youngster, S.K., McKeown, K.A. and Singer, T.P. (1988) Importance of monoamine oxidase A in the bioactivation of neurotoxic analogs of 1-methyl-4-phenyl-1,2,3,6-tetrahydropyridine. *Proc. Natl. Acad. Sci. USA*, 85: 6172–6176.

Hornykiewicz, O. and Kish, S.J. (1986) Biochemical pathophysiology of Parkinson's disease. *Adv. Neurol.*, 45: 19–34.

Javitch, J.A., Blaustein, R.O. and Synder, S.H. (1984) [³H]Mazindol binding associated with neuronal dopamine and norephrine uptake sites. *Mol. Pharmacol.*, 26: 35.

Jonsson, G., Sundstrom, E., Nwanze, E., Hallman, H. and Luthman, J. (1986) Mode of action of MPTP on catecholaminergic neurons in the mouse. In: S.P. Markey, N. Castagnoli Jr., A.J. Trevor and I.J. Kopin (Eds.), *MPTP–A Neurotoxic Producing a Parkinsonian Syndrome*, Academic Press, New York, pp. 253–272.

Kardos, V., Patthy, M., Kollár, E., Gaál, J., Solti, M. and Sziráki, I. (1992) Deprenyl protects against neurotoxicity induced by 2'-CH_3-MPTP in mice. *Neurosci. Int.*, 21(Abstract No. 38): D10.

Karoum, D.F. and Wyatt, R.J. (1982) Metabolism of (−)deprenyl's therapeutic benefit: A biochemical assessment. *Neurology*, 32: 503–509.

Knoll, J. (1988) The striatal dopamine dependency of life span in male rats: Longevity study with (−)deprenyl. *Mech. Ageing Dev.*, 46: 237–262.

Lai, C.T., Zuo, D.M. and Yu, P.H. (1994) Is brain superoxide dismutase activity increased following chronic treatment with l-deprenyl? *J. Neural Transm.*, 41: 221–229.

Langston, J.W., Ballard, P., Tetrud, J.W. and Irwin, I. (1983) Chronic parkinsonism in humans due to a product of meperidine-analog synthesis. *Science*, 219: 979–980.

Marshall, J.F. and Navarrete, R.J. (1990) Contrasting tissue factors predict heterogeneous striatal dopamine neurotoxicity after MPTP or methamphetmaine treatment. *Brain Res.*, 534: 348–351.

Mayer, R.A., Kindt, M.V. and Heikkila, R.E. (1986) Prevention of the nigrostriatal toxicity of 1-methyl-4-phenyl-1,2,3,6-tetrahydropyridine by inhibitors of 3,4-dihydroxyphenylethyl-amine transport. *J. Neurochem.*, 47: 1073–1079.

Mohanakumar, K.P., De Bartolomeis, A., Wu, R.-M., Yeh, K.J., Sternberger, L., Peng, S.-Y., Murphy, D.L. and Chiueh, C.C. (1994) Ferrous-citrate complex and nigral degeneration: evidence for free-radical formation and lipid peroxidation. *Ann. N.Y. Acad. Sci.*, 738: 25–36.

Oh, C., Murray, B., Bhattacharya, N., Holland, D. and Tatton, W.G. (1994) (−)-Deprenyl alters the survival of adult murine facial motoneurons after axotomy: increases in vulnerable C57BL strain but decreases in motor neuron degeneration mutants. *J. Neurosci. Res.*, 38: 64–74.

Parkes, J.D., Tarsy, D., Marsden, C.D., Bovill, K.T., Phipps, J.A., Rose, P. and Asselman, P. (1975) Amphetamines in the treatment of Parkinson's disease. *J. Neurol. Neurosurg. Psychiatry*, 38: 232–237.

Parkinson Study Group (1989) Effect of deprenyl on the progression of disability in early Parkinson's disease. *N. Engl. J. Med.*, 321: 1364–1371.

Parkinson Study Group (1993) Effects of tocopherol and deprenyl on the progression of disability in early Parkinson's disease. *N. Engl. J. Med.*, 328: 176–183.

Patthy, M. and Gyenge, R. (1988) Perfluorinated acids as ion-pairing agent in the determination of monoamine transmitters and some prominent metabolites in rat brain by high-performance liquid chromatography with amperometric detection. *J. Chromatogr.*, 449: 191–205.

Philips, R.S. (1981) Amphetamine, parahydroxy-amphetamine and beta-phenylethylamine in mouse brain and urine after (−)- and (+)-deprenyl administration. *J. Pharm. Pharmacol.*, 33: 739–741.

Reinhard, J.F. and Nichol, C.A. (1986) Neurotoxin MPTP decreases striatal dopamine and tetrahydrobiopterin levels and increases striatal dopamine turnover in mice. In: S.P. Markey, N. Castagnoli Jr, A.J. Trevor and I.J. Kopin (Eds.), *MPTP–A Neurotoxic Producing a Parkinsonian Syndrome*, Academic Press, New York, pp. 473–479.

Reynolds, G.P., Elsworth, J.D., Blau, K., Sandler, M., Lees, A.J. and Stern, G.M. (1978) Deprenyl is metabolized to methamphetamine and amphetamine in man. *Br. J. Clin. Pharmacol.*, 6: 542–544.

Sershen, H., Mason, M.F., Hashim, A. and Lajtha, A. (1985) Effect of N-methyl-4-phenyl-1,2,3,6-tetrahydropyridine (MPTP) on age-related changes in dopamine turnover and transporter function in the mouse striatum. *Eur. J. Pharmacol.*, 113: 135–136.

Sershen, H., Mason, M.F., Reith, M.E.A., Hashim, A. and Lajtha, A. (1986a) Effect of amphetamine on 1-methyl-4-phenyl-1,2,3,6-tetrahydrop yridine (MPTP) neurotoxicity in mice. *Neuropharmacology*, 25: 927–930.

Sershen, H., Mason, M.F., Reith, M.E.A., Hashim, A. and Lajtha, A. (1986b) Effect of nicotine and amphetamine N-methyl-4-phenyl-1,2,3,6-tetrahydropyridine (MPTP) neurotoxicity in mice. *Neuropharmacology*, 25: 1231–1234.

Shahi, G.S., Moochhala, S.M., Das, N.P., Sunamoto, J. and Tajima, K. (1990) The neurotoxin 1-methyl-4-phenyl-1,2,3,6-tetrahydropyridine (MPTP) induces changes in the heme spin state of microsomal cytochrome P-450. *Biochem. Int.*, 22(5): 895–902.

Sonsalla, D.K., Yougster, S.K., Kindt, M.V. and Heikkila, R.E. (1987) Characteristics of 1-methyl-4-(2'methylphenyl)-1,2,3,6-tetrahydropyrid ine-induced neurotoxicity in the mouse. *J. Pharmacol. Exp. Ther.*, 242: 850–857.

Spina, M.B. and Cohen, G. (1989) Dopamine turnover and glutathione oxidation: implications for Parkinson disease. *Proc. Natl. Acad. Sci. USA*, 86: 1398–1400.

Sundstrom, E. and Jonsson, G. (1986) Differential time course of protection by monoamine oxidase inhibition and uptake inhibition against MPTP neurotoxicity on central catecholamine neurons in mice. *Eur. J. Pharmacol.*, 122: 275–278.

Sziráki, I. (1989) A mouse model of parkinsonism: differential neurotoxicity of MPTP in two inbred strains with genetic differences in central dopaminergic systems. 19th Meeting of the Federation of European Biochemical Societies, Rome, Abstract, TH91L.

Sziráki, I., Juhász, M., Kóbor, Gy., Lajtha, A. and Vadász, Cs. (1986) Regional differences in the effect of MPTP on tyrosine hydroxylase activity in mice. *Soc. Neurosci. Abstr.*, 12: 609.

Sziráki, I., Kardos, V., Patthy, M., Pátfalusi, M., Gaál, J., Solti, M. and Kollár, E. (1992) Complex mode of action of deprenyl in protection against MPTP-parkinsonism in mice. *Neurosci. Int.*, 21(Abstract No. 69): D18.

Sziráki, I., Kardos, V., Patthy, M., Pátfalusi, M., Gaál, J., Solti, M., Kollár, E. and Tömösközi, Z.S. (1993) Metabolites of deprenyl are involved in protection against the neurotoxicity of MPTP and its analogs in mice. *J. Neurochem.*, 61: S64.

Sziráki, I., Kardos, V., Patthy, M., Pátfalusi, M. and Budai, G. (1994a) Methamphetamine protects against MPTP neurotoxicity in C57BL mice. *Eur. J. Pharmacol.*, 251: 311–314.

Sziráki, I., Kardos, V., Patthy, M., Pátfalusi, M., Gaál, J., Solti, M., Kollár, E. and Singer, J. (1994b) Amphetamine-metabolites of deprenyl involved in protection against neurotoxicity induced by MPTP and 2′-methyl-MPTP. *J. Neural Transm.*, 41: 207–219.

Tatton, W.G. (1993) Selegiline can mediate neuronal rescue rather than neuronal protection. *Mov. Disord.*, 8: 520–530.

Tatton, W.G. and Greenwood, C.E. (1991) Rescue of dying neurons: A new action for deprenyl in MPTP parkinsonism. *J. Neurosci. Res.*, 30: 666–672.

Tatton, W.G., Ju, W.Y.L., Holland, D.P., Tai, C. and Kwan, M. (1994) (−)-Deprenyl reduces PC12 cell apoptosis by inducing new protein synthesis. *J. Neurochem.*, 63: 1572–1575.

Tetrud, J.W. and Langston, J.W. (1989) The effect of deprenyl (Selegiline) on the natural history of Parkinson's disease. *Science*, 245: 519–522.

Tipton, K.F. and Singer, T.P. (1993) Advances in our understanding of the mechanisms of the neurotoxicity of MPTP and related compounds. *J. Neurochem.*, 61: 1191–1206.

Vizuete, M.L., Steffen, V., Ayala, A., Cano, J. and Machado, A. (1993) Protective effect of deprenyl against 1-methyl-4-phenylpyridinium neurotoxicity in rat striatum. *Neurosci. Lett.*, 152: 113–116.

Wu, R.-M., Chiueh, C.C., Pert, A. and Murphy, D.L. (1993) Apparent antioxidant effect of l-deprenyl on hydroxyl radical formation and nigral injury elicited by MPP + in vivo. *Eur. J. Pharmacol.*, 243: 241–247.

Wu, R.-M., Murphy, D.L. and Chiueh, C.C. (1995) Neuronal protective and rescue effects of deprenyl against MPP + dopaminergic toxicity. *J. Neural Transm. (Gen. Sect.)*, 100: 53–61.

Youngster, S.K., Duvoisin, R.C., Hess, A., Sonsalla, P.K., Kindt, M.V. and Heillika, R.E. (1986) 1-methyl-4-(2′-methylphenyl)-1,2,3,6-te trahydropyridine (2′-CH_3-MPTP) is a more potent dopaminergic neurotoxin than MPTP in mice. *Eur. J. Pharmacol.*, 122: 283–287.

Peter M. Yu, Keith F. Tipton and Alan A. Boulton (Eds.)
Progress in Brain Research, Vol 106

CHAPTER 17

Effects of transient global ischemia and a monoamine oxidase inhibitor ifenprodil on rat brain monoamine metabolism

Takeshi Tadano[1], Akihiko Yonezawa[1], Katsuyuki Oyama[1], Kensuko Kisara[1], Yuichiro Arai[2], Mitsunori Togashi[3] and Hiroyasu Kinemuchi[3]

[1] *Department of Pharmacology, Tohoku College of Pharmacy, Aobaku, Sendai 981,* [2] *Department of Pharmacology, School of Medicine, Showa University, Tokyo 141, and* [3] *Laboratory of Biological Chemistry, Faculty of Sciences and Engineering, Ishinomaki Senshu University, Ishinomaki 986, Japan*

Introduction

It is well documented that certain brain regions and specific neuronal cell types are highly susceptible to brief periods of transient cerebral ischaemia. Although cerebral ischaemia inhibits brain energy metabolism and protein biosynthesis (Kleihues and Hossmann, 1971; Morimoto et al., 1978), the selective susceptibility of these regions and/or cell types to the ischaemia cannot be fully explained by regional blood flow changes or energy depletion. Some other mechanisms may thus be responsible. Brain l-glutamate is an endogenous excitatory amino acid (EAA) neurotransmitter that contributes to excitatory input to a majority of synapses in the CNS (for review, see Monaghan et al., 1989; Wroblewski and Danysz, 1989; Headley and Grillner, 1990). It has been postulated that the neurotoxicity of glutamate plays an important role in the pathogenesis of the neuronal degeneration associated with several neurological disease states, including ischaemia (see Meldrum and Garthwaite 1990). The *N*-methyl-D-aspartate (NMDA) receptor plays a crucial role in glutamate-induced cytotoxicity in cortical neurons (Hartley and Choi, 1989). A strong correlation between the neurotoxic and excitatory potencies of different EAA analogues suggests a convergence in the mechanism underlying these two actions (Meldrum and Garthwaite, 1990).

Recent studies suggest that the levels of EAAs, such as glutamate and aspartate, are markedly elevated in the ischaemic brain. Excitotoxic mechanisms triggered by the ischaemia-induced EAA release may constitute a major factor determining selective vulnerability. Studies with NMDA receptor antagonists have led to the suggestion that this receptor plays a major role in the selective neuronal loss occurring after cerebral ischaemia. The activity of NMDA receptors is influenced by a number of endogenous substances, such as divalent cations (Mg^{2+}, Zn^{2+}), glycine (Wroblewski and Danysz, 1989), and polyamines (spermine and spermidine) (Ransom and Stec, 1988). These latter two groups of substances potentiate the effects of NMDA agonists, suggesting that selective antagonists for these two modulatory sites may result in a neuroprotective action against the NMDA complex-mediated neurotoxicity.

Ifenprodil was originally reported as an effective cerebral vasodilator (Carron et al., 1971). Recently, however, this agent has been evaluated as a cerebral anti-ischaemic agent, since it is a noncompetitive NMDA antagonist, and has protective effects in animal models of focal cerebral ischaemia (Gotti et al., 1988; Carter et al., 1988). The protective effect of ifenprodil was thought to act directly against NMDA-induced acute excitotoxicity (Zeevalk and Nicklas, 1990). Polyamines selectively bind to the modulatory site linked to the NMDA receptor complex and potentiate the excitatory action of glutamate on the NMDA receptor. It is now becoming clear that ifenprodil interacts mainly with this polyamine modulatory site (Carter et al., 1988, 1990; Sprosen and Woodruff, 1990). Ifenprodil can also alter cerebral blood flow, probably by an α-adrenoceptor blocking action (Carron et al., 1971) and/or by acting as a Ca^{2+} antagonist (Honda and Sakai, 1987). These actions may potentiate the efficacy of ifenprodil as an anti-ischaemic agent.

Changes in the levels and turnover of neurotransmitter monoamines and their metabolites have recently been implicated in the pathogenesis of ischaemic brain injury in animal models (Harik et al., 1986). These monoamine changes during ischaemia and after reperfusion may contribute, at least in part, to neuronal cell death (Globus et al., 1988; Slivka et al., 1988). For instance, brain dopamine (DA) is involved in ischaemia-induced cell damage in the striatum, probably due to the marked activation of the nigro-striatal DAergic system after the ischaemic insult (Globus et al., 1987b, 1988). Administration of the selective MAO-B inhibitor pargyline was found to increase the survival rate of rats subjected to ischaemia (Damsma et al., 1990). This effect might be due to the protection of brain tissue from the MAO-mediated, potentially neurotoxic product hydrogen peroxide (H_2O_2) and/or free radicals (Globus et al., 1987a,b; Damsma et al., 1990; Arai et al., 1991; Kinemuchi et al., 1993).

Our previous studies reported the inhibition of both MAO-A and MAO-B activity by ifenprodil with a slightly higher selectivity for MAO-A. In this study we have measured the levels of some monoamines and their metabolites in various brain regions following transient ischaemia in rats; we have also evaluated the effects of ifenprodil on these brain amine levels.

Materials and methods

Male Wistar rats, weighing 250 ± 10 g, were used. Animals were housed in cages with free access to food and water under conditions of constant temperature ($23.0 \pm 0.1°C$), humidity ($55 \pm 5\%$) and a 12 h light/dark cycle (9:00 h–21:00 h). Cerebral ischaemia was produced as described previously by Pulsinelli and Brierley (1979), by temporary occlusion of the bilateral common carotid arteries. Under light ether anesthesia, the bilateral carotid arteries were occluded for 20 min. Ifenprodil was then administered (10 mg/kg, i.p., as the salt) and blood reperfusion re-started. Rats were killed 1 h after the injection of ifenprodil and DA, NE, 3MT, 5HT and Dopac, HVA and 5HIAA assessed. The rat brain was dissected into eight regions (cortex, hippocampus, hypothalamus, thalamus, midbrain, P-M oblongata, cerebellum and striatum) on an ice-cold glass plate and each region was homogenized in ice-cold 0.1 M perchloric acid containing 0.1 mM EDTA using an ultrasonic cell disruptor. The homogenates were centrifuged at $12\,000 \times g$ for 10 min and aliquots of the supernatants were used for assay of amines and the metabolites by high-performance liquid chromatography with electro-chemical detection (Murai et al., 1988).

The in vitro assay of MAO-A and MAO-B activity in rat forebrain homogenates was carried out radiochemically, as reported previously (Kinemuchi et al., 1985; Arai et al., 1991) using 0.1 mM [^{14}C]5-HT and [^{14}C]benzylamine (BZ) as respective substrates. As also reported previously (Kinemuchi et al., 1985), the oxidation of 5-HT (by MAO-A) and BZ (by MAO-B) at the concentrations used in the homogenates was completely inhibited by 0.1 μM clorgyline and l-deprenyl, respectively. Semicarbazide-sensitive amine oxidase (SSAO) activity in rat lung homogenates was also determined radiochemically as previously reported (Morikawa et al., 1986) using 0.01 mM

[^{14}C]BZ as substrate. To investigate changes in the extent of inhibition of MAO and SSAO by ifenprodil, the respective enzyme preparations were preincubated with ifenprodil at 37°C for various times, as indicated in the text. After preincubation, the remaining activities of MAO-A, MAO-B and SSAO were determined, as described above. The results were compared with those obtained without preincubation.

Ifenprodil tartrate was kindly supplied by Grelan Pharmaceutical Co., Tokyo, Japan. Radioactively labelled 5-HT as creatinine sulfate and BZ as its hydrochloride were purchased from Amersham International plc, UK. Other agents used in this study were of the highest grade commercially available. The data were analyzed using analysis of variance (ANOVA) and the critical difference of the means was calculated by Dunnett's test.

Results

As described in our preliminary report (Arai et al., 1991), some vasodilators and cerebral metabolic activators that have been clinically used, such as ifenprodil, dilazep, ergotamine, homopantothenic acid, pantothenic acid, γ-aminobutyric acid, γ-amino-β-hydroxybutyric acid, pentoxifylline and centrol phenoxine, were tested to determine whether or not they affect MAO and SSAO activities. Of the agents tested, only ifenprodil inhibited both forms of MAO activity, albeit with different sensitivities. Preincubation of MAO-A or MAO-B in the homogenate with ifenprodil at 37°C for 30 min did not change the extent of inhibition of either form of MAO. No other clinically used agent tested affected either MAO-A or MAO-B in the concentration range 0.01 μM to 1 mM, with or without preincubation for up to 60 min. Double reciprocal plots of inhibition of both forms of MAO by ifenprodil showed that the inhibitions were competitive towards both MAO-A (5-HT) and MAO-B (BZ) with K_i values of 75 μM for MAO-A and 110 μM for MAO-B, determined from linear slope replots against various concentrations of ifenprodil. These results clearly indicate that only

ifenprodil significantly inhibited MAO, with a slightly higher reversible inhibition potency on MAO-A. Despite inhibition of rat brain MAO, ifenprodil did not cause any change in rat lung SSAO activity either after preincubation at 37°C for up to 60 min, or without preincubation. This absence of effect on SSAO was also observed for other clinically used agents tested.

Levels of monoamines and their main metabolites in the eight brain regions (only striatum and hippocampus shown in Figs. 1 and 2) were measured 60 min after injection of ifenprodil (10 mg/kg) and the start of the blood reperfusion in rats subject to a 20 min cerebral ischaemia insult. Global ischaemic treatment caused a severe reduction of local cerebral blood flow in cortex, hippocampus, thalamus, and striatum, and an increase of extracellular glutamate in these brain regions. At end of the 20 min ischaemia insult, histopathological injury in these brain regions, especially in the striatum, is induced (Globus et al., 1988). In the present study, amines and their metabolite levels were estimated in eight regions and compared with those in two control groups, i.e. sham-operated and ischaemia untreated group. In comparison to the sham-operated rats, the cerebral ischaemic treatment induced an increase in DA, 3,4-dihydroxyphenylacetic acid (DOPAC) and homovanillic acid (HVA) and a decrease in 3MT in striatum (see Fig. 1). An increase in HVA in the cortex and P-M oblongata was also seen (results not shown). This treatment also increased 5-HT in striatum and cerebellum and increased 5-hydroxyindoleacetic acid (5-HIAA) in the striatum, cortex, hippocampus, midbrain and P-M oblongata. NE levels decreased only in the cerebellum after this treatment. The striatal DA and DOPAC levels elevated by the ischaemic treatment were substantially reversed and returned toward the levels of the sham-operated group after treatment with ifenprodil (see Fig. 1). The increased 5-HT and 5-HIAA levels, however, were less substantially decreased, whilst HVA was even further increased after ifenprodil treatment (Fig. 1). In contrast to the striatum, hippocampal levels of

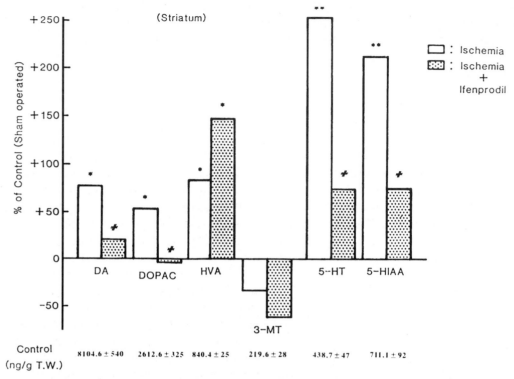

Fig. 1. Effects of ischemia and ifenprodil treatment on rat striatal monoamines and their principal metabolites. Results obtained are expressed as percentages of control (sham-operated group). Below the columns the absolute values of each substance are expressed in ng/g of tissue. $*P < 0.05$, $**P < 0.01$, significantly different from the sham-operated group. $P < 0.01$, significantly different from the ischaemic group.

DA and HVA were markedly increased, while DOPAC and 5-HT were not much changed after ifenprodil treatment (Fig. 2). 5HT and 5HIAA, whilst increased by the ischaemia, were not much affected by ifenprodil.

Discussion

There is increasing evidence that the release of synaptic EAAs and the consequently prolonged activation of excitatory receptors mediate the death of anoxic neurons. An increased glutamate release has been observed during both cerebral anoxia and ischaemia. The neurotoxic action of ischaemia has been postulated to be the result of receptor-mediated increases in ionic permeability linked to EAA's potent excitatory actions, involv-

ing Na^+ entry which then leads to passive Cl^- and water influx, and consequent cell swelling and lysis (Rothman and Olney, 1986). This system also includes Ca^{2+} entry which mediates neurotoxicity. EAA receptor agonists of the NMDA site may induce selective neuronal death of discrete brain regions, such as the hippocampus, striatum and cortex, since these regions are the most sensitive to ischaemia (for review, see Meldrum and Garthwaite, 1990). Higher sensitivity was confirmed in the present study, where even 60 min after reperfusion some neurotransmitter monoamines and their metabolites were found to be increased in these brain regions in the ischaemic animals. Except for HVA and 3-MT, these increased levels of amines and metabolites in striatum were reversed after injection of ifen-

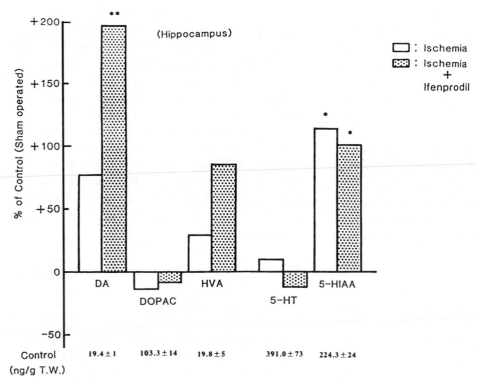

Fig. 2. Effects of ischaemia and ifenprodil treatment on rat hippocampus monoamines and their metabolites. Results, absolute values and significance are as in Fig. 1.

prodil. This agent, however, failed to reverse the levels of these substances in cortex and hippocampus (results not shown). A number of studies have confirmed the anti-ischaemic potential of NMDA antagonists.

Although ifenprodil was originally thought to act as a cerebral vasodilator that improved cerebrovascular disease and/or dementia (Carron et al., 1971) it has also recently been reported to be a potent anti-ischaemic agent where it effectively blocks neuronal cell death induced by activating the NMDA receptor complex. More recent reports have shown that this agent mainly binds to the polyamine modulatory site with consequent protection towards the NMDA receptor complex (Schoemaker et al., 1990; Baker et al., 1991; Shalaby et al., 1992; Tamura et al., 1993). In addition to these EAAs, other neurotransmitters or neuro-

modulators have also been proposed to cause or modulate cerebral ischaemic or anoxic neuronal death (Globus et al., 1987a,b).

We confirm here that the brain levels of some monoamine transmitters and their metabolites are markedly changed by transient cerebral ischaemia. These monoamine changes may also contribute to neuronal cell death (Globus et al., 1987a, 1988; Slivka et al., 1988). Regional changes in DA and 5-HT, and their metabolites, in ischaemia groups were observed even at 60 min after the ischaemia (Globus et al., 1988; Baker et al., 1991). After ifenprodil treatment, DA, DOPAC, 5-HT and 5-HIAA levels were greatly reduced almost to the levels of the sham-operated controls, but in cortex and hippocampus this tendency was not observed (Figs. 2–4). As previously reported (Arai et al., 1991), and in the present in vitro studies, ifenprodil competitively and reversibly inhibited both MAO-A and MAO-B activity with slightly higher potency towards MAO-A. MAO activity depends on oxygen tension (Tipton, 1972) and the A-form of this enzyme is mainly responsible for metabolism of these amines (Kinemuchi et al., 1984). Following perfusion the increased DA (Baker et al., 1991) and 5-HT (Sarna et al., 1990) rapidly (within 10 min) returned toward baseline. The inhibition of MAO by ifenprodil failed to increase DA and 5-HT in the striatum, but instead decreased their levels towards baseline (Fig. 1). One of the possible explanations for this finding might be the depletion of these transmitters in the releasable pools during ischaemia.

Recent reports have shown that the nigrostriatal DAergic system is activated by transient cerebral ischaemia. This may indicate that DA is involved in ischaemia-induced cell damage in the striatum (Globus et al., 1988; Slivka et al., 1988). An increase in DA and 5-HT turnovers in the rat striatum after ischaemia was confirmed in this present study, by the increase in their metabolite levels. The deleterious DA effects might be due to the production of the MAO-mediated, potentially neurotoxic product, hydrogen peroxide. MAO may also play an important role in other neurodegenerative disorders, because of its ability to produce cytotoxic free radicals (hydroxyl radicals and other reactive species, derived from hydrogen peroxide produced during oxidative deamination) (Kinemuchi et al., 1993). Free radical formation also increases EAA release from rat hippocampus slices (Pellegrini-Giampietro et al., 1988). This release was found for Fe^{2+}-catalyzed free radicals playing a role in tissue damage (Liu et al., 1994). Taken together, we should consider that free radicals and EAA may form a feedback loop that produces secondary damage in brain regions. Inhibition of brain MAO by ifenprodil, therefore, may result in a decrease in the rate of hydrogen peroxide formation following cerebral ischaemia, as found for pargyline

(Damsma et al., 1990). It is interest to note that ifenprodil not only acts as an NMDA receptor antagonist by binding at the polyamine site, but also inhibits MAO activity, thus reducing the formation of neurotoxic free radicals.

At present, however, because of the design of our study, it is not yet possible to conclude whether ifenprodil prevents neuronal damage or facilitates the recovery of the neuron injured by experimental ischaemia. The possible role of inhibition of brain MAO by this agent in the improvement of symptoms remains to be elucidated.

Summary

Ifenprodil, a cerebral vasodilator and non-competitive glutamate antagonist, is also an anti-ischaemic agent; it has been shown to inhibit both forms of MAO in rat brain and lung (with slightly greater potency towards MAO-A), but it does not inhibit SSAO. The effects of ifenprodil on rat brain regional levels of monoamines and their principal metabolites following transient global ischaemia have been investigated 1 h after reperfusion. Among the three most ischaemically vulnerable brain regions (striatum, hippocampus and cortex), striatal DA, DOPAC, HVA, 5-HT and 5-HIAA levels were the most markedly increased. Simultaneous treatment with ifenprodil during reperfusion reversed the increases in the striatum, except for HVA, to the level similar to those of sham-operated controls. In contrast to the striatum, ifenprodil failed to reverse the increases seen in the cortex and hippocampus.

References

Arai, Y., Nakazato, K., Kinemuchi, H., Tadano, T., Satoh, N., Oyama, K. and Kisara, K. (1991) Inhibition of rat brain monoamine oxidase activity by cerebral anti-ischemic agent, ifenprodil. *Neuropharmacology*, 30: 809–812.

Baker, M.H.M., McKernan, R.M., Wong, E.H.F. and Foster, A.C.(1991) [³H]MK-801 binding to N-methyl-D-aspartate receptors solubilized from rat brain; Effects of glycine site ligands, polyamines, ifenprodil, and desipramine. *J. Neurochem.*, 57: 39–45.

Carron, C., Jullian, A. and Butcher, B. (1971) Synthesis and pharmacological properties of a series of 2-piperidinoalkanol derivatives. *Arznei. Forsch.*, 21: 1992–1998.

Carter, C.J., Benavides, J., Legendre, P., Vincent, J.D., Noel, F., Thuret, F., Lloyd, K.G., Arbilla, S., Zivkovic, B., MacKenzie, E.T., Scatton, B. and Langer, S.Z. (1988) Ifenprodil and SL 82.0715 as cerebral anti-ischemic agent. II. Evidence for *N*-methyl-D-aspartate receptor antagonist properties. *J. Pharmacol. Exp. Ther.*, 247: 1222–1232.

Carter, C. J., Lloyd, K.G., Zivkovic, G. and Scatton, B (1990) Ifenprodil and SL 82.0715 as cerebral anti-ischemic agent. III. Evidence for antagonistic effects at the polyamine site of the *N*-methyl-D-aspartate receptor complex. *J. Pharmacol. Exp. Ther.*, 253: 475–482.

Damsma, G., Boisvert, D.P., Mudrick, D., Wenkstern, D. and Fibiger. H.C. (1990) Effects of transient forebrain ischemia and pargyline on extracellular concentrations of dopamine, serotonin, and their metabolites in the rat striatum as determined by in vivo microdialysis. *J. Neurochem.*, 54: 801–808.

Globus, M.Y.-T., Ginsberg, M.D., Harik, S.I., Busto, R. and Dietrich, W.D. (1987a) Role of dopamine in ischemic striatal injury; Metabolic evidence. *Neurology*, 37: 1712–1719.

Globus, M.Y.-T., Ginsberg, M.D., Dietrich, W.D., Busto, R. and Scheinberg, P. (1987b) Substantia nigra lesion protect against ischemic damage in the striatum. *Neurosci. Lett.*, 80: 251–256.

Globus,M.Y.-T., Busto, R., Dietrich, W.D., Martinez, E., Valdes, I. and Ginsberg, M.D. (1988) Effect of ischemic on the in vivo release of striatal dopamine, glutamate, and gamma-aminobutyric acid studied by intracerebral microdialysis. *J. Neurochem.*, 51: 1455–1461.

Gotti, B., Duverger, D., Bertin, J., Carter, C., Dupont,R., Frost, J., Gaudilliere, B., MacKenzie, E.T., Rousseau, J., Scatton, B. and Wick. A. (1988) Ifenprodil and SA 82.0715 as cerebral anti-ischemic agent. *I. Evidence for efficacy in models of focal cerebral ischemia. J. Pharmacol. Exp. Ther.*, 247: 1211–1222.

Harik, S.I., Yoshida, S., Busto, R. and Ginsberg, M.D. (1986) Monoamine neurotransmitters in diffuse reversible forebrain ischemia and early recirculation. Increased dopaminergic activity. *Neurology*, 36: 971–976.

Hartley, D.M. and Choi, D.W. (1989) Delayed rescue of *N*-methyl-D-aspartate receptors mediated neuronal injury in cortical culture. *J. Pharmacol. Exp. Ther.*, 250: 752–758.

Headley, P.M. and Grillner, S. (1990) Excitatory amino acids and synaptic transmission; The evidence for a physiological function. *Trends Pharmacol. Sci.*, 11: 205–211.

Honda, H. and Sakai, Y. (1987) The mode of action of ifenprodil tartarate in isolated canine cerebral and femoral arteries. *Arch. Int. Pharmacodyn.*, 285: 211–225.

Kinemuchi, H., Fowler, C.J. and Tipton, K.F. (1984) Substrate specificities of the two forms of monoamine oxidase. In: K.F. Tipton, P. Dostert and M. Strolin Benedetti (Eds.), *Monoamine Oxidase and Disease*, Academic Press, New York, pp. 53–62.

Kinemuchi, H., Arai, Y. and Toyoshima, Y.(1985) Participation of brain monoamine oxidase-B form in the neurotoxicity of 1-methyl-4-phenyl-1,2,3,6-tetrahydropyridine; Relationship between the enzyme inhibition and the neurotoxicity. *Neurosci. Lett.*, 58: 195–200.

Kinemuchi, H., Arai, Y. and Fowler, C.J. (1993) A role for monoamine oxidase in the development of Parkinson's disease ? In: H. Yasuhara, S.H. Parvez, K. Oguchi, M. Sandler and T. Nagatsu (Eds.), *Monoamine Oxidase: Basic and Clinical Aspects*, VSP, Utrecht, pp. 127–135.

Kleihues, P. and Hossmann, K.-A. (1971) Protein synthesis in the cat after prolonged cerebral ischemia. *Brain Res.*, 35: 409–418.

Liu, D., Yang, R., Yan, X. and McAdoo, D.J. (1994) Hydroxycal radicals generated in vivo kill neurons in the rat spinal cord; Electrophysiological, histological, and neurochemical results. *J. Neurochem.*, 62: 37–44.

Meldrum, B. and Garthwaite, J. (1990) Excitatory amino acid neurotoxicity and neurodegenerative disease. *Trends Pharmacol. Sci.*, 11: 379–387.

Monaghan, D.T., Bridges, R.T. and Cotman, C.W. (1989) The excitatory amino acid receptor; Their classes, pharmacology and distinct properties in the function of the central nervous system. *Annu. Rev. Pharmacol. Toxicol.*, 29: 365–402.

Morikawa, F., Ueda, T., Arai, Y. and Kinemuchi, H. (1986) Inhibition of monoamine oxidase A-form and semicarbazide-sensitive amine oxidase by selective and reversible monoamine oxidase-A inhibitors, amiflamine and FLA 788(+). *Pharmacology*, 32: 38–45.

Morimoto, K., Brengman, J. and Yanagihara, T. (1978) Further evaluation of polypeptide synthesis in cerebral anoxia, hypoxia and ischemia. *J. Neurochem.*, 31: 1277–1282.

Murai, S., Saito, H., Masuda, Y. and Itoh, T. (1988) Rapid determination of norepinephrine, dopamine, serotonin, their precursor amino acids, and related metabolites in discrete brain areas of mice with ten minutes by HPLC with electro-chemical detection. *J. Neurochem.*, 50: 473–479.

Pellegrini-Giampietro, D.E., Cherici,G., Alesiani, M., Carla, V. and Moroni, F. (1988) Excitatory amino acid release from rat hippocampus slices as a consequences of free radical formation. *J. Neurochem.*, 51: 1960–1963.

Pulsinelli, W.A. and Brierley, J.B. (1979) A new model of bilateral hemispheric ischemia in the unanesthetized rat. *Stroke*, 10: 267–272.

Ransom, R.W. and Stec, N.L. (1988) Cooperative modulation of [^{3}H]MK-801 binding to the *N*-methyl-D-aspartate receptor-ion channel complex by L-glutamate, glycine, and polyamines. *J. Neurochem.*, 51: 830–836.

Rothman, S.M. and Olney, J.W. (1986) Glutamate and the pathophysiology of hypoxic-ischemic damage. *Ann. Neurol.*, 19: 105–111.

Sarna, G.S., Obrenovitch, T.P., Matsumoto, T., Symon, L. and Curzon, G. (1990) Effect of transient cerebral ischemia and cardiac arrest on brain extracellular dopamine and serotonin as determined by in vivo dialysis in the rat. *J. Neurochem.*, 55: 937–940.

Schoemaker, H., Allen, J. and Langer, S.Z. (1990) Binding of [3]Hifenprodil, a novel NMDA antagonist, to a polyamine-sensitive site in the rat cerebral cortex. *Eur. J. Pharmacol.*, 176: 249–250.

Shalaby, I.A., Chenard, B.L., Prochniak, M.A. and Butler, T.W. (1992) Neuroprotective effects of the *N*-methyl-D-aspartate receptor antagonists ifenprodil and SL-82,0715 on hippocampus cells in culture. *J. Pharmacol. Exp. Ther.*, 260: 925–932.

Slivka, A., Brannan, T.S., Weinberger, J., Knott, P.J. and Cohen, G. (1988) Increase in extracellular dopamine in the striatum during cerebral ischemia; A study utilizing cerebral microdialysis. *J. Neurochem.*, 50: 1714–1718.

Sprosen, T. S. and Woodruff, G.N. (1990) Polyamines potentiate NMDA induced whole cell currents in cultured striatal neurons. *Eur. J. Pharmacol.*, 179: 477–478.

Tamura, Y., Sato, Y., Yokota, T., Akaike, A., Sasa, M. and Takaori, S (1993) Ifenprodil prevents glutamate cytotoxicity via polyamine modulatory site of *N*-methyl-D-aspartate receptors in cultured cortical neuron. *J. Pharmacol. Exp. Ther.*, 265: 1017–1025.

Tipton, K.F. (1972) Some properties of monoamine oxidase. In: E.Costa and M. Sandler (Eds.), *Monoamine Oxidase–New Vistas*, Vol. 5, Raven Press, New York, pp. 11–24.

Wroblewski, J.T. and Danysz, W. (1989) Modulation of glutamate receptors; Molecular mechanisms and functional implications. *Annu. Rev. Pharmacol. Toxicol.*, 29: 441–474.

Zeevalk, G.D. and Nicklas, W.J. (1990) Action of the anti-ischemic agent ifenprodil on *N*-methyl-D-aspartate and kinate-mediated excitotoxicity. *Brain Res.*, 522: 135–139.

Peter M. Yu, Keith F. Tipton and Alan A. Boulton (Eds.)
Progress in Brain Research, Vol 106

CHAPTER 18

Effects of the MAO inhibitor phenelzine on glutamine and GABA concentrations in rat brain

T.M. Paslawski[1], B.D. Sloley[2] and G.B. Baker[1]

[1]*Neurochemical Research Unit, Department of Psychiatry, and* [2]*Department of Zoology, University of Alberta, Edmonton, Alberta, Canada T6G 2B7*

Introduction

The monoamine oxidase (MAO) inhibitor phenelzine (2-phenylethylhydrazine, PLZ) is used extensively in treating depression and panic disorder (Johnson et al., 1994; Martin et al., 1994). In addition to being a potent MAO inhibitor, PLZ also causes marked increases in brain levels of the neurotransmitter amino acid γ-aminobutyric acid (GABA) (Popov and Matthies, 1969; Baker et al., 1991; McKenna et al., 1991; Mc-Manus et al., 1992). There is a growing body of evidence implicating GABA in the etiology and pharmacotherapy of depression and panic disorder (Breslow et al., 1989; Lloyd et al., 1989; Petty et al., 1993), and it is possible that this effect on GABA may contribute to the therapeutic effects of PLZ.

It is assumed that the elevation of GABA by PLZ is the result of inhibition of GABA-T (Popov and Matthies, 1969; Perry and Hansen, 1973; McKenna et al., 1991). However, it has been reported that inhibition of GABA-T is considerably less than that of MAO at the same drug doses (Baker et al., 1991; McManus et al., 1992). Popov and Matthies (1969) found that intraperitoneally administered PLZ could not produce greater than 50% inhibition of GABA-T, and findings in our laboratory agree with this observa-tion. These findings suggest that additional mechanisms may be contributing to the effect on GABA. In order to investigate this situation further, we have studied the effects of PLZ on glutamine (GLN), an important substance whose formation is known to be involved in GABA metabolism (McGeer and McGeer, 1989; De-Lorey and Olsen, 1994).

PLZ is a rather unusual drug in that it is a substrate for, as well as an inhibitor of, MAO (Clineschmidt and Horita, 1969a,b). Experiments utilizing pretreatment of rats with other MAO inhibitors before administering PLZ suggest that a metabolite of PLZ formed by the action of MAO may contribute to the GABA-elevating action of this drug (Popov and Matthies, 1969; Todd and Baker, 1993). Therefore we included studies on pretreatment with the MAO inhibitor tranyl-cypromine (TCP) in the current investigation.

Methods

In a preliminary study, PLZ (15 mg kg^{-1} i.p.) was administered to male Sprague Dawley rats. Groups of rats ($n = 5$–6 per group) were killed by decapitation 1 or 6 h after drug administration. The brains were dissected out, frozen immediately in isopentane on solid carbon dioxide, then removed to a set of tubes and frozen at -60°C.

At the time of analysis, the brains were thawed on ice and the hypothalamus dissected out and homogenized in ice-cold HPLC-grade methanol. A modification of the procedure of Sloley et al. (1992) was used to determine GABA and GLN levels in hypothalamus by HPLC with fluorometric detection after formation of *o*-phthalaldehyde (OPT) derivatives of the amino acids. In the studies utilizing TCP pretreatment, TCP (5 mg kg^{-1}) or vehicle (saline) was administered i.p. followed 1 h later by an injection of PLZ at a dose of either 15 or 30 mg kg^{-1}. At 3 h after the injection of PLZ, the rats were killed and the brain tissue removed and frozen as described above prior to dissection of the hypothalamus and HPLC analysis. The resulting data were analyzed using analysis of variance and multiple *F* comparisons using an α-level of 0.05.

All procedures involving the handling of rats were approved by the Health Sciences Animal Welfare Committee, University of Alberta.

Results and discussion

In the preliminary study, PLZ produced a marked increase in hypothalamic levels of GABA at 6 h (Fig. 1). An increase in whole brain GABA was evident at both 1 and 6 h, in agreement with previous findings in whole brain (Baker et al., 1991). Conversely, levels of GLN were significantly decreased from control levels at 6 h after PLZ administration in hypothalamus and at 1 and 6 h in whole brain (Fig. 1). The effects of two doses of PLZ (3 h after injection) on GABA and GLN levels in hypothalamus were blocked by pretreatment of the rats with the MAO inhibitor TCP (Figs. 2 and 3); a similar pattern was observed in whole brain (data not shown).

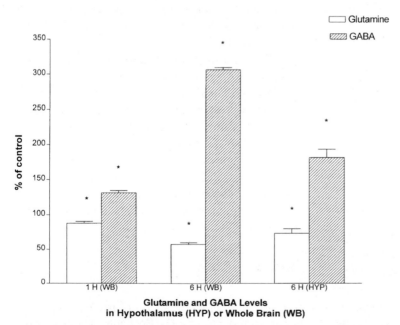

Fig. 1. Effects of administration of PLZ (15 mg kg^{-1}) on GLN and GABA levels in hypothalamus at 6 h post administration and in whole brain at 1 and 6 h. Values are expressed as mean % ($\pm$SEM) of vehicle-treated controls ($n = 5$ or 6). *$P < 0.05$ compared to vehicle-treated control group. GABA and GLN levels were not significantly different from control levels in the hypothalamus at 1 h. Control values (μg/g) were: 528 ± 39 and 438 ± 26 for GLN and GABA, respectively, in hypothalamus; GLN, whole brain, 485 ± 15, 543 ± 23 at 1 and 6 h, respectively; GABA, whole brain, 229 ± 13 and 224 ± 11 at 1 and 6 h, respectively.

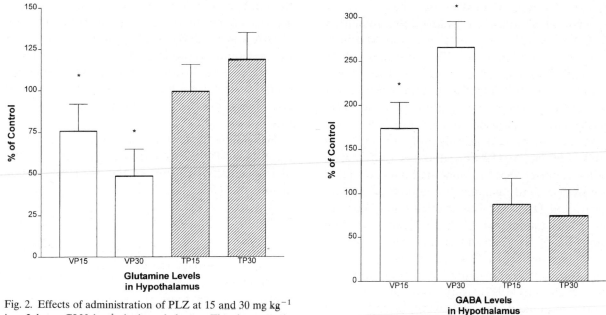

Fig. 2. Effects of administration of PLZ at 15 and 30 mg kg^{-1} i.p., 3 h on GLN levels in hypothalamus. The decreases in GLN levels were blocked by pretreatment with TCP (5 mg kg^{-1}) 1 h prior to PLZ administration. Results are expressed as mean % ($\pm$ SEM) of values in vehicle-treated controls. VP, vehicle, followed 1 h later by PLZ (15 or 30 mg kg^{-1}), and rats were killed 3 h later. TP, tranylcypromine (5 mg kg^{-1}), followed 1 h later by PLZ (15 or 30 mg kg^{-1}), and rats were killed 3 h later. *$P < 0.05$ compared to vehicle-treated control group.

Fig. 3. Effects of administration of PLZ at 15 and 30 mg kg^{-1} i.p., 3 h on GABA levels in hypothalamus. The increases in GABA levels were blocked by pretreatment with TCP (5 mg kg^{-1}) 1 h prior to PLZ administration. Results are expressed as mean % ($\pm$ SEM) of values in vehicle-treated controls. VP, vehicle, followed 1 h later by PLZ (15 or 30 mg kg^{-1}), and rats were killed 3 h later. TP, tranylcypromine (5 mg kg^{-1}), followed 1 h later by PLZ (15 or 30 mg kg^{-1}), and rats were killed 3 h later. *$P < 0.05$ compared to vehicle-treated control group.

GABA is formed in the metabolic pathway commonly referred to as the GABA shunt (McGeer and McGeer, 1989), but formation of GLN is closely associated with the GABA shunt through another loop in which GABA is picked up by glial cells and acted upon by GABA-T. Since the glial cells lack glutamate decarboxylase (GAD), the glutamate formed in the transamination reaction is transformed by glutamine synthetase into GLN, which can be returned to the nerve ending to be converted back to glutamate by the enzyme glutaminase (McGeer and McGeer, 1989). It is possible that PLZ (and/or its metabolite(s)) inhibits glutamine synthetase or stimulates glutaminase, but such effects on these enzymes would probably be expected to also affect levels of glutamate. A

small decrease in glutamate levels was observed in these investigations at the higher dose of PLZ and was also reversible by pretreatment with TCP; this effect is being investigated further. Comprehensive studies are currently under way to examine the effects of PLZ, after both acute and chronic administration, on both glutaminase and glutamine synthetase in rat brain. Such studies should consider actions of PLZ in both neurons and glia, since glutamine synthetase is present only in glia and glutaminase occurs in both neurones and glia (McGeer and McGeer, 1989; Makar et al., 1994; Yudkoff et al., 1994).

As mentioned above, the mechanisms involved

in the elevation of GABA are not yet clearly understood, although it is assumed that inhibition of GABA-T plays a role (Popov and Matthies, 1969; Perry and Hansen, 1973; McManus, 1992). Yu and Boulton (1992), in an in vitro study, reported that PLZ inhibited several pyridoxal-dependent enzymes, including aromatic amino acid decarboxylase, tyrosine amino transferase and GABA-T. In ex vivo investigations in rat brain, Dyck and Dewar (1986) and Baker and Martin (1989) reported that PLZ inhibited tyrosine amino transferase and alanine transaminase, respectively, and Dyck and Dewar (1986) and Wong et al. (1990) found that PLZ produced a marked elevation of tyrosine and alanine levels, respectively. However, the effect of PLZ may not just be a general effect on amino acid transaminases, since McManus (1992), using a dose of PLZ which produced marked elevations of rat brain levels of GABA and alanine, found no changes in levels of leucine, isoleucine and valine, amino acids which are also substrates for transaminases.

The ability of TCP to block the effects of PLZ on GABA lends further support to the suggestion of Popov and Matthies (1969) that a metabolite of PLZ may be contributing to the GABA-elevating effects of PLZ. Popov and Matthies (1969) reported that pretreatment with TCP blocked the effects of PLZ on GABA but had no effect on the GABA-elevating effects of aminooxyacetic acid (a drug known to inhibit GABA-T). It is well known that PLZ is a substrate for, as well as an inhibitor of, MAO (Clineschmidt and Horita, 1969a,b), but the nature of the metabolite(s) responsible for the GABA-elevating effect of PLZ is still not known. Phenylacetic acid and 4-hydroxyphenylacetic acid are identified metabolites of PLZ (Clineschmidt and Horita, 1969b; Dyck et al., 1985; Robinson et al., 1985), but neither of these compounds inhibits GABA-T in vitro (Baker, Leung and McKenna, unpublished results). Some workers have suggested that phenylacetaldehyde hydrazone and/or phenylethyldiimide may be formed (Tipton and Spires, 1972; Patek and Hellerman, 1974; Yu and Tipton, 1989), but this has not been confirmed by other researchers, nor are the effects of these possible metabolites on GABA known. Perry et al. (1981) suggested that the metabolite responsible for the GABA-elevating effect is a hydrazine-containing compound, even hydrazine itself, which they demonstrated does inhibit GABA-T and elevate brain GABA in rats.

The results of the present study indicate that a metabolite of PLZ is contributing to the GLN-depleting effects as well as the GABA-elevating actions of PLZ.

Summary

Phenelzine (PLZ), a frequently prescribed monoamine oxidase (MAO) inhibitor, is used as an antidepressant/antipanic drug and has been shown to cause marked increases in rat brain levels of the amino acids γ-aminobutyric acid (GABA) and alanine. In an extension of previous studies related to GABA metabolism, we investigated the effects of PLZ on rat brain levels of glutamine (GLN). At 1, 3 or 6 h after injection of PLZ (15 mg kg^{-1} i.p.), rats were killed and the brains removed. Analyses (using HPLC with fluorescence detection of OPT derivatives) of whole brain or hypothalamus revealed a decrease in brain levels of GLN and an increase in GABA levels at 3 and 6 h after PLZ injection. The effects of PLZ on GLN and GABA were blocked by prior treatment of the rats with tranylcypromine, a MAO inhibitor that had been shown previously to have no direct effect itself on GABA levels in rat brain. Since PLZ is known to be a substrate (as well as an inhibitor) of MAO, the studies with tranylcypromine pretreatment suggest that the effects on GLN and GABA are caused, at least in part, by a metabolite of PLZ.

Acknowledgements

Funding was provided by the MRC of Canada and the U. of A. Scholarship Fund. The assistance of Ms. S. Omura in typing this manuscript is greatly appreciated.

References

Baker, G.B. and Martin, I.L. (1989) The antidepressant phenelzine and metabolism of γ-aminobutyric acid and alanine in rat brain. *Soc. Neurosci. Abstr.*, 15: 853.

Baker, G.B., Wong, J.F.T., Yeung, J.M. and Coutts, R.T. (1991) Effects of the antidepressant phenelzine on brain levels of γ-aminobutyric acid (GABA). *J. Affec. Disorders*, 21: 207–211.

Breslow, M.F., Faukhauser, M.P., Potter, R.L., Meredith, K.E., Misiaszek, J. and Hope, D.G. (1989) Role of γ-aminobutyric acid in antipanic drug efficacy. *Am. J. Psychiatry*, 146: 353–356.

Clineschmidt, B.V. and Horita, A. (1969a) The monoamine oxidase catalyzed degradation of phenelzine-1-^{14}C, an irreversible inhibitor of monoamine oxidase. I. Studies in vitro. *Biochem. Pharmacol.*, 18: 1011–1020.

Clineschmidt, B.V. and Horita, A. (1969b) The monoamine oxidase catalyzed degradation of phenelzine-1-^{14}C, an irreversible inhibitor of monoamine oxidase. II. Studies in vivo. *Biochem. Pharmacol.*, 18: 1021–1028.

DeLorey, T.M. and Olsen, R.W. (1994) GABA and Glycine. In: G.J. Seigel, B.W. Agranoff, R.W. Albers and P.B. Molinoff (Eds.), *Basic Neurochemistry: Molecular, Cellular, and Medical Aspects*, 5th edn., Raven Press, New York, pp. 389–399.

Dyck, L.E. and Dewar, K.M. (1986) Inhibition of aromatic l-amino acid decarboxylase and tyrosine aminotransferase by the monoamine oxidase inhibitor phenelzine. *J. Neurochem.*, 46: 1899–1903.

Dyck, L.E., Durden, D.A. and Boulton, A.A. (1985) Formation of β-phenylethylamine from the antidepressant, β-phenylethylhydrazine. *Biochem. Pharmacol.*, 34: 1925–1929.

Johnson, M.R., Lydiard, R.B. and Ballenger, J.C. (1994) MAOIs in panic disorder and agoraphobia. In: S.H. Kennedy (Ed.), *Progress in Psychiatry, Vol. 43, Clinical Advances in Monoamine Oxidase Inhibitor Therapies*, American Psychiatric Press, Washington, DC, pp. 205–224.

Lloyd, K.G., Zivkovic, B., Scatton, B., Morselli, P.L. and Bartholini, G. (1989) The GABAergic hypothesis of depression. *Prog. Neuropsychopharmacol. Biol. Psychiatry*, 13: 341–351.

Makar, T.K., Nedergaard, M., Preuss, A., Hertz, L. and Cooper, A.J.L. (1994) Glutamine transaminase K and ω-amidase activities in primary cultures of astrocytes and neurons and in embryonic chick forebrain: marked induction of brain glutamine transaminase K at time of hatching. *J. Neurochem.*, 62: 1983–1988.

Martin, L., Bakish, D. and Joffe, R. (1994) MAOI treatment of depression. In: S.H. Kennedy (Ed.), *Progress in Psychiatry, Vol. 43, Clinical Advances in Monoamine Oxidase Inhibitor Therapies*, American Psychiatric Press, Washington, DC, pp. 147–180.

McGeer, P.L. and McGeer, E.G. (1989) Amino Acid Neurotransmitters. In: G.J. Seigel, B.W. Agranoff, R.W. Albers and P.B. Molinoff (Eds.), *Basic Neurochemistry: Molecular, Cellular, and Medical Aspects*, 4th edn., Raven Press, New York, pp. 311–332.

McKenna, K.F., Baker, G.B. and Coutts, R.T. (1991) N^2-Acetylphenelzine: effects on rat brain GABA, alanine and biogenic amines. *Naunyn-Schmeid. Arch. Pharmacol.*, 343: 478–482.

McManus, D.J. (1992) Effects of chronic antidepressant drug administration on GABAergic mechanisms in rat brain. PhD Thesis, University of Alberta, Edmonton, Canada.

McManus, D.J., Baker, G.B., Martin, I.L., Greenshaw, A.J. and McKenna, K.F. (1992) Effects of the antidepressant/antipanic drug phenelzine on GABA concentrations and GABA-transaminase activity in rat brain. *Biochem. Pharmacol.*, 43: 2486–2489.

Patek, D.R. and Hellerman, L. (1974) Mitochondrial monoamine oxidase. Mechanism of inhibition by phenylhydrazine and by aralkylhydrazines. Role of enzymatic oxidation. *J. Biol. Chem.*, 249: 2373–2380.

Perry, T.L. and Hansen, S. (1973) Sustained drug-induced elevation of brain GABA in the rat. *J. Neurochem.*, 21: 1167–1175.

Perry, T.L., Kish, S.J., Hansen, S., Wright, J.M., Wall, R.A., Dunn, W.L. and Bellward, G.D. (1981) Elevation of brain GABA content by chronic low-dosage administration of hydrazine, a metabolite of isoniazid. *J. Neurochem.*, 37: 32–39.

Petty, F., Kramer, G.L. and Hendrickse, W. (1993) GABA and depression. In: J.J. Mann and D.J. Kupfer (Eds.), *Biology of Depressive Disorders, Part A: A Systems Perspective*, Plenum Press, New York, pp. 79–108.

Popov, N. and Matthies, H. (1969) Some effects of monoamine oxidase inhibitors on the metabolism of γ-aminobutyric acid in rat brain. *J. Neurochem.*, 16: 899–907.

Robinson, D.S., Cooper, T.B., Jindal, S.P., Corcella, J. and Lutz, T. (1985) Metabolism and pharmacokinetics of phenelzine: lack of evidence for acetylation pathway in humans. *J. Clin. Psychopharmacol.*, 5: 333–337.

Sloley, B.D., Kah, O., Trudeau, V.L., Dulka, J.G. and Peter, R.E. (1992) Amino acid neurotransmitters and dopamine in brain and pituitary of the goldfish: involvement in the regulation of gonadotropin secretion. *J. Neurochem.*, 58: 2254–2262.

Tipton, K.F. and Spires, I.P.C. (1972) Oxidation of 2-phenylethylhydrazine by monoamine oxidase. *Biochem. Pharmacol.*, 21: 268–270.

Todd, K.G. and Baker, G.B. (1993) Elevation of rat brain GABA levels following administration of the antidepressant/antipanic drug phenelzine: effects of pretreatment with selective inhibitors of MAO-A and MAO-B. *Proc. 16th Annu. Meet. Can. Coll. Neuropsychopharmacol.*, M-11.

186

Wong, J.T.F., Baker, G.B., Coutts, R.T. and Dewhurst, W.G. (1990) Long-lasting elevation of alanine in brain produced by the antidepressant phenelzine. *Brain Res. Bull.*, 25: 179–181.

Yu, P.H. and Boulton, A.A. (1992) A comparison of the effect of brofaromine, phenelzine and tranylcypromine on the activities of some enzymes involved in the metabolism of different neurotransmitters. *Res. Commun. Chem. Path. Pharmacol.*, 16: 141–153.

Yu, P.H. and Tipton, K.F. (1989) Deuterium isotope effect of phenelzine on the inhibition of rat liver mitochondrial monoamine oxidase activity. *Biochm. Pharmacol.*, 38: 4245–4251.

Yudkoff, M., Daikhin, Y., Nissim, I., Pleasure, D., Stern, J. and Nissim, I. (1994) Inhibition of astrocyte glutamine production by α-ketoisocaproic acid. *J. Neurochem., 63:* 1508–1515.

Peter M. Yu, Keith F. Tipton and Alan A. Boulton (Eds.)
Progress in Brain Research, Vol 106
© 1995 Elsevier Science BV. All rights reserved.

CHAPTER 19

Metabolism of agmatine (clonidine-displacing substance) by diamine oxidase and the possible implications for studies of imidazoline receptors

Andrew Holt and Glen B. Baker

Neurochemical Research Unit, Department of Psychiatry, and Faculty of Pharmacy and Pharmaceutical Sciences, University of Alberta, Edmonton, Alberta, Canada T6G 2B7

Introduction

Clonidine (Fig. 1) belongs to the general class of imidazoline α-adrenergic receptor agonists and was originally developed in the hope that it would cause peripheral vasoconstriction and could thus be included in shaving soaps to prevent bleeding from razor cuts (Bowman and Rand, 1980). However, administration of clonidine lowers blood pressure and this effect is thought to result from decreased sympathetic nerve activity in the central nervous system (see Kobinger, 1978). While clonidine is most efficacious in lowering blood pressure and has been marketed as an antihypertensive for more than two decades, many undesired side-effects such as daytime sedation and dry mouth have resulted in a steady loss of popularity for this agent in recent years. The accepted view has been that the hypotensive effect of clonidine is a consequence of its affinity for α_2-adrenergic receptors. However, agents such as guanabenz, while displaying much higher affinity for α_2-receptors than does clonidine, are less potent antihypertensive agents and yet display similar side-effect profiles (Weber et al., 1990).

More recently, it has been established that, while many of its side effects result from α_2-receptor stimulation (Harron, 1992), the hypotensive action of clonidine is mediated through novel,

non-adrenergic binding sites in the ventrolateral medulla (Bousquet et al., 1984; Ernsberger et al., 1987). These binding sites have a high affinity for imidazolines such as clonidine and rilmenidine (Sannajust and Head, 1994), and the term "imidazoline sites" has thus been accepted by consensus to distinguish them from α-adrenergic receptors (Michel and Ernsberger, 1992). Two subtypes of imidazoline sites have already been described (Michel and Insel, 1989). Sites which show high affinity for [^{3}H]clonidine have been classed as I_1 sites, while those showing high affinity for [^{3}H]idazoxan have been termed I_2 sites (Michel and Insel, 1989; see Ernsberger et al., 1994). I_2 sites may be further subdivided based on relative affinities for the diuretic, amiloride (Fig. 1; Michel and Insel, 1989; see Regunathan et al., 1993).

Demonstrating the presence of an endogenous ligand for imidazoline sites has proved problematic. In 1984, a low molecular weight substance which could displace clonidine from α_2-receptors in human platelets (Diamant et al., 1987) and p-[^{3}H]aminoclonidine from imidazoline sites in the rat ventrolateral medulla (Ernsberger et al., 1988) was isolated and partially purified from calf brain (Atlas and Burstein, 1984). Only recently did attempts to identify this clonidine-displacing substance prove successful when, by mass spectrometry, Li et al. (1994a) determined the struc-

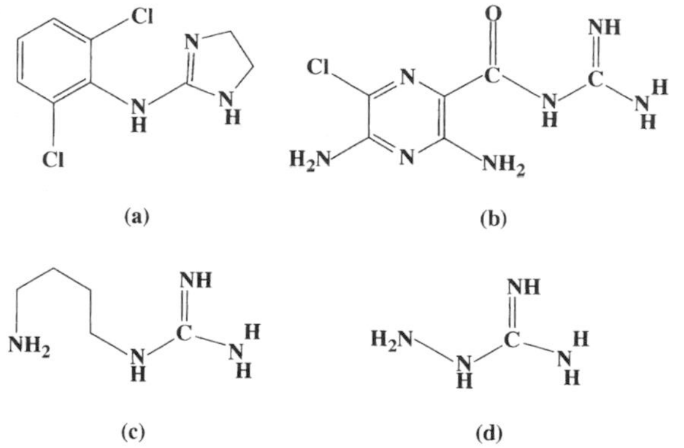

Fig. 1. Structures of clonidine (a), amiloride (b), agmatine (c) and aminoguanidine (d).

ture of the purified compound to be that of agmatine (1-amino-4-guanidinobutane; Fig. 1). Agmatine is known to occur endogenously as a decarboxylation product of arginine and both arginine decarboxylase and agmatine are present in mammalian brain and in plants and bacteria (White et al., 1973; Tabor and Tabor, 1984; Li et al., 1994a). In bacteria at least, agmatine can be further metabolised to putrescine by agmatine ureohydrolase (White et al., 1973). However, doubt surrounds the importance of such a pathway in mammals, since it is generally accepted that the intermediate in putrescine formation in higher organisms is ornithine (Pegg and McCann, 1982; Tabor and Tabor, 1984). Thus, the fate of mammalian agmatine remains unclear.

It has been demonstrated that agmatine shares with clonidine-displacing substance the ability to release adrenaline and noradrenaline from adrenal chromaffin cells via an interaction with imidazoline binding sites (Regunathan et al., 1991; Li et al., 1994a). Agmatine also induces a concentration-dependent release of insulin from rat pancreatic islet cells (Sener et al., 1989) while a number of agmatine derivatives, as well as agmatine itself, mimic the effect of insulin on isolated fat cells (Weitzel et al., 1980). Furthermore, clonidine-displacing substance contracts rat gastric fundus strips in a dose-dependent manner (Felsen et al., 1987). If agmatine does indeed have a rôle

as an endogenous transmitter or neuromodulator, some means must exist whereby its action can be rapidly terminated.

Agmatine is classed as a polyamine, although only two of its four amino groups are primary in nature. Early reports in the literature provided evidence that agmatine might be a substrate for some diamine oxidase (DAO) enzymes, such as those derived from pig kidney (Zeller, 1938, 1941; Zeller et al., 1956) and cockroach Malpighian tubules (Boadle and Blaschko, 1968), but not for the enzymes isolated from cephalopod liver, renal appendage or pancreas (Boadle, 1969). Unfortunately, some of the enzymes examined were insensitive to recognised DAO inhibitors, observations inconsistent with the assumption that DAO was exclusively responsible for amine metabolism in these studies.

Diamine oxidase (amine:oxygen oxidoreductase [deaminating] [pyridoxal containing]; EC 1.4.3.6) has been detected in a variety of mammalian tissues, including brain, kidney and liver (see Buffoni, 1966, and references therein). In porcine kidney at least, the enzyme does not contain pyridoxal as cofactor, but rather the quinone of trihydroxyphenylalanine (topaquinone; Janes et al., 1992; see Klinman and Mu, 1994). DAO is a member of the copper-containing amine oxidase family which constitutes a subgroup of the semicarbazide-sensitive amine oxidase (SSAO) enzymes (see Callingham et al., 1990, 1991). SSAO enzymes are sensitive to inhibition by carbonyl reagents, for example semicarbazide, benserazide, iproniazid (Lyles, 1984), procarbazine and methylhydrazine (Holt et al., 1992a,b). While semicarbazide-sensitive monoamine oxidase enzymes can also be inhibited by the antidepressant, phenelzine (Lyles, 1984), this compound does not, to our knowledge, appear in the exhaustive lists of drugs which have been shown to inhibit DAO (for example Buffoni, 1966; Sattler and Lorenz, 1990).

The aims of the project were thus to demonstrate that agmatine is a substrate for purified porcine kidney DAO in vitro and that inhibition of this enzyme could reduce metabolism of the amine. The effects of phenelzine as a potential inhibitor were compared with those of aminoguanidine (Fig. 1), a compound recognised to be highly potent against DAO (Burkard et al., 1960; Shore and Cohn, 1960; Sattler and Lorenz, 1990). In light of the recent observations that porcine kidney DAO is the amiloride-binding protein detected in that species (Mu et al., 1994; Novotny et al., 1994), the possible implications of these findings are discussed, as they relate to radioligand binding studies of imidazoline binding sites.

Methods

Colorimetric assay for diamine oxidase

The method used to measure DAO activity was the plasma amine oxidase assay described by Elliott et al. (1991), a more sensitive version of the technique first described by Yamada et al. (1979). This method detects the hydrogen peroxide produced during oxidative deamination of an amine substrate in a peroxidase-linked colorimetric assay and has been used previously to measure activities of both tissue-bound (A. Holt, unpublished observations) and plasma SSAO activities. Classical MAO enzymes cannot be measured with the technique as described here (A. Holt and D.F. Sharman, unpublished observations) and it has not been used previously to measure DAO. In the reaction (Fig. 2), 4-aminoantipyrine acts as the proton and electron donor in the peroxidase reaction and then condenses with 2,4-dichlorophenol to form a red quinoneimine dye, the formation of which can be measured by following the absorbance change at 492 nm.

Purified porcine kidney DAO was prepared in potassium phosphate buffer (0.2 M, pH 7.8) at a concentration of 0.6 units ml^{-1}, where 1 unit is defined as that amount of DAO which will oxidise 1 μmol of putrescine per hour at 37°C. Assays were performed in disposable glass test tubes which were placed on ice for the addition of assay reagents. Fifty μl of enzyme solution were preincubated in quadruplicate with water (controls, blanks) or aqueous inhibitor solutions for 20 min

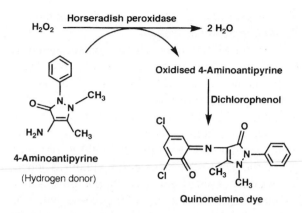

Fig. 2. Reaction scheme for the peroxidase-linked colorimetric assay for DAO activity.

at 37°C. To each tube were then added 200 μl water (blanks) or aqueous agmatine at 5-times the desired final concentration and 700 μl of a colorimetric reagent mixture: this mixture contained 2,4-dichlorophenol, 4-aminoantipyrine and horseradish peroxidase (EC 1.11.1.7; Sigma Type II), all at 0.2 mg ml^{-1} in water. Samples were then further incubated at 37°C for an appropriate period (usually 1 h) and the reaction was stopped by removing samples onto ice and adding aminoguanidine (10 μl, 100 μM).

Absorbance values at 492 nm were read in a Pye Unicam SP1700 UV spectrophotometer and the blank values were subtracted. A standard curve for hydrogen peroxide was constructed by the addition of known amounts of peroxide (standardised by titration with potassium permanganate) to tubes in which blank assays had been performed. This allowed calculation of the control enzyme specific activity in μmol agmatine metabolised h^{-1} (unit DAO activity)$^{-1}$.

Inhibitor IC$_{50}$ values were determined by preincubating DAO with phenelzine (0.3 μM–1 mM) or aminoguanidine (3 nM–1 μM) before addition of agmatine (final concentration 100 μM). Sigmoid curves were fitted to the data using the nonlinear regression facility of GraphPad Prism, Version 1.0 (GraphPad Software, San Diego, CA).

Radiochemical assay of the effects of agmatine on MAO and SSAO activities

In order to determine whether or not agmatine might be a substrate either for rat brain monoamine oxidase (MAO)-A or -B or for rat interscapular brown adipose tissue SSAO, radio-labelled substrates of these enzymes were incubated with homogenates of tissues from naive male Sprague-Dawley rats (280–300 g, obtained from the University of Alberta Health Sciences Laboratory Animal Services) in the presence of agmatine. An interaction of agmatine with the active site of any of these enzymes would be manifested as a reduction in the rate of metabolism of the radiolabelled substrates. The assay method used was based on that of Lyles and Callingham (1982). Assays, carried out in triplicate, were set up in ice-cooled disposable glass test tubes containing 25 μl of homogenate, 25 μl of water or agmatine (final concentration 50 μM) and 50 μl of appropriate radiolabelled substrate. Samples were oxygenated and incubated for 10 min at 37°C. Enzyme activity was terminated by plunging the tubes into ice and adding HCl (3 M, 10 μl) to each. Blanks had HCl added before incubation with substrate. Deaminated metabolites were extracted into 1 ml ethyl acetate/toluene (1:1 v/v, saturated with water) and 700 μl of the organic phase were counted in 4 ml Ready Safe liquid scintillation cocktail for radioactive metabolites, with quench correction by external standardisation, in a scintillation spectrometer (Beckman model LS 6000SC). Substrates used were, for MAO-A, [^{3}H]5-hydroxytryptamine (250 μM, spec. act. 1 μCi μmol^{-1}), for MAO-B, [^{14}C]phenylethylamine (50 μM, spec. act. 1 μCi μmol^{-1}) and for tissue-bound SSAO, [^{14}C]benzylamine (10 μM, spec. act. 10 μCi μmol^{-1}). Protein contents of homogenates were determined by the method of Lowry et al. (1951), with bovine serum albumin as standard.

Drugs and reagents

Porcine kidney DAO, 2,4-dichlorophenol, 4-aminoantipyrine, horseradish peroxidase, agmatine sulphate, phenelzine sulphate, aminoguanidine hemisulphate, benzylamine hydrochloride, β-phenylethylamine hydrochloride and 5-hydroxytryptamine creatinine sulphate were all obtained from Sigma Chemical Company, St. Louis, MO, USA. 5-Hydroxy[G-^{3}H]tryptamine creatinine sulphate and [7-^{14}C]benzylamine hydrochloride were purchased from Amersham International plc, Amersham, Bucks, UK, and β-[ethyl-1-^{14}C]phenylethylamine hydrochloride from Du Pont, Markham, Ontario, Canada. Ready Safe liquid scintillation cocktail was obtained from Beckman Instruments Inc., Fullerton, CA, USA. All other reagents were of analytical grade, where possible.

Results

Diamine oxidase inhibition in vitro

Figure 3 illustrates the concentration-dependent inhibition of DAO-catalysed agmatine deamination by aminoguanidine and phenelzine. The IC$_{50}$ values obtained following fitting of sigmoid curves to the data were 14.9 nM (aminoguanidine) and 1.95 μM (phenelzine). Control DAO activity in these experiments was estimated to be 0.8 μmol agmatine h^{-1} (unit DAO activity)$^{-1}$, with approx. 24% substrate depletion occurring in control samples during the incubation period.

The metabolism of a range of concentrations of agmatine was also examined in an attempt to obtain estimates of kinetic constants for the reaction. Between 100 μM and 50 μM agmatine, the enzyme appeared initially to be saturated. At lower concentrations of agmatine, substantial substrate depletion occurred during the incubation period, and when incubation times were reduced in order to limit substrate depletion, absorbance (colour) changes were neither visible nor detectable by spectrophotometry.

Effects of agmatine on MAO and tissue-bound SSAO activities in vitro

Following incubation of tissue homogenates with radiolabelled amine substrates in the presence of agmatine (50 μM), initial rates of amine metabolism were calculated and expressed as a

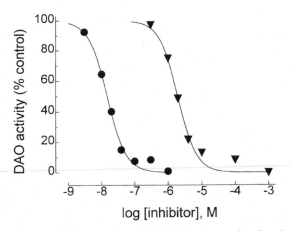

Fig. 3. Inhibitor plots for the inhibition of agmatine deamination by aminoguanidine (●) and phenelzine (▼). Purified porcine kidney diamine oxidase was preincubated with aminoguanidine (3 nM–1 μM) or phenelzine (0.3 μM–1 mM) at 37°C for 20 min before incubation with agmatine (100 μM) for 1 h. Values shown are from a single experiment, performed in quadruplicate. IC$_{50}$ values, obtained by nonlinear regression of the data, are 14.9 nM (aminoguanidine) and 1.95 μM (phenelzine).

percentage of control values. These were, for MAO-A, 90.6 ± 10.6%, for MAO-B, 101.6 ± 3.6 % and for SSAO, 96.2 ± 2.8% (mean ± S.E., n = 3). Control enzyme activities (expressed as nmol product formed h^{-1} (mg protein)$^{-1}$) were 64.0 ± 7.0 (MAO-A), 19.7 ± 0.5 (MAO-B) and 7.12 ± 0.34 (SSAO). Thus, agmatine, at a concentration sufficient to saturate DAO, was without significant effect on rates of amine metabolism by monoamine-oxidising enzymes, suggesting that agmatine is probably not a substrate for these enzymes.

Discussion

The results presented here confirm earlier observations (Zeller, 1938, 1941; Zeller et al., 1956; Boadle and Blaschko, 1968; Boadle, 1969) that agmatine is a substrate for DAO. Although the aldehyde product of agmatine deamination has not been identified, the most likely candidate would seem to be 4-guanidinobutanal. The inability of agmatine to reduce the deamination of

5-hydroxytryptamine or β-phenylethylamine by rat brain MAO-A or -B respectively is not surprising since diamines and polyamines are not substrates for MAO enzymes (see Blaschko, 1974). However, although no interaction of agmatine was seen with tissue-bound SSAO in the present study, some copper-containing plasma SSAO enzymes are able to metabolise the polyamines, spermine and spermidine (Blaschko, 1974), and one may not preclude the possibility that agmatine might also be a substrate for such plasma enzymes.

The peroxidase-linked colorimetric assay for DAO activity proved too insensitive to determine kinetic constants for the deamination of agmatine by porcine kidney DAO, although preliminary experiments suggested that the enzyme was no longer saturated when the concentration of agmatine dropped much below 50 μM. In order to obtain a K_M value in the absence of a more sensitive direct assay method, it would be relatively straightforward to instead determine a K_i value for agmatine as a competitive inhibitor of [^{14}C]putrescine deamination by DAO (Kusche et al., 1973). A K_i value obtained in this way provides a good approximation to the K_M for metabolism of the competing substrate by the same enzyme.

Aminoguanidine was shown to inhibit the DAO-catalysed metabolism of agmatine with an IC$_{50}$ of 14.9 nM. The potency of this compound as an inhibitor of DAO is well established, both in vitro (Burkard et al., 1960) and in vivo (Shore and Cohn, 1960). Although aminoguanidine is not used clinically, drugs such as dihydralazine, chloroquine and cycloserine are potent inhibitors in vitro of porcine and human intestinal DAO (Sattler and Lorenz, 1990). The present study has demonstrated that the antidepressant, phenelzine displays an IC$_{50}$ (1.95 μM) comparable with the most potent of other clinically used drugs versus DAO and it is likely that other hydrazine-based drugs will also inhibit DAO to a similar degree (see Lyles, 1984). Thus, the possibility exists that inhibition of DAO in vivo may increase levels of agmatine in tissues and in blood. It has been demonstrated that chronic administration of idazoxan to rabbits causes a substantial decrease in the number of renal imidazoline binding sites (Yakubu et al., 1990). On the other hand, chronic administration of idazoxan to rats increased the density of central imidazoline sites (Olmos et al., 1992). Such observations indicate that imidazoline sites may be subject to physiological regulation and therefore that changes in endogenous agmatine levels may alter imidazoline binding site densities.

In a preliminary study (results not shown), rats were administered saline, aminoguanidine (20 mg kg^{-1}) or phenelzine (60 mg kg^{-1}) i.p. and were killed 2 h later. Agmatine levels were determined in whole brain by gas chromatography with electron-capture detection after derivatisation with pentafluoropropionic anhydride (A. Holt and G.B. Baker, unpublished observations). Although, at the drug doses used, we can be reasonably certain that inhibition of DAO would be substantial, if not complete (see Shore and Cohn, 1960; Kusche et al., 1975), neither drug caused an increase in brain agmatine levels. It is possible that the turnover of agmatine by DAO is sufficiently slow that brain agmatine levels may not have changed significantly within 2 h of drug administration. Furthermore, rat brain does not possess high DAO activity (see Buffoni, 1966). Assuming that agmatine can cross the blood–brain barrier, increased brain agmatine levels may occur largely as a consequence of increased agmatine in the plasma following inhibition of peripheral DAO. Thus, chronic inhibition of DAO may be necessary before a measurable increase in brain agmatine takes place. This view is supported by the observation that whole brain levels of spermine and spermidine also did not change following administration of aminoguanidine or phenelzine to rats (results not shown). The effects of chronic drug administration on rat brain agmatine levels are currently under investigation in our laboratory. Clearly, in the event that changes in agmatine levels are found, it will be important to establish whether or not such changes are associated with altered imidazoline binding site densities.

I_1 Imidazoline sites have been detected in the medulla oblongata of various species, where they are probably associated with neurons (see Ernsberger et al., 1994 and references therein). In human brain, both I_1 and I_2 sites are widely distributed throughout the grey matter, although the significance of non-medullary sites is not known (De Vos et al., 1994). I_1 Sites are also present in a variety of peripheral tissues such as kidney, trachea and prostate, where they may be involved with epithelial cell ion transport (Bidet et al., 1990; Felsen et al., 1994). A number of functional responses have been attributed to the actions of agonists at I_1 sites and these binding sites may therefore represent functional receptors. For example, the affinities of clonidine analogues for I_1 sites show a strong correlation with the antihypertensive potencies of these compounds (Ernsberger et al., 1990). Selective agonists such as moxonidine are also able to lower intraocular pressure (Campbell and Potter, 1994), either administered intracerebroventricularly or applied topically, and both moxonidine and rilmenidine, another I_1 agonist, increase urinary flow and osmolar clearance when infused into the rat renal artery (Li et al., 1994b; Penner and Smyth, 1994). It is apparent that many of the effects of I_1 receptor agonists and antagonists studied thus far might be linked to control of blood pressure and/or electrolyte balance. Thus, one might speculate that altered imidazoline receptor density resulting from increased agmatine levels may be manifested as alterations in the control of such systems. Clearly, this represents a very promising area of research, but a great deal of work will still be necessary before the effects of pharmacological manipulation of I_1 receptors can be predicted with any degree of certainty.

Rather less is known regarding the pharmacology and physiology of I_2 sites. They are thought to be present on mitochondrial membranes of bovine adrenal medullary chromaffin cells (Regunathan et al., 1993), human and rabbit hepatocytes (Tesson et al., 1991) and on rabbit adipocyte membranes (Langin and Lafontan, 1989). Agmatine stimulates the release of catecholamines from adrenal chromaffin cells (Regunathan et al., 1991; Li et al., 1994a) and mimics the antilipolytic effects of insulin in rat epididymal fat cells (Weitzel et al., 1980), probably through an interaction with I_2 sites. However, rather less evidence exists to support the view that all I_2 sites correspond to functional receptors when the available data are compared with what is known concerning the I_1 receptor in this respect. The picture is further confused by the apparent presence of multiple I_2 site subtypes in the same tissue. For example, in bovine adrenal chromaffin cells, the inhibition curve for the displacement of [^{3}H]idazoxan from I_2 sites by agmatine has a Hill slope of 0.5 (Li et al., 1994a). Similarly, of 29 compounds incubated with guinea pig kidney membranes in the presence of [^{3}H]idazoxan, 22 generated biphasic or shallow competition curves (Wikberg et al., 1992) and ligand binding was not affected by non-hydrolysable guanine nucleotides. Interestingly, these workers found that histamine appeared to have substantially different affinities for the two sites: it was thus included in some competition experiments at an appropriate concentration in an attempt to block one site so that K_i values might be determined for other competing ligands at the second site. Kidney membranes were incubated with pargyline beforehand to inactivate MAO and thus, supposedly, to prevent metabolism of histamine during the binding equilibration period. However, histamine is metabolised not by MAO but by DAO and pargyline does not inhibit DAO (Kusche et al., 1975). These and other data have been interpreted to suggest the existence of different interacting I_2 subtypes or different affinity states for a single receptor. In a number of tissues, these subtypes or different affinity forms are separable on the basis of widely differing affinities for amiloride (see Michel and Insel, 1989). However, a second possible explanation becomes apparent if the pharmacology of amiloride is examined more closely.

Amiloride is thought to exert a diuretic and natriuretic effect by binding to Na^+ channels in the distal tubule and collecting duct of the kidney, thereby preventing Na^+ reabsorption and K^+ excretion (see Barbry et al., 1990a). The amiloride binding protein, assumed to be a component of the amiloride-sensitive Na^+ channel, has been photoaffinity labelled (Kleyman et al., 1986), isolated and purified (Barbry et al., 1989, 1990a,b). However, Kleyman et al. (1986) found that [^{3}H]bromobenzamil, a photoactive amiloride analogue, bound to three peptides of differing molecular weights in bovine kidney and that binding in each case could be prevented by the presence of amiloride. Similarly, [^{3}H]phenamil, another amiloride derivative, along with amiloride itself, recognised two binding sites in porcine kidney which were assumed to be isoforms of the apical Na^+ channel (Barbry et al., 1989). The affinities of amiloride for these putative channels were 100 nM and 4 μM. It is thus clear that the so-called amiloride binding protein does not represent a single peptide, but more likely two or more proteins which may or may not constitute part or all of a Na^+ channel.

Recently, the cDNA isolated for one human kidney amiloride binding protein was found not to encode for a Na^+ channel, but for a human kidney DAO enzyme (Mu et al., 1994; Novotny et al., 1994).

The K_i value of 9.1 μM for amiloride versus putrescine metabolism by purified porcine kidney DAO, obtained by Mu et al. (1994), is very similar to the K_D of amiloride (4.2 μM) for dissociation from purified porcine kidney amiloride binding protein obtained by Barbry et al. (1989). However, when K_i values for amiloride versus [^{3}H]idazoxan binding to I_2 site subtypes are also considered, constants almost identical to those above have been determined. For example, the K_i versus a high affinity [^{3}H]idazoxan site in guinea pig kidney is 3.3 μM (Wikberg et al., 1992); versus a low affinity site in rabbit cerebral cortex, 3.8 μM (Renouard et al., 1993) and versus I_2 sites in human, rat and porcine kidney, 1.1, 7.8 and 3.0 μM, respectively (Michel and Insel, 1989). Similarly, guanabenz was shown to bind to two I_2 sites in rabbit cerebral cortex, with K_i values of 12.9 nM and 1.9 μM (Wikberg et al., 1992) and to one site in porcine kidney (K_i value 18 nM;

Michel and Insel, 1989). To our knowledge, inhibition of DAO by guanabenz has not been reported. However, guanabenz is simply a terminal N-substituted analogue of aminoguanidine, the latter inhibiting porcine kidney DAO in the present study with an IC_{50} of 14.9 nM.

Data such as those presented above provide support for the idea that, in tissues where more than one idazoxan-preferring (I_2) site has been demonstrated, this may indicate ligand binding not only to an I_2 site but also to DAO. The possibility that rabbit cerebral cortex I_2 sites might correspond to the active site of MAO had been examined previously by Renouard et al. (1993). The affinities of clorgyline, pargyline and deprenyl for the I_2 site were not compatible with that binding site being the MAO active site, although the possibility that binding was to a modulatory site cannot be discounted. Nevertheless, a similarity between K_i or IC_{50} values for a series of I_2 site ligands and their inhibitor constants versus DAO would provide further evidence in favour of the hypothesis that some I_2 sites may represent DAO. It is important in such studies to determine whether or not the ligand under examination is both competitive and reversible, since it is inappropriate to convert an IC_{50} to a K_i value by way of the Cheng-Prusoff relationship if the ligand binds irreversibly. Unfortunately, K_i values have been quoted almost universally for ligand interactions with I_2 receptors (for example, Wikberg et al., 1992), although, where compounds such as aminoguanidine and probably guanabenz are concerned, such K_i values may have been derived from IC_{50} values for irreversible interactions with DAO. One should also bear in mind that, unlike K_i values, IC_{50} values determined for inhibitors or antagonists may depend upon the concentration of substrate or radioligand present in the assay. Consistency in the choice of radioligand concentration is thus important if comparisons of IC_{50} values are to be made between experiments. Corpus et al. (1994) determined IC_{50} values for a series of guanidinium compounds, including aminoguanidine, versus [^{3}H]idazoxan binding to I_2 sites. However, these studies were performed with rabbit kidney membranes and, in the periphery at least, DAO is found in the rabbit intestine but not in other tissues such as kidney or liver (Kusche et al., 1975). This observation may explain the apparent lack of multiple I_2 sites in the rabbit when compared with human, rat, porcine and bovine tissues (Michel and Insel, 1989). It would thus be inappropriate to compare the IC_{50} value obtained by those workers (390 μM) with that obtained in the present study versus porcine kidney DAO.

It is possible that a compound such as agmatine might initiate a cellular response which appears to be receptor-mediated, simply by binding to DAO on the cell membrane, and such a response would be independent of any second-messenger system. For example, both insulin and agmatine induce glucose oxidation in rat adipocytes (Weitzel et al., 1980). The effects of insulin are probably initiated by oxidation of sulphydryl groups on the insulin receptor (Czech et al., 1974a), caused by H_2O_2 produced within the cell membrane on binding of insulin (Mukherjee and Mukherjee, 1982). The effects of insulin upon glucose metabolism can be mimicked by H_2O_2 or N-ethylmaleimide (Czech et al., 1974b) and hydrogen peroxide is a product of amine metabolism by DAO at the cell membrane (see Buffoni, 1966). Thus, if what is assumed to be an I_2 receptor on the adipocyte membrane instead corresponds to DAO, then binding and metabolism of agmatine and subsequent production of H_2O_2 could lead to sulphydryl group oxidation and increased glucose metabolism. Although such a scenario is little more than speculation at present, it serves to underline the importance of establishing the signal transduction mechanisms responsible for cellular effects evoked by imidazoline binding site ligands.

In conclusion, we have demonstrated that agmatine, known previously as clonidine-displacing substance and thought to be the endogenous agonist at imidazoline binding sites/receptors, is a substrate for porcine kidney diamine oxidase. Aminoguanidine and phenelzine are both inhibitors of agmatine metabolism, and administration of hydrazine-based drugs to animals or human subjects may thus increase endogenous agmatine levels, thereby altering densities of imidazoline binding sites. The similarities between dissociation constants for guanabenz and, in particular, amiloride, obtained for amiloride binding protein, DAO and subtypes of I_2 receptors, suggest that some idazoxan-preferring sites may actually represent DAO enzymes. The fact that agmatine, the proposed endogenous ligand for these binding sites, is a substrate for this enzyme further supports this view, as do the differences in tissue DAO distribution seen between rabbits and other mammals. Examinations of the effects of a series of I_2-preferring ligands on DAO activity in vitro, and of the effects of DAO inhibition in vivo on endogenous agmatine levels, are currently under way in our laboratory.

Summary

Clonidine-displacing substance, thought to be the endogenous ligand for imidazoline receptors, has been identified recently as agmatine (1-amino-4-guanidinobutane). The similarity of this compound's structure to that of the diamine oxidase (DAO) inhibitor, aminoguanidine, led us to investigate the possibility that agmatine might be a substrate for this enzyme. The metabolism of agmatine by purified porcine kidney DAO was measured by a peroxidase-linked colorimetric assay. Agmatine was a substrate for this enzyme and, under the experimental conditions used here, was metabolised at a rate of 0.8 μmol agmatine h^{-1} (unit DAO activity)$^{-1}$. In contrast, agmatine was a substrate neither for rat brain monoamine oxidase (MAO) -A or -B, nor for rat brown adipose tissue semicarbazide-sensitive amine oxidase (SSAO). The metabolism of agmatine by DAO was inhibited by aminoguanidine (IC_{50} 14.9 nM) and by the antidepressant, phenelzine (IC_{50} 1.95 μM). These results suggest that administration of DAO inhibitors may increase endogenous agmatine levels and thus alter imidazoline receptor densities. A review of the literature documenting ligand affinities for idazoxan-preferring (I_2) imidazoline binding site subtypes and drug affinities for DAO enzymes indicates that some of the I_2 sites described elsewhere may correspond to DAO and not to an imidazoline receptor.

Acknowledgements

We wish to thank Gail Rauw for her technical assistance. Funding was provided by the Medical Research Council of Canada and salary support for A.H. was provided by Ciba-Geigy Pharmaceuticals.

References

Atlas, D. and Burstein, Y. (1984) Isolation and partial purification of a clonidine-displacing endogenous brain substance. Eur. J. Biochem., 144: 287–293.

Barbry, P., Chassande, O., Duval, D., Rousseau, B., Frelin, C. and Lazdunski, M. (1989) Biochemical identification of two types of phenamil binding sites associated with amiloride-sensitive Na^+ channels. Biochemistry, 28: 3744–3749.

Barbry, P., Champe, M., Chassande, O., Munemitsu, S., Champigny, G., Lingueglia, E., Maes, P., Frelin, C., Tartar, A., Ullrich, A. and Lazdunski, M. (1990a) Human kidney amiloride-binding protein: cDNA structure and functional expression. Proc. Natl. Acad. Sci. USA, 87: 7347–7351.

Barbry, P., Chassande, O., Marsault, R., Lazdunski, M. and Frelin, C. (1990b) [^{3}H]Phenamil binding protein of the renal epithelium Na^+ channel. Purification, affinity labeling, and functional reconstitution. Biochemistry, 29: 1039–1045.

Bidet, M., Poujeol, P. and Parini, A. (1990) Effect of imidazolines on Na^+ transport and intracellular pH in renal proximal tubule cells. Biochim. Biophys. Acta, 1024: 173–178.

Blaschko, H. (1974) The natural history of amine oxidases. Rev. Physiol. Biochem. Pharmacol., 70: 83–148.

Boadle, M.C. (1969) Observations on a histaminase of invertebrate origin: a contribution to the study of cephalopod amine oxidases. Comp. Biochem. Physiol., 30: 611–620.

Boadle, M.C. and Blaschko, H. (1968) Cockroach amine oxidase: classification and substrate specificity. Comp. Biochem. Physiol., 25: 129–138.

Bousquet, P., Feldman, J. and Schwartz, J. (1984) Central cardiovascular effects of alpha adrenergic drugs: Differences between catecholamines and imidazolines. J. Pharmacol. Exp. Ther., 230: 232–236.

Bowman, W.C. and Rand, M.J. (1980) Textbook of Pharmacology, 2nd edn., Blackwell, Oxford, 23.47 pp.

Buffoni, F. (1966) Histaminase and related amine oxidases. Pharmacol. Rev., 18: 1163–1199.

Burkard, W.P., Gey, K.F. and Pletscher, A. (1960) Inhibition of diamine oxidase in vivo by hydrazine derivatives. *Biochem. Pharmacol.*, 3: 249–255.

Callingham, B.A., Holt, A. and Elliott, J. (1990) Some aspects of the pharmacology of semicarbazide-sensitive amine oxidases. *J. Neural Transm.*, 32 (Suppl.): 279–290.

Callingham, B.A., Holt, A. and Elliott, J. (1991) Properties and functions of the semicarbazide-sensitive amine oxidases. *Biochem. Soc. Trans.*, 19: 228–233.

Campbell, W.R. and Potter, D.E. (1994) Potential role of imidazoline (I_1) receptors in modulating aqueous humor dynamics. *J. Ocular Pharmacol.*, 10: 393–402.

Corpus, V.M., Bressie, S.M., Stillwell, L.I. and Olins, G.M. (1994) Interaction of guanidinium compounds and K^+ channel modulators with imidazoline binding sites in rabbit kidney. *Eur. J. Pharmacol.*, 266: 197–200.

Czech, M.P., Lawrence, J.C. and Lynn, W.S. (1974a) Evidence for the involvement of sulphydryl oxidation in the regulation of fat cell hexose transport by insulin. *Proc. Natl. Acad. Sci. USA*, 71: 4173–4177.

Czech, M.P., Lawrence, J.C. and Lynn, W.S. (1974b) Hexose transport in isolated brown fat cells. A model system for investigating insulin action on membrane transport. *J. Biol. Chem.*, 249: 5421–5427.

De Vos, H., Bricca, G., De Keyser, J., De Backer, J. -P., Bousquet, P. and Vauquelin, G. (1994) Imidazoline receptors, non-adrenergic idazoxan binding sites and α_2-adrenoceptors in the human central nervous system. *Neuroscience*, 59: 589–598.

Diamant, S., Eldor, A. and Atlas, D. (1987) A low molecular weight brain substance interacts, similarly to clonidine, with α_2-adrenoceptors of human platelets. *Eur. J. Pharmacol.*, 144: 247–255.

Elliott, J., Fowden, A.L., Callingham, B.A., Sharman, D.F. and Silver, M. (1991) Physiological and pathological influences on sheep blood plasma amine oxidase: effect of pregnancy and experimental alloxan-induced diabetes mellitus. *Res. Vet. Sci.*, 50: 334–339.

Ernsberger, P., Meeley, M.P., Mann, J.J. and Reis, D.J. (1987) Clonidine binds to imidazole binding sites as well as α_1-adrenoceptors in the ventrolateral medulla. *Eur. J. Pharmacol.*, 134: 1–13.

Ernsberger, P., Meeley, M.P. and Reis, D.J. (1988) An endogenous substance with clonidine-like properties: selective binding to imidazole sites in the ventrolateral medulla. *Brain Res.*, 441: 309–318.

Ernsberger, P., Giuliano, R., Willette, R.N. and Reis, D.J. (1990) Role of imidazole receptors in the vasodepressor response to clonidine analogs in the rostral ventrolateral medulla. *J. Pharmacol. Exp. Ther.*, 253: 408–418.

Ernsberger, P., Haxhiu, M.A., Graff, L.M., Collins, L.A., Dreshaj, I., Grove, D.L., Graves, M.E., Schäfer, S.G. and Christen, M.O. (1994) A novel mechanism of action for hypertension control: moxonidine as a selective I_1-imidazoline agonist. *Cardiovasc. Drugs Ther.*, 8: 27–41.

Felsen, D., Ernsberger, P., Meeley, M.P. and Reis, D.J. (1987) Clonidine displacing substance is biologically active on smooth muscle. *Eur. J. Pharmacol.*, 142: 453–455.

Felsen, D., Ernsberger, P., Sutaria, P.M., Nejat, R.J., Nguyen, P., May, M., Breslin, D.S., Marion, D.N. and Vaughan, E.D. (1994) Identification, localization and functional analysis of imidazoline and alpha-adrenergic receptors in canine prostate. *J. Pharmacol. Exp. Ther.*, 268: 1063–1071.

Harron, D.W.G. (1992) Clinical pharmacology of imidazolines and related compounds. *Fundam. Clin. Pharmacol.*, 6 (Suppl. 1): 41s–44s.

Holt, A., Sharman, D.F., Callingham, B.A. and Kettler, R. (1992a) Characteristics of procarbazine as an inhibitor in vitro of rat semicarbazide-sensitive amine oxidase. *J. Pharm. Pharmacol.*, 44: 487–493.

Holt, A., Sharman, D.F. and Callingham, B.A. (1992b) Effects in vitro of procarbazine metabolites on some amine oxidase activities in the rat. *J. Pharm. Pharmacol.*, 44: 494–499.

Janes, S.M., Palcic, M.M., Scaman, C.H., Smith, A.J., Brown, D.E., Dooley, D.M., Mure, M. and Klinman, J.P. (1992) Identification of topaquinone and its consensus sequence in copper amine oxidases. *Biochemistry*, 31: 12147–12154.

Kleyman, T.R., Yulo, T., Ashbaugh, C., Landry, D., Cragoe, E., Karlin, A. and Al-Awqati, Q. (1986) Photoaffinity labelling of the epithelial sodium channel. *J. Biol. Chem.*, 261: 2839–2843.

Klinman, J.P. and Mu, D. (1994) Quinoenzymes in biology. *Annu. Rev. Biochem.*, 63: 299–344.

Kobinger, W. (1978) Central α-adrenergic systems as targets for hypotensive drugs. *Rev. Physiol. Biochem. Pharmacol.*, 81: 40–100.

Kusche, J., Richter, M., Hesterberg, J., Schmidt, J. and Lorenz, W. (1973) Comparison of the ^{14}C-putrescine assay with the NADH test for the determination of diamine oxidase: description of a standard procedure with a high precision and an improved assay. *Agents Actions*, 3: 668–672.

Kusche, J., Richter, H., Schmidt, J., Hesterberg, R., Friedrich, A. and Lorenz, W. (1975) Diamine oxydase in rabbit small intestine: separation from a soluble monoamine oxidase, properties and pathophysiological significance in intestinal ischemia. *Agents Actions*, 5: 431–439.

Langin, D. and Lafontan, M. (1989) [^{3}H]Idazoxan binding at non-α_2-adrenoceptors in rabbit adipocyte membranes. *Eur. J. Pharmacol.*, 159: 199–203.

Li, G., Regunathan, S., Barrow, C.J., Eshraghi, J., Cooper, R. and Reis, D.J. (1994a) Agmatine: an endogenous clonidine-displacing substance in the brain. *Science*, 263: 966–969.

Li, P., Penner, S.B. and Smyth, D.D. (1994b) Attenuated renal response to moxonidine and rilmenidine in one kidney-one clip hypertensive rats. *Br. J. Pharmacol.*, 112: 200–206.

Lowry, O.H., Rosebrough, N.J., Farr, A.L. and Randall, R.J. (1951) Protein measurement with the Folin phenol reagent. *J. Biol. Chem.*, 193: 265–275.

Lyles, G.A. (1984) The interaction of semicarbazide-sensitive amine oxidase with MAO inhibitors. In: K.F. Tipton, P. Dostert and M. Strolin-Benedetti (Eds.), *Monoamine oxidase and disease. Prospects for therapy with reversible inhibitors*, Academic Press, London, pp. 547–556.

Lyles, G.A. and Callingham, B.A. (1982) In vitro and in vivo inhibition by benserazide of clorgyline-resistant amine oxidases in rat cardiovascular tissues. *Biochem. Pharmacol.*, 31: 1417–1424.

Michel, M.C. and Ernsberger, P. (1992) Keeping an eye on the I site: imidazoline-preferring receptors. *Trends Pharmacol. Sci.*, 13: 369–370.

Michel, M.C. and Insel, P.A. (1989) Are there multiple imidazoline binding sites? *Trends Pharmacol. Sci.*, 10: 342–344.

Mu, D., Medzihradszky, K.F., Adams, G.W., Mayer, P., Hines, W.M., Burlingame, A.L., Smith, A.J., Cai, D. and Klinman, J.P. (1994) Primary structures for a mammalian cellular and serum copper amine oxidase. *J. Biol. Chem.*, 269: 9926–9932.

Mukherjee, S.P. and Mukherjee, C. (1982) Similar activities of nerve growth factor and its homologue proinsulin in intracellular hydrogen peroxide production and metabolism in adipocytes. Transmembrane signalling relative to insulin-mimicking cellular effects. *Biochem. Pharmacol.*, 31: 3163–3172.

Novotny, W.F., Chassande, O., Baker, M., Lazdunski, M. and Barbry, P. (1994) Diamine oxidase is the amiloride binding protein and is inhibited by amiloride analogues. *J. Biol. Chem.*, 269: 9921–9925.

Olmos, G., Miralles, A., Barturen, F. and García-Sevilla, J.A. (1992) Characterization of brain imidazoline receptors in normotensive and hypertensive rats: differential regulation by chronic imidazoline drug treatment. *J. Pharmacol. Exp. Ther.*, 260: 1000–1007.

Pegg, A.E. and McCann, P.P. (1982) Polyamine metabolism and function. *Am. J. Physiol.*, 243: C212-C221.

Penner, S.B. and Smyth, D.D. (1994) Central and renal I_1 imidazoline preferring receptors: two unique sites mediating natriuresis in the rat. *Cardiovasc. Drugs Ther.*, 8: 43–48.

Regunathan, S., Meeley, M.P. and Reis, D.J. (1991) Clonidine-displacing substance from bovine brain binds to imidazoline receptors and releases catecholamines in adrenal chromaffin cells. *Mol. Pharmacol.*, 40: 884–888.

Regunathan, S., Meeley, M.P. and Reis, D.J. (1993) Expression of non-adrenergic imidazoline sites in chromaffin cells and mitochondrial membranes of bovine adrenal medulla. *Biochem. Pharmacol.*, 45: 1667–1675.

Renouard, A., Widdowson, P.S. and Cordi, A. (1993) [^{3}H]-Idazoxan binding to rabbit cerebral cortex recognises multiple imidazoline I_2-type receptors: pharmacological charac-

terization and relationship to monoamine oxidase. *Br. J. Pharmacol.*, 109: 625–631.

Sannajust, F. and Head, G.A. (1994) Rilmenidine-induced hypotension in conscious rabbits involves imidazoline-preferring receptors. *J. Cardiovasc. Pharmacol.*, 23: 42–50.

Sattler, J. and Lorenz, W. (1990) Intestinal diamine oxidases and enteral-induced histaminosis: studies on three prognostic variables in an epidemiological model. *J. Neural Transm.*, 32 (Suppl.): 291–314.

Sener, A., Lebrun, P., Blachier, F. and Malaisse, W.J. (1989) Stimulus-secretion coupling of arginine-induced insulin release. Insulinotropic action of agmatine. *Biochem. Pharmacol.*, 38: 327–330.

Shore, P.A. and Cohn, V.H. (1960) Comparative effects of monoamine oxidase inhibitors on monoamine oxidase and diamine oxidase. *Biochem. Pharmacol.*, 5: 91–95.

Tabor, C.W. and Tabor, H. (1984) Polyamines. *Annu. Rev. Biochem.*, 53: 749–790.

Tesson, F., Prip-Buus, C., Lemoine, A., Pegorier, J.-P. and Parini, A. (1991) Subcellular distribution of imidazoline-guanidinium-receptive sites in human and rabbit liver. *J. Biol. Chem.*, 266: 155–160.

Weber, M.A., Graettinger, W.F. and Cheung, D.G. (1990) Centrally acting sympathetic inhibitors. In: J.H. Laragh and B.M. Brenner (Eds.), *Hypertension: Pathophysiology, Diagnosis, and Management*, Raven Press, New York, pp. 2251–2261.

Weitzel, G., Pfeiffer, B. and Stock, W. (1980) Insulin-like partial effects of agmatine derivatives in adipocytes. *Hoppe-Seyler's Z. Physiol. Chem.*, 361: 51–60.

White, A., Handler, P. and Smith, E.L. (1973) *Principles of Biochemistry*, 5th edn., McGraw-Hill, Kogakusha, 674 pp.

Wikberg, J.E.S., Uhlén, S. and Chhajlani, V. (1992) Evidence that drug binding to non-adrenergic [^{3}H]-idazoxan binding sites (I-receptors) occurs to interacting or interconvertible affinity forms of the receptor. *Pharmacol. Toxicol.*, 70: 208–219.

Yakubu, M.A., Deighton, N.M., Hamilton, C.A. and Reid, J.L. (1990) Differences in the regulation of [^{3}H]idazoxan and [^{3}H]yohimbine binding sites in the rabbit. *Eur. J. Pharmacol.*, 176: 305–311.

Yamada, H., Isobe, K., Tani, Y. and Hiromi, K. (1979) A differential determination procedure for spermine and spermidine with beef plasma amine oxidase. *Agric. Biol. Chem.*, 43: 2487–2491.

Zeller, E.A. (1938) Über den enzymatischen Abbau von Histamin und Diaminen. *Helv. Chim. Acta*, 21: 880–890.

Zeller, E.A. (1941) Zur Kenntnis der Mono- und Diaminoxydase. *Helv. Chim. Acta*, 24: 539–548.

Zeller, E.A., Fouts, J.R., Carbon, J.A., Lazanas, J.C. and Voegtli, W. (1956) Über die Substratspezifität der Diaminoxydase. *Helv. Chim. Acta*, 39: 1632–1644.

Peter M. Yu, Keith F. Tipton and Alan A. Boulton (Eds.)
Progress in Brain Research, Vol 106
© 1995 Elsevier Science BV. All rights reserved.

CHAPTER 20

Increase of survival of dopaminergic neuroblastoma in co-cultures with C-6 glioma by R-(−)-deprenyl

Dongmei Zuo and Peter H. Yu

Neuropsychiatry Research Unit, Department of Psychiatry, University of Saskatchewan, Saskatoon, Saskatchewan, Canada S7N 0W0

Introduction

R-(−)-Deprenyl (selegiline) is the archetypical selective inhibitor of type B monoamine oxidase (MAO) (Knoll and Magyar, 1972). It has been used as a co-drug to increase the efficacy of levo-dopa therapy in the treatment of Parkinson's Disease (PD) (Birkmayer et al., 1975). The mode of action of R-(−)-deprenyl has been initially ascribed to its attenuation of dopamine (DA) catabolism by MAO-B (Birkmayer et al., 1983) or potention of DA action (Paterson et al., 1990). More recently, it has been suggested that R-(−)-deprenyl alone can slow down the progression of movement deficits in PD (Parkinson Study Group, 1989, 1993; Tetrud and Langston, 1989) and cognitive decline in Alzheimers Disease (AD) (Mangoni et al., 1991; Tariot et al., 1987). The mechanisms underlying the drug action are not yet well understood (Langston, 1990).

It has been suggested that R-(−)-deprenyl protects dopaminergic neurons against toxic oxidative damage by reducing free-radical formation derived from excessive deamination (Cohen, 1986). Recently R-(−)-deprenyl has been shown to rescue neurons that have been damaged by MPTP and wash out of the neurotoxin (Tatton and Greenwood, 1991) or reduce the death of motoneurons after facial axotomy in young rats (Salo and Tatton, 1992). The death of the motor neurons in the facial nuclei after axotomy is thought to reflect the dependency of the immature motoneurons on trophic support axonally-transported from the muscles they innervate (Crews and Wigston, 1990). A reduction in motoneuronal death produced by axotomy in immature rats can be seen after treatment with neurotrophic factors, such as ciliary neuronotrophic factor (Sendtner et al., 1990) or basic fibroblast growth factor (Grothe and Unsicker, 1992). R-(−)-Deprenyl can apparently compensate somewhat for the loss of target-derived trophic support in this model. R-(−)-deprenyl-mediated reduction in motoneuron death does not seem to involve inhibition of MAO-B activity (Ansari et al., 1993).

R-(−)-Deprenyl has recently been shown to increase the survival of tyrosine hydroxylase positive neurons in rat mesencephalic cultures (Roy and Bedard, 1993). It is, however, unknown whether or not R-(−)-deprenyl acted directly towards neurons or via trophic effects from astrocytes. We have, therefore, investigated the effects of R-(−)-deprenyl on neuronal survival in a co-culture of dopaminergic neuroblastoma and glioma cells.

Materials and methods

Materials

The glioma (C-6) cell line was obtained from ATCC (Rockville, MA, USA) and SH-SY5Y neuroblastoma cells (a human dopaminergic neuroblastoma cell line) were kindly provided by Dr. C. Haymen (Regeneron Pharmaceuticals, Tarrytown, New York, USA). [methyl-^{3}H]Thymidine was obtained from Amersham (Oakville, Ontario, Canada). All other chemicals were of analytical grade.

Cell cultures

SH-SY5Y cells were cultured in RPMI 1640 medium containing 10% fetal bovine serum (FBS, Sigma, St. Louis, MS, USA); C-6 glioma cells were maintained in RPMI 1640 medium with 10% horse serum and 5% new-born calf serum. All cells were maintained in a humidified atmosphere of 5% CO_2 and 95% air at 37°C. Media usually contained sodium bicarbonate (14.3 mM), streptomycin (75 units/ml), penicillin (100 units/ml) and L-glutamine (20 mM). The medium was replaced with fresh medium twice a week. For subculture the medium was removed and 0.01% EDTA and 0.1% collagenase were added; the cells were then incubated at room temperature for 10 min until cell detachment. Fresh medium was then added, aspirated and dispensed into new flasks. The subcultivation ratios were maintained at 1:3 to 1:8.

Preparation of tritium-labelled SH-SY5Y cells and assessment of neuronal survival

Subconfluent SH-SY5Y cells were labelled by incubating the cells in a 75 cm^2 flask containing 20 ml media and 20 μCi [methyl-^{3}H]thymidine for 24 h. The cells were removed from the flasks and suspended by repeated pipetting using a Pasteur pipette and then centrifuged (600 × g, 5 min). The cells were resuspended and the suspension was washed twice with the culture medium. A total of about (3–5) × 10^5 viable cells in 1 ml medium (viability was determined by trypan blue staining) were then transferred to each 60 mm Petri-dish that either contained or did not contain a monolayer of C-6 glioma cells (24 h after seeding), in the presence or absence of 6-hydroxy-

dopamine. The cultures were then maintained for 24 h and surviving SH-SY5Y cells, i.e. radioactively labelled intact cells, were washed and collected by a cell harvester (Brandel, Gaithersburg, MD, USA); the amount of radioactivity was estimated in a scintillation counter (Beckmann, LS 5000TD).

Results

Effect of R-(−)-deprenyl on the viability of neuroblastoma and glioma cells

Both SH-SY5Y and C-6 cells were grown for 24 h, the media of these cultured cells were replaced by media containing different concentrations of R-(−)-deprenyl and serum which was replaced and further maintained for 48 or 72 h. R-(−)-Deprenyl does not affect the viability of either type of cell in media containing 1% or 15% serum (see Fig 1).

Effect of R-(−)-deprenyl on neuronal survival in co-culture

Freshly prepared, viable, tritium-labelled SH-SY5Y cells were subcultured to culture dishes containing a monolayer of C-6 glioma cells, which were maintained in media containing either 15% or 1% serum. Microscopic examination revealed that an extensive cell-cell adhesion occurred between the neuroblastoma cells and the glioma cells. As can be seen in Fig. 2A, the survival of SH-SY5Y cells in co-culture with C-6 grown in 1% serum media after 48 h was lower in comparison with those grown in 15% serum (see left group of columns). R-(−)-Deprenyl was found to increase significantly the survival of SH-SY5Y in the C-6 cells culture maintained in 1% serum. Such a R-(−)-deprenyl effect on SH-SY5Y was, however, not detected in the coculture with higher density of C-6 cells (see Fig. 2B).

We have also investigated the effect of R-(−)-deprenyl on 6-hydroxydopamine (6-OHDA)-induced neurotoxicity towards SH-SY5Y in the cocultures. SH-SY5Y cells alone are very sensitive

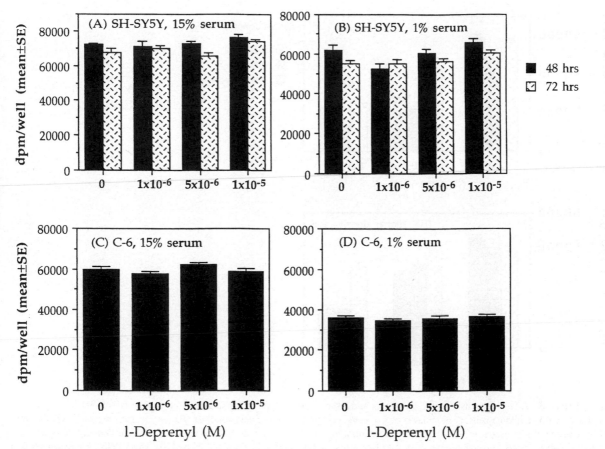

Fig. 1. Effect of R-$(-)$-deprenyl on the viability of SH-SY5Y neuronal and C-6 glioma cells. Cells were grown for 48 or 72 h on plates of 96-wells ($n = 6$) in the presence of different concentrations of l-deprenyl in media containing either 15% or 1% bovine fetal serum. [^{3}H]Thymidine (0.5 μCi/well) was added and following incubation for 4 h the cells were collected and washed with a cell harvester. The amount of incorporated radioactivity was assessed in a scintillation counter (Beckmann, LS 5000TD). (A) SH-SY5Y in 15% serum; (B) SH-SY5Y in 1% serum; (C) C-6 in 15% serum; (D) C-6 in 1% serum. Results are means $\pm$ SE (bars) ($n = 6$). All treated groups were not significantly different (according to ANOVA).

towards 6-OHDA; in monocultures less than 15% of the neuroblastoma cells survive in media containing 1×10^{-4} M 6-OHDA (Fig. 3), which is consistent with previous observations (Zuo and Yu, 1994). The survival of SH-SY5Y cells in co-culture with C-6 cells against 6-OHDA is enhanced. Although more SH-SY5Y cells survived in C-6 cultures grown in 15% serum or at high C-6 density than those cells maintained in 1% serum and low density of C-6 cells (Fig. 2), there was no evidence that R-$(-)$-deprenyl improved

survival of neurons damaged by 6-OHDA in the co-cultures.

Dose-dependent effect of R-$(-)$-deprenyl on survival of SH-SY5Y

R-$(-)$-Deprenyl at different concentrations was included in the C-6 cultures in the presence of either 1% or 15% serum for 24 h. The increase in neuronal survival was only observed in the C-6 cultures with low serum and in the presence of R-$(-)$-deprenyl from 1×10^{-6} to 1×10^{-5} M

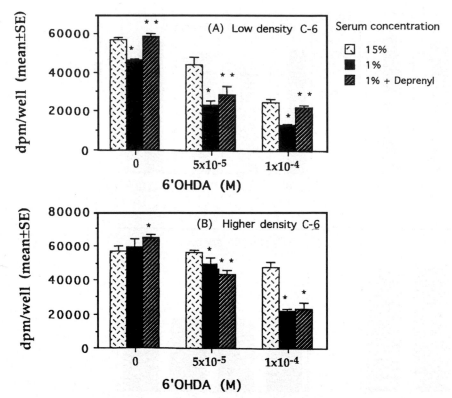

Fig. 2. Effect of R-$(-)$-deprenyl, in the presence and absence of 6-hydroxydopamine, on the survival of SH-SY5Y cells in co-culture with C-6 glioma cells. A monolayer of C-6 cells, i.e. (A) 1×10^5 (upper panel) or (B) 2×10^5 (lower panel) cells/60 mm dish were seeded and grown in RPMI 1640 media containing 15% serum for 24 h. The media were then changed to fresh 15% serum, 1% serum, or 1% serum containing 10^{-6} M l-deprenyl. After 24 h [^{3}H]thymidine-labelled SH-SY5Y cells (3×10^5 cells/dish) were seeded into the C-6 cultures. Followimg a further 24 h incubation, 6-hydroxydopamine was added and the cells were then harvested and washed 24 h later with a Brandel cell harvester. The viability, i.e. the amount of radioactivity retained and attached to the plates, was then assessed. Results are means ± SE (bars) of independent triplicate experiments. * and ** denote significant differences ($P < 0.01$, Newman-Keuls test) compared to control groups (without l-deprenyl) in media containing 10% and 1% serum, respectively.

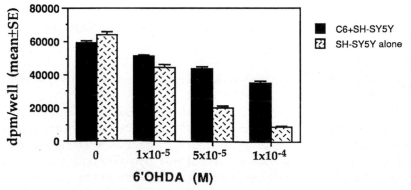

Fig. 3. Effect of 6-OHDA on the survival of SH-SY5Y cells in monoculture or in co-culture with the primary astrocytes. For experimental details see Fig. 2.

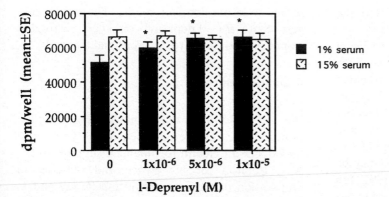

Fig. 4. Dose-dependent effect of R-($-$)-deprenyl on the survival of SH-SY5Y cells in co-culture with C-6 glioma cells. Monolayers of C-6 cells (1×10^5 cells/60 mm dish, in RPMI 1640 media containing 15% or 1% serum for 24 h) were prepared and [^{3}H]thymidine-labelled SH-SY5Y cells (3×10^5 cells/dish) were then seeded onto the C-6 cultures. The co-cultures were maintained for 48 h and the labelled neuroblastoma cells were then collected and washed by a Brandel cell harvester. The viability (i.e. amount of radioactivity retained) was then assessed. Results are means $\pm$ SE (bars) of triplicate independent experiments. Asterisks denote significant differences ($P < 0.01$, Newman-Keuls test) compared to control group (without R-($-$)-deprenyl) in 1% serum media.

(Fig. 4). R-($-$)-Deprenyl does not affect the survival of SH-SY5Y in C-6 co-culture in the presence of 15% serum.

Discussion

R-($-$)-Deprenyl has been shown to be capable of increasing neuronal survival in some animal models (Salo and Tatton, 1992; Tatton et al., 1991). Recently it has been shown that the survival of rat fetal nigral tyrosine hydroxylase-positive neurons in mesencephalic culture is enhanced by R-($-$)-deprenyl (Roy and Bedard, 1993). This cell culture study is consistent with the in vivo results, although it remains unclear just how the R-($-$)-deprenyl increases neuronal survival. In this present study we were unable to detect any significant effect of R-($-$)-deprenyl on the viability (based on DNA synthesis) of either neuroblastoma or glioma cells cultured in either high or low serum conditions. When the neuroblastoma cells were seeded into C-6 glioma cultures, however, the neuronal cells adhered closely to the glioma cells. The morphology of the neuronal cells changed slightly, especially in confluenced C-6 cultures. The survival of SH-SY5Y cells was

decreased when they were co-cultured with glioma cells in 1% serum as compared with 10% serum. R-($-$)-Deprenyl enhanced neuronal survival of SH-SY5Y cells in the C-6 cultures, but only when the serum concentration was low (i.e. 1%). This effect is dependent not only on the concentration of serum, but also on the density of the SH-SY5Y cells seeded into each dish and on the concentration of the R-($-$)-deprenyl. Since R-($-$)-deprenyl does not directly affect the viability or survival of SH-SY5Y or C-6 cells grown separately, the increase in survival of the neuroblastoma cells by R-($-$)-deprenyl in co-culture with C-6 cells must be due to some kind of interaction occurring between the two types of cell. This could involve a modification in the state of the C-6 cells, such as, for example, an increase in trophic effects without significant change in the viability of the glioma cells. We have recently observed that R-($-$)-deprenyl is capable of inhibiting the expression of statin and this has been proposed to act on the G_1-G_0 boundary of the cell cycle by preventing astroglial cells from entering the nonproliferative phase of the cycle under unfavorable cultural conditions, such as in media containing low serum (Skibo et al., 1992). Such an effect of R-($-$)-deprenyl on the glioma cells may be related the increase of survial of neuroblastoma cells.

Cell–cell interactions are considered to be of prime importance during neuronogenesis. Such interactions are responsible for the co-ordinated morphogenetic steps: neural induction, cell proliferation, migration, aggregation, cytodifferentiation, synapse formation, cell death and synapse elimination (Abbott, 1991). Several trophic factors, such as bFGF, BDNF and GDNF, may be supported by astrocytes (Hyman et al., 1991; Lin et al., 1993). Astroglial CNTF gene expression has been recently found to be augmented by R-($-$)-deprenyl (Seniuk et al., 1994). A strong adhesion occurs between SH-SY5Y and C-6 cells. Our study cannot rule out the possibility that the enhancement of SH-SY5Y cell survival by R-($-$)-deprenyl may be related to an effect of specific cell–cell adhesion and the subsequent biochemical cascade related to cell survival. Specific adhesion among different neural cell types at different development stages can transduce cell surface events to intracellular signals in axonal membranes, which might provide neuroprotective and neurorescue effects (Gloor et al., 1990; Schuch et al., 1989).

The present study has shown that R-($-$)-deprenyl is capable of increasing survival of neuroblastom cells when co-cultured with glioma cells in serum-deprived and low-cell-density conditions. R-($-$)-deprenyl affects astrocytes and subsequently provides favorable conditions to support neurons. This may be relevant to the neurorescue effect of R-($-$)-deprenyl in the treatment of neurodegenerative illnesss, such as Parkinson's disease.

Summary

We have observed that the survival of dopamine neuroblastoma (SH-SY5Y) cells in co-cultures with C-6 glioma in serum-deprived media is slightly but significantly enhanced by R-($-$)-deprenyl, a selective monoamine oxidase B inhibitor. This drug, however, does not directly affect the viability of SH-SY5Y cells or glioma cells in serum or serum-deprived media. The results suggest that R-($-$)-deprenyl enhances astroglial trophic support in favor of neuronal survival.

Acknowledgements

We are grateful to the Canadian Parkinsonian Foundation, Deprenyl Research Ltd. and Saskatchewan Health for financial support, to Dr. A.A. Boulton for his advice and criticism in preparation of the manuscript and K. Jay and T. Yu for their technical assistance.

References

Abbott, N.J. (Ed.) (1991) *Glial-Neuronal Interactions*, Vol. 633, New York Academy of Sciences, New York.

Ansari, K.S., Tatton, W.G., Yu, P.H. and Kruck, T.X. (1993) Death of axotomized immature rat facial motoneurons: Stereospecificity of deprenyl-induced rescue. *J. Neurosci.*, 13: 4042–4053.

Birkmayer, W., Riederer, P., Youdim, M.B.H. and Linauer, W. (1975) The potentiation of the anti-akinetic effect after L-dopa treatment by an inhibitor of MAO-B, deprenyl. *J. Neural Transm.*, 36: 303–336.

Birkmayer, W., Knoll, J., Riederer, P. and Youdim, M.B.H. (1983) ($-$)-Deprenyl leads to prolongation of L-dopa efficacy in Parkinson's disease. *Mod. Prob. Pharmacopsychiatry*, 19: 170–176.

Cohen, G. (1986) Monoamine oxidase, hydrogen peroxide, and Parkinson's disease. *Adv. Neurol.*, 45: 119–125.

Crews, L.L. and Wigston, D.J. (1990) The dependence of motoneurons on their target muscle during postnatal development of the mouse. *J. Neurosci.*, 10: 1643–1653.

Gloor, S., Antonicek, H., Sweadner, K.J., Pagliusi, S., Moos, M., and Schachner M. (1990) The adhesion moleculue on glia (AMOG) is a homogologue of the β subunit of the Na,K-ATPase. *J. Cell Biol.*, 110: 165–174.

Grothe, C. and Unsicker, K. (1992) Basic fibroblast growth factor in the hypoglossal system: specific retrograde transport, trophic and lesion-related responses. *J. Neurosc. Res.*, 32: 317–328.

Hyman, C., Hofer, C., Barde, Y.A., Juhasz, M., Yancopoulos, G.D., Squinto, S.P. and Lindsay, R.M. (1991) BDNF is a neurotrophic factor for dopaminergic neurons of the substantia nigra. *Nature*, 350: 230–232.

Knoll, J. and Magyar, K. (1972) Some puzzling pharmacological effects of monoamine oxidase inhibitors. Monoamine oxidase. Adv. Biochem. Psychopharmacol, 5: 393–408.

Langston, J.W. (1990) Selegiline as neuroprotective therapy in

Parkinson's disease: concepts and controversies. *Neurology*, 40 (Suppl.): 61–66.

Lin, L.F.H., Doherty, D.H., Lile, J.D., Bektesh S. and Collins, F. (1993) GDNF: A glial cell line-derived neurotrophic factor for midbrain dopaminergic neurons. *Science*, 260: 1130–1132.

Mangoni, A., Grassi, M.P., Frattola, L., Piolti, R., Bassi, S., Motta, A., Marcone, A. and Smirne, S. (1991) Effects of a MAO-B inhibitor in the treatment of Alzheimer disease. *Eur. Neurol.*, 31: 100–107.

Parkinson Study Group, USA (1989) Effect of deprenyl on the progression of disability in early Parkinson's disease. *N. Engl. J. Med.*, 321: 1364–1371.

Parkinson Study Group, USA (1993) Effects of tocopherol and deprenyl on the progresssion of disability in early Parkinson's disease. *N. Engl. J. Med.*, 328: 176–183.

Paterson, I.A., Juorio, A.V. and Boulton, A.A. (1990) Possible mechanism of action of deprenyl in Parkinsonism. *Lancet*, 36: 183.

Roy, E. and Bedard, P.J. (1993) Deprenyl increases survival of rat foetal nigral neurones in culutre. *NeuroReport*, 4: 1183–1186.

Salo, P.T. and Tatton, W.G. (1992) Deprenyl reduces the death of motoneurons caused by axotomy. *J. Neursci. Res.*, 31: 394–400.

Schuch, U., Lohse, M.J. and Schachner, M. (1989) Neural cell adhesion molecules influence second messenger systems. *Neuron*, 3: 13–20.

Sendtner, M., Kreutzberg, G.W. and Thoenen, H. (1990) Ciliary neurotrophic factor prevents the degeneration of motor neurons after axotomy. *Nature*, 345: 440–441.

Seniuk, N.A., Henderson, J.T., Tatton, W.G. and Roder J.C. (1994) Increased CNTF gene expression in processs-bearing astrocytes folowing injury is augmented by *R*-(−)-deprenyl. *J. Neurosci. Res.*, 37: 278–286.

Skibo, G., Ahmed, I., Yu, P.H., Boulton, A.A. and Fedoroff, S. (1992) l-Deprenyl, a monoamine oxidase-B (MAO-B) inhibitors, acts on the astroglia cell cycle at the G1/G0 boundary. *Proc. Am. Soc. Cell Biol.*, 12: 532.

Tariot, P.N., Sunderland, T., Weingartner, H., Murphy, D.L., Welkowitz, J.A., Thompson, K. and Cohen, R.M. (1987) Cognitive effects of l-deprenyl in Alzheimer's disease. *Psychopharmacology*, 91: 489–495.

Tatton, W.G. and Greenwood, C.E. (1991) Rescue of dying neurons: A new action for deprenyl in MPTP Parkinsonism. *J. Neurosci. Res.*, 30: 666–672.

Tetrud, J.W. and Langston, J.W. (1989) The effect of deprenyl (selegiline) on the natural history of Parkinson's disease. *Science*, 245: 519–522.

Zuo, D.M. and Yu, P.H. (1994) Increase in the survival of neuroblastoma cells treated with 6-hydroxydopamine in co-culutres with primary astrocytes: Possible involvement of specific cell-cell adhesion. *Trans. Am. Soc. Neurochem.*, 25: 118.

Peter M. Yu, Keith F. Tipton and Alan A. Boulton (Eds.)
Progress in Brain Research, Vol 106
© 1995 Elsevier Science BV. All rights reserved.

CHAPTER 21

Canine pituitary-dependent hyperadrenocorticism: a spontaneous animal model for neurodegenerative disorders and their treatment with 1-deprenyl

David S. Bruyette[1], William W. Ruehl[2,3] and Theresa L. Smidberg[2]

[1]*Department of Clinical Sciences, College of Veterinary Medicine, Kansas State University, Manhattan, KS 66502,* [2]*Deprenyl Animal Health, Inc., Overland Park, KS 66210, and* [3]*Department of Pathology, Stanford University, Palo Alto, CA, USA*

Introduction

Canine hyperadrenocorticism is a common disorder in the dog and probably the most common endocrinopathy encountered in geriatric patients. The majority of cases (90%) occur as the result of pituitary hypersecretion of ACTH (pituitary-dependent hyperadrenocorticism (PDH); Cushing's disease) which results in bilateral adrenal hyperplasia and overproduction of cortisol. Histologically, adenoma formation and/or areas of hyperplasia of ACTH-producing cells within the pars distalis and/or pars intermedia are the most frequently encountered findings. The remaining cases occur as the result of a functional adrenal tumor (AT). The clinical signs of PDH include polyuria and polydipsia (PU/PD), polyphagia, obesity, abdominal distention, hepatomegaly and alopecia. Behavioral abnormalities including decreased activity, increased sleeping and decreased interaction with owners are also observed. Common laboratory abnormalities include an elevated white blood cell count, increased serum alkaline phosphatase activity, and loss of urine-concentrating ability (Feldman, 1989).

The average age at the time of diagnosis is 14 years. There is no sex predilection but there are definite breed predilections. Dachshunds, poodles, beagles, boxers and Boston terriers are the most commonly affected breeds. Familial cases of PDH have also been reported.

The diagnosis of hyperadrenocorticism is confirmed by evaluation of the hypothalamic-pituitary-adrenal axis (HPA). The urine cortisol to creatinine ratio (UCCR) is often used as an initial screening test in dogs, as cortisol production and urinary excretion are elevated with hyperadrenocorticism. Unfortunately, a number of other non-adrenal disorders can also result in an elevated UCCR as the result of a generalized stress response. Therefore, an elevated UCCR is followed by additional endocrinologic testing. Dogs with hyperadrenocorticism demonstrate an exaggerated serum cortisol response to exogenously administered adrenocorticotropic hormone (ACTH) and/or a failure of serum cortisol concentrations to suppress in response to low dose dexamethasone administration (low-dose dexamethasone suppression test; LDDS test). The

—————
Address reprint requests to: William W. Ruehl, VMD, PhD, Deprenyl Animal Health, Inc., Overland Park, KS 66210, USA.

LDDS test is more sensitive and specific than the ACTH stimulation test in establishing a diagnosis of hyperadrenocorticism (Feldman, 1989). In addition, it also demonstrates dysregulation of the HPA axis through loss of the normal negative feedback mechanism that exists between circulating cortisol concentrations and ACTH. PDH is distinguished from functional adrenal neoplasia by evaluating serum cortisol response to a high dose of dexamethasone (high-dose dexamethasone suppression test; HDDS) or via endogenous plasma ACTH concentrations. Approximately 70% of dogs with PDH will demonstrate a fall in cortisol concentration of at least 50% during the course of the HDDS test, while dogs with AT show no suppression. Thirty percent of dogs with PDH will fail to suppress on the HDDS test for reasons to be discussed below. Plasma ACTH levels are normal or elevated in the face of hypercortisolemia in dogs with PDH and low to nondetectable in dogs with AT (Feldman, 1983).

Current medical treatment options for dogs with PDH include the adrenolytic agent 1,1-dichloro-2-(o-chlorophenyl)-2-(p-chlorophenyl) ethane (o,p'-DDD, mitotane, Lysodren, Bristol-Myers) and the adrenal enzyme inhibitor ketoconazole (Nizoral, Janssen) (Bruyette et al., 1988; Feldman et al., 1989b, 1990). Lysodren is the most commonly used medication. While efficacy rates of up to 80% can be expected with either medication, significant side-effects occur in 25–35% of patients during either induction or long-term maintenance therapy. These side-effects may necessitate withdrawal of the medication. Toxicities include gastrointestinal upset, hepatotoxicity and transient (ketoconazole) or permanent (o,p'-DDD) hypoadrenocorticism. During maintenance therapy, approximately 80% of patients treated with o,p'-DDD will experience a relapse within the first 12 months of therapy (Kintzer and Peterson, 1991). These treatments, while resulting in palliation of the clinical signs of PDH as the result of decreasing cortisol secretory capacity, do not address the underlying pathophysiology of PDH and in fact result in further dysregulation of the HPA axis.

PDH is a relentlessly progressive disease that, if left untreated, is eventually fatal. The prognosis for dogs with well controlled PDH is favorable, with an average life expectancy of 26 months.

Pathophysiology

Currently, two hypotheses exist with respect to the pathogenesis of pituitary adenomas. One theory ("hypothalamic" hypothesis) supports the role of altered hypothalamic control mechanisms (overstimulation, loss of inhibitory factors) leading to pituitary tumorigenesis and hormonal overproduction. In the second theory ("pituitary" hypothesis), a primary intrinsic defect in the pituitary cells leads to tumor formation (Faglia, 1994). These theories need not be mutually exclusive if we view the development of tumorigenesis as consisting of both an initiation (pituitary) and a promotion (hypothalamic) stage.

Several studies have indicated that most if not all pituitary tumors in man are monoclonal in origin, based on X chromosome inactivation analysis confirming that these tumors originate from a single cell. While few initiating mutations have been identified, initiating events may be quite common, as the incidence of occult pituitary adenomas ranges from 11 to 23% in autopsy studies. The incidence of clinically evident tumors in the general population is estimated at 0.020%, indicating that factors promoting tumor growth are present in only a minority of cases (Faglia, 1994). While X-linked studies have not been performed in dogs with PDH, we have recently reported a very high incidence of pituitary tumors (10%) in a colony of geriatric beagle dogs. Unlike the apparent situation in man, 51% of the animals with a pituitary tumor did show clinically evident disease (PDH) (Berry and Bruyette, 1994). This may indicate that while the initiation of tumor formation in man and dogs may be similar, factors leading to the promotion of tumorigenesis appear to be much more common in the dog. This may explain why the incidence of PDH is much higher in dogs than in man.

What are the factors that may lead to promotion of either tumor development or hyperplasia within the ACTH-producing cells of the dog pituitary, leading eventually to PDH? In normal dogs regulation of ACTH secretion differs depending on which lobe of the pituitary one is considering. In the pars distalis (PD), ACTH secretion is regulated by a positive-feedback mechanism mediated via corticotropin-releasing hormone (CRH), and a negative-feedback mechanism mediated via cortisol and dexamethasone (Kemppainen et al., 1992). Currently, about 70% of cases of PDH appear to arise from abnormalities within the PD (Peterson et al., 1982). ACTH release from the pars intermedia (PI) appears to be primarily regulated via a negative-feedback mechanism involving dopamine, although CRH-containing fibers have been observed in the canine PI (Stolp et al., 1987; Zerbe et al., 1993). Approximately 30% of cases of canine PDH are thought to arise from the PI.

Hypothalamic overstimulation of pituitary ACTH secretion could occur as a result of abnormalities in CRH production or secretion, and/or problems related to CRH receptor function or signal transduction. In the dog, little evidence exists to implicate CRH as a factor in the development of PDH. CRH concentrations within the paraventricular nucleus and median eminence (as well as a preparation composed of the entire hypothalamus) were normal or low in dogs with PDH when compared to normal dogs (Meijer et al., 1978; Peterson et al., 1989). In addition, CRH levels in the cerebrospinal fluid were also low in dogs with PDH when compared to normal dogs (Van Wijk et al., 1992). Other studies have also failed to show any appreciable differences between normal dogs and dogs with PDH with respect to other neurotransmitters such as norepinephrine, when specific hypothalamic nuclei were studied (Meijer et al., 1981; Peterson et al., 1989).

The role of dopamine in canine PDH

An increasing body of evidence points to hypothalamic dopamine deficiency playing a role in the pathogenesis of PDH in the dog. In normal dogs, while dopamine appears to primarily inhibit ACTH secretion from the PI, it also appears to affect ACTH release from the PD. Dogs treated with the dopamine antagonist domperidone had enhanced CRH-mediated ACTH release and this response was only partially blocked when the animals were pre-treated with dexamethasone (Zerbe et al., 1993). Several reports have indicated that acute or chronic administration of dopamine antagonists (domperidone, haloperidol, metoclopramide) increases secretion of proopiomelanocortin (POMC) peptides from the PD of dog, rat and man (Sharp et al., 1982; Kemppainen et al., 1989; Zerbe et al., 1993). Under the influence of dopaminergic blockade (and/or dopamine deficiency) an increase in ACTH responsiveness from the PD may be related to recruitment of previously non-secreting corticotrophs or increased responsiveness to CRH (Jia et al., 1991). Dopamine concentrations were also found to be significantly decreased in the median eminence of dogs with PDH when compared to control dogs and dogs treated with dexamethasone (Peterson et al., 1993).

Other lines of evidence also suggest a role for dopamine deficiency in PDH. The dopamine agonist bromocriptine has been shown to result in a decrease in ACTH and cortisol concentrations in some human patients with PDH (Lamberts et al., 1980). In studies in dogs, a few animals have also experienced both a hormonal and a clinical response to therapy with bromocriptine (Rijnberk et al., 1988). Unfortunately, side-effects in dogs have precluded its routine clinical use. Treatment of normal dogs with l-dopa following pre-treatment with carbidopa resulted in significant reductions in plasma ACTH and cortisol concentrations (Reid et al., 1986).

The neurotoxin 1-methyl-4-phenyl-1,2,3,6-tetrahydropyridine (MPTP) results in parkinsonian signs and symptoms in many species, including man and dogs. MPTP is converted to the active metabolite MPP^+ via oxidation through monoamine oxidase B (MAO-B). MPP^+ then results in damage to nigrostriatal dopaminergic neurons, resulting in signs identical to those observed with spontaneous Parkinson's disease.

ACTH and cortisol levels were found to increase 40 and 60%, respectively, in dogs treated with a single intravenous injection of MPTP (Mizobuchi, 1993).

We recently reported the efficacy of l-deprenyl therapy in seven dogs with PDH. The dogs were treated with 2.0 mg/kg of l-deprenyl orally once a day. The dose was chosen based on MAO-B inhibition data obtained in normal dogs. Five of the seven dogs showed amelioration or elimination of their clinical signs and normalization or a return towards normal in their LDDS test results. Two of the dogs have been on medication for more than 2 years (Bruyette et al., 1993).

Effects of l-deprenyl in geriatric dogs

We have studied the effects of chronic administration of l-deprenyl on the HPA axis in a group of geriatric (6–17 years) beagle dogs. Tests were performed on pairs matched by age, sex and weight. One member of each pair had been treated orally with 1 mg/kg of l-deprenyl every 24 h orally for 1 year; the other member received placebo. All dogs were judged to be healthy at the time of testing. All tests were performed between 0800 and 1000 hours, prior to administration of the daily l-deprenyl dose. ACTH stimulation tests were performed on 58 animals (29 pairs). Baseline and 2 h serum cortisol concentrations were obtained following the i.m. administration of 2.2 units/kg of ACTH (Acthar Gel, Organon). There was no statistical difference in the baseline (59 ± 29 nmol/l; 56 ± 29 nmol/l) or 2 h post-stimulation cortisol concentrations (400 ± 90 nmol/l; 456 ± 236 nmol/l) between the l-deprenyl and placebo group, respectively. These results indicated that chronic therapy with l-deprenyl does not result in glucocorticoid insufficiency (hypoadrenocorticism).

CRH stimulation tests were performed on 58 animals (29 pairs). All tests were started between 0800 and 1000 hours, prior to administration of the daily l-deprenyl dose. Plasma ACTH and cortisol concentrations were determined at times 0, 15, 30, 45, 60, 120 and 180 min following the IV administration of oCRH (1 μg/kg). Mean plasma cortisol concentrations were consistently lower in the l-deprenyl-treated group at every time point and were significantly lower at 120 and 180 min. No significant differences in plasma ACTH concentrations between the placebo and l-deprenyl groups were detected at any time point, although mean ACTH levels were lower in the l-deprenyl group at times 0, 15, 60, 120 and 180 min. The area under the curve (AUC) for plasma cortisol concentration was significantly lower for the l-deprenyl treated group when compared to placebo ($P < 0.05$). No difference in AUC for ACTH was detected. The results of the CRH stimulation tests complement earlier studies in which dopaminergic blockade resulted in enhanced CRH-mediated ACTH release in normal dogs.

In addition to the effects on the HPA axis, we have also examined the safety of chronic l-deprenyl treatment in the same group of geriatric beagle dogs. During the 2 years of treatment, no clinically relevant differences between the l-deprenyl and placebo groups were seen with respect to routine laboratory parameters (complete blood counts, serum biochemistry profiles, which included alkaline phosphatase, alanine aminotransferase, total protein, albumin, total and direct bilirubin, cholesterol, urea nitrogen, creatinine, phosphorus, glucose, calcium, iron and iron-binding capacity), liver function tests (bile acids), neurological and behavioral examinations, ophthalmic examinations and blood pressure measurements (i.e., no "cheese" effect was detected). We have also evaluated the safety of chronic l-deprenyl therapy in over 200 geriatric pet dogs on doses ranging from 0.5 to 2.0 mg/kg, with no significant adverse events thought to be drug-related.

Effects of l-deprenyl in dogs with PDH

We recently conducted a large-scale study evaluating the efficacy of l-deprenyl in the treatment of PDH in dogs. This was an open-label study in which 30 privately owned pet dogs with PDH were consecutively enrolled throughout a 9-month period. Dogs ranged in age from 6 to 16 years. None of the dogs had been treated with systemic corticosteroids during the 6 months prior to enrollment, nor had they been treated with topical, ophthalmic or otic corticosteroids within the prior 2 months. Hyperadrenocorticism was suspected, owing to the clinical manifestations of the disease, including polyuria, polydipsia, abdominal distention, increased appetite, dermatological changes (hyperpigmentation, thin skin, alopecia), decreased level of activity, panting, sleep-wake cycle disturbances, and characteristic laboratory findings including results of a CBC (lymphopenia, eosinopenia), serum biochemical profile (elevated alkaline phosphatase) and urinalysis (low urine specific gravity). A diagnosis of hyperadrenocorticism was established based on the results of an LDDS test, and the diagnosis of PDH was confirmed by an HDDS test and/or assay of plasma ACTH concentration. Each of the dogs was confirmed to be free of other concurrent endocrine or systemic diseases by the procedures noted above. The drug was administered orally at a dosage of 2 mg/kg every 24 h. Efficacy and toxicity were determined based on clinical, hormonal and biochemical responses to l-deprenyl therapy. Owners completed a daily observation form. The dogs were evaluated by the attending veterinarian approximately every 30 days. Monthly evaluations consisted of a review of the owner daily observation form, an owner questionnaire to evaluate the clinical status of the dogs, a physical examination focusing on manifestations of PDH, routine laboratory testing (CBC, serum chemistry profile) and an LDDS test. Response to therapy was based on remission or amelioration of clinical signs (as assessed by responses on the owner questionnaire, physical examination) and LDDS testing (normalization or a return towards normal in the post-LDDS cortisol concentration). Any animal which failed to respond to l-deprenyl therapy or developed life-threatening complications of Cushing's disease (e.g., diabetes mellitus, pulmonary thromboembolism) was removed from the study and alternative therapies were discussed with the owner. Each dog served as its own con-

trol and was studied for as long as 6 months. Eight dogs were unavailable for analysis at the 4–6 month time points because they had not yet progressed to that point in the trial. Other dogs were excluded from analysis at certain time points due to development of concurrent disease, treatment with corticosteroids, or inability of the owner to continue with the study procedures. Four dogs were dismissed after 3 months of therapy due to inadequate response. Animals responding to therapy at the end of the 6-month study were continued on medication on a compassionate-use basis.

Assessment of clinical and hormonal response to l-deprenyl therapy was determined by comparing the monthly post-LDDS cortisol concentrations and the scores obtained from the owner questionnaire and the veterinary physical examination form to those obtained at enrollment using a one-sided paired t-test and a Wilcoxon signed rank test, respectively. A P value of less than or equal to 0.05 was considered significant.

l-Deprenyl therapy resulted in a decrease in the post-LDDS cortisol concentration which was statistically significant ($P < 0.05$) at months 4, 5 and 6 (Fig. 1). In contrast, a separate group of 25 dogs with PDH who remained untreated during a 1-month period exhibited a mean 13% increase in LDDS test results ($0.05 < P < 0.1$, data not shown), perhaps reflecting the progressive nature of the untreated disease.

Owners of dogs treated with l-deprenyl reported statistically significant improvement in all clinical parameters (Table 1) and statistically significant improvement in the physical examination parameters was also observed with l-deprenyl therapy (see Table 1; significance at $P < 0.05$ is indicated by an asterisk at each time point). Adverse events thought to be related to the medication were uncommon.

Canine PDH as a neurodegenerative disorder

There are many similarities between canine PDH and human Parkinson's disease. Both are related to dopamine deficiency within specific areas of the brain, with attendant disruption of normal

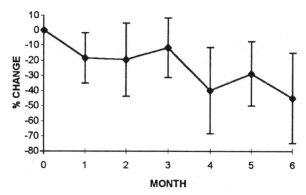

Fig. 1. Eight hour post-dexamethasone serum cortisol concentrations in dogs with PDH treated with 2.0 mg/kg/day of l-deprenyl expressed as the percent change from enrollment at each time point (mean ± SE). The number of dogs available at each time point was 29, 28, 27, 17, 16 and 9, respectively; see text for details. Mean cortisol levels were significantly lower ($P < 0.05$) than enrollment at months 4, 5 and 6.

function. In the case of Parkinson's disease, it is loss of dopaminergic cells within the nigrostriatal area resulting in decreased neurotransmission throughout the basal ganglia (Calne, 1993). Loss of normal neurotransmission results in the bradykinesias and dyskinesias associated with parkinsonism. In canine PDH, dopaminergic depletion occurs in the median eminence and paraventricular nuclei associated with an increased secretion of POMC peptides (including ACTH) from the PD and PI. The hypersecretion of ACTH results in overproduction of cortisol and leads to the clinical signs and laboratory abnormalities characteristic of PDH. The clinical signs of Parkinson's disease can be ameliorated by treatment with l-deprenyl. The use of l-deprenyl in dogs with PDH results in an amelioration of clinical signs and a return of post-dexamethasone (LDDS) cortisol levels towards or into the normal reference range.

The administration of the dopaminergic neurotoxin MPTP not only results in a parkinsonian state in man and dogs but also results in a state of functional hyperadrenocorticism (elevated ACTH and cortisol concentrations) in normal dogs. Additional studies are required in order to establish whether MPTP administration can result in clinical signs of hyperadrenocorticism in dogs and whether the effect of MPTP on the HPA axis can be prevented by pre-treatment with l-deprenyl, or remedied following MPTP administration.

It would appear that l-deprenyl has therapeutic benefit in both Parkinson's disease and canine PDH. Presumably, this benefit is due, at least in part, to the MAO-B inhibitory effects of l-deprenyl resulting in increased concentrations of dopamine in the synaptic cleft. MAO-B levels are known to increase in age, particularly in certain neurodegenerative disorders such as Parkinson's disease and Alzheimer's disease. However, a variety of additional effects of l-deprenyl may also play a role, including a reduction in free radical formation, increased clearance of free radicals, modulation of NMDA receptor, and a neuroprotective action independent of MAO-B inhibition (Tatton et al., 1991; Gerlach et al., 1993). l-Deprenyl has been used both as monotherapy in early cases of Parkinson's disease and in combination with l-dopa (Birkmayer et al., 1985; Parkinson Study Group, 1989, 1993; Elizan, 1993). Combination therapy results in symptomatic improvement and at the same time allows for lowering of the l-dopa dose, thereby reducing troubling side-effects. When used as early monotherapy, l-deprenyl may extend the life of the patient and delay the need for initiation of l-dopa therapy. As the disease progresses, monotherapy can be augmented by l-dopa or other appropriate medications. A similar strategy can be envisioned for the management of canine PDH. Once the clinical signs of the disease appear and the diagnosis is confirmed, therapy with l-deprenyl would begin. Additional medications (o,p'-DDD, ketoconazole) could be added, if necessary, should the patient show a poor initial response or if the beneficial effect of the l-deprenyl is lost following further loss of dopaminergic neurons. In some patients l-deprenyl therapy alone may be sufficient indefinitely.

Canine PDH is a geriatric-onset disorder, as are Parkinson's disease, Alzheimer's disease and

TABLE I

Clinical response of dogs with PDH treated with 2.0 mg/kg/day of l-deprenyl

Months of treatment: Parameter	1	2	3	4	5	6
Thickness of skin	I	I*	I*	I	I	I
Pyoderma	D	D	D	D*	D	D
Alopecia	D*	D*	D	D	D*	D
Regrowth of clipped hair	R**	R**	R**	R**	R**	R**
Abdominal conformation	Im**	Im**	Im**	Im**	Im**	Im**
Abdominal circumference	D**	D**	D*	D*	D	D
Ground clearance	I	I*	I	I*	I	I*
Water drinking	D**	D**	D*	D*	D**	D*
Signaling to go out	D*	D	D	D	D*	D*
Appetite	Im	Im	Im	Im	Im	Im*
Activity	I**	I**	I**	I**	I**	I**
Sleep	D**	D**	D**	D**	D**	D**
Panting	D**	D*	D*	D*	D	D
General health	Im**	Im**	Im**	Im**	Im**	Im**

The population exhibited improvement in each parameter at each time point; the improvement was statistically significant (*$P < 0.05$) or highly significant (**$P < 0.01$) at numerous time points.

I, increased towards normal since treatment began, with respect to thickness of skin, ground clearance (distance between ground and lowest point of abdomen) and activity.

D, decreased towards normal since treatment began, with respect to pyoderma, alopecia, abdominal circumference, amount of water drinking daily, signaling to go outdoors (to urinate, on a daily basis), sleep (during daytime) and panting.

R, indicates measurable hair regrowth; the hair was clipped at enrollment.

Im, improved compared to pre-treatment, with respect to abdominal conformation, appetite and change in general health.

other human neurodegenerative disorders. Recent studies have demonstrated that geriatric dogs have increased basal secretion of ACTH and cortisol, elevated urine cortisol to creatinine ratios (UCCR) and exaggerated responses to stress and exogenously administered CRH (Rothuizen et al., 1991). This hyperadrenal state is not necessarily accompanied by the clinical signs of PDH. This overactivation is mediated, at least in part, by alterations in glucocorticoid receptor concentrations. Two types of glucocorticoid receptor exist in the brain. Mineralocorticoid receptors (MR) are located in the hippocampus. Glucocorticoids, acting via MR receptors, exert a tonic inhibitory effect on the activity of the HPA axis and the threshold for HPA responsiveness. Glucocorticoid receptors (GR) exist in both the hippocampus and the hypothalamus. In the hippocampus, glucocorticoids acting through the GR appear to antagonize the MR-mediated effects. In the hypothalamus and pituitary, glucocorticoids act via the GR to terminate the HPA response to stress. In the dog, aging appears to be associated with a 60% reduction in MR concentration in the hippocampus. GR concentration appears unchanged. This alteration in the MR/GR ratio contributes to the chronic overstimulation of the HPA axis (Ruthuizen et al., 1991).

It is interesting to take this information together with what we know regarding pituitary tumorigen-

214

esis and dopamine deficiency. Canine PDH may be seen to result from one of the following scenarios. (1) Aging results in chronic overstimulation of the HPA axis. Hypothalamic dopamine deficiency also leads to ACTH overproduction and hyperplasia of corticotrophs and, in combination with the normal aging changes, results in further hyperplasia and ultimately progression to adenoma formation. This scenario would explain why not all cases of canine PDH are found to have a well identified pituitary adenoma. (2) Alternatively, some dogs may develop PDH as the result of prior initiation of pituitary adenoma formation which occurred as the result of spontaneous or acquired mutations. This initiation may in some cases be genetically based, perhaps accounting for the breed predisposition observed in PDH. Promotion then occurs via dopamine deficiency, glucocorticoid receptor imbalances, or both, which serve to transform a silent adenoma into a functional adenoma complete with all the signs typical of PDH.

Aging in the dog is also associated with a decline in cognitive function, which may result from amyloid accumulation in the brain in a pattern similar to that seen in Alzheimer's disease. Cognitive dysfunction in geriatric canine patients has also been successfully managed with l-deprenyl (see Chapter 22 in this volume). It is interesting to speculate on the relationship between aging, amyloid accumulation in the brain, cognitive dysfunction and hyperadrenocorticism. Hyperactivity of the HPA axis has been observed in human patients suffering from Alzheimer's disease (DeLeon et al., 1988) and basal cortisol levels have been shown to correlate with cognitive dysfunction in aged humans (Lupien et al., 1994). Behavioral changes have been well described in humans with PDH. A number of the clinical signs seen in dogs with cognitive dysfunction are also seen in dogs with PDH. It is possible that the mechanisms responsible for amyloid deposition resulting in cognitive dysfunction may also result in amyloid deposition which may affect the hippocampus (MR/GR receptors) or hypothalamus (dopamine), resulting in PDH. Furthermore, chronic exposure to steroids may predispose to Alzheimer's-like lesions leading to cognitive dysfunction. Additional clinical and morphological studies are required to investigate these mechanisms and to further assess the efficacy of l-deprenyl therapy with respect to progression of disease and amelioration of clinical signs.

References

Berry, M. and Bruyette, D.S. (1994) A retrospective study of pituitary and adrenal neoplasia and the incidence of hyperadrenocorticism in a geriatric beagle colony. *J. Vet. Int. Med.*, 8: 163 (abs).

Birkmayer, W., Knoll, J., Riederer, P., et al. (1985) Increased life expectancy resulting from addition of l-deprenyl to Madopar treatment in Parkinson's disease: a longterm study. *J. Neurol. Transm.*, 64: 113–127.

Bruyette, D.B. and Feldman, E.C (1988) Ketoconazole and its use in the management of canine Cushing's disease. *Compend. Cont. Educ. Pract. Vet.*, 10: 1379–1386.

Bruyette, D.S, Ruehl, W.W. and Smidberg, T.L. (1993) Therapy of canine pituitary dependent hyperadrenocorticism with l-deprenyl. *J. Vet. Int. Med.*, 7: 114 (abstr).

Calne, D.B. (1993) Treatment of Parkinson's disease. *N. Engl. J. Med.*, 329: 1021–1027.

DeLeon, M., McRae, T., Tsai, J., et al. (1988) Abnormal cortisol response in Alzheimer's disease linked to hippocampal atrophy. *Lancet*, 2: 391–392.

Elizan, T.S. (1993) (-)-Deprenyl combined with l-dopa in the treatment of Parkinson's disease. In: I. Szelenyi (Ed.), *Inhibitors of Monoamine Oxidase B. Pharmacology and Clinical Use in Neurodegenerative Disorders*, Birkhauser, Basel, pp. 277–289.

Faglia, G. (1994) Epidemiology and pathogenesis of pituitary adenomas. *Acta Endocrinol.*, 129: 1–5.

Feldman, E.C. (1983) Distinguishing dogs with functioning adrenocortical tumors from dogs with pituitary-dependent hyperadrenocorticism. *J. Am. Vet. Med. Assoc.*, 183: 195–200.

Feldman, E.C. (1989) Adrenal gland disease. In: S.J. Ettinger (Ed.), *Textbook of Veterinary Internal Medicine*, 3rd Edition, W.B. Saunders, Philadelphia, pp. 1721–1777.

Feldman, E.C., Bruyette, D.S. and Nelson, R.W (1989) Therapy for spontaneous canine hyperadrenocorticism. In: R.W. Kirk (Ed.), *Current Veterinary Therapy X*, W.B. Saunders, Philadelphia, pp. 1024–1031.

Feldman, E.C., Bruyette, D.S., Nelson, R.W., et al. (1990) Plasma cortisol response to ketoconazole administration in dogs with hyperadrenocorticism. *J. Am. Vet. Med. Assoc.*, 197: 71–78.

Gerlach, M., Riederer, P. and Youdim, M.H. (1993) The mode of action of MAO-B inhibitors. In: I. Szelenyi (Ed.), *Inhibitors of Monoamine Oxidase B. Pharmacology and Clinical Use in Neurodegenerative Disorders*, Birkhauser, Basel, pp. 183–201.

Jia, L.G., Canny, B.J., Orth, D.N., et al. (1991) Distinct classes of corticotropes mediate corticotropin-releasing hormone and arginine vasopressin-stimulated adrenocorticotropin release. *Endocrinology*, 128: 197–203.

Kemppainen, R.J., Zerbe, C.A. and Sartin, J.L. (1989) Regulation and secretion of proopiomelanocortin peptides from isolated perifused dog pituitary pars intermedia cells. *Endocrinology*, 124: 2208–2217.

Kemppainen, R.J., Clark, T.P., Sartin, J.L., et al. (1992) Regulation of the adrenocorticotropin secretion from cultured canine anterior pituitary cells. *Am. J. Vet. Res.*, 53: 2355–2358.

Kintzer, P.P. and Peterson, M.E. (1991) Mitotane (*o,p'*-DDD) treatment of 200 dogs with pituitary-dependent hyperadrenocorticism. *J. Vet. Int. Med.*, 5: 182–190.

Lamberts, S.W., Klijn, J.G., De Quijada, M., et al. (1980) The mechanism of the suppressive action of bromocriptine on adrenocorticotropin secretion in patients with Cushing's disease and Nelson's syndrome. *J. Clin. Endocrinol. Metab.*, 51: 307–311.

Lupien, S., LeCours, A., Lussier, I., et al. (1994) Basal cortisol levels and cognitive deficits in human aging. *J. Neurosci.*, 14: 2893–2903.

Meijer, J.C., Mulder, G.H., Rijnberk, A., et al. (1978) Hypothalamic corticotrophin-releasing factor activity in dogs with pituitary-dependent hyperadrenocorticism. *J. Endocrinol.*, 79: 209–213.

Meijer, J.C., Croughs, R.M., Rijnberk, A., et al. (1981) Hypothalamic catecholamine levels in dogs with spontaneous hyperadrenocorticism. *Neuroendocrinology*, 32: 197–201.

Mizobuchi, M., Hineno, T., Kakimoto, Y., et al. (1993) Increase of plasma adrenocorticotrophin and cortisol in 1-methyl-4-phenyl-1,2,3,6-tetrahydropyridine (MPTP)-treated dogs. *Brain Res.*, 612: 319–321.

Parkinson Study Group (1989) Effect of deprenyl on the progression of disability in early Parkinson's disease. *N. Engl. J. Med.*, 321: 1363–1371.

Parkinson Study Group (1993) Effects of tocopherol and de-prenyl on the progression of disability in early Parkinson's disease. *N. Engl. J. Med.*, 328: 176- 183.

Peterson, M.E., Krieger, D.T., Drucker, W.D., et al. (1982) Immunocytochemical study of the hypophysis in 25 dogs with pituitary-dependent hyperadrenocorticism. *Acta Endocrinol.*, 101: 15–24.

Peterson, M.E., Palkovits, M., Chiueh, C.C., et al. (1989) Biogenic amine and corticotropin-releasing factor concentrations in hypothalamic paraventricular nucleus and biogenic amine levels in the median eminence of normal dogs, chronic dexamethasone treated dogs, and dogs with naturally-occurring pituitary-dependent hyperadrenocorticism (canine Cushing's disease). *J. Neuroendocrinol.*, 1: 169–171.

Reid, I.A., Chou, L., Chang, D., et al. (1986) Role of dopamine in the inhibition of vasopressin secretion by l-dopa in carbidopa-treated dogs. *Hypertension*, 8: 890–896.

Rijnberk, A., Mol, J.A., Kwant, M.M., et al. (1988) Effects of bromocriptine on corticotrophin, melanotrophin, and corticosteroid secretion in dogs with pituitary-dependent hyperadrenocorticism. *J. Endocrinol.*, 118: 271–277.

Rothuizen, J., Reul, J.M., Rijnberk, A., et al. (1991) Aging and the hypothalamus-pituitary-adrenocortical axis, with special reference to the dog. *Acta Endocrinol. (Copenh.)*, 125: 73–76.

Sharp, B., Ross, R., Levin, E., et al. (1982) Dopamine regulates canine plasma β-endorphin-immunoreactivity levels. *Endocrinology*, 110: 1828–1830.

Stolp, R., Steinbusch, H.M., Rijnberk A., et al. (1987) Organization of ovine corticotropin-releasing factor immunoreactive neurons in the canine hypothalamo-pituitary system. *Neurosci. Lett.*, 74: 337–342.

Tatton, W.G. and Greenwood, C.E. (1991) Rescue of dying neurons: A new action for deprenyl in MPTP parkinsonism. *J. Neurosci. Res.*, 30: 666–672.

Van Wijk, P.A., Rijnberk, A., Croughs, R.M., et al. (1992) Corticotrophin-releasing hormone and adrenocorticotropic hormone concentrations in cerebrospinal fluid of dogs with pituitary-dependent hyperadrenocorticism. *Endocrinology*, 231: 2659–2662.

Zerbe, C.A., Clark, T.P., Sartin, J.L., et al. (1993) Domperidone treatment enhances corticotropin-releasing hormone stimulated ACTH release from the dog pituitary. *Neuroendocrinology*, 57: 282–288.

Peter M. Yu, Keith F. Tipton and Alan A. Boulton (Eds.)
Progress in Brain Research, Vol 106

CHAPTER 22

Canine cognitive dysfunction as a model for human age-related cognitive decline, dementia and Alzheimer's disease: clinical presentation, cognitive testing, pathology and response to 1-deprenyl therapy

W.W. Ruehl[1,2], D.S. Bruyette[3], A. DePaoli [1], C.W. Cotman[4], E. Head[5], N.W. Milgram[5] and B.J. Cummings[4]

[1]*Deprenyl Animal Health, Inc., Overland Park, KS,* [2]*Department of Pathology, School of Medicine, Stanford, CA,* [3]*College of Veterinary Medicine, Kansas State University, Manhattan, KS,* [4]*University of California, Irvine, CA, and* [5]*University of Toronto, Toronto, Canada*

Introduction

Severe cognitive dysfunction (CD) or dementia is an important clinical syndrome in people which increases in incidence from 1–3% in people 65–70 years old to as high as 47% in the very elderly (> 85 yr) (Jorm et al., 1987; Evans et al., 1989). It is one of the most common causes for institutionalization of elderly individuals, and more than half of nursing home residents are intellectually impaired. Practicing veterinarians have long been aware of geriatric behavioral changes in pet dogs, often described by the pet owners as "normal aging" or "senility". In this chapter we discuss these phenomena and explore the potential of the canine as a model of human age-related cognitive decline (ARCD), dementia and Alzheimer's dis-

Address correspondence to: W.W. Ruehl, Deprenyl Animal Health, Inc., Overland Park, KS 66210, USA.

ease (AD). We also discuss a number of studies which indicate that some people with dementia and dogs with cognitive dysfunction respond to therapy with the monoamine oxidase inhibitor 1-deprenyl (selegiline HCl).

The definition of dementia in human patients has continued to evolve, with a common theme that the syndrome involves a general mental deterioration or global decline of intellectual ability sufficient to produce functional disability (Hensel, 1990). The criteria by which the syndrome or disorder of dementia is diagnosed have been formally defined and recently updated in the Diagnostic and Statistical Manual of Mental Disorders, 4th Edition (DSM IV) (Frances et al., 1994). Briefly, these criteria require that to make the diagnosis of dementia in an individual who was previously fully functional the existence of multiple cognitive deficits must be present, which in aggregate "cause significant impairment in social or occupational functioning and represent a significant decline from a previous level of functioning". The multiple deficits include memory impairment plus one or more of the following: language disturbance; impaired ability to carry out motor tasks despite intact motor function; failure to recognize or identify familiar objects despite intact sensory function; decreased ability to perform complex tasks, planning, organizing or abstract thought.

One important challenge for clinicians and investigators is the differentiation of mild dementia from the cognitive dysfunction associated with aging in otherwise healthy individuals, which in people is termed age-related cognitive decline (ARCD) or age-associated memory impairment (AAMI) (Reisberg and Ferris, 1991; Frances et al., 1994). One of our goals is to develop such guidelines for elderly canines.

There are more than 60 diseases or conditions which cause dementia in people, the most common of which are Alzheimer's disease (AD) and vascular dementia (Katzman, 1986). Although there have been recent advances in diagnosing AD, especially with respect to imaging techniques, for most clinicians the diagnosis of AD remains one of exclusion (Frances et al., 1994).

Inadequacy of current animal models

Animal models have been utilized in the continually increasing research on aging and associated cognitive dysfunction at levels from the molecular to the epidemiological. However, progress has been hampered by the lack of a completely adequate animal model. The majority of studies on the effects of aging on learning and memory have been conducted in rodents and primates, each of which have specific advantages and limitations. Elderly rats exhibit cognitive dysfunction and offer the convenience and reduced expense of a short life span. However, rats do not appear to develop extensive age-related neuropathological changes or naturally occurring Alzheimer's-like pathology in their brains (Brizzee et al., 1978). It is not clear that results from rat studies can be extrapolated

to other species such as dogs, humans or other primates.

Primates also exhibit age-related cognitive dysfunction (Arnsten, 1993) and, in contrast to rodents, primates also exhibit age-related changes in neuropathology, including all human plaque subtypes (Wisniewski et al., 1973; Struble et al., 1985). In studies of elderly rhesus monkeys involving several tests of cognition two factors thought to influence cognitive performance were the number of abnormal neurons and the number of senile plaques, although the relation with cognitive impairment was less convincing for the latter (Walker et al., 1988; Cork, 1993). Primates are difficult to handle and expensive to maintain compared to canines or rodents. In addition, primate tissue can be as difficult to obtain as human tissue, and pathological changes are not usually observed until a monkey is at least 20 years of age.

We have been investigating the elderly canine as a model for aging in general, and more specifically as a model for ARCD, dementia and Alzheimer's disease. The dog is an excellent model in many respects.

Clinical similarities: observations of geriatric onset behavior problems

There have been no formal definitions or reports of cognitive dysfunction or ARCD in dogs and no consensus as to the occurrence or definition of canine dementia. Recognition of a problem has been based on a variety of clinical signs, such as reduced reaction to stimuli, partial loss of responsiveness to sensory input, incontinence, irritability, slowness in obeying commands, and problems with orientation and learned behaviors (Mosier, 1989; Hunthausen, 1994). One form of canine cognitive problem resembling human dementia has been characterized as retirement from participation with kennel mates, confusion upon presentation of simple routine tasks, deficits in conditioned learning, inappropriate responses, decreased affection, reduced vitality, loss of bearing, inability to localize sound, difficulty locating food trays, loss of fastidious eating habits, and decreased exploratory behavior (Koppang, 1973). Taken together these observations suggest that elderly dogs may exhibit multiple behavioral or cognitive problems indicative of cognitive dysfunction, and which in some canine patients is sufficiently severe to disrupt the dog's function. These dogs fulfill a canine equivalent of the DSM IV definition for dementia.

Pathological similarities

There are also similarities between human and canine with respect to age-related neuropathology. The pathology of human AD has been extensively studied, especially with respect to β-amyloid accumulation, neurofibrillary tangles, formation of plaques and other changes (Cotman et al., 1993). Canines experience Alzheimer's-like neuropathology within the same brain regions as humans (Cummings et al., 1993a), including age-related cerebral vascular changes (Uchida et al., 1992), thickening of the meninges and dilatation of the ventricles, and age-related reactive gliosis (Shimada et al., 1992). Other investigators have also documented Alzheimer-like pathology in aged canine brains (Giaccone et al., 1990; Uchida et al., 1993). At least some of the pathology present within aged canine brains may be genetically linked, since in a study of laboratory beagles Russell et al. (1992) found congruence of pathology within 15 of 16 litters. The plaques observed in all but one animal were of the diffuse subtype. Recently, some of us (Cummings et al., 1993a) studied the pathology of elderly dog brains, focusing on plaque morphology and patterns of amyloid deposition, and proposed that the dog provides a model of early plaque formation in AD. Typical lesions of Alzheimer's-like pathology in human and canine brain are compared in Fig. 1. One study of brains obtained from elderly pet dogs with urinary incontinence, disorientation and various other geriatric-onset behavioral problems demonstrated meningeal fibrosis, lipofuscinosis, generalized gliosis, and ubiquitin-containing granules in white matter (Ferrer et al., 1993).

Pathophysiological and pharmacological considerations

The enzyme monoamine oxidase B (MAOB) catalyzes dopamine breakdown, with the secondary production of free radicals. In a variety of species brain MAOB activity is higher in the aged than in the young, and MAOB activities can be very high in patients with neurodegenerative disorders such as Parkinsonism and Alzheimer's disease (Tariot et al., 1993). In addition to increased MAOB activity, there is dopamine depletion and loss of dopaminergic neurons in the nigrostriatal region of the parkinsonian brain. A variety of neurotransmitter abnormalities, including dopaminergic imbalances, have been described in Alzheimer's patients. Dopaminergic depletion in the prefrontal cortex has been correlated to cognitive dysfunction in monkeys (Arnsten, 1993).

Cognitive deficits have recently been demonstrated in people with imbalance of the hypothalamic pituitary adrenal (HPA) axis (Lupien et al., 1994). Dysregulation of the HPA axis in both humans and dogs is associated with hypothalamic dopamine depletion (see Chapter 21 of this volume). Dogs with pituitary-dependent hyperadrenocorticism (PDH, Cushing's disease) also exhibit behavioral or cognitive signs, such as lethargy and decreased interaction with their owners. Further work is needed to determine the extent to which cortisol excess and dopamine depletion contribute to the cognitive dysfunction of these patients.

Cognitive tests of laboratory dogs

Since Pavlov's pioneering studies on classical conditioning at the beginning of this century, canines have been studied in a variety of cognitive tests, including tone discrimination (Chorazyna, 1967), intermediate size problem (Ebel and Werbott, 1967), same/different problem (Pierzykowska and

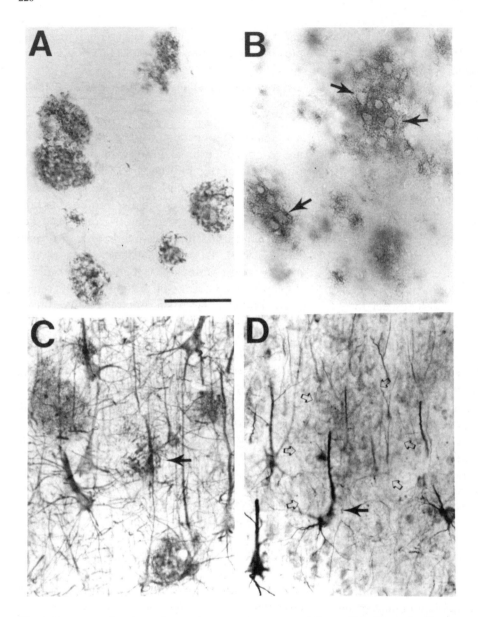

Fig. 1. Representative photomicrographs comparing neuropathology within the aged canine versus the human Alzheimer's disease (AD) brain. (A) In the AD brain, β-amyloid immunocytochemistry following formic acid pretreatment reveals numerous senile plaques typically measuring less than 50 μm in diameter. (B) In the aged canine brain, β-amyloid immunoreactivity demonstrates extensive amyloid deposition surrounding neurons (arrows). Plaques within the canine brain are often greater than 100 μm in diameter. In C and D, β-amyloid immunocytochemistry has been followed by a different colored label for phosphorylated neurofilaments (SMI-311). (C) In a very early case of AD, many neurons can be detected within deposits of amyloid, although their morphology is sometimes abnormal (arrow). (D) In the aged canine brain, while neurons are often found within clouds of β-amyloid, some appear abnormal (arrow). A diffuse β-amyloid-positive plaque is outlined with open arrows. All sections were processed in parallel.

Soltysik, 1975), odor discrimination (Lubow et al., 1976), time discrimination (Rosenkilde and Lawicka, 1977), and visual discrimination (Frank et al., 1989).

In spite of the considerable research with canine subjects and cognition, an extensive search of the literature failed to identify any experimental studies of aging and cognitive function in dogs other than those conducted by members of our group. An age-related decline of function in dogs has been established in a variety of cognitive tests, including object discrimination, object discrimination reversal, object recognition memory (Milgram et al., 1993, 1994) and spatial memory (Head et al., 1993; Cummings et al., 1993b). The findings confirmed that dogs, like other species, suffer age-dependent cognitive deterioration. The extent of the deterioration is also a function of task and prior experience, and at least part of the deterioration is a result of increased behavioral rigidity (Milgram et al., 1994). Additional work has established that cognitive dysfunction on some tasks, but not others, correlates with increasing age, and that such dysfunction correlates even more strongly with the amount of β-amyloid present in the brain (Cummings et al., 1993a and unpublished observations). A greater variance in individual cognitive performance occurs with increasing age, as previously reported for aged nonhuman primates and humans.

Effects of l-deprenyl

l-Deprenyl, by inhibiting MAOB and thus increasing dopamine levels, should theoretically help restore dopaminergic balance in the prefrontal cortex and other brain regions of an individual with cognitive dysfunction and thus reverse or slow the progression of clinical signs. Furthermore, l-deprenyl is thought to decrease the production of free radicals, enhance clearance of free radicals and to exert protective and "rescue" effects on damaged neurons (Tatton and Greenwood, 1991). Rats exhibit age-related cognitive dysfunction,

which can be reversed at least in part by administration of l-deprenyl (Brandeis et al., 1991). A recent review of 12 clinical trials of l-deprenyl in demented people noted that overall the results were encouraging (Tariot et al., 1993); further study in both AD patients and animals therefore seems warranted.

We explored the effects of l-deprenyl on cognitive performance of laboratory-housed canines as a model system for treatment of cognitive dysfunction. Administration of l-deprenyl was found to have a beneficial effect on spatial short-term memory in aged dogs but not in young dogs (Head et al., 1994). In another study, l-deprenyl therapy improved the performance of dogs which exhibited cognitive dysfunction as documented by poor baseline performance in object discrimination reversal testing, but not those dogs that were relatively unimpaired with respect to performance on this test (Milgram et al., 1993).

Prospective clinical study

There is little information available on behavioral problems in elderly pet dogs (Chapman and Voith, 1992; Hunthausen, 1994), virtually none of which is presented in the context of neuropathology or cognitive dysfunction. We have conducted a clinical trial in pet dogs, therefore, in which, the goals were to: (a) identify clinical signs and behavioral problems of cognitive dysfunction, (b) evaluate the safety and efficacy of l-deprenyl for treatment of such canine problems, and (c) evaluate the utility of elderly pet dogs with cognitive dysfunction as a model system of age-related cognitive decline, dementia, Alzheimer's disease and other neurodegenerative disorders.

Dogs nominated by their owners based on dysfunction in one or more of the parameters listed in Table 1 were studied. To determine eligibility for enrollment, each dog was evaluated by signalment, anamnesis, physical and neurological examinations, complete blood count and serum biochemistry profile. Dogs were excluded if they

TABLE 1

Incidence, severity and response to 0.5 mg/kg once daily l-deprenyl treatment of behavioral and cognitive problems in 69 elderly dogs, as reported by their owners

Problem	Percent of dogs affected at enrollment				Response to 1-deprenyl
	Mild	Moderate	Severe	Total	
Housetraining	18	22	27	67	**
Interest in food	26	12	4	42	**
Activity, or attention to environment, including people or other animals	26	26	25	77	**
Awareness or/orientation to surroundings	17	28	23	68	**
Ability to recognize familiar places, people or other animals	25	22	16	63	**
Ability to recognize/respond to commands or when called by name	17	19	44	80	**
Hearing	7	12	68	87	**
Climbing up or down stairs	22	31	25	78	**
Tolerance to being alone	19	16	9	44	
Development of compulsive behavior	25	32	12	69	*
Circling	13	10	6	29	**
Tremor or shaking	16	28	13	57	**
Wakes owner more at night &/or sleeps more in daytime	16	19	32	67	*
Inappropriate, persistent vocalization	19	7	16	42	
Increased stiffness or weakness	16	29	30	75	**

$*P < 0.05$; $**P < 0.01$.

exhibited evidence of a concurrent, non-neurological systemic or debilitating condition. The owner of each enrolled subject completed a written questionnaire in which s/he recorded the pet's status with respect to each parameter in Table 1 as: excellent or normal; good or mildly affected; fair or moderately affected; poor or severely affected. The owner also noted which of the dog's problems caused the owner greatest concern. Sixty-nine dogs fulfilled the enrollment criteria and were administered 0.5 mg/kg l-deprenyl tablets once daily in open-label fashion by their owners. Subjects were re-evaluated monthly during the 3-month study in a fashion identical to that performed at enrollment, and the owner completed a questionnaire pertaining to the pet's response to therapy. Performance on each parameter during the prior month was scored by the owner numerically, as well as by the code "Improved", "Same" or "Worse".

Primary measures of the population's response to therapy were based on comparison of the parameters listed in Table 1 at enrollment (pre treatment) and at each of the 3 monthly re-examinations. Individual response to therapy was also evaluated, by tabulating an over-all cumulative response score for each patient at each re-examination.

In this study population the occurrence of behavioral or cognitive problems was rare in dogs less than 9 years old, despite the fact that enrollment was not restricted by a minimum age. Average age was 13.5 yr (range 7–19 yr), and there was an increase in the number of dogs per year between the ages of 9 and 15. Few dogs were enrolled above this age. Mean body weight was 13.8 kg (range 3.6–36.3 kg).

All of the dogs exhibited multiple problems, with 46% exhibiting 11 or more problems. The most commonly reported problems were decrements of hearing, activity, attention and ability to navigate stairs. Many of the problems reported in these dogs were similar to those noted in people with cognitive dysfunction and, as in people, the average number and severity of abnormalities per subject tended to increase with increasing age.

The population responded to l-deprenyl therapy with improvement in every parameter by month 1, with the relation being significant ($P < 0.05$) in 13 of 15 parameters (Table 1). Benefits were generally maintained in the population at months 2 and 3. The proportions of individuals who improved with respect to global function were 77% at 1 month, 76% at 2 months and 78% at 3 months. There was deterioration (progression of clinical signs or behavioral problems) despite l-deprenyl therapy noted in 5% of dogs at 1 month, 16% at 2 months and 15% at 3 months. There were no reported serious adverse events thought to be related to drug therapy, and no reported adverse drug interactions.

Discussion

Our results indicate that elderly pet dogs exhibit multiple behavioral or cognitive problems indicative of cognitive dysfunction, which in some canine patients are sufficiently severe to disrupt the dog's function as an adequate pet (i.e., fulfilling a canine equivalent of the DSM IV definition for dementia). In some affected pet dogs the change in behavior was found to be due to the presence of systemic, non-neurological disease; however, in numerous cases no such general medical condition was identified, suggesting that the behavioral or cognitive dysfunction may be due to brain pathology. Whether clinical signs of cognitive dysfunction in pet dogs is causally related to Alzheimer's-like pathology requires further study; however, our studies in laboratory-housed canines

(see above) indicate that some cognitive deficits, but not others, are correlated with age and with amyloid accumulation. Screening tests might be developed to use in pet dogs to predict amyloid accumulation and/or response to therapy. If so, this information might be extrapolated to cognitively impaired people. The dogs in this study responded quite favorably to once-daily therapy with 0.5 mg/kg l-deprenyl. Similarly, human patients with dementia of the Alzheimer's type have responded to l-deprenyl therapy (Tariot et al., 1993).

Dogs have moderate life spans of approx. 12–20 yr depending on the breed and are considered by veterinarians to be elderly at approx. 7.5–12 yr depending on size (Goldston, 1989). Importantly, pet dogs live with people and share common environmental (and often nutritional) risk factors for aging and age-associated disorders. In contrast to primates, dogs are easier to obtain and handle and can be specially bred for research, thus obtaining a genetically homogeneous population. Their nutrition and husbandry are consistent and controlled. Furthermore, dogs are highly motivated to perform consistently on tests of cognitive function using food reward, and deprivation paradigms are not prerequisites.

Comparison of results of cognitive testing in laboratory-housed dogs with clinical studies of cognitive dysfunction in pet dogs provides a unique and valuable opportunity to develop improved methods of field detection of clinically significant cognitive dysfunction in dogs, facilitating epidemiological and clinical studies in pet dogs and perhaps in people. Toward this end, we have augmented laboratory cognitive testing of research dogs with clinical studies in elderly pet dogs.

Conclusions

Information from the studies noted above and other sources establishes that elderly dogs with cognitive dysfunction provide an excellent spontaneously occurring animal model of dementia, Alzheimer's disease, and other neurodegenerative disorders. Some similarities include: (a) increasing incidence with increasing age; (b) occurrence of clinically relevant behavioral and cognitive problems; (c) deterioration of performance on formal cognitive tests with increasing age; (d) increasing Alzheimer's like pathology with increasing age; and (e) response to l-deprenyl therapy. The population of pet dogs who exhibit behavioral or cognitive dysfunction may also offer an additional clinical trial system for the evaluation of cognitive enhancer drugs.

References

Arnsten, A.F.T. (1993) Catecholamine mechanisms in age-related cognitive decline. *Neurobiol. Aging*, 14: 639–641.

Brandeis, R., Dapir, M., Kapon, Y., Borelli, G., Cadel, S. and Valsecchi, B. (1991) Improvement of cognitive function by MAO-B inhibitor l-deprenyl in aged rats. *Pharm. Biochem. Behav.*, 39: 297–304.

Brizzee, K.R., Ordy, J.M., Hofer, H. and Kaack, B. (1978) Animal models for the study of brain disease and aging changes in the brain. In: *Alzheimer's Disease: Senile Dementia and Related Disorders*, Raven Press, New York, pp. 515–554.

Chapman, B.L. and Voith, V.L. (1990) Behavioral problems in old dogs. *J. Am. Vet. Med. Assoc.*, 196: 944–946.

Chorazyna, H. (1967) Differentiation between same tone compound vs. low-high tone compound in dogs. *Acta. Biol. Exp.*, 27: 199–206.

Cork, L.C. (1993) Plaques in prefrontal cortex of aged, behaviorally tested rhesus monkeys: incidence, distribution and relationship to task performance. *Neurobiol. Aging*, 14: 675–676.

Cotman, C.W., Cummings, B.J. and Pike, C.J. (1993) Molecular cascades in adaptive versus pathologic plasticity. In: A. Gloria (Ed.), *Neuroregeneration*, Raven Press, New York, pp. 217–240.

Cummings, B.J., Su, J.H., Cotman, C.W., White, R. and Russell, M.J. (1993a) β-Amyloid accumulation in aged canine brain: a model of early plaque formation in Alzheimer's disease. *Neurobiol. Aging*, 14: 547–560.

Cummings, B.J., Honsberger, P.E., Afagh, A.J., Head, E., Ivy, G., Milgram, N.W. and Cotman, C.W. (1993b) Cognitive function and Alzheimer's like pathology in the aged canine: II. neuropathology (abstract). *Soc. Neurosci.*, 19: 1046.

Ebel, H. and Werboff, J. (1967) Transposition in dogs: successive reversals of the intermediate size problem. *Percept. Motor Skills*, 24: 507–511.

Evans, D.A., Funkenstein, H.H., Albert, M.S. (1989) Prevalence of Alzheimer's disease in a community population of older persons. *J. Am. Med. Assoc.*, 262: 2551–2556.

Ferrer, I., Pumarola, M., Rivera, R., Zujar, M.J., Cruz-Sanchez, F., and Vidal, A. (1993) Primary central white matter degeneration in old dogs. *Acta Neuropathol.*, 86: 172–175.

Frances, A., Pincus, H.A. and First, M.B. (1994) *Diagnostic and Statistical Manual of Mental Disorders*, 4th. Edn., American Psychiatric Association, Washington, DC, pp. 133–143.

Frank, H., Frank, M., Hasselbach, L. and Littleton, D. (1989) Motivation and insight in wolf (*Canis lupus*) and Alaskan malamute (*Canis familiaris*): visual discrimination learning. *Bull. Psychonomic Soc.*, 27: 455–458.

Giaccone, G., Verga, L., Finazzi, M. Pollo, B., Tagliavini, F., Frangione, B. and Bugiani, O. (1990) Cerebral preamyloid deposits and congophilic angiopathy in aged dogs. *Neurosci. Lett.*, 114: 178–183.

Goldston, R.T. (1989) Preface. In: R.T. Goldston (Ed.), *Geriatrics and Gerontology, The Veterinary Clinics of North America, Small Animal Practice*, Vol. 19, No. 1, Saunders, Philadelphia, pp. ix–x.

Head, E., Ivy, G., Cummings, B.J., Cotman, C.W. and Milgram, N.W. (1993) Cognitive function and Alzheimer's like pathology in the aged canine: I. spatial learning and memory (abstract). *Soc. Neurosci.*, 19: 1046.

Head, E., Hartley, J., Mehta, R., Kameka, A.M., Ivy, G., Ruehl, W.W., and Milgram, N.W. (1994) The effects of l-deprenyl on spatial short term memory in the dog (abstract). *Soc. Neurosci.*, 20: 152.

Hensel, W.R. (1990) *Stedman's Medical Dictionary*, 25th Edn., Williams & Wilkins, Baltimore, p. 410.

Hunthausen, W. (1994) Identifying and treating behavior problems in geriatric dogs. *Vet. Med., Suppl.*, 688–700.

Jorm, A.F., Kosten, A.E. and Henderson, A.S. (1987) The prevalence of dementia: a quantitative integration of the literature. *Acta Psychiatr. Scand.*, 76: 465–479.

Koppang, N. (1973) Canine ceroid lipofuscinsosis — a model for human neuronal ceroid lipofuscinosis and aging. *Mech. Ageing Dev.*, 2: 421–445.

Katzman, R. (1986) Alzheimer's disease. *N. Engl. J. Med.*, 314: 964–973.

Lubow, R.E., Kahn, M. and Frommer, R. (1976) Information processing of olfactory stimuli by the dog: II. stimulus control and sampling strategies in simultaneous discrimination learning. *Bull. Psychonomic Soc.*, 8: 323–326.

Lupien, S., LeCours, A., Lussier, I., et al. (1994) Basal cortisol levels and cognitive deficits in human aging. *J. Neurosci.*, 14: 2893–2903.

Milgram, N.W., Ivy, G.O., Head, E., Murphy, P., Wu, P.H., Ruehl, W.W., Yu, P.H., Durden, D.A., Davis, B.A., Paterson, I.A. and Boulton, A.A. (1993) The effect of l-deprenyl on behavior, cognitive function and biogenic amines in the dog. *Neurochem. Res.*, 18: 1211–1219.

Milgram, N.W., Head, E., Weiner, E. and Thomas, E. (1994) Cognitive functions and aging in the dog: acquisition of nonspatial visual tasks. *Behav. Neurosci.*, 108: 57–68.

Mosier, J.E. (1989) Effects of aging on body systems of the

dog. In: R.T. Goldston (Ed.), *Geriatrics and Gerontology, The Veterinary Clinics of North America, Small Animal Practice*, Vol. 19, No. 1, Saunders, Philadelphia, pp. 1–12.

Pierzykowska, B. and Soltysik, S. (1975) Transfer of the "same–different" differentiation task in dogs. *Acta Neurobiol. Exp.*, 35: 33–50.

Reisberg, B. and Ferris, H. (1991) In: T. Crook and S. Gershon (Eds.), *Diagnosis and Treatment of Adult Onset Cognitive Disorders (AOCD)*, Psymark Communications, Old Saybrook, CN, pp. 37–48.

Rosenkilde, C. and Lawicka, W. (1977) Effects of medial and dorsal prefrontal ablations on a go left—go right time discrimination task in dogs. *Acta Neurobiol. Exp.*, 37: 209–221.

Russell, M.J., White, R., Patel, E., Markesbery, W.R., Watson, C.R., and Geddes, J.W. (1992) Familial influence on plaque formation in the beagle brain. *Neuroreport*, 3: 1093–1096.

Shimada, A., Kuwamura, M., Awakura, T., Umemura, T., Takada, K., Ohama, E. and Itakura, C. (1992) Topographic relationship between senile plaques and cerebrovascular amyloidosis in the brain of aged dogs. *J. Vet. Med. Sci.*, 54: 137–144.

Struble, R.G., Price, D.J., Cork, L.C. and Price, D.L. (1985) Senile plaques in cortex of aged normal monkeys. *Brain Res.*, 361: 267–275.

Tatton, W.G. and Greenwood, C.E. (1991) Rescue of dying neurons: a new action for deprenyl in MPTP parkinsonism. *J. Neurosci. Res.*, 30: 666–672.

Tariot, P.N., Schneider, L.S., Patel, S.V. and Goldstein, B. (1993) Alzheimer's disease and l-deprenyl: rationales and findings. In: I. Szelenyi (Ed.), *Inhibitors of Monoamine Oxidase B*, Birkhauser Verlag, Basel, pp. 301–317.

Uchida, K., Nakayama, H., Tateyama, S. and Goto, N. (1992) Immunohistochemical analysis of constituents of senile plaques and cerebro-vascular amyloid in aged dogs. *J. Vet. Med. Sci.*, 54: 1023–1029.

Uchida, K., Okuda, R., Yamaguchi, R., Tateyama, S., Nakayama, H. and Goto, N. (1993) Double labeling immunohistochemical studies on canine senile plaques and cerebral amyloid angiopathy. *J. Vet. Med. Sci.*, 55: 637–642.

Walker, L.C., Kitt, C.A., Struble, R.G., Wagster, M.V., Price, D.L., and Cork, L.C. (1988) The neuronal basis of memory decline in aged monkeys. *Neurobiol. Aging*, 9: 657–666.

Wisniewski, H.M., Ghetti, B. and Terry, R.D. (1973) Neuritic (senile) plaques and filamentous changes in aged rhesus monkeys. *J. Neuropathol. Exp. Neurol.*, 32: 566–584.

Peter M. Yu, Keith F. Tipton and Alan A. Boulton (Eds.)
Progress in Brain Research, Vol 106
© 1995 Elsevier Science BV. All rights reserved.

CHAPTER 23

Dopamine-derived 6,7-dihydroxy-1,2,3, 4-tetrahydroisoquinolines; oxidation and neurotoxicity

M. Naoi[1], W. Maruyama[2] and P. Dostert[3]

[1]*Department of Biosciences, Nagoya Institute of Technology, Gokiso-cho, Showa-ku, Nagoya 466, Japan,* [2]*Department of Neurology, Nagoya University School of Medicine, Tsurumai-cho 65, Showa-ku, Nagoya 466, Japan, and* [3]*Pharmacia-Farmilitalia Carlo Erba, Research and Development, Milan, Italy*

Introduction

A dopamine-derived alkaloid, 1-methyl-6,7-dihydroxy-1,2,3,4-tetrahydroisoquinoline (salsolinol), was found for the first time in urine of patients treated with L-DOPA (Sandler et al., 1973), and then in human brain (Sjoequist et al., 1982a,b; Ung-Chhun et al., 1985). Salsolinol has an asymmetric center at C-1 position and the non-enzymatic Pictet-Spengler reaction of dopamine with acetaldehyde yields the racemic form of salsolinol. However, in human urine the *R*-enantiomer of salsolinol is predominant, whereas the *S*-enantiomer is detected predominantly in foods, such as Port wine (Strolin Benedetti et al., 1989). As an alternative biosynthesis pathway, dopamine can condense with pyruvic acid, followed by enzymatic decarboxylation (Collins and Cheng, 1988) and reduction to yield the *R*-enantiomer of salsolinol (Brossi, 1982; Dostert et al., 1991). The enzyme involved in the asymmetric biosynthesis of salsolinol, if any, has not been identified. The origin of this alkaloid and its occurrence in the brain suggest that catechol isoquinolines may be involved in some neurological and psychiatric disorders (Dostert et al., 1988). To examine the effects of salsolinol on the brain functions, in vivo experiments should be the most adequate methods, but

the results reported so far were contradictory (Melchior et al., 1982). This may be due to the fact that salsolinol does not cross the blood–brain barrier into the brain (Origitano et al., 1981), or to its very short half-life in the brain (Melchior et al., 1980).

The discovery of the potent dopaminergic neurotoxin 1-methyl-4-phenyl-1,2,3,6-tetrahydropyridine (MPTP) has suggested that endogenous or xenobiotic toxins may induce Parkinson's disease in humans. The essential characteristics of MPTP-like dopaminergic neurotoxins in animal models have been established (for reviews see Singer et al., 1987; Tipton and Singer, 1993). MPTP is oxidized by type B monoamine oxidase [monoamine:oxygen oxidoreductase (deaminating), EC 1.4.3.4, MAO] into 1-methyl-4-phenyl-pyridinium ion (MPP^+). The selective uptake of MPP^+ by dopamine neurons is thought to cause the death of dopamine neurons in the substantia nigra. The inhibition of oxidative phosphorylation at the site of Complex I in the mitochondrial respiratory chain has been proposed as the possible mechanism of MPTP cytotoxicity. Increases in the selectivity and potency of MPP^+ cytotoxicity by oxidation from MPTP suggest that endogenous or xenobiotic compounds may also enhance the neurotoxicity to specific neurons by the oxidation and other reactions in the brain. The contribution of the metabolic bioactivation process to the occurrence of neurotoxicity has been shown for isoquinolines with and without catechol structure (Naoi et al., 1993a, 1994b) and β-carbolines (Matsubara et al., 1993).

Considering these results, naturally occurring compounds have been intensively examined for their potential neurotoxicity to dopaminergic neurons. This paper presents some data on the metabolism of salsolinol in the brain and discusses the possible involvement of salsolinol metabolism in the induced cytotoxicity. The catechol isoquinolines administered into the rat brain induced behavioral changes, which were very similar to those observed in patients with Parkinson's disease. Biochemical and pathological findings suggest that this approach might be used as an animal model of Parkinson's disease. The oxidation of the catechol isoquinolines was found to be a prerequisite for the selective and potent neurotoxicity to dopamine neurons to occur. The oxidation of $N(2)$-methylated catechol isoquinolines was found to be enzymatic and non-enzymatic. The properties of the (R)NMSal oxidase are partially characterized. The enzyme activity was found to be insensitive to clorgyline and deprenyl, typical inhibitors of type A and B MAO, respectively.

N-Methylation of salsolinol in the brain

As shown in Fig. 1, N-methyl salsolinol is structurally similar to MPTP, and 1,2-dimethyl-6,7-dihydroxyisoquinolinium ion (DiMeDHIQ$^+$), formed from salsolinol by two reactions, N-methylation and oxidation, to MPP$^+$. Salsolinol was perfused in several brain regions of the rat by in vivo microdialysis (Maruyama et al., 1992, 1993). The dialysate was analyzed by high-performance liquid chromatography (HPLC) connected to a multi-electrochemical detection (ECD) system (ESA, Bedford, MA) (Naoi et al., 1993b). As shown in Fig. 2, N-methylsalsolinol (NMSal) was formed from (R)-salsolinol. Both the (R)- and (S)-enantiomers of salsolinol were N-methylated

with almost the same velocity. In the substantia nigra, the enzymatic activity was about 3-fold that in the other brain regions examined: the striatum, hypothalamus and hippocampus. The N-methyltransferase of salsolinol is localized in the cytosol fraction of the human brain, and may be identical to that reported previously for the N-methylation of 1,2,3,4-tetrahydroisoquinoline (Naoi et al., 1989). The identity of NMSal in the microdialysate was further confirmed by gas chromatography–mass spectrometry (GC-MS) (Niwa et al., 1992). In the human brain, the occurrence of 2-methyl-6,7-dihydroxy-1,2,3,4-tetrahydroisoquinoline and NMSal was also established by GC-MS (Niwa et al., 1991).

Oxidation of N-methylsalsolinol

Enzymatic oxidation

The enzymatic oxidation of (R)NMSal was examined by use of a sample prepared from human brain mitochondria by solubilization with Triton X-100. The mitochondrial fraction was prepared from human brain gray matter by the method of Gray and Whittakar (1962); the mitochondria were washed with 10 mM Tris-HCl buffer, pH 7.4, containing 1 mM EDTA, then suspended in 1% n-octyl β-D-glucoside solution of 10 mM Tris-HCl buffer, pH 7.4, stirred for 30 min in an ice bath, and centrifuged at 150 000 × g for 30 min. The mitochondria were re-suspended in 10 mM Tris buffer, pH 7.4 containing 1% Triton X-100, stirred for 60 min and centrifuged. The supernatant was passed through a column of SM beads and a Sephadex G-25 column, successively. This enzyme sample was endowed with type A and B MAO activities. The values of the Michaelis constant, K_m, and of the maximal velocity, V_{max}, were as follows; for type A 166 ± 35.9 μM and 2.43 ± 0.49 nmol/min per mg protein, and for type B 46.2 ± 2.5 μM and 6.17 ± 0.27 nmol/min per mg protein, respectively, when kynuramine was used as a substrate.

The enzyme sample was incubated with 1 mM (R)NMSal in 100 μl of 25 mM potassium phosphate buffer, or other buffers, at pH 7.4, contain-

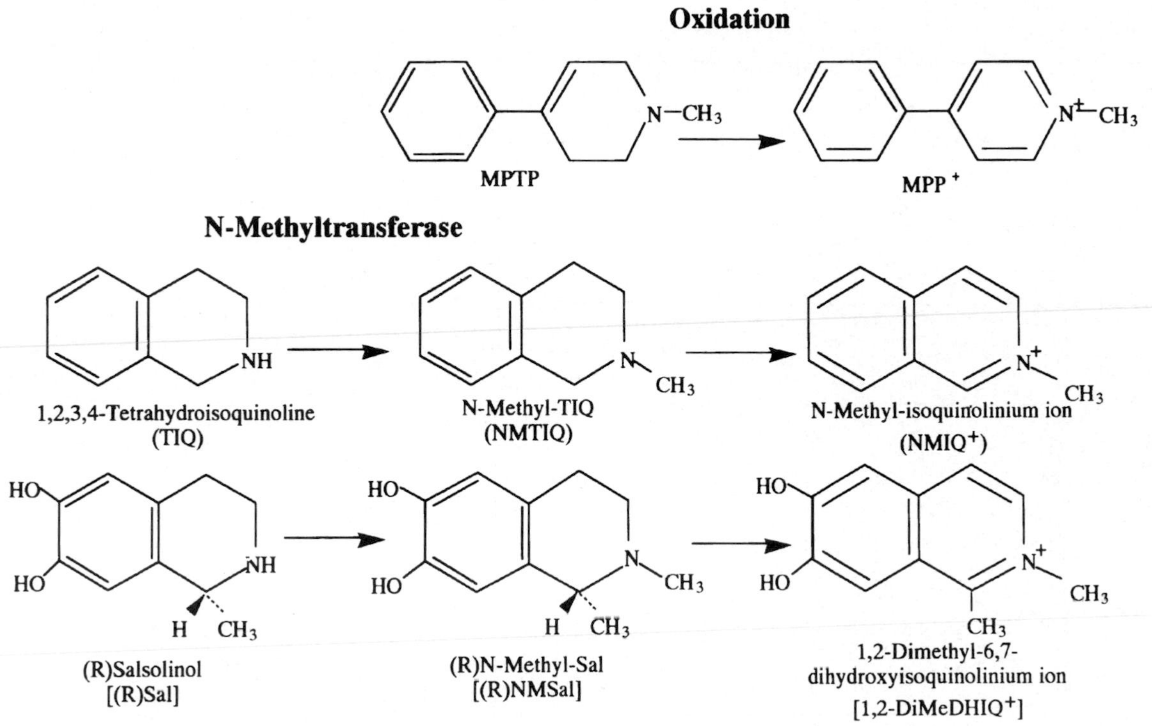

Oxidation

N-Methyltransferase

Fig. 1. Metabolic pathway of MPTP and isoquinolines with and without catechol structure in the brain.

ing 1 mM EDTA at 37°C for 20 min. Then, the reaction mixture was mixed with 25 μl of 0.1 M perchloric acid containing 0.1 mM EDTA and 0.1 mM sodium metabisulfite, and centrifuged at 22 000 × g for 10 min. The oxidation product, 1,2-DiMeDHIQ$^+$, was quantitatively analyzed by HPLC with fluorometric detection (FD). The column was a reversed-phase ODS column and the mobile phase was 90 mM sodium acetate/35 mM citric acid buffer, pH 4.35, containing 130 μM EDTA and 230 μM sodium octanesulfonate, and methanol was added to be 16.6%. The fluorescence at 500 nm was measured with the excitation at 355 nm. As summarized in Table 1, the non-enzymatic oxidation of (R)NMSal was high in phosphate buffer, but the oxidation was significantly higher upon incubation with the enzyme sample (statistically significant; $P < 0.05$ by ANOVA). Thus the oxidation was partly enzymatic, as shown by comparison of the amount of

oxidized product formed in the presence of the enzyme sample with that formed when the denatured enzyme sample after boiling for 3 min was used. The oxidation was dependent linearly on the reaction time up to 20 min at 37°C and on the enzyme sample up to 500 μg protein. The effects of clorgyline, deprenyl and semicarbazide on (R)NMSal were examined (Fig. 3). The enzymatic oxidation, calculated from 1,2-DiMeDHIQ$^+$ production increased in the presence of the enzyme sample, was completely inhibited by semicarbazide at 1 mM, and 57% inhibition was observed at 100 μM. With 1 mM clorgyline the oxidation was inhibited about to 53% of the control, and no significant inhibition was detected with clorgyline at lower than 100 μM. Deprenyl did not inhibit the oxidation at all even at 1 mM. These results suggest that (R)NMSal is not oxidized by B MAO, and that the oxidase activity is rather sensitive to semicarbazide.

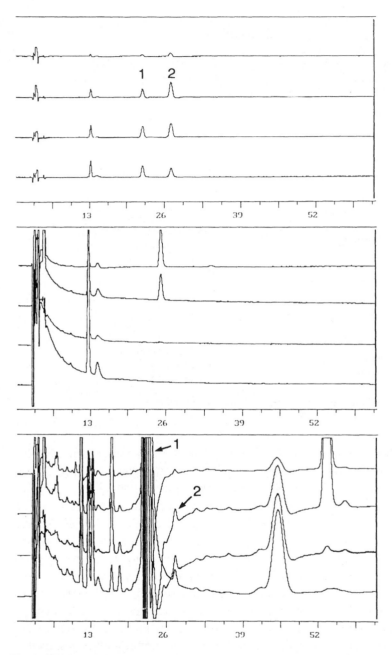

Fig. 2. HPLC-multi-ECD pattern of the samples obtained by microdialysis in the rat striatum. The upper chromatogram; the standard of (R)-salsolinol (1) and (R)NMSal (2). The middle; the dialysate before (R)-salsolinol perfusion. The lower; the dialysate after 100 min perfusion of 1 mM (R)-salsolinol.

The kinetics of (R)NMSal oxidation by the brain sample are as follows: the K_m value is $160.7 \pm 29.7\,\mu$M and the V_{max} value 291.1 ± 32.4 pmol/min per mg protein. The optimal pH of the oxidation was around 8.75, as shown in Fig. 4. The characterization of this oxidase is now under way.

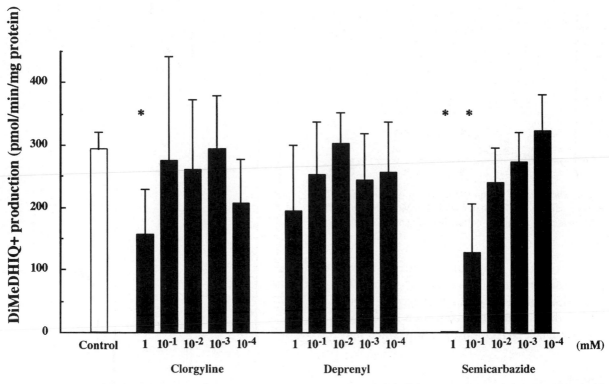

Fig. 3. The effects of clorgyline, deprenyl and semicarbazide on the oxidation of (R)NMSal. The enzyme sample was incubated with 1 mM (R)NMSal in 25 mM potassium phosphate buffer, pH 7.4, in the presence of 1 mM to 100 nM of each inhibitor. Column and bar represent the mean and SD of triplicate measurements of two experiments. ignificantly different from control; $P < 0.05$ by ANOVA.

In the brain of rat intraventricularly injected with (R)NMSal, the oxidized isoquinolinium ion was detected as shown by HPLC-FD (Fig. 5).

Non-enzymatic oxidation

By analogy with the catecholamines, (R)NMSal was oxidized also non-enzymatically into 1,2-Di-MeDHIQ$^+$. As described above, the production of the catechol isoquinolinium ion was measured by HPLC-FD. Hydroxyl radicals were found to be concomitantly produced, and trapped as 2,3- and 2,5-dihydroxybenzoic acid (2,3- and 2,5-DHBA) derivatives with detection by HPLC-ECD. The non-enzymatic production of the catechol isoquinolinium ion was decreased in the presence of ascorbic acid and reduced glutathione. The formation of hydroxyl radicals was also inhibited

by addition of the reducing agents, and partly by catalase and superoxide dismutase. These results indicate that hydrogen peroxide and superoxide radicals are involved in the oxidation of (R)NMSal. Hydroxyl radicals may be produced from hydrogen peroxide, which is further accelerated by superoxide radicals by iron-catalyzed Haber-Weiss reaction.

Production of an animal model of Parkinson's disease

The effects of the catechol isoquinolines were examined in vivo after injection in the rat brain. After administration of (R)NMSal and 1,2-Di-MeDHIQ$^+$, the rat showed behavioral changes, such as akinesia, rotation, postural disturbance

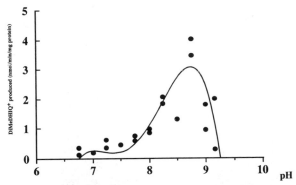

Fig. 4. The effect of pH on the oxidation of (R)NMSal. The enzyme sample was incubated with 1 mM (R)NMSal in 50 mM potassium phosphate buffer, pH from 6.75 to 9.16.

and involuntary movement, whereas other catechol isoquinolines, (R)- and (S)-salsolinol and (S)NMSal, did not cause any behavioral changes. Three days after single injection of (R)NMSal and 1,2-DiMeDHIQ$^+$, the rat was killed and the

TABLE 1

Oxidation of (R)NMSal into 1,2-DiMeDHIQ$^+$

	1,2-DiMeDHIQ$^+$ produced (pmol/min)	
	With the brain enzyme sample	Without the sample
Potassium phosphate buffer	865.3 ± 51.3*	586.5 ± 102.9*
Denatured sample[a]	437.7 ± 60.7	
Tris-HCl buffer	11.6 ± 1.8	8.26 ± 0.8.
HEPES buffer	15.3 ± 0.18	13.3 ± 1.6

(R)NMSal (1 mM) was incubated in 200 μl of 25 mM buffer, pH 7.4, with the enzyme sample (1 mg protein) for 20 min at 37°C. To the reaction mixture were added 20 μl of 1 M perchloric acid containing 1 mM EDTA and sodium metabisulfite, vortexed and centrifuged at 22000 × g for 10 min. The sample was filtered and applied to HPLC-FD.
The values represent the means ± SD of triplicate measurements of two experiments.
* Significantly different between the value with and without enzyme sample, P < 0.05 by ANOVA.
[a] The enzyme sample was boiled for 3 min before with (R)NMSal.

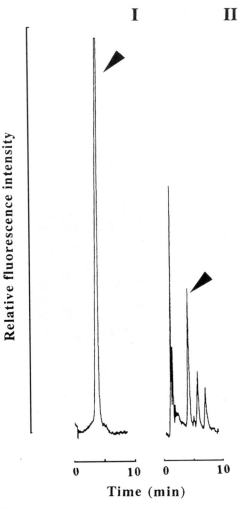

Fig. 5. HPLC-FD pattern of a standard sample of 1,2-DiMeDHIQ$^+$ (I) and of a brain sample after perfusion of (R)NMSal (II). Three days after perfusion of (R)NMSal in the ventricle, the brain sample was analyzed by HPLC-FD.

brain was taken out and sliced in coronal section with a Brain Matrix (Activational System) in 2 mm thickness. The amounts of biogenic amines, (R)NMSal and 1,2-DiMeDHIQ$^+$ were quantitatively analyzed by HPLC-multi-ECD and HPLC-FD. In the brain of rats administered 1,2-DiMeDHIQ$^+$, the catechol isoquinolinium ion was detected in the brain slices (Nos. 2 and 3) including the striatum. In the Nos. 1–3 slices of the rat injected with (R)NMSal, considerable amounts of (R)NMSal were detected. However, the oxidized product, 1,2-DiMeDHIQ$^+$, was also detected and its amount was higher than that of the reduced catechol isoquinoline. In slice No. 2, the amount of (R)NMSal was 1.71 pmol/mg wet weight, while that of 1,2-DiMeDHIQ$^+$ was 3.86 pmol/mg wet weight. It should be emphasized that definite amounts of 1,2-DiMeDHIQ$^+$ were also found in the brain slices Nos. 6 and 7, which should include substantia nigra material with concentrations of 0.45 and 0.48 pmol/mg wet weight, for No. 6 and No. 7, respectively. The amounts of catecholamines and indoleamines and their metabolites were reduced in the brain slices No. 2 and No. 7 by perfusion of (R)NMSal and DiMeDHIQ$^+$ in the striatum (No. 2). Dopamine was markedly reduced in the two brain regions by both (R)NMSal and 1,2-DiMeDHIQ$^+$, and the reduction was more manifest in the substantia nigra region than in the striatum region. The concentrations of the dopamine metabolites, 6,7-dihydroxyphenylacetic acid (DOPAC) and homovanillic acid (HVA), were less modified. The levels of norepinephrine and its metabolite, 4-methyl-4-hydroxyphenylethyleneglycol (MHPG), were also reduced in both the striatum and substantia nigra, but serotonin and its metabolite 5-hydroxyindoleacetic acid (5-HIAA) remained unchanged. The activity of the rate-limiting enzyme of catecholamine synthesis, tyrosine hydroxylase (tyrosine, tetrahydropteridine:oxygen oxidoreductase (3-hydroxylating), EC 1.14. 16.2), was also reduced in the striatum and substantia nigra. The reduction was most manifest in the substantia nigra with (R)NMSal.

Involvement of metabolic bioactivation in dopaminergic neurotoxicity

Selective uptake into dopaminergic cells

To elucidate the selective dopaminergic cytotoxicity, the transport of catechol isoquinolines was examined by use of a human dopaminergic neuroblastoma cell line, SH-SY5Y. Only (R)NMSal was found to be transported into the cells by dopamine transporter (Takahashi et al., 1994). As shown in Fig. 6, the uptake of (R)NMSal

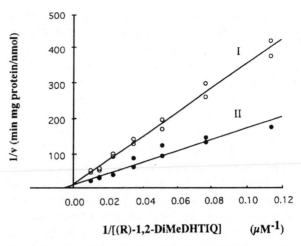

Fig. 6. Kinetics of the uptake of 1,2-DiMeDHIQ$^+$ into SH-SY5Y cells and the effect of dopamine. The cells were incubated with 7 concentrations of (R)NMSal in the absence (II) and presence of 1 mM dopamine (I).

was competitively inhibited by dopamine. The values of K_m and V_{max} of the uptake of (R)NMSal into the cells are 102.6 ± 36.9 μM and 66.0 ± 2.8 pmol/min per mg protein. The involvement of the selective transport of (R)NMSal was clearly shown by the effect on intracellular ATP level of SH-SY5Y cells. The incubation of SH-SY5Y cells with 100 μM catechol isoquinolines reduced the intracellular ATP level, and (R)NMSal was found to be most potent among the catechol isoquinolines. Pre-treatment of the cells with the inhibitors of dopamine transporter, mazindol and nomifensine, protected the cells from the ATP reduction by (R)NMSal. These results further suggest the view that the transport of (R)NMSal into dopamine cells is the first step of the selective cytotoxicity.

Accumulation of the oxidized catechol isoquinolinium ion in dopamine cells

The oxidation of (R)NMSal into the isoquinolinium ion and its accumulation in cells were found to be another important step in the selective toxicity of (R)NMSal towards dopaminergic cells. The above-mentioned data on the localization of (R)NMSal and 1,2-DiMeDHIQ$^+$

in the brain regions after injection of (R)NMSal in the rat brain demonatrate that (R)NMSal is taken up into the nerve terminals in the striatum, and that the oxidized catechol isoquinolinium ion is accumulated in the cell bodies in addition to the nerve terminals, where these catechol isoquinolines were injected. The accumulation of catechol isoquinolinium ion was much higher than that of the reduced form. The fact that the cate-chol isoquinolinium ion accumulates more markedly than the reduced isoquinoline was proved also by culture of another type of do-pamine cell model, the rat pheochromocytoma PC12h cells. As shown in Table 2, in the cells cultured in the presence of (R)NMSal, 1,2-Di-MeDHIQ$^+$ was also detected, and in the cells cultured with the isoquinolinium ion a larger amount of 1,2-DiMeDHIQ$^+$ was accumulated than when the reduced form was used.

The studies using MPTP and MPP$^+$ suggest that the accumulation in or binding to the intra-cellular components, such as melanin and mito-chondria, is essential for the cytotoxicity to occur. Recently, it was found that 1,2-DiMeDHIQ$^+$ se-lectively binds to melanin (Naoi et al., 1994a). The binding has two components with low and high affinity, as shown in Fig. 7. The high-affinity binding site has a dissociation constant, K_D, value of 2.12 ± 1.63 nM and a binding capacity, B_{max},

value of 103.0 ± 80.3 pmol/min per mg melanin, while the low-affinity binding site has a K_D value of 79.4 ± 100.1 nM and a B_{max} value of 1336 ± 1052 pmol/min per mg melanin. In addition, the binding of 1,2-DiMeDHIQ$^+$ was found to be reg-ulated by the concentration of Fe(II) and Fe(III). Fe(II) increased the binding markedly, whereas Fe(III) released the bound isoquinolinium ion from melanin. As previously reported, in the brain the ratio of the Fe(III)/Fe(II) concentrations is increased with aging and also in parkinsonian brains (Riederer et al., 1989). This suggests that, in the aged brain, the bound catechol isoquinolin-ium ion might be released at once, when the ratio of Fe(III) to Fe(II) passes a critical threshold value.

These results demonstrate that after the selec-tive uptake of (R)NMSal into dopamine cells, the oxidation into the isoquinolinium ion is an impor-tant step for the intracellular accumulation.

Potent cytotoxicity of the oxidized catechol isoquinolinium ion

The oxidation of (R)NMSal produces hydroxyl radicals and the isoquinolinium ion, which is a more potent cytotoxic agent than the reduced form. Histological studies revealed that 1,2-Di-MeDHIQ$^+$ is much more cytotoxic than (R)NMSal. Massive necrosis was observed in the

TABLE 2

Accumulation of (R)-salsolinol, (R)NMSal and 1,2-DiMeDHIQ$^+$ in PC12h cells after 3 day culture with 100 μM isoquinolines

	Accumulation isoquinolines (pmol/culture flask)		
	(R)Salsolinol	(R)NMSal	1,2-DiMeDHIQ$^+$
Cells cultured with			
(R)Salsolinol	47.9 ± 0.1	N.D.	N.D.
(R)NMSal	N.D.	719 ± 28	35.6 ± 5.6
1,2-DiMeDHIQ$^+$	N.D.	N.D.	60700 + 20600

PC12h cells were cultured with 100 μM isoquinoline for 3 days in a 20 cm^2 flask, then washed with phosphate-buffered saline and centrifuged three times. The precipitated cells were suspended in 200 μl of 0.1 M perchloric acid containing 0.1 mM EDTA and sodium metabisulfite. After mixing, centrifugation and filtration, (R)-salsolinol and (R)NMSal were analyzed by HPLC-ECD and 1,2-DiMeDHIQ$^+$ by HPLC-FD.
The values represent the means ± SD of triplicate measurements of three experiments.

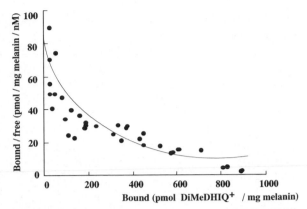

Fig. 7. The Scatchard plot of the binding of 1,2-DiMeDHIQ$^+$ to melanin. The catechol isoquinolinium ion was incubated with melanin and the free unbound isoquinolinium ion was measured by HPLC-FD. The line is the theoretical values simulated using the K_D and B_{max} values obtained by the non-linear square method.

injected region with the catechol isoquinolinium ion, while with the reduced catechol isoquinoline, only limited cell damage due to mechanical injury was observed. The potent cytotoxicity of 1,2-DiMeDHIQ$^+$ suggests that the isoquinolinium ion might be a true neurotoxin eliciting PD in humans. As a mechanism of the cytotoxicity, 1,2-DiMeDHIQ$^+$ was found to inhibit mitochondrial oxidative phosphorylation, and the effects of these catechol isoquinolines on the mitochondrial enzymes are now being examined (Mizuno et al., in preparation). The currently available results indicate that the oxidation of (R)NMSal increases the cytotoxicity by ATP depletion, in addition to the oxidative stress through hydroxyl radical generation, as described above.

Effects of catechol isoquinolines on monoamine metabolism in the brain

Recent results established that dopamine-derived isoquinolines perturb monoamine metabolism in the brain by two mechanisms: inhibition of the activity of enzymes involved in catecholamine and indoleamine metabolism, and release of biogenic monoamines from the nerve terminals.

Effects of catechol isoquinolines on the activity of monoamine oxidase, tyrosine hydroxylase and tryptophan hydroxylase

Using in vivo and in vitro experiments, the effects of the isoquinolines on the activity of MAO, tyrosine hydroxylase, and tryptophan hydroxylase (L-tryptophan, tetrahydropteridine:oxygen oxidoreductase (5-hydroxylating), EC 1.14.16.4) were examined.

Catechol isoquinolines were found to be potent and competitive inhibitors of type A MAO, as summarized in Table 3 (Minami et al., 1993; Naoi et al., 1994c). Among the isoquinolines and isoquinolinium ions examined, the most potent inhibitor of type A MAO is 1,2-DiMeDHIQ$^+$, followed by another catechol isoquinolinium ion, 2(N)-methyl-6,7-dihydroxyisoquino linium ion (Naoi et al., 1994c). To type B MAO, the catechol isoquinolines were poor inhibitors and the values of K_i were much higher than for type A.

The activity of tyrosine hydroxylase was found to be regulated by positive allostery by its biopterin cofactor, (6R)-L-erythro-5,6,7,8-tetrahydrobiopterin [(6R)BH$_4$] (Minami et al., 1992b). The allostery disappeared in the presence of (R)- and (S)-salsolinol with reduction of its affinity for (6R)BH$_4$, suggesting that salsolinols induce conformational change in the hydroxylase. At the biopterin concentrations in the brain, (R)- and (S)-enantiomers of salsolinol were found to inhibit the activity of tyrosine hydroxylase markedly (Minami et al., 1992a). A similar type of inhibition of tyrosine hydroxylase activity was found with MPP$^+$ (Maruyama and Naoi, 1994).

These catechol isoquinolines also inhibit the activity of tryptophan hydroxylase, the key enzyme in the biosynthesis of serotonin (Ota et al., 1992). The inhibition was non-competitive to the substrate, L-tryptophan. In term of the biopterin cofactor (6R)BH$_4$, (R)- and (S) enantiomers of salsolinol inhibited the hydroxylase, competitively and non-competitively according to the biopterin concentration. More recently, the structure−activity relation of isoquinolines on the inhibition of tryptophan hydroxylase was studied (Matsubara

TABLE 3

Kinetics of type A and type B monoamine oxidase and the effects of isoquinolines

Isoquinoline	K_m (μM)	V_{max} (nmol/min per mg protein)	K_i (μM)
Type A monoamine oxidase			
Control	32.0 ± 2.2	0.285 ± 0.015	
1,2-DiMeDHIQ$^+$	404.1 ± 86.7	0.144 ± 0.083	9.21 ± 6.36
(R)Salsolinol	78.5 ± 18.0	0.173 ± 0.035	75.9 ± 21.0
(R)NMSal	69.9 ± 8.58	0.277 ± 0.030	86.4 ± 23.3
Type of inhibition; competitive in terms of substrate			
Type B monoamine oxidase			
Control	53.3 ± 6.0	2.67 ± 0.16	
1,2-DiMeDHIQ$^+$	85.1 ± 19.3	2.11 ± 0.43	77.8 ± 14.4
(R)Salsolinol	86.9 ± 22.6	2.14 ± 0.50	68.3 ± 14.4
(R)NMSal	67.4 ± 7.12	3.00 ± 0.19	433.3 ± 262.7
Type of inhibition; non-competitive in terms of substrate			

The MAO activity was measured with kynuramine as substrate and the activities of type A and of type B were differentiated by use of 1 μM deprenyl or clorgyline. K_m and V_{max} values were obtained in terms of a substrate, kynuramine.
Each value represents the mean $\pm$ SD of duplicate measurements of two experiments.

et al., 1994). Among catechol isoquinolines examined, 1,2-DiMeDHIQ$^+$ was the most potent inhibitor of tryptophan hydroxylase with a K_i value of 0.88 ± 0.17 and 0.64 ± 0.08 μM, in terms of the substrate and ($6R$)BH$_4$, respectively. The requirement of catechol structure for inhibition of tryptophan hydroxylase was also shown for two isoquinolines derived from cigarette smoke. 6,7-Dihydroxy-N-cyanomethyl-1,2,3,4-tetrahydroi oquinoline inhibits the activity of tryptophan hydroxylase, whereas 6-hydroxy-N-cyanomethyl-tetrahydro-β-carbolin , a cyanomethyl derivative of serotonin, does not (Minami et al., 1993b).

These results indicate isoquinolines and especially isoquinolinium ions inhibit the enzymes participating in the biosynthesis and catabolism of catecholamines and indoleamines and perturb their metabolism in the brain.

Release of monoamines from the nerve terminals by catechol isoquinolines

MPP$^+$ was shown to release dopamine from the nerve terminals. Then, dopamine is oxidized non-enzymatically or enzymatically with production of hydroxyl radicals and oxidative stress as a result (Chiueh et al., 1992). Upon perfusion in the rat striatum catechol isoquinolines were found to release monoamine massively. In vivo microdialysis studies demonstrate that (R)- and (S)-salsolinol release marked amounts of serotonin (Maruyama et al., 1993), and also dopamine and norepinephrine in the brain regions where dopamine and noradrenaline neurons are distributed (Fig. 8). The structural studies on the production of hydroxyl radicals in the brain were carried out in vivo and in vitro (Maruyama et al., 1994). Among catechol isoquinolines perfused in the rat striatum by in vivo microdialysis, (R)-salsolinol and 1,2-DiMeDHIQ$^+$ were found to reduce hydroxyl radical levels, whereas (R)NMSal increased hydroxyl radical production. In vitro experiments showed also that catechol isoquinolines and 2(N)-methyl-1,2,3,4-tetrahydroisoquinoline produce hydroxyl radicals, but tetrahydroisoquinolines without a catechol structure did not. These results suggest that the presence of a

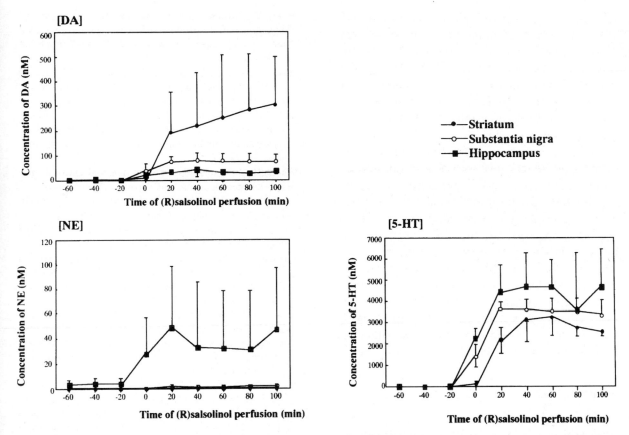

Fig. 8. The release of dopamine, norepinephrine and serotonin in rat brain regions. Dopamine (DA), norepinephrine (NE) and serotonin (5-HT) were measured in the microdialysate after perfusion of 1 mM (R)-salsolinol in the striatum, substantia nigra and hippocampus.

methyl group at the 2(N)-position favors oxidation and hydroxyl radical formation.

The present results suggest that catechol isoquinolines can release dopamine and other monoamines and that they may be neurotoxic or neuroprotective depending on their promotion or reduction of hydroxyl radical production.

Conclusion

As a whole these data show that an endogenous isoquinoline, (R)-salsolinol, increases its potency and selectivity as a neurotoxin for dopamine neurons by N-methylation and oxidation. The metabolic bioactivation appears to be a common feature observed in neurotoxins, such as isoquino-

lines (Naoi et al., 1994a) and β-carbolines (Matsubara et al., 1994). The N-methylation is the first reaction for the selective uptake into dopamine neurons by the dopamine transporter. The selective uptake of (R)NMSal into dopaminergic cells was clearly demonstrated by dopamine cell models, SH-SY5Y and PC12h cells.

Enzymatic and non-enzymatic oxidation seems to determine the selective neurotoxicity toward dopamine neurons. The oxidation of (R)NMSal into the isoquinolinium ion is essential for the accumulation into dopamine cells and enhanced cytotoxicity. As shown by injection in the rat striatum, the oxidized product, 1,2-DiMeDHIQ$^+$, was found to accumulate more than the reduced isoquinoline, particularly in the region including substantia nigra. Histological observation indicates the isoquinolinium ion is more cytotoxic than (R)NMSal and (R)-salsolinol. The enzyme involved in this bioactivation for MPTP is mainly type B MAO (Chiba et al., 1984; Heikkila et al., 1984), whereas the oxidase involved in the transformation of (R)NMSal into 1,2-DiMeDHIQ$^+$ is sensitive to neither clorgyline nor deprenyl, but is sensitive to semicarbazide. The characterization of this oxidase may give us a clue to the selective neurotoxicity of this endogenous catechol isoquinoline. On the other hand, the results reported here suggest that autoxidation of endogenous catechol isoquinolines might be also involved in the cytotoxicity. Not only in Parkinson's disease, but also in the aged brain, the gradual cell loss in the dopaminergic system is recognized (Hornykiewica and Kish, 1986). The involvement of the dopamine-derived isoquinolines in dopaminergic neuronal death should be further clarified.

Acknowledgment

This work was supported by a Grant-In-Aid for Scientific Research on Priority Area from the Ministry of Education, Science and Culture, Japan.

References

Brossi, A. (1982) Mammalian TIQs; products of condensation with aldehydes or pyruvic acids? *Prog. Clin. Biol. Res.*, 90: 123–133.

Chiba , K., Trevor, A.J. and Castagnoli, N. (1964) Metabolism of the neurotoxic amine MPTP by brain monoamine oxidase. *Biochem. Biophys. Res. Commun.*, 120: 574–578.

Chiueh, C.C., Kristhna G., Tulsi, P., Obata, T., Lanh, K., Huang, S.-H. and Murphy, D.L. (1992) Intracranial microdialysis of salicylic acid to detect hydroxyl radical generation through dopamine autooxidation in the caudate nucleus: effects of MPP$^+$. *Free Radical Biol. Med.*, 13: 581–583.

Collins, M.A. and Cheng B.Y. (1988) Oxidative decarboxylation of salsolinol-1-carboxylic acid to 1,2-dehydrosalsolinol: Evidence for exclusive catalysis by particular factors in rat kidney. *Arch. Biochem. Biophys.*, 263: 86–96.

Dostert, P., Strolin Beneditti, M. and Dordain, G. (1988) Dopamine-derived alkaloids in alcoholism and in Parkinson's and Huntington's diseases. *J. Neural Transm.*, 74: 61–74.

Dostert, P., Strolin Beneditti, M., Dordain, G. and Vernay, D. (1991) Urinary elimination of salsolinol enantiomers in alcoholics. *J. Neural Transm. (Gen. Sect.)*, 85: 51–59.

Gray, E.G. and Whittakar, V.P. (1962) The isolation of nerve endings from brain: an electron-microscopic study of cell fragments derived by homogenization and centrifugation. *J. Anat.*, 96: 79–87.

Heikkila, R.E., Manzino, L., Cabbat, F.S. and Duvoisin, R.C. (1994) Protection against the dopaminergic neurotoxicity of 1-methyl-4-phenyl-1,2,3,6-tetrahydropyridine by monoamine oxidase inhibitor. *Nature*, 311: 467–469.

Hornykiewicz, O. and Kish, S. (1986) Biochemical pathophysiology of Parkinson's disease. *Adv. Neurol.*, 45: 19–32.

Maruyama, W. and Naoi, M. (1994) Inhibition of tyrosine hydroxylase by a dopamine neurotoxin, 1-methyl-4-phenylpyridinium ion: Depletion of allostery to the biopterin cofactor. *Life Sci.*, 55: 207–212.

Maruyama, W., Nakahara, D., Ota, M., Takahashi, T., Takahashi, T., Nagatsu, T. and Naoi, M. (1992) *N*-Methylation of dopamine-derived 6,7-dihydroxy-1,2,3,4-tetrahydroisoquinoline, (R)-salsolinol, in rat brains; in vivo microdialysis. *J. Neurochem.*, 59: 395–400.

Maruyama, W., Nakahara, D. Dostert, P., Hashiguchi, H. Ohta, S., Hirobe, M., Takahashi, A., Nagatsu, T. and Naoi, M. (1993) Selective release of serotonin by endogenous alkaloids, 1-methyl-6,7-dihydroxy-1,2,3,4-tetrahydroisoquinolines, (R)- and (S)salsolinol, in the rat striatum; in vivo microdialysis study. *Neurosci. Lett.*, 149: 115–118.

Maruyama, W., Nakahara, D., Dostert, P., Takahashi, T. and Naoi, M. (1994) Dopamine-derived isoquinolines as dopaminergic neurotoxins and oxidative stress. *Alzheimer's and Parkinson's Diseases; Recent Developments*. Plenum, New York and London, pp. 575–581.

Matsubara, K., Collins, M.A., Akane, A., Ikebuchi, J., Neafsey, E.J., Kagawa, M. and Shiono, H. (1993) Potential bioactivated neurotoxins, *N*-methylated β-carbolinium ions, are present in human brain. *Brain Res.*, 610: 90–96.

Matsubara, K., Ota, M., Takahashi, T., Maruyama, W. and Naoi, M. (1994) Structural studies of condensation products of biogenic amines as inhibitors of tryptophan hydroxylase. *Brain Res.*, 655: 121–127.

Melchior, C. and Collins, M.A. (1982) The route and significance of endogenous synthesis of alkaloids in animals. *CRC Critical Reviews in Toxicology*, CRC Press, Boca Rotan, pp. 313–356.

Melchior, C.L., Mueller, A. and Detrich, R.A. (1980) Half-lives of salsolinol and tetrahydropapaveroline hydrobromide following intracerebroventricular injection. *Biochem. Pharmacol.*, 29: 657–658.

Minami, M., Maruyama, W., Dostert, P., Nagatsu, T. and Naoi, M. (1993a) Inhibition of type A and B monoamine oxidase by 6,7-dihydroxyisoquinolines and their N-methylated derivatives. *J. Neural Transm. (Gen. Sect.)*, 92: 125–135.

Minami, M., Takahashi, T., Maruyama, W., Takahashi, A., Dostert, P., Nagatsu, T. and Naoi, M. (1992a) Inhibition of tyrosine hydroxylase by R and S enantiomers of salsolinol, 1-methyl-6,7-dihydroxy-1,2,3,4-tetrahydroisoquinoline. *J. Neurochem.*, 58: 2097–2101.

Minami, M., Takahashi, T., Maruyama, W., Takahashi A., Nagatsu, T. and Naoi, M. (1992b) Allosteric effect of tetrahydrobiopterin cofactor on tyrosine hydroxylase activity. *Life Sci.*, 50: 15–20.

Minami, M., Yu, P.H., Davis, B.A., Takahashi, T., Shimomura, Y. and Naoi, M. (1993b) Inhibition of tryptophan hydroxylase by 6,7-dihydroxy-N-cyanomethyl-1,2,3,4-tetrahydroisoquinoline, a cyanomethyl derivative of dopamine formed from cigarette smoke. *Neurosci. Lett .*, 160: 217–220.

Naoi, M., Dostert, P., Yoshida, M. and Nagatsu, T. (1993a) N-Methylated tetrahydroisoquinolines as dopaminergic neurotoxins. *Adv. Neurol.*, 60: 212–217.

Naoi, M., Maruyama, W., Acworth, I.N., Nakahara, D. and Parvez, H. (1993b) Multi-electrode detection system for determination of neurotransmitters. *Methods in Neurotransmitter and Neuropeptide Research, Part 1*, Elsevier, Amsterdam, pp. 1–39.

Naoi, M., Maruyama, W. and Dostert, P. (1994a) Binding of 1,2(N)-dimethyl-6,7-dihydroxy-isoquinolinium ion to melanin: effects of ferrous and ferric ion on the binding. *Neurosci. Lett.*, 171: 9–12.

Naoi, M., Maruyama W., Nakahara, D., Dostert, P. and Nagatsu, T. (1994b) Metabolic bioactivation of endogenous isoquinolines as dopaminergic neurotoxins to elicit Parkinson's disease, *Alzheimer's and Parkinson's Diseases: Recent Developments*, Plenum, New York and London, pp. 553–559.

Naoi, M., Maruyama, W., Sasuga, S., Deng, Y., Dostert, P., Ohta, S. and Takahashi, T. (1994c) Inhibition of type A monoamine oxidase by 2(N)-methyl-6,7-dihydroxy-isoquinolinium ions. *Neurochem. Int.*, 25: 475–481.

Naoi, M., Matsuura, S., Takahashi, T. and Nagatsu, T. (1989) An N-methyltransferase in human brain catalyzes N-methylation of 1,2,3,4-tetrahydroisoquinoline into N-methyl-1,2,3,4-tetrahydroisoquinoline, a precursor of a dopaminergic neurotoxin, N-methylisoquinolinium ion. *Biochem. Biophys. Res. Commun.*, 161: 1213–1219.

Niwa, T., Maruyama, W., Nakahara, D., Takeda, N., Yoshizumi, H., Tatematsu, A., Takahashi, A., Dostert, P., Naoi, M. and Nagatsu, T. (1992) Endogenous synthesis of N-methylsalsolinol, an analogue of 1-methyl-4-phenyl-1,2,3,6-tetrahydropyridine, in rat brain during in vivo microdialysis with salsolinol, as demonstrated by gas chromatography-mass spectrometry. *J. Chromatogr.*, 578: 109–115.

Niwa, T., Takeda, N., Yoshizumi, H., Tatematsu, A. Yoshida, M., Dostert, P., Naoi, M. and Nagatsu, T. (1991) Presence of 2-methyl-6,7-dihydro-1,2,3,4-tetrahydroisoquinoline and 1,2-dimethyl-6,7-dihydroxy-1,2,3,4-tetrahydroisoquinoline, novel endogenous amines, in parkinsonian and normal human brains. *Biochem. Biophys. Res. Commun.*, 177: 603–609.

Origitano, T., Hannigan, J. and Collins, M.A. (1981) Rat brain salsolinol and blood-brain barrier. *Brain Res.*, 224: 446–451.

Ota, M., Dostert, P., Hamanaka, T., Nagatsu, T. and Naoi, M. (1992) Inhibition of tryptophan hydroxylase by (R)- and (S)-1-methyl-6,7-dihydroxy-1,2,3,4-tetrahydroisoquinolines (salsolinols). *Neuropharmacology*, 31: 337–341.

Riederer, P., Sofic, E., Rausch, W.-D., Schmidt, B., Reynolds, G.P., Jellinger, K. and Youdim, M.B. H. (1989) Transition metals, ferritin, glutathione and ascorbic acid in parkinsonian brains. *J. Neurochem.*, 52: 515–520.

Sandler, M., Carter, S.B., Hunter, K.R. and Stern, G.M. (1973) Tetrahydroisoquinoline alkaloids; in vivo metabolites of L-DOPA in man. *Nature*, 241: 439–443.

Singer, T.P., Castagnoli, J.N., Jr., Ramsay, R.R. and Trevor, A.J. (1987) Biochemical events in the development of parkinsonism induced by 1-methyl-4-phenyl-1,2,3,6-tetrahydropyridine. *J. Neurochem.*, 49: 1–8.

Sjoequist, B., Eriksson, A. and Winblad, B. (1982a) Brain salsolinol levels in alcoholism. *Lancet*, i: 675–676.

Sjoequist, B., Eriksson, A. and Winblad, B. (1982b) Salsolinol and catecholamines in human brain and their relation to alcoholism. *Prog. Clin. Biol. Res.*, 90: 56–67.

Strolin Beneditti, M., Bellotti, V., Poanezola, E., Carminati, P. and Dostert, P. (1989) Ratio of the R and S enantiomers of salsolinol in food and human urine. *J. Neural Transm.*, 77: 47–53.

Takahashi, T., Y. Deng, Maruyama, W., Dostert, P., Kawai, M. and Naoi, M. (1994). Uptake of a neurotoxin-candidate, (R)-1,2-dimethyl-6,7-dihydroxy-1,2,3,4-tetrahydroisoquinoline into human dopaminergic neuroblastoma SH-SY5Y cells by dopamine transport system. *J. Neural Transm. (Gen. Sect)*, 98: 107–118

Tipton, K.F. and Singer T.P. (1993) Advances in our understanding of the mechanisms of the neurotoxicity of MPTP and related compounds. *J. Neurochem.*, 61: 1191–1206.

Ung-Chhun, N., Cheng, B.Y., Pronger, D.A., Serrano, P., Chave, B., Pere, R.F., Morles, J. and Collins, M.A. (1985) Alkaloid adducts in human brain: Coexistence of 1-carboxylated and noncarboxylated isoquinolines and β-carbolines in alcoholics and nonalcoholics. *Prog. Clin. Biol. Res.*, 183: 125–136.

Peter M. Yu, Keith F. Tipton and Alan A. Boulton (Eds.)
Progress in Brain Research, Vol 106

Monoamines, cytoskeletal elements and psychiatric disorders: a neurochemical fugue

J. Harris[1], M.E. Knight[2] and M.M. Rasenick[2,3]

[1]*Department of Chemistry and Biochemistry, Arizona State University, Box 871604, Tempe, AZ 85287-1604, USA, and*
[2]*Department of Physiology and Biophysics, University of Illinois at Chicago, Chicago, IL 60612-7342, USA*

Introduction

Pharmacological studies with psychoactive drugs such as monoamine oxidase inhibitors and anti-depressants have led to the formulation of a biogenic amine neurotransmitter (aminergic) hypothesis of psychiatric disorders (Schildkraut, 1965; Schildkraut and Kety, 1967; Snyder et al., 1974). The catecholamine hypothesis has profoundly influenced neurochemical research in psychiatry, especially into depression, mania and other mood disorders. Disturbances in signal transduction at the level of receptors and second messengers have been implicated in the pathophysiology of bipolar affective disorder (Klyner et al., 1987; Ebstein et al., 1988; Ozawa and Rasenick, 1989, 1991). Well documented decreases in the number of adrenergic receptors and reduced sensitivity of stimulated adenylyl cyclase have been found in rodent brain after chronic administration of anti-depressant drugs or electroconvulsive shock (Sulser et al., 1978; Bergstrom and Kellar, 1979). Although a disparity between receptor density and the responsiveness of the adenylyl cyclase system has been reported (Manier et al., 1989; Chen and Rasenick, 1994), we are led to the suggestion that the site of action may also be located beyond the aminergic receptors and their second messengers. In terms of receptor-effector cascade of signal transduction,

other sites would include the protein kinases, the targets beyond the receptors and second messengers that function to amplify signal transduction (Nestler et al., 1989). In this manner, the cell is altered in a variety of ways, from changing gene transcription to altering electrical conditions leading to a well orchestrated network of activity and physiological functions in the body. Importantly, the mechanism by which spatial information can be communicated from membrane to nucleus lies in the key role of the cytoskeletal system. The concept related to the action of hormones and neurotransmitters through the reorientation of the cytoskeleton was first suggested in 1956 by Sir Rudolph Peters and, unacceptable at that time, now has come full circle. This discussion attempts to enlarge on this concept.

The disruption of neuronal cytoarchitecture has long been implicated in the pathophysiology that produces a spectrum of neurobehavioral deficits. In this discussion salient features of both earlier and recent work are given to support the view that the cytoskeleton and, in particular, tubulin and microtubules are involved in cellular communications subserving normal behavior and psychiatric disease. We impart a view of the cytoskeletal system as serving in the role of a third messenger in conjunction with first-messenger biogenic amines, receptors and second messengers, affording the mechanism to account for the heterogeneous etiology of psychiatric disorders. This encompasses structural (anatomic), biochemical and genetic abnormalities. This interaction and the resultant effects on effector systems is not a simplistic domino cascade network, but rather that of a neurochemical fugue. Analogous to a musical fugue, a neurochemical fugue combines the several parts from the dynamic changes in receptors, second-messenger systems and the cytoskeletal system, each responsive to one another, that result in the development of a global theme underlying neurobehavioral deficits.

Tubulin and microtubules

Based on the use of anti-mitotic alkaloid substances which affect microtubule stability, a progression of reports make it evident that cytoskeletal restructuring is involved in synaptic transmission. In the 1960s the anti-mitotic agents colchicine and vinblastine provided the first evidence that tubulin was involved in nerve function by interference with the intraaxonal transport of amine storage granules (Dahlstrom et al., 1966). In other laboratories evidence was obtained for a possible role of microtubules in catecholamine release from adrenal medulla (Poisner et al., 1971). In that decade details were filled in to reveal that uptake and release of the various neurotransmitters, namely, noradrenaline (NE), dopamine (DA), 5-hydroxytryptamine (5HT) and acetylcholine (ACh) and more recently γ-aminobutyric acid (GABA), involved microtubules (Thoa et al., 1972; Nicklas et al., 1973; Wooten et al., 1974; Nomura et al., 1975; Segawa et al., 1978; O'Leary et al., 1983; Ashton et al., 1991).

Cytoskeletal-modifying drugs also affect the mobility of membrane receptors, not only the lateral mobility of molecules in the membrane but also the shape and motility of the cell surface. In addition, dendritic transport of newly synthesized RNA has been found to be dependent upon microtubules (Kleiman et al., 1992).

While the early work with colchicine focused on growth, differentiation, and transport in cell and tissue changes, recent reports show that colchicine injections induced both behavioral and neurochemical hypersensitivity associated in schizophrenia (Klancnik et al., 1993) with dopamine release and hyperactivity.

In addition to the complex anti-mitotic alkaloid molecules, a structurally simple neuro-modulator, 2-phenethylamine, was found to affect tubulin. The observation led to the suggestion that in addition to the current mechanism of signal transduction, namely, (a) receptor, (b) second messenger, there should be considered (c) tubulin/microtubules (Knight and Harris, 1993).

Adenylyl cyclase

At the time that Peters (1956) hypothesized that cytoskeletal reorganization was involved in hormone action, Rall et al. (1956) proposed that cAMP could act as a second messenger of hormonal action. Slowly data began to accumulate and reveal that the cytoskeleton system has a role in the regulation of the hormonal sensitive adenylyl cyclase system. Among the early studies were observations of a potentiation in hormone-stimulated cAMP with a decrease in microtubule polymerization in leukocytes (Rudolf et al., 1979), lymphoma cells (Kennedy and Insel, 1979); macrophages (Hagmann et al., 1980) and cerebral cortex synaptic membranes (Rasenick et al., 1981).

Further evidence of a cytoskeletal involvement with adenylyl cyclase was obtained by Sayhoun et al. (1981) and Levine et al. (1982). In addition, adenylyl cyclase activation by GTP-binding proteins was enhanced by long-term anti-depressant treatment (Menkes et al., 1983). Related to this is the finding that chronic lithium enhances cAMP levels in human platelets and in the nucleus accumbens (Kelley et al., 1993).

Tubulin–G protein interactions

The G proteins, widely distributed, membrane-bound proteins, serve as receptor-effector couplers in a large number of signal transduction processes. The state of microtubule assembly as well as dimeric tubulin itself can modulate G protein responsiveness. Tubulin modifies neuronal signaling through the association of G proteins (Hatta et al., 1992) wherein tubulin regulates G protein activation by transfer of guanine nucleotide to G_s and G_i. (Both β-adrenergic and DA-D_2 receptors are affected.) The interaction of G proteins with tubulin involves microtubule polymerization domains (Wang and Rasenick, 1991). The binding of tubulin is specific to the signal transduction proteins G_s and $G_{i\alpha}1$ (Wang et al., 1990) and, in the process of activating G_s and G_i1, modulates their function. The transfer and hydrolysis of GTP from tubulin to $G_{\alpha}s$ and $G_{\alpha i}1$ would provide a mechanism for cross-talk among signal transduction mechanisms (Roychowdhury and Rasenick, 1993).

Similarities of both function and amino acid sequence appear to exist between tubulin and signal transducing G proteins (Linse and Mandelkow, 1988; Sternlicht et al., 1987; Yan and Rasenick, 1990). Such similarities evoke the possibility that tubulin, which is associated, perhaps intrinsically, with synaptic membranes (Stephens, 1986; Zisapel et al., 1980) may interact with other synaptic membrane G proteins, including G_s and G_i. Thus, there may exist an interdependence between synaptic shape and response to neurotransmitters. Recently, it has been demonstrated that in rat cerebral cortex post-synaptic densities, tubulin and $G_{\alpha}s$ or $G_{\alpha i}1$ exist in preformed complexes (Cohen et al., 1993). Perhaps this interaction is related to the absence of microtubules associated with synaptic membrane despite the abundance of tubulin there. Sustained neural transmission has been reported to modify synaptic form in *Aplysia* (Schacher, et al., 1993) as well as the formation of dendritic spines in the hippocampus (Lisman and Harris, 1993). Thus, increased activity at a given synapse may modify the form of that synapse via a series of interactions between G proteins and tubulin.

Evidence predicts that microtubules and microtubule associated proteins (MAPs) provide a network for signaling and processing information (Vassilev et al., 1985). MAPs are well established as important regulators of microtubule dynamics

as well as contributing to regulating neuronal morphology, neurite outgrowth and regeneration and may be considered as a major structural component of the neuronal skeleton.

MAP_2 is linked to signal transduction in that it is an in vitro substrate for cAMP-dependent protein kinase (Perez et al., 1993) and is rapidly phosphorylated in response to activation of glutamate receptors. The NMDA receptors are coupled to a pathway which targets MAPs for rapid and long-lasting dephosphorylation. The pathway is mediated by the calcium-dependent protein phosphatase calcineurin (Halpain and Lister, 1993). The microtubule-stabilizing agent taxol attenuates glutamate receptor-mediated neurite swelling (Goldberg and Bateman, 1992).

Alterations in G protein are observed in cocaine self-administering rats. There is a decrease in G proteins in several mesolimbic nuclei. G_i1 is decreased in nucleus accumbens but not in the ventral tegmental area. The view presented is that long-term G protein change in the nucleus accumbens may be related to the long-term expression of cocaine sensitization (Striplin and Kalivas, 1993). Future work should involve cytoskeletal microtubule changes with the observed changes in G protein and resultant initiation of transcription factors.

Calcium as a second messenger

Ca^{2+}, an intracellular second messenger with calmodulin as the intracellular receptor, may act as a physiological regulator of the dynamic state of microtubules (Weisenberg, 1972; Keith et al., 1986). Ca^{2+}/calmodulin-dependent protein kinase (CaM kinase II) is associated with the neuronal cytoskeleton and may play a role in mediation of Ca^{2+} effects on cytoskeletal function (Vallano et al., 1986). Ca^{2+} depolymerization of microtubules and regulation of phosphorylation of synapsin 1 via a Ca^{2+}-calmodulin-dependent protein kinase (Sikra et al., 1989) indicate a role for microtubules in neurotransmitter release. Recently, Greengard et al. (1993) reported a role of CaM kinase II in the regulation of neurotransmitter release via phosphorylation of cytoskeletal synapsin I.

MARCKS, a myristoylated alanine-rich phosphorylated protein and a substrate of protein kinase C (PKC), plays a role as a critical effector molecule in cytoskeletal restructuring, Ca^{2+} regulation and synaptic transmission (Hartwig et al., 1992). Some insight into this was reported by Kim et al. (1993). Neuromodulin and the MARCKS protein bind calmodulin with high affinity and are thus able to sequester cellular calmodulin. PKC phosphorylation decreases the affinities of these proteins for calmodulin. Calcium concentration in the cell is thus regulated; the cytoskeletal restructuring signaling pathway is controlled.

Interest in MARCKS increased, as noted by the report that chronic administration of lithium reduces significantly the level of hippocampal MARCKS and this reduction persists after cessation of treatment. The result parallels the clinical efficacy of lithium in the treatment of bipolar disorder (Lenox et al., 1992).

Depression

Two major neurotransmitter systems are implicated in depression: NE and 5HT. All anti-depressants diminish levels of tyrosine hydroxylase (TH) (rate-limiting enzyme for catecholamine synthesis) as well as decreasing messenger RNA for the enzyme (Nestler et al., 1990). Anti-depressant effects are region- and enzyme-specific. The finding that 5HT-reuptake inhibitors are also capable of reducing mRNA expression for TH suggests that there could be an interaction between NE and 5HT systems (in the locus coeruleus). It is noteworthy that stress, which precipitates or coevolves with some forms of depression, affects the mRNA expression of TH in the opposite direction, i.e. increases mRNA (Richard et al., 1988). It must be considered that effects on mRNA levels occur within hours, while changes in the copies of protein take weeks. The clinical efficacy of anti-depressants resembles more closely the latter course.

Chronic, but not acute, tricyclic anti-depressants affect G_s protein, resulting in increased G_s-activated adenylyl cyclase without change in G-protein content, indicative of a tighter interaction between G_s and adenylyl cyclase (Ozawa and Rasenick, 1989, 1991). It is hypothesized that G_s-adenylyl cyclase activity is more readily translocated from the membrane and in the cytoskeleton as a result of treatment. Recently, it was demonstrated that chronic treatment of C6 glioma cells with amitripytline or iprindole caused a similar increase of coupling between $G_{\alpha s}$ and adenylyl cyclase. This suggests that the effects of anti-depressants may not require a presynaptic component (Chen and Rasenick, 1995). In another report chronic anti-depressant treatment with amitriptyline altered tubulin function in a manner that resulted in increased adenylyl cyclase activity (Kamada et al., 1993). The amount of tubulin was not altered by the treatment and thus it was the altered tubulin function that contributed to the increased adenylyl cyclase activity in chronic anti-depressant administration.

Earlier mention was made of long-term anti-depressant treatment enhancing GTP-activation of brain adenylyl cyclase (Menkes et al., 1983). Subsequent work as noted above relates to the need to determine the nature of the changes in tubulin to understand the resultant effect on adenylyl cyclase.

Bipolar affective disorder

Current therapeutic regimes are directed to the motor and affective symptomatology of manic-depressive disorders. Behavioral evidence has been obtained by alterations in G-protein activity in nucleus accumbens induced by chronic administration of Li^+ to rats. Studies in humans report enhanced cAMP levels in platelets and in nucleus accumbens (Kelley et al., 1993) following Li^+ treatment. The association of tubulin with G proteins relates to this alteration in signal transduction. Increased levels of cAMP may reflect a long-term upregulation via G-protein stimulation.

Disturbances in G-protein function in bipolar affective disorder have gained greater attention recently. An increased $G_{\alpha s}$ immunoreactivity was found in post mortem brain of individuals with bipolar affective disorder (Young et al., 1991). In another study, enhanced agonist-stimulated GTP binding was observed in the lymphocytes of patients with bipolar affective disorder.

More recently Young et al. (1993) extended earlier studies and found that increased levels of G proteins occur in peripheral cells in bipolar affective disorder but not in major depressive disorder. G-protein subunit, namely $G_{i\alpha}$, levels were altered by cocaine. Amygdala kindling decreased $G_{i1/2}$ in a manner that was regionally specific and time-dependent (Cutz et al., 1993). Studies showing changes in G-protein expression must be interpreted with caution, since it is not clear that small changes in the number of G proteins would alter G-protein-mediated signal transduction.

Schizophrenia

Multiple lines of evidence indicate that the prefrontal cortex is a site of dysfunction in schizophrenia associated with an altered organization in certain synaptic connections in the brain. Glantz and Lewis (1993) investigated the current concept in human post mortem brain by measuring immunoreactivity for synaptophysin, an integral membrane protein of small synaptic vesicles. Decreased density was found in Brodman areas 9 and 46 and no change in a control area 17 of schizophrenics, findings consistent with the concepts outlined.

Schizophrenia has been proposed to be a hypoglutamatergic-based syndrome. Among the many views is that of an altered GABA-ergic transmission, a view buttressed by the finding of an upregulation of GABA-A receptors and decreased GABA uptake in the cerebral cortex of schizophrenics. Bunney et al. (1993) attempted to obtain evidence for a decreased production of the GABA transmitter, by measurement of mRNA for glutamic acid decarboxylase (GAD), the key enzyme in GABA synthesis. A significant decrease in the gene expression for GAD mRNA was found, leading to the hypothesis of a deficit for gene expression of GAD in prefrontal cortex as an etiological factor in schizophrenia. The hypoglutamatergic syndrome which could fit in with the Bunney et al. GAD gene deficit is unresolved. A decreased availability of glutamate would also reduce the need for GAD and hence result in reduced GABA formation. A reduced GAD gene expression could result. The inclusion of a microtubule involvement is a consideration that would encompass the informational network from receptor to nucleus which would control the levels of glutamate, GABA, GAD enzyme and transcription factors for GAD mRNA.

Kinases and phosphokinase

In terms of the aminergic hypothesis, the protein kinases and the serine-threonine protein phosphatases are of particular interest as targets beyond the receptor and second-messenger level. Modulation of synaptic activity may be regulated by a balance between kinase and phosphatase activities considered as a molecular switch of phosphorylation in signal transduction (Tan, 1993). Kinases as active modulators and phosphatases as passive counter-modulators maintain the state of phosphorylation in the cell. Tubulin polarized domains have properties which permit them also to serve as flip-flop switches in the polymerization-depolymerization process.

The catecholamine hypothesis proposed a quarter of a century ago formed the basis of neurochemical research in affective disorders and has been extended to include other biogenic amines, indolamines, other neurotransmitters, neuropeptides, hormones and ionic changes.

Studies continue with utilization of neuroendocrine challenge strategies, peripheral blood cell receptors, and various biochemical assays yielding a reductionistic single-focus view of a very complex biological condition. Ultimately, there will be the need to formulate an understanding of the processes that involve the simultaneous effects of the neurotransmitters, neuropeptides and ionic changes, etc.

We suggest in this presentation that among the important pathways underlying the mechanism of mood disorders should be included the cytoskeletal element tubulin and its role in signal transduction. There is a rich historical literature supporting this. The biogenic amine neurotransmitters, NE, serotonin and dopamine, dominated current biochemical theories of mental illness. Recently, amino acid neurotransmitters, especially GABA, have been included. These have led to clinically useful drugs for the treatment of schizophrenia, depression and drug addiction. Receptors have commanded attention in keeping with the current scientific thrusts, to which have been added G proteins associated with the receptors.

Long-term changes in behavior underlying psychiatric disorders imply concomitant changes in the CNS. At the cellular level changes range from alterations in receptor expression to receptor interactions with intracellular signalling molecules, including pre-translational and post-translational alterations in expression or activity of such molecules.

The picture of a simple domino cascading network of receptor to effector communication is misleading. A more accurate picture may be described as regulation by committee, a series of members of various families, all interacting with one another. Perhaps it is not as messengers in tightly linked signaling systems but as "housekeepers" regulating the response of cellular metabolism to particular changes in conditions. Nevertheless, as in the case of an orchestral fugue, a series of events and responses occur with precise coordination. Cytoskeletal elements may serve as the conductor.

References

Ashton, A.C. and Dolly, J.O. (1991) Microtubule-dissociating drugs and A23187 reveal differences in the inhibition of synaptosomal transmitter release by botulinum neurotoxin types A and B. *J. Neurochem.*, 56: 827–835.

Bergstrom, D.A. and Kellar, K.J. (1979) Effect of electrocon-vulsive shock on monoaminergic receptor binding sites in rat brain. *Nature*, 278: 464–466.

Bunney, Jr., W.E., Akbarian, S., Kim, J.J., Hagman, J.O., Potkin, S.G. and Jones, E.G. (1993) Gene expression for glutamic acid decarboxylase is reduced in prefrontal cortex of schizophrenia. *Soc. Neurosci. Abstr.*, 19: 199.

Chen, J. and Rasenick, M.M. (1995) Chronic anti-depressant treatment changes G-protein functional interactions without altering G-protein content. *J. Neurochem.*, 64(2) 724–732.

Cohen, R.S., Rasenick, M.M. and Manning, D.R. (1993) Subsynaptic localization of GTP-binding proteins. *Soc. Neurosci. Abstr.*, 19(2): 939.

Cutz, J.C., Li, P.P., Burnham, W.M. and Warsh, J.J. (1993) Effect of amygdala kindling on G-protein subunit levels. *Biol. Psychiatr.*, 33(6A): 135A.

Dählstrom, A. and Häggendahl, J. (1966) Studies on the transport and life-span of amine storage granules in a peripheral adrenergic neuron system. *Acta Physiol. Scand.*, 67: 278–288.

Ebstein, R.P., Lerer, B., Shapira, B., Shemesk, Z., Moscovich, D.G. and Kindler, S. (1988) Cyclic AMP second messenger signal amplification in depression. *Br. J. Psychiatry*, 152: 665–669.

Glantz, E.A. and Lewis, D.A. (1993) Synaptophysin immunoreactivity is selectively decreased in prefrontal cortex of schizophrenic subjects. *Soc. Neurosci. Abstr.*, 19: 201.

Goldberg, M.P. and Bateman, M.C. (1993) Taxol attenuates glutamate receptor-mediated neurite swelling. *Soc. Neurosci. Abstr.*, 19(1): 26.

Greengard, P., Valtorta, F., Caernik, A.J. and Benfenati, F. (1993) Synaptic vesicles, phosphoproteins and regulation of synaptic function. *Science*, 259: 780–785.

Hagmann, J. and Fishman, P.H. (1980) Modulation of adenylate cyclase in intact macrophages by microtubules. *J. Biol. Chem.*, 255: 2659–2662.

Halpain, S. and Lister, A.E. (1993) Glutamate receptor-stimulated dephosphorylation of the cytoskeletal protein MAP$_2$. *Soc. Neurosci. Abstr.*, 19: 273.

Hartwig, J.H., Thelen, M., Rosen, A., Janmey, P.A., Navin, A.C. and Aderem, A. (1992) MARCKS is an actin filament crosslinking protein regulated by protein kinase C and calcium-calmodulin. *Nature*, 356: 618–622.

Hatta, S., Amemiga, N., Oshika, H., Saito, T. and Ozawa, H. (1992) Tubulin modifies neuronal signal transduction through the association with G-proteins in rat cerebral cortex and striatum. *Soc. Neurosci. Abstr.*, 18: 285.

Kamada, H., Saito, T., Ozawa, H., Hatta, S., Hashimoto, E., Ashizawa, T., Rasenick, M.M. and Takahata, N. (1993) Effect of chronic anti-depressant treatment in tubulin function in rat brain. *Soc. Neurosci. Abstr.*, 19: 939.

Keith, C.H., Bajer, A.S., Ratan, R., Maxfield, F.R. and Schelanski, M.L. (1986) Calcium calmodulin in the regulation of the microtubular cytoskeleton. *Ann. N.Y. Acad. Sci.*, 466: 375–391.

Kelley, A.E., Finn, M., Cunningham, S.T., Renshaw, P. and Sachs, X. (1993) Lithium enhances behavioral response to cholera toxin infusion into nucleus accumbens. *Soc. Neurosci. Abstr.*, 19: 310.

Kennedy, M.S. and Insel, P.A. (1979) Inhibitors of microtubule assembly enhance β-adrenergic and prostaglandin E_1-stimulated c-AMP accumulation in S49 lymphoma cells. *Mol. Pharmacol.*, 16: 215–223.

Kim, J., Blackshear, P.J., Johnson, J.D. and McLaughlin, S. (1993) Phosphorylation by PKC reverses the association of peptides that mimic the calmodulin-binding domains of MARCKS and neuromodulin. *Biophys. J.*, 64: A59.

Klancnik, J.M. and Abercrombie, E.D. (1993) The effects of colchicine lesions of the dentate gyrus of the rat on dopamine release in the nucleus accumbens and on behavioural activity. *Soc. Neurosci. Abstr.*, 19: 487.

Kleiman, R., Banker, G. and Steward, Q. (1992) Dendritic transport of newly synthesized RNA is disrupted by microtubule poisons. *Soc. Neurosci. Abstr.*, 18: 66.

Klyner, R., Geisler, A. and Rosenberg, R. (1987) Enhanced histamine and β-adrenoreceptor mediated cyclic AMP formation in leukocytes from patients with endogenous depression. *J. Affect. Disord.*, 13: 227–232.

Knight, M.E. and Harris, J. (1993) Biochemical basis of neuromodulation by 2-phenylethylamine: effect on microtubule protein. *Neurochem. Res.*, 18: 1221–1229.

Lenox, R.H., Watson, D.G., Patel, J. and Ellis, J. (1992) Chronic lithium administration alters a prominent PKC substrate in rat hippocampus. *Brain Res.*, 570: 333–340.

Levine, I.H., Sayhoun, N.E. and Cuattrecasas, P. (1982) Properties of erythrocyte membrane cytoskeletal structures produced by digitonin extraction: digitonin-insoluble β-adrenergic receptor, adenylate cyclase and cholera toxin substrate. *J. Mem. Biol.*, 64: 225–231.

Linse, K. and Mandelkow, E.M. (1988) The GTP-binding peptide of β-tubulin. *J.Biol. Chem.*, 263: 15205–15210.

Lisman, J.E. and Harris, K.M. (1993) Quantal analysis and synaptic anatomy-integrating two views of hippocampal plasticity. *Trends Neurosci.*, 16: 141–147.

Manier, D.H., Gillespie, D.D. and Sulser, F. (1989) Dual aminergic regulation of central beta-adrenoceptors: effect of atypical anti-depressants and 5-hydroxytryptophan. *Neuropsychopharmacology*, 2: 89–95.

Menkes, D., Rasenick, M.M., Wheeler, M. and Bitensky, M. (1983) GTP activation of brain adenylate cyclase: enhancement by long-term anti-depressant treatment. *Science*, 219: 65–67.

Nestler, E.J., McMahan, A., Sabban, E.L., Tallman, J.E. and Duman, R.S. (1990) Chronic anti-depressant administration decreases the expression of tyrosine hydroxylases in rat locus conucleus. *Proc. Natl. Acad. Sci. USA*, 87: 7522–7526.

Nestler, E.J., Terwilliger, R.Z. and Duman, R.S. (1989) Chronic anti-depressant administration alters the subcellular distribution of cyclic AMP-dependent protein kinase in rat frontal cortex. *J. Neurochem.*, 53: 1644–1647.

Nicklas, W.J., Puszkin, S. and Berl, S. (1973) Effects of vinblastine and colchicine on uptake and release of putative transmitters by synaptosomes and on brain actinomysin-like protein. *J. Neurochem.*, 20: 109–121.

Nomura, Y. and Segawa, T. (1975) Influences of colchicine and vinblastine on the uptake of 5HT and NE by synaptosomes and small vesicle fractions. *J. Neurochem.*, 24: 1257–1259.

O'Leary, M.E. and Susgkiw, J.B. (1983) Effect of colchicine on Ca^{2+} and choline uptake and ACh release in synaptosomes. *J. Neurochem.*, 40: 1192–1195.

Ozawa, H. and Rasenick, M.M. (1989) Coupling of the stimulatory GTP-binding protein G_s to rat synaptic membrane adenylate cyclase is enhanced subsequent to chronic anti-depressant treatment. *Mol. Pharmacol.*, 36: 803–808.

Ozawa, H. and Rasenick, M.M. (1991) Chronic electroconvulsive treatment augments coupling of the GTP-binding protein G_s to the catalytic moiety of adenylate cyclase in a manner similar to that seen with chronic anti-depressant drugs. *J. Neurochem.*, 56: 330–338.

Perez, J., Tinelli, D., Cagnoli, C., Mori, S., Magloavaces, E. and Racagni, G. (1993) Microtubule associated protein 2 is an *in vitro* substrate for a GMP protein kinase. *Soc. Neurosci. Abstr.*, 19: 22.

Peters, R.A. (1956) Hormones and the cytoskeleton. *Nature*, 77: 426.

Poisner, A.M. and Bernstein, J. (1971) A possible role for microtubules in catecholamine release from the adrenal medulla: effect of colchicine, vinca alkaloids. *J. Pharm. Exp. Ther.*, 177: 102–108.

Rall, T.W., Sutherland, E.W. and Wasilant, W.O. (1956) The relationship of epinephrine and glucogen to liver phosphorylase. III. *J. Biol. Chem.*, 218: 483.

Rasenick, M.M., Stein, P.J. and Bitensky, M.W. (1981) The regulatory subunit of adenylate cyclase interacts with cytoskeletal components. *Nature*, 294: 560–562.

Richard, E., Faucon-Biguet, M., Lobatul, E., Rollet, D., Mallet, J. and Buda, M. (1988) Modulation of tyrosine hydroxylase gene expression in rat brain and adrenals by exposure to cold. *J. Neurosci. Res.*, 20: 32–37.

Roychowdhury, S. and Rasenick, M.M. (1994) Tubulin G-protein complex formation stabilizes the GTP binding and promotes GTPase: cytoskeletal participation in neuronal signal transduction. *Biochemistry*, 33: 9800–9805.

Rudolf, S.A., Hegstrand, L.R., Greengard, P. and Malawista, S.E. (1979) The interaction of colchicine with hormone-sensitive adenylate cyclase in human leucocytes. *Mol. Pharmacol.*, 16: 805–812.

Sahyoun, N.E., LeVine, I.H., Hebdon, G.M., Kouri, R.K. and Cuattrecasas, P. (1981) Evidence for cytoskeletal associations of the adenylate cyclase system obtained by differential extraction of erythrocyte ghosts. *Biochem. Biophys. Res. Commun.*, 101: 1003–1010.

Schacher, S., Kandel, E.R. and Montarolo, P. (1993) cAMP and arachidonic acid simulate long-term structural and functional changes produced by neurotransmitters in *Aplysia* sensory neurons. *Neuron*, 10(6):1079–1088.

Schildkraut, J.J. (1965) The catecholamine hypothesis of affective disorders: a review of supporting evidence. *Am. J. Psychiatry*, 122: 509–522.

Schildkraut, J.J. and Kety, S.S. (1967) Biogenic amines and emotion. *Science*, 156: 21–30.

Segawa, T., Muakami, H., Inouye, A. and Tanaka, Y. (1978) Influences of solchicine, vinblastine, and cytochalasin on the release of 5HT from synaptosomes. *J. Neurochem.*, 30: 175–180.

Sikra, T.S., Wang, J.K. T., Gorelick, F.S. and Greengard, P. (1989) Translocation of synapsin 1 in response to depolarization of isolated nerve terminals. *Proc. Natl. Acad. Sci. USA*, 86: 8108–8112.

Snyder, S.H., Banerjee, S.P., Yamamura, H.I. and Greenberg, D. (1974) Drugs, neurotransmitters and schizophrenia. *Science*, 184: 1243–1253.

Stephens, R.E. (1986) Membrane tubulin. *Biol. Cell*, 57: 95–110.

Sternlicht, H., Yaffe, M.B. and Farr, G.W. (1987) A model of the nucleotide binding site in tubulin. *FEBS Lett.*, 214: 223–235.

Striplin, C. and Kalivas, P.W. (1993) G-Protein alterations in cocaine self-administrating rats. *Soc. Neurosci. Abstr.*, 19: 309.

Sulser, F., Vetulani, J. and Mobley, P.L. (1978) Mode of action of anti-depressant drugs. *Biochem. Pharmacol.*, 27: 257–271.

Tan, Y.H. (1993) Yin-Yang of phosphorylation in cytokine signalling. *Science*, 262: 376–377.

Thoa, N.B., Wooten, G.F., Axelrod, J. and Kopin, I. (1972) Inhibition of release of dopamine-β-hydroxylase and NE from symphatic nerves by colchicine, vinblastine or cytochalasin-β. *Proc. Natl. Acad. Sci. USA*, 69: 520–522.

Vallano, M.L., Goldenring, J.R., Lasher, R.S. and Delorenzo, R.J. (1986) Association of Ca^{2+}/calmodulin-dependent kinase with cytoskeletal preparations: phosphorylation of tubulin, neurofilament and MAPs. *Ann. N.Y. Acad. Sci.*, 466: 357–374.

Vassilev, P., Kanazirska, M. and Titien, H. (1985) Intermediate linkage mediated by tubulin. *Biochem. Biophys. Res. Commun.*, 126: 559–565.

Wang, N. and Rasenick, M.M. (1991) Tubulin-G-protein interactions involve microtubule polymerization domains. *Biochemistry*, 30: 10957–10965.

Wang, N., Yan, K. and Rasenick, M.M. (1990) Tubulin binds specifically to the signal transducing proteins $G_{s\alpha}$ and $G_{i\alpha}1$. *J. Biol. Chem.*, 265: 1239–1242.

Weisenberg, R.C. (1972) Microtubule formation in vitro in solution containing low calcium concentrations. *Science*, 177: 1104–1105.

Wooten, G.F., Kopin, I.J. and Axelrod, J. (1974) Effects of colchicine and vinblastine on axonal transport and transmitter release in sympathetic nerves. *Ann. N.Y. Acad. Sci.*, 253: 528–534.

Yan, K. and Rasenick, M.M. (1990) Cytoskeletal participation in the spinal transuction process: Tubulin-G protein interaction in the regulation of adenylate cyclase in cultured glioma cells. In: J. Vanderhock (Ed.), *Biology of Cellular Signal Transducers*, Plenum Press, Amsterdam, pp. 163–172.

Young, L.T., Li, P.P., Kish, S.J., Liu, K.P., Karmble, A., Hornykiewiz, O. and Warsh, J.J. (1991) Cerebral cortex G-proteins and cAMP formation in bipolar affective disorders. *Soc. Neurosci. Abstr.* 18: 1596.

Young, L.T., Li, P.P., Kamble, A., Siu, K.P. and Warsh, J.J. (1993) Increased lymphocyte membrane $G_{\alpha s}$ and $G_{\alpha i}$ in bipolar but not major depressive disorder. *Soc. Neurosci. Abstr.*, 19: 34.

Zisapel, N., Levi, M. and Gozes, I. (1980) Tubulin: an integral protein of mammalian synaptic vesicle membranes. *J. Neurochem.*, 34: 26–32.

Peter M. Yu, Keith F. Tipton and Alan A. Boulton (Eds.)
Progress in Brain Research, Vol 106
© 1995 Elsevier Science BV. All rights reserved.

CHAPTER 25

Pharmacology and molecular biology of octopamine receptors from different insect species

T. Roeder, J. Degen, C. Dyczkowski and M. Gewecke

University of Hamburg, Zoological Institute, Neurophysiology, Martin-Luther-King-Platz 3, 20146 Hamburg, Germany

Introduction

The biogenic monoamine octopamine (OA), which was discovered in the salivary glands of octopus (Erspamer and Boretti, 1951), is the best-studied neuroactive substance in invertebrates. Its modulatory effects on most peripheral organs have been studied in great detail (Axelrod and Saavedra, 1977; Orchard, 1982; Evans, 1985; Saavedra, 1989). Not only are different muscles, such as the locust extensor-tibiae-muscle (Evans, 1981), the locust flight muscle (Lafon-Cazal and Bockaert, 1985), the locust lateral oviducts (Orchard and Lange, 1986), or the cockroach hyperneural muscle (Penzlin, 1994), targets of octopamine action, but also the fat body (Orchard and Lange, 1984) and endocrine organs such as the corpora cardiaca (Pannabecker and Orchard, 1986) and the corpora allata are modulated by this biogenic amine. In addition, the sensitivity of most, if not all sense organs is modulated by octopamine application. Among them are the optic pathway and the cricket auditory system (Lühr and Wiese, 1994). In both cases, it appears that the modulation takes place at the level of identified interneurons. In addition, proprioreception (Ramirez and French, 1990; Ramirez and Pearson, 1990) and olfaction as well as taste perception are modulated by this multipotent neuromodulator (Linn and Roelofs, 1986). This kind of modulation appears to be very important because it enables the insect to achieve optimal performance of these sensory systems, even when the sensory inputs vary strongly.

Nevertheless our knowledge about the physiological role of octopamine in the central nervous system is limited to very few examples (Bicker and Menzel, 1989), octopaminergic neuromodulation is, in comparison with other types of neuromodulation, much better characterized. The first example of a putative physiological role of OA in the central nervous system of insects derived from studies dealing with the flight motor system of locusts. Injection of OA into defined regions of the metathoracic ganglion leads to initiation of flight motor activity (Sombati and Hoyle, 1984). Comparable results were obtained using a similar approach in *Manduca sexta* (Claassen and Kammer, 1986) and in first instar larvae of locusts (Stevenson and Kutsch, 1988). A possible cellular substrate for this phenomenon was shown recently. Ramirez and Pearson (1991) were able to show that the bursting properties of an identified neuron that is involved in the flight motor generation is changed by OA application. In addition to the modulation and initiation of various rhythmic behaviors, this biogenic amine is also involved in complex processes such as learning and memory. Local injection of octopamine into defined areas of the honeybee brain was able to increase their learning ability as well as the retrieval of learned information (Menzel et al. 1989). A single pair of octopaminergic neurones that have their somata in the suboesophageal ganglion of the honeybee appears to be essential for associative olfactory learning. Electrical stimulation of these neurons substitutes the unconditioned stimulus in an associative olfactory learning paradigm (Hammer, 1993).

The various actions of octopamine are mediated through a set of at least four different octopamine receptor subtypes. All OA receptors characterized so far belong to the class of G-protein-coupled receptors. Most of them are positively coupled to adenylate cyclase. In the periphery, three OA receptors could be distinguished due to pharmacological differences (Evans, 1981). One of them, the so-called OA 2A receptor, appears to be the most abundant one (Evans, 1985). In the central nervous system of insects, a peculiar OA receptor class is present. It shows pharmacological features that are distinct from those of the peripheral OA receptors (Roeder, 1992; Roeder and Nathanson, 1993). It appears to be restricted in its occurrence to the nervous tissue. This receptor, which is responsible for the transmission of the various actions of octopamine in the nervous system, is positively coupled to adenylate cyclase (Nathanson and Greengard, 1973). Electrophysiological studies using isolated locust somata could confirm the peculiar pharmacology of this receptor type (Kaufmann and Benson, 1991).

Octopamine and noradrenaline

Although octopamine and noradrenaline are chemically not identical, it appears that octopaminergic systems of invertebrates and noradrenergic systems of vertebrates are homologous. OA, the neuroactive substance of invertebrates, has no known physiological role in vertebrates. On the other hand, NA, the important neurotransmitter of vertebrates, has no known physiological role in invertebrates. Therefore, it was speculated that octopamine is the "adrenergic" transmitter of invertebrates. This assumption is supported by the similar chemical structures of both substances, which are distinguished only by the hy-droxyl group at position 3 of the phenolic ring. Interestingly, octopaminergic and adrenergic systems have additional common features (Table 1). In the periphery, both NA and OA are thought to act as "stress hormones". The contractability of various muscles as well as glycogenolysis are increased in response to NA release. The actions of NA could be interpreted as part of the organism's adaptation to energy-demanding situations such as startle behavior. The physiological situation found in insects is similar. OA is also released in response to stress. This leads to a modification of the contraction properties of various muscles. In addition, the metabolism of the fat body, the major storage organ of insects, is activated by application of octopamine. This enables the insect to cope with energy-demanding situations such as long-term flight (Orchard and Lange, 1984).

This homology is also evident for the respective systems within the central nervous system. In both systems only relatively few neurons contain the respective neurotransmitter. In vertebrates, the locus coeruleus is the area where most somata of noradrenergic neurons are located. In man, only 24,000 neurones supply most other parts of the brain with noradrenaline (Foote, 1987). It is believed that each locus coeruleus neuron has synaptic contact with more than 10,000 other neurones. In insects, a small number of octopamine-containing neurons supply most neuropiles of the insect brain (Bräunig, 1991). Among the 40–50 octopaminergic neurons are the so called DUM (dorsal unpaired median) and VUM (ventral unpaired median) neurons (Konings et al., 1988). Both, NA and OA are thought to be involved in the regulation of the general neuronal activity, the "motivation" of the organism. In addition to these functional and structural homologies, the respective receptors share some common features. All adrenergic and octopaminergic receptors are G-protein-coupled. Pharmacological similarities are evident between α-adrenergic receptors on the one hand and octopaminergic receptors on the other hand. β-Adrenergic receptors are thought to be related to insect

TABLE 1

Comparison of adrenergic systems from vertebrates and octopaminergic systems from invertebrates

Adrenergic system of vertebrates	Octopaminergic system of invertebrates

Structure of the transmitters

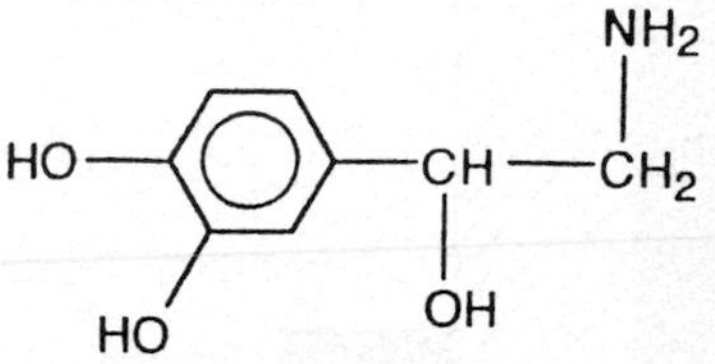

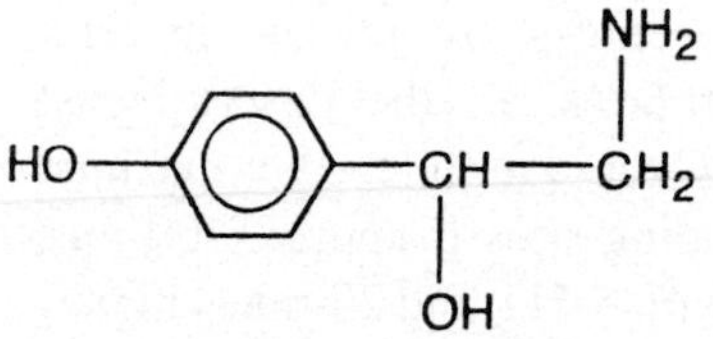

Structure and function of the transmitter systems

Periphery

acts as "stress" hormone; leads to -glycogenolysis -increase in muscle contraction preparation for energy demanding situations such as startle behaviour	"stress" hormone in peripheral tissues leads to -liberation of diacylglycerols from the fat body -increase in muscle contraction preparation for energy demanding situations such as startle behaviour and long term flight

Central nervous system

NA release leads to changes in the motivational state	octopamine release appears to be necessary for the initiation and maintenance of various behaviours
arousal appears to be regulated by NA	OA regulates "arousal" in the CNS
only few neurones contain noradrenaline Locus coeruleus (24 000 neurones in man)	very few cells in each ganglion contain octopamine DUM, VUM and very few other neurones (~ 40–50 cells in the brain)
all major parts of the brain are supplied with NA	all major neuropiles are densely innervated with octopaminergic projections

Receptors

G-protein coupled receptors α-adrenergic receptors β-adrenergic receptors coupled to adenylate cyclase	G-protein coupled receptors octopamine receptors tyramine receptors coupled to adenylate cyclase

tyramine receptors.

Pharmacology of insect neuronal octopamine receptors

The structure and pharmacology of octopamine receptors were studied using two different radioligands. In addition to the natural agonist octopamine, the phenlyiminoimidazolidine derivative ^{3}H-NC-5Z served as the second radioligand (Fig. 1; Dudai, 1982; Roeder and Gewecke, 1990; Nathanson et al., 1989; Roeder and Nathanson,

1993). Because it has a higher affinity and it is not degraded by endogenous enzymes, it is much better suited for ligand-binding studies (Nathanson, 1989). Using these radioligands, the octopamine receptor of the locusts *Schistocerca gregaria* and *Locusta migratoria* and the honey bee *Apis mellifera* were studied in detail. In all these preparations octopamine receptors are present in relatively high concentrations. In the desert locust *Schistocerca gregaria* for example, the maximal concentration of binding sites is approx. 10-times higher if compared with 5-HT and 20-times higher if compared with dopamine receptors (Fig. 2). Only the neuronal histamine H1-like receptor has a slightly higher concentration of binding sites. This indicates the important role of octopamine in the nervous system of insects.

Most pharmacological studies of insect neuronal octopamine receptors were performed using locusts. High-affinity antagonists are well suited

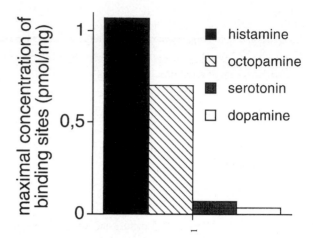

Fig. 2. The maximal concentration of binding sites of histamine, octopamine, serotonin and dopamine receptors in the locust central nervous system.

for physiological studies (Roeder, 1991). The most important among them are the tetracyclic substances mianserin (K_i = 1.2 nM) and, with even higher affinity, the structurally related substance maroxepine (K_i = 1.07 nM; Roeder, 1991). In recent experiments, another antagonist with interesting properties was characterized. It is a tetracyclic substance and has an affinity below 1 nM. Epinastine is perhaps the most important antagonist for octopamine receptors characterized so far (Fig. 3). It has, in contrast to all other high-affinity octopaminergic antagonists, only low-affinity properties for other receptors for biogenic amines in the central nervous system of insects. Its affinity for the neuronal 5-HT receptor, for example, is at least 5 orders of magnitude lower than that for the octopamine receptor. This is also true for the insect dopamine, tyramine, and histamine receptor. Therefore, this antagonist appears to be ideally suited for the specific blocking of octopaminergic neurotransmission in the insect nervous system which is a prerequisite for the physiological dissection of the various actions of octopamine.

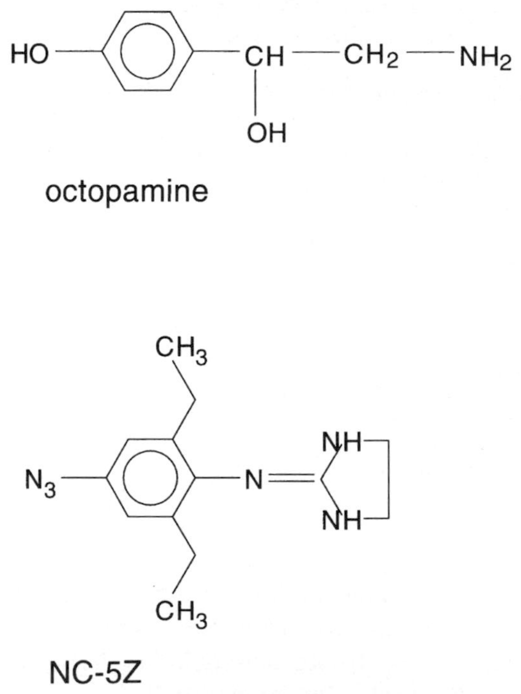

In comparison with octopamine receptor antagonists, agonists are much better characterized. Beside the natural agonist octopamine, biogenic

HO — ⬡ — CH — CH$_2$ — NH$_2$
　　　　　|
　　　　　OH

octopamine

CH$_3$

N$_3$ — N=⟨NH / NH⟩

CH$_3$

NC-5Z

Fig. 1. Structure of octopamine and NC-5Z used as radioligands for the characterization of neuronal octopamine receptors.

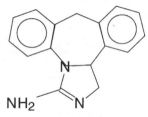

Fig. 3. Chemical structure of the high-affinity octopaminergic antagonist epinastine.

amines with a similar structure also have high-affinity properties. Two of them, the *N*-methylated analogue of octopamine synephrine and the biological precursor of OA tyramine, are of major interest. In most preparations, synephrine has an affinity that is higher than that of octopamine itself (in locusts $K_i = 3.3$ nM compared with 7 nM of OA). In honeybees, however, octopamine has a slightly higher affinity than synephrine. Tyramine, itself a neurotransmitter candidate in the insect nervous system (Saudou et al., 1991) has, in the locust nervous tissue, an affinity that is approx. 6-times lower than that of octopamine (Roeder and Gewecke, 1990).

Other agonists derived from different classes of compounds are of even greater importance. Among them are the so-called formamidines that were widely used as potent octopaminergic insecticides. The insecticide chlordimeform has a relatively low affinity if compared with octopamine (in locusts $K_i = 137$ nM). It is believed that chlordimeform is metabolized in the insect into the much more potent demethylchlordimeform, which is among the most potent agonists for octopamine receptors characterized so far (K_i in locusts $= 3.3$ nM). The study of structure-activity relationship using differentially substituted formamidines revealed some pharmacological features that could also be seen for other classes of compounds such as the phenyliminoimidazolidines (PIIs). In addition to the formamidines, substances with insecticidal activity such as amitraz or the aminooxazoline derivative AC-6 also have high-affinity properties (K_i in the locust nervous tissue $= 0.95$ nM; in the honey bee brain

$K_i = 0.52$ nM). This coincidence of high affinity with insecticidal activity led to the assumption that the insecticidal activity of these substances is the result of interaction with the octopamine receptor.

One of the most important classes of compounds, the phenyliminoimidazolidines (PIIs), are characterized by their high-affinity properties for octopamine receptors in general (Nathanson, 1985; Evans, 1987; Roeder and Gewecke, 1990). A variety of different compounds are available that are distinguished only by different substituents at the phenolic ring (Table 2). Although they have high-affinity properties for most OA receptors, different receptors have different substitution preferences. The OA receptor in the firefly lantern has a preference for 2,6-disubstituted PIIs (Nathanson, 1985). In contrast, substitution at position 6 of the phenolic ring has a negative effect on the affinity for the locust neuronal octopamine receptor preparation. In the locust nervous tissue, substitutions at the positions 2 and 4 of the phenolic ring gave maximal affinity. The same is true for the honeybee central nervous system octopamine receptor. Therefore, this differential substitution preference might reflect pharmacological differences between central OA receptors that belong to the OA class 3 and peripheral class 2A receptors (Table 2).

The study of structure-activity relationships of octopaminergic antagonists revealed some interesting features. At position 1 of the phenolic ring some substituents are preferred. Highest affinity was observed with heterocyclic substituents as present in the PIIs or the aminooxazolines. The heterocyclic ring needs a spacing group to the phenolic ring to have maximal affinity. If the spacing group is omitted, the affinity drops by 3 orders of magnitude (tolazoline $K_i = 18.5$ nM; phenyliminoimidazolidine $K_i = 23.4$ nM; 2-phenyl-2-imidazolidine $K_i = 16,200$ nM). The substitution that characterizes the natural agonist octopamine has an intermediate affinity (phenylethanolamine $K_i = 115$ nM). As mentioned above, substitutions at the positions 2 and 4 of the phenolic ring always have positive effects on

TABLE 2

Affinity of phenyliminoimidazolidines (PIIs) for the locust neuronal octopamine receptor

Substance	Substitution	K_1(nM)	K_{loc}/K_{lx}
NC 7	4-chlor-2-methyl-	0.3 ± 0.04	26.4
St 92	2,4,6-triethyl-	0.56 ± 0.14	14.2
NC 8	2,4-dichlor-	0.81 ± 0.18	9.73
NC 5	2,6-diethyl-	0.87 ± 0.32	9.04
NC 9	2,4-dimethyl-	1.02 ± 0.42	7.75
NC-5Z	4-azido-2,6-dimethyl-	1.05 ± 0.47	7.52
NC 3	2,4,5-trichlor-	2.27 ± 0.89	3.48
NC 13	2,4,6-trimethyl-	4.38 ± 1.3	1.8
NC 12	4-bromo-	14.9 ± 3.3	0.53
NC 11	2,4,6-trichlor-	18.7 ± 3	0.42
NC 4	2,6-dimethyl-	19.8 ± 6.5	0.4
NC 10	—	23.4 ± 4.7	0.34
p-Azidoclonidine	4-azido-2,6-dichlor-	44.5 ± 7.1	0.18
Clonidine	2,6-dichlor-	47.4 ± 17.5	0.17
p-Aminoclonidine	4-amino-2,6-dichlor-	58 ± 16.2	0.14
NC 20	2,6-diisopropyl-	132 ± 35.6	0.06

the affinity for the locust neuronal octopamine receptor (Fig. 4). At position 2, alkyl substitutions are more effective than chloride substitutions. The opposite is true for the position 4 of the phenolic ring. Interestingly, even bulky substitutions at position 4 of the phenolic ring are tolerated without loss in affinity (2,6-dichlor-PII (clonidine) K_i = 47.4 nM; 4-azido-clonidine K_i = 44.5 nM). This kind of substitution preference appears to be a more general feature of insect neuronal octopamine receptors, because in the honeybee brain similar observations were made. The use of other ligands that have a comparable structure, but whose spacing between the phenolic ring and the heterocycle is increased by an additional group, gave slightly different results. The substitution preference in the cockroach brain appears to be changed. XAMI which is a 2,3-di-methyl-substituted substance, has highest affinity

in this preparation (Orr et al., 1991). In the locust nervous tissue, another class of compounds appears to have comparable properties. The 2-ben-zyl-amino-thiazolines are a class of compounds that are also characterized by a spacing between the phenolic ring and the heterocycle that consists of two functional groups. As for XAMI, the positions 2 and 3 of the phenolic ring are most interesting. This is in contrast to the situation found using PIIs or formamidines. This different substitution preference might reflect changes in the steric situation of the agonist in the receptor binding site, caused by the increased length of the molecule.

Photoaffinity-labeling of octopamine receptors

The molecular characterization of octopamine receptors using classical methods was hampered by

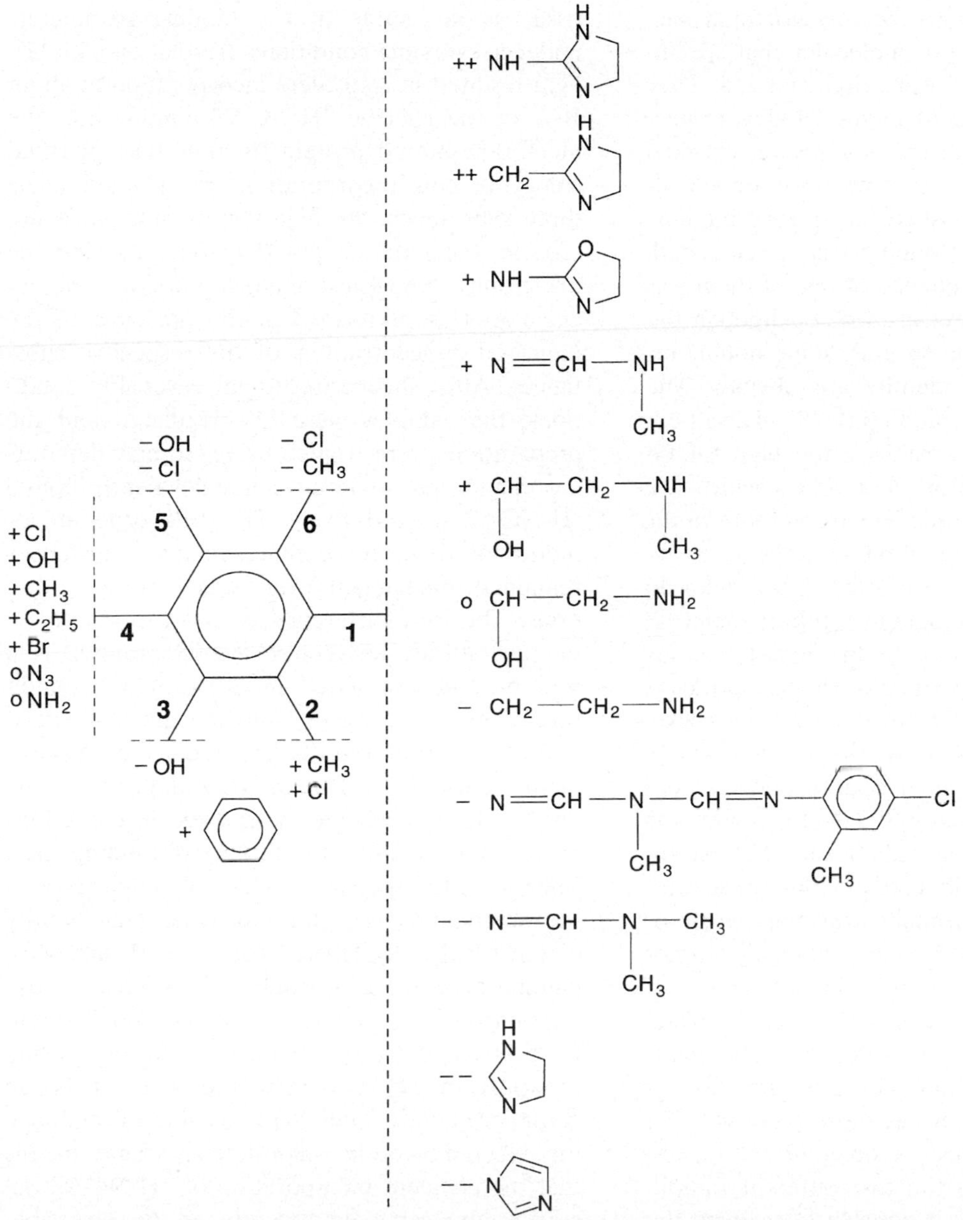

Fig. 4. Structure-activity relationship of agonists for the locust neuronal octopamine receptor. At each position, the effect of a given substitution is listed. + +, increase in affinity by more than 10-times; +, increase in affinity between 2- and 10-times; o, no effect on the affinity; − −, decrease in affinity by more than 10-times; −, decrease in affinty between 2- and 10-times.

the inability to solubilize the receptor molecule in an active state. This was a prerequisite for the further biochemical treatment with the goal of isolating the pure receptor molecule. As an alternative, photoaffinity-labeling was successfully used. A new photoaffinity label, the PII derivative ^{3}H-NC-5Z, was introduced by Nathanson and co-workers (Nathanson et al., 1989; Nathanson, 1989). It combines high affinity for octopamine receptors with its ability to bind covalently, if activated by UV light, to the receptor molecule. In the firefly lantern, two molecules that specifically bound ^{3}H-NC-5Z were characterized. They have molecular weights of 75 and 79 kDa, respectively. The specificity of the binding was checked by incubation with octopamine prior to UV illumination, which abolished the specific binding. Both molecules were found to be glycosylated, and the N-terminal sequence of one of them was evaluated (Nathanson et al., 1989). Although the binding appeared to be specific, some doubts regarding the receptor identity are obvious. The labeled protein represented up to 3% of a salt-extractable fraction. This value is too high for G-protein-coupled receptors and values which are even 1 order of magnitude less are not known for any tissue studied. Therefore, it appears to be possible that the specifically labeled molecules do not represent the octopamine receptor molecule (Nathanson et al., 1989). In the locust nervous tissue a well characterized octopamine receptor is present (Roeder, 1992; Roeder and Gewecke, 1990). It occurs in relatively high concentrations (Fig. 2) and shows peculiar pharmacological features. In this preparation [^{3}H]octopamine was successfully used as the radioligand. The photo-affinity label ^{3}H-NC-5Z binds in this tissue with high affinity to the neuronal octopamine receptor. Its affinity ($K_i = 1.5$ nM) is approximately 5-times that of octopamine. To study the interaction of this ligand with the octopamine receptor, pharmacological studies were performed. The pharmacological features that are seen with this ligand are exactly the same as those seen with the tritiated natural agonist octopamine. If the K_i values obtained using the two different radioligands are compared, it is possible to evaluate the homology between both labeled binding sites. The pharmacological profiles obtained from both studies are more or less congruent because the respective K_i values were almost the same. Therefore, it is reasonable that ^{3}H-NC-5Z could be used as a radioligand for the study of neuronal octopamine receptors under reversible conditions. The next step towards the molecular characterization of octopamine receptors from locust nervous

tissue is the study of the binding parameters under irreversible conditions. Irradiation with UV light resulted in a covalent incorporation of about 10% of the specific ^{3}H-NC-5Z binding into the membrane-bound protein fraction. The pharmacology of this incorporation was studied using three substances, the high-affinity antagonist mianserin, the natural agonist octopamine and the low-affinity antagonist metoclopramide. The incubation was performed in the presence of the indicated concentrations of the respective substances. After incubation under reversible conditions, the samples were UV-irradiated and the preparations were treated using strongly denaturing conditions, to remove non-covalently bound ^{3}H-NC-5Z quantitatively. The rank order of affinities of these three representative substances remained unchanged even under these conditions. The only difference is that the affinity of the low-affinity antagonist metoclopramide is a little bit underestimated under irreversible conditions. This could result from the quick dissociation of low-affinity substances under these experimental conditions. This pharmacological identity under either reversible or irreversible conditions mirrors the identity of both labeled binding sites. Therefore, the specific covalent labeling occurs at the octopamine receptor molecule. The identity of the specifically labeled protein with the octopamine receptor could only be proven by those pharmacological studies. The labeled protein fraction could not be solubilized effectively using a variety of classical detergents such as Triton X-100 or cholate. Only SDS was able to solubilize the labeled protein quantitatively. That means that the covalent incorporation of ^{3}H-NC-5Z occurs at the same binding site as the reversible binding, the octopamine receptor molecule. Using SDS-electrophoresis it was possible to further characterize the specifically labeled octopamine receptor molecule. Incubation was performed in the absence (normal) and in the presence of 10 mM octopamine (control) prior to illumination with UV light, to covalently cross-link the label with the receptor molecule. The two samples were run in parallel, and the gel was sliced subse-

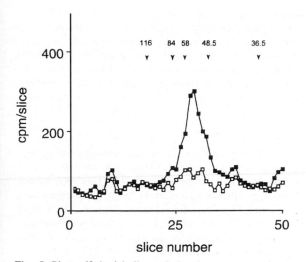

Fig. 5. Photoaffinity-labeling of the locust neuronal octopamine receptor using ³H-NC-5Z as the radio-ligand. Samples were incubated with ³H-NC-5Z in the presence (●) and absence (□) of 10 mM octopamine prior to irradiation with UV light. The solubilized samples were run in parallel in an SDS-PAGE and the gel was subsequently sliced (1.5 mm). Each slice was resolubilized and the radioactivity was quantified. To determine the molecular weight, standard proteins were run in parallel.

quently into 1.5 mm slices. The gel slices were resolubilized and the radioactivity was measured. Whereas the control shows a relatively low activity over the whole range, a marked increase in the non-control situation could be seen. This increase occurred at a molecular weight of approx. 53 kDa. This peak in activity corresponds with the locust neuronal octopamine receptor molecule (Fig. 5). 53 kDa is a value that fits well with the estimated molecular weights of various G-protein-coupled receptors.

In addition to the estimation of the molecular weight, some other features of this molecule were studied. If the receptor is solubilized using nonionic detergents such as Nonidet P-40 it is possible to study the glycosylation of the receptor molecule. Although this kind of solubilization is not as effective as SDS solubilization, the solubilized material is sufficient for subsequent studies. If applied to immobilized lectins, its glycosyla-

tion pattern could easily be studied. Most lectins did not bind any solubilized activity at all. Among them are well known lectins such as the lectin of *Ricinus communis*, the lectin of *Glycine maximus*, or wheat germ agglutinin. Only two lectins, the lentil lectin and the Con A lectin, bound solubilized receptors in reasonable amounts. Con A was much more effective than the lentil lectin. Both lectins are known to bind specifically to mannose-like terminal sugars. The higher binding capacity was expected because Con A binds with greater affinity to these sugars than the lentil lectin does. Specific elution was performed using high concentrations of the sugar α-D-mannopyranoside. The amount of activity that could be eluted using this sugar was more than two times higher for the lentil lectin than for the Con A lectin, which might be due to the lower affinity of the lentil lectin for the mannose-like sugar structures.

Using molecular biological techniques it should be possible to characterize octopamine receptors in more detail. This is a prerequisite for the further characterization of octopaminergic systems.

Acknowledgements

The work in our group was supported by grants from the DFG (Ge 249/12–1) and the GTZ (integrated biological control of grasshoppers and locusts).

References

Axelrod, J. and Saavedra, J.M. (1977) Octopamine. *Nature*, 265: 501–504.

Bicker, G. and Menzel, R. (1989) Chemical codes for the control of behaviour in arthropods. *Nature*, 337: 33–39.

Bräunig, P. (1991) Suboesophageal DUM neurons innervate the principal neuropiles of the locust brain. *Phil Trans. R. Soc. Lond. B*, 332: 221–240.

Claassen, D.E. and Kammer, A.E. (1986) Effects of octopamine, dopamine, and serotonin on production of flight motor output by thoracic ganglia of *Manduca sexta*. *J. Neurobiol.*, 8: 49–63.

Dudai, Y. (1982) High-affinity octopamine receptors revealed in *Drosophila* by binding of [^{3}H]octopamine. *Neurosci. Lett.*, 28: 163–178.

Erspamer, V. and Boretti, G. (1951) Idenfication and characterization by paper chromatography of enteramine, octopamine, tyramine, histamine, and allied substances in extracts of posterior salivary glands of Octopoda and in other tissue extracts of vertebrates and invertebrates. *Arch. Int. Pharmacodyn.*, 88: 296–332.

Evans, P.D. (1981) Multiple receptor types for octopamine in the locust. *J. Physiol.*, 318: 99–122.

Evans, P.D. (1985) Octopamine. In: G.A. Kerkut and C. Gilbert (Eds.), *Comprehensive Insect Phsiology, Biochemistry and Pharmacology*, Pergamon Press, London, pp. 499–530.

Evans, P.D. (1987) Phenyliminoimidazolidine derivatives activate both octopamine1 and octopamine2 receptor subtypes in locust skeletal muscle. *J. Exp. Biol.*, 129: 239–250.

Foote, S.L. (1987) Locus coeruleus. In: G. Adelman (Ed.), *Encyclopedia of Neuroscience*, Birkhäuser, Stuttgart, pp. 596–597.

Hammer, M. (1993) An identified neuron mediates the unconditioned stimulus in associative olfactory learning in honeybees. *Nature*, 366: 59–63.

Kaufmann, L. and Benson, J.A. (1991) Characterization of a locust neuronal octopamine response. *Soc. Neurosci. Abstr.*, 17: 277.

Konings, P.N.M., Vullings, H.G.B., Geffard, M., Buijs, R.M., Diederen, J.H.B. and Jansen, W.F. (1988) Immunocytochemical demonstration of octopamine-immunoreactive cells in the nervous system of *Locusta migratoria* and *Schistocerca gregaria*. *Cell Tiss. Res.*, 251: 371–379.

Lafon-Cazal, M. and Bockaert, J. (1985) Pharmacological characterization of octopamine-sensitive adenylate cyclase in the flight muscle of *Locusta migratoria* L. *Eur. J. Pharmacol.*, 119: 53–59.

Linn, C.E. and Roelofs, W.L. (1986) Modulatory effects of octopamine and serotonin on male sensitivity and periodicity of response to sex pheromone in the cabbage looper moth, *Trichuplusia ni*. *Arch. Insect Biochem. Physiol.*, 3: 161–171.

Lühr, B. and Wiese, K. (1994) Octopaminergic modulation of the auditory pathway in the cricket *Gryllus bimaculatus*. In: N. Elsner and H. Breer (Eds.), *Göttinger Neurobiology Report*, Thieme, Stuttgart, p. 329.

Menzel, R., Wittstock, S. and Sugawa, M. (1989) Chemical codes of learning and memory in the honey bees. In: L.R. Squirre and E. Lindenlaub (Eds.), *The Biology of Memory*, Schattauer, Stuttgart, pp. 335–355.

Nathanson, J.A. (1985) Characterization of octopamine-sensitive adenylate cyclase: elucidation of a class of potent and selective octopamine-2 receptor agonists with toxic effects in insects. *Proc. Natl. Acad. Sci. USA*, 82: 599–603.

Nathanson, J.A. (1989) Development of a photoaffinity ligand for octopamine receptors. *Mol. Pharmacol.*, 35: 34–43.

Nathanson, J.A. and Greengard, P.A. (1973) Octopamine-sensitive adenylate cyclase: evidence for a biological role of octopamine in nervous tissue. *Science*, 180: 308–310.

Nathanson, J.A., Kantham, L. and Hunnicutt, E.J. (1989) Isolation and N-terminal amino acid sequence of an octopamine ligand binding protein. *FEBS Lett.*, 259: 117–120.

Orchard, I. (1982) Octopamine in insects: neurotransmitter, neurohormone, and neuromodulator. *Can. J. Zool.*, 60: 659–669.

Orchard, I. and Lange, A.B. (1984) Cyclic AMP in locust fat body: correlation with octopamine and adipokinetic hormones during flight. *J. Insect Physiol.*, 30: 901–904.

Orr, N., Orr, G.L. and Hollingworth R.M. (1991) Characterization of a potent agonist of the insect octopamine-receptor-coupled adenylate cyclase. *Insect Biochem.*, 21: 335–340.

Pannabecker, T. and Orchard, I. (1986) Pharmacologcial properties of octopamine-2 receptors in locust neuroendocrine tissue. *J. Insect Physiol.*, 32: 909–915.

Penzlin, H. (1994) Antagonistic control of the hyperneural muscle in *Periplaneta americana* (L). *J. Insect Physiol.*, 40: 39–51.

Ramirez, J.-M. and French, A.S. (1990) Phentolamine selectively affects the fast sodium component of sensory adaptation in an insect mechanoreceptor. *J. Neurobiol.*, 21: 893–899.

Ramirez, J.-M. and Pearson, K.G. (1990) Chemical deafferentation of the locust flight system by phentolamine. *J. Comp. Physiol.*, 167A: 485–494.

Ramirez, J.-M. and Pearson, K.G. (1991) Octopamine induces bursting and plateau potentials in insect neurones. *Brain Res.*, 549: 332–337.

Roeder, T. (1991) High-affinity anatgonists of the locust neuronal octopamine receptor. *Eur. J. Pharmacol.*, 191: 221–224.

Roeder, T. (1992) A new class of octopamine receptors, the octopamine 3 (OAR3) receptor. *Life Sci.*, 50: 21–28.

Roeder, T. and Gewecke, M. (1990) Octopamine receptors in locust nervous tissue. *Biochem. Pharmacol.*, 39: 1793–1797.

Roeder, T. and Nathanson, J.A. (1993) Characterization of insect neuronal octopamine receptors (OA3 receptors). *Neurochem. Res.*, 18: 921–925.

Saavedra, J.M. (1989) β-Phenylethylamine, phenylethanolamine, tyramine and octopamine. *Handbook Exp. Pharmacol.*, 90: 181–210.

Saudou, F., Amlaiky, N., Plassat, J.-L., Borelli, E. and Hen, R. (1991) Cloning and characterization of a *Drosophila* tyramine receptor. *EMBO J.*, 9: 3611–3617.

Sombati, S. and Hoyle, G. (1984) Generation of specific behaviours in a locust by local release into neuropil of the natural neuromodulator octopamine. *J. Neurobiol.*, 6: 481–506.

Stevenson, P.A. and Kutsch, W. (1986) Basic circuitry of an adult-specific motor program completed with embryogenesis. *Naturwissenschaften*, 73: 741–743.

Peter M. Yu, Keith F. Tipton and Alan A. Boulton (Eds.)
Progress in Brain Research, Vol 106

Agonist-specific coupling of G-protein-coupled receptors to second-messenger systems

Peter D. Evans[1], Sandra Robb[1], Timothy R. Cheek[1], Vincenzina Reale[1], Frances L. Hannan[1], Lesley S. Swales[1], Linda M. Hall[2] and John M. Midgley[3]

[1]*The Babraham Institute Laboratory of Molecular Signalling, Department of Zoology, University of Cambridge Downing Street, Cambridge CB2 3EJ, UK,* [2]*Department of Biochemical Pharmacology, School of Pharmacy, State University of New York, Buffalo, NY 14260, USA, and* [3]*Department of Pharmaceutical Sciences, University of Strathclyde, Royal College, 204 George Street, Glasgow G1 1XW, UK*

Introduction

Single agonists can effect changes in the levels of multiple second messengers in cells by a number of different pathways (Fig. 1). It has been known for some considerable time that single agonists can interact with different subtypes of G-protein-coupled receptors, each of which can be coupled to a specific second-messenger system (Bylund, 1992; Hosey, 1992). However, the use of cloned receptors has shown recently that single G-protein-coupled receptors may potentially couple to multiple second-messenger systems (Thompson, 1992). Thus, the cloned muscarinic-M2 (Lai et al., 1991) and α_2-adrenergic (Cotecchia et al., 1990) receptors both stimulate phosphoinositide hydrolysis and inhibit adenylate cyclase activity, whilst the cloned receptors for thyrotropin (Van Sande et al., 1990), calcitonin (Chabre et al., 1992), parathyroid hormone (Abou-Samra et al., 1992) and three classes of tachykinin receptor (Mitsuhashi et al., 1992; Nakajima et al., 1992) all stimulate both pathways. Evidence is now emerging for a third class of interactions between agonists and second-messenger systems, where naturally occurring structurally related agonists, which act on a single receptor, can induce different conformatio-

nal changes in the receptor when bound, which allows the receptor to preferentially activate different G-protein-mediated second-messenger pathways (Evans and Robb, 1993; Spengler et al., 1993; Robb et al., 1994). The present paper will review the current evidence for the concept of agonist-specific coupling of G-protein-coupled receptors to multiple second-messenger systems. It will also discuss the related concept of synthetic ligand-specific coupling of G-protein-coupled receptors to second-messenger systems. The important general implications of these concepts for pharmacology and signalling mechanisms will be examined.

Expression studies on a cloned *Drosophila* octopamine / tyramine receptor

A putative seven transmembrane-spanning receptor (Fig. 2) which can be activated by both octopamine and tyramine has been cloned from *Drosophila* (Arakawa et al., 1990; Saudou et al., 1990). A comparison of its deduced amino acid sequence with those of a range of mammalian receptors reveals that it has the highest homology with vertebrate α_2 adrenergic receptors. However, the *Drosophila* receptor has a much longer third in-

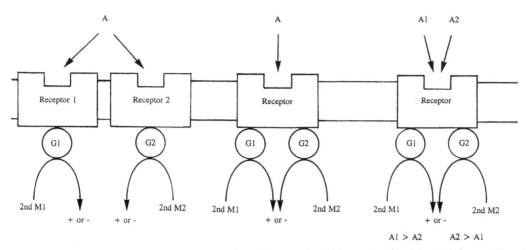

Fig. 1. Schematic diagram showing a number of possible ways in which agonists (A, A1 and A2) can effect changes in different second-messenger systems (M1 and M2) by interactions with independent G-protein-coupled pathways (G1 and G2). The scheme on the left shows the interaction of a single agonist with different receptor subtypes, each of which is coupled to a different second-messenger system. The middle scheme shows an agonist activating a single receptor which is directly coupled to two second-messenger systems. The scheme on the right shows agonist-specific coupling of a single receptor to two second-messenger systems.

tracellular loop between membrane-spanning elements five and six than any cloned α-adrenergic receptor.

The pharmacology of this receptor has been studied using [³H]yohimbine, the α_2-adrenergic antagonist, in radioligand binding studies on membranes prepared from a Chinese hamster ovary (CHO) K1 cell line permanently transfected with the *Drosophila* octopamine/tyramine receptor (Arakawa et al., 1990; Robb et al., 1994). The fact that tyramine was a much more potent displacer of [³H]yohimbine binding than octopamine suggests that this receptor represents a novel class of receptor, despite sharing some pharmacological similarities with the OCTOPAMINE$_1$ subtype of receptor from locust skeletal muscle (Evans, 1981; Arakawa et al., 1990). This finding is in agreement with those from an independent isolation of the same gene expressed in a different vertebrate cell line (Saudou et al., 1990). In addition, the receptor expressed in the CHO cell line showed little or no stereoselectivity between the (+)- and (−)-enantiomers of the most potent structural isomers of octopamine and synephrine.

This contrasts with previous studies on the pharmacological characterization of other insect octopamine receptors using physiological and biochemical studies, where the (−)-isomers were much more potent than the (+)-isomers of octopamine and synephrine (Evans, 1980, 1981, 1984a,b, 1993; Evans et al., 1988). The rank order of potency of both the (+)- and (−)-enantiomers of the positional isomers of octopamine (*o*-octopamine = *p*-octopamine > *m*-octopamine) is also different from that found for locust octopamine receptors (Evans et al., 1988) and for vertebrate α- and β-adrenergic receptors (Jordan et al., 1987; Brown et al., 1988). The finding of a [³H]yohimbine binding site in a membrane preparation from *Drosophila* heads with a similar pharmacology to that of the cloned receptor suggests that the unusual pharmacological properties of the latter receptor are not due to its expression in a vertebrate cell line (Robb et al., 1994).

The *Drosophila* octopamine/tyramine receptor can couple to multiple second-messenger systems when expressed in the CHO cells (Arakawa et al., 1990; Robb et al., 1991, 1994). When activated by

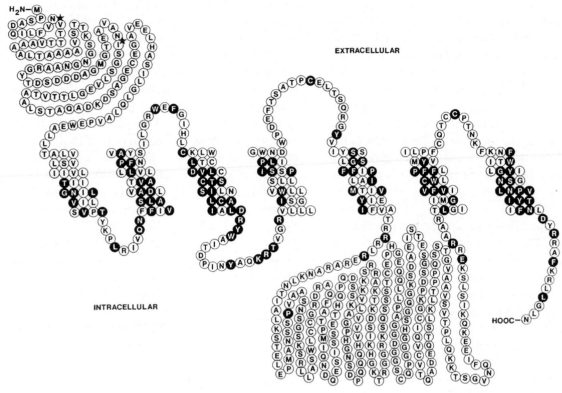

Fig. 2. Structural motif of the cloned *Drosophila* octopamine/tyramine receptor based on its deduced amino acid sequence as determined by Arakawa et al. (1990). Amino acids conserved between this receptor and α_2-adrenergic sequences are shown in black.

either octopamine or tyramine it can inhibit the forskolin-induced accumulation of cyclic AMP levels in the cells by a mechanism which is blocked by pretreatment of the cells with pertussis toxin and which is also blocked by low concentrations of yohimbine. This effect is again non-stereospecific for the (+)- and (−)-enantiomers of the positional isomers of octopamine and the pharmacology of the effect closely parallels the [^{3}H]yohimbine binding studies, with tyramine being two orders of magnitude more potent than octopamine. The *Drosophila* receptor can also transiently raise intracellular Ca^{2+} levels in single transfected CHO cells when activated by either octopamine or tyramine (Robb et al., 1991, 1994). The effect is transient even in the presence of a prolonged exposure to the agonist and is medi-

ated via a pertussis toxin insensitive pathway. The Ca^{2+} transients initiated in the cells by either tyramine or octopamine are dose-dependent and both the lag time before the onset of a Ca^{2+} response and the time to the peak of a Ca^{2+} transient decrease over the range 0.1–100 μM for both DL-octopamine and tyramine. Previous single-cell studies have shown a similar relationship between ligand concentration and the latency of the response (Millard et al., 1988; Monck et al., 1988; Corps et al., 1989). It is known that a range of other cloned G-protein-coupled receptors when expressed in CHO cells can activate phospholipase C, leading to a production of inositol trisphosphate (IP$_3$) and a release of intracellular Ca^{2+} from IP$_3$-sensitive stores (e.g. human 5-HT$_{1A}$ receptors, Raymond et al., 1992; three tachykinin receptors, Nakajima et al., 1992). However, in parallel experiments with the CHO cell line transfected with the *Drosophila* octopamine/tyramine receptor, we have not been able to demonstrate any agonist-specific increases in inositol phosphate levels (Robb, Cheek and Evans, unpublished observations). Nevertheless, in single-cell Ca^{2+} imaging experiments (Cheek, Robb and Evans, unpublished observations) depletion of the ryanodine-sensitive Ca^{2+} stores, by exposure of the cells to caffeine in the presence of ryanodine, substantially blocked the responses of the cells to applied octopamine or tyramine. Thus, the *Drosophila* octopamine/tyramine receptor when expressed in CHO cells appears to produce a transient elevation of intracellular Ca^{2+} levels by a mechanism involving the release of Ca^{2+} from ryanodine-sensitive stores. This could occur by two possible mechanisms. A direct second messenger, for instance cyclic ADP ribose (Berridge, 1994), could couple the receptor to release of Ca^{2+} from ryanodine-sensitive Ca^{2+} stores. A second possible mechanism could involve the receptor-mediated production of extremely small, undetectable, amounts of IP_3 which could then release small amounts of Ca^{2+} from IP_3-sensitive stores, which in turn could induce a massive efflux of Ca^{2+} from the ryanodine-sensitive stores by a calcium-induced calcium release mechanism. These possibilities are currently being investigated.

The coupling of the cloned *Drosophila* octopamine/tyramine receptor to the changes in cyclic AMP levels is direct and not a secondary consequence of changes in intracellular Ca^{2+} levels (Robb et al., 1994). Neither the cell-permeant Ca^{2+} chelator 1,2-bis-(2-aminophenoxy)-ethane-N,N,N',N'-tetraacetic acid (BAPTA), or externally applied lanthanum, affects the agonist-induced changes in cyclic AMP levels. In addition, the time courses of the two second-messenger events are different, with the changes in cyclic AMP levels being maintained for as long as the cells are exposed to the agonist, in contrast to the transient nature of the induced changes in Ca^{2+} levels. Thus, the cloned *Drosophila* octopamine/tyramine receptor appears to be one of a growing list of receptors that can potentially couple to more than one second-messenger system (see Milligan, 1993), indicating that this phenomenon is shared by certain groups of both vertebrate and invertebrate G-protein-coupled receptors. The majority of cases reported to date have been found in studies on cloned receptors expressed in cell lines, and the criticism has been raised that the results from such studies may be a function of the overexpression of the receptor in the cell line and not necessarily an indication of its physiological action in its normal environment (Taylor, 1990). However, an increasing number of observations of the same phenomenon are now being reported for endogenously expressed G-protein-coupled receptors (Chakraborty et al., 1991; Crawford et al., 1992; Wolsing and Rosenbaum, 1993). The *Drosophila* octopamine/tyramine receptor inhibition of forskolin-stimulated increases in cyclic AMP levels is mediated by a pertussis toxin-sensitive G-protein-coupled pathway, whilst its elevation in intracellular Ca^{2+} levels is mediated via an independent pathway which is pertussis toxin-insensitive. It remains to be demonstrated whether the receptor can be coupled to both second-messenger pathways in an individual *Drosophila* neurone or whether the observed phenomenon reflects the ability of this receptor to couple to different second-messenger systems when expressed in different cells with different complements of G-proteins. Further, it seems possible that factors that control the expression of G-proteins themselves could switch the second-messenger responses induced by this receptor in a single cell.

An additional level of complexity in the coupling of the cloned *Drosophila* octopamine/tyramine receptor to the two second-messenger pathways was revealed in detailed studies of the relative potency of octopamine and tyramine in inducing the transient changes in

Ca^{2+} levels in single transfected CHO cells (Evans and Robb, 1993; Robb et al., 1994). Unlike both the ligand binding studies and cyclic AMP attenuation studies where tyramine was almost two orders of magnitude more potent than octopamine, in the single-cell Ca^{2+} imaging experiments octopamine was equipotent with tyramine when the peak amplitudes of the Ca^{2+} transients were compared. The measurement of peak Ca^{2+} responses from cells, however, is complex and can be strongly influenced by the degree of Ca^{2+} loading of the internal stores in individual cells. Thus, we also examined the kinetics of the induced Ca^{2+} responses and found that octopamine consistently produced effects with shorter lag times and shorter times to peak Ca^{2+} responses.

We have recently examined the expression of the *Drosophila* octopamine/tyramine receptor in *Xenopus* oocytes to see if its coupling to calcium-release mechanisms differs when it is expressed in different cell types (Reale, Hannan, Midgley and Evans, unpublished observation). In voltage-clamped oocytes expressing this receptor both octopamine and tyramine application leads to the production of oscillatory currents superimposed upon a maintained inward current. The induced current is due to the activation of the endogenous oocyte calcium-sensitive chloride current. The expressed receptor exhibits a similar pharmacological profile to that described above for its expression in CHO cells. Tyramine and octopamine are also equipotent in initiating the current responses in expressing oocytes, with thresholds for the induction of inward currents occurring between 10^{-7} and 10^{-6} M for both amines. In addition, the responses showed no stereospecificity for the (+)- and (−)- enantiomers of *p*-octopamine. Further studies are currently under way to evaluate the nature of the oocyte G-proteins involved in the coupling of this receptor to the calcium signals when it is activated by either octopamine or tyramine.

The above expression studies reopen the debate as to whether this cloned *Drosophila* aminergic receptor is really an octopamine (Arakawa et al., 1990) or a tyramine (Saudou et al., 1990) receptor, but the resolution of this question must await the demonstration of its endogenous ligand at specific cellular locations. However, it could be a multifunctional receptor that is activated by octopamine at some locations and by tyramine at other locations, depending upon the identity of the amine released presynaptically. Equally, the receptor may be involved in a novel form of modulation, whereby agents that can alter the ratio of octopamine and tyramine (the immediate biochemical precursor of octopamine) released from octopaminergic neurones in insects could bias the postsynaptic responses of an effector cell to favour one second-messenger system over another.

An important point to consider in the above expression studies on the *Drosophila* octopamine/tyramine receptor in the CHO cells is that the results observed are not likely to be the result of the production of multiple receptors due to alternative splicing, since our binding studies indicate a single binding site for our ligand and since a polymerase chain reaction (PCR) analysis of transfected CHO cell mRNA using closely spaced overlapping primer pairs gave no evidence for the production of multiple transcripts (Robb et al., 1994). Equally, it is unlikely that our results can be explained by a differential post-translational modification of some of the receptor population, by for instance a differential glycosylation. Recent Western blot studies of transfected CHO cell membrane proteins, using a range of antibodies raised against peptides corresponding to different regions of the receptor, only give rise to a single positive product of the expected molecular weight for the receptor (unpubished observation). In general terms, it would appear that agonists differing by only a single hydroxyl in their side chain may be able to bias the interactions of a single G-protein-coupled receptor with multiple second-messenger systems by inducing specific conformational changes which enable it to couple

264

preferentially to separate G-proteins (Fig. 3). Thus, a single receptor may have a different pharmacological profile depending on which second-messenger system is used to assay its efficacy.

Expression studies on cloned vertebrate G-protein-coupled receptors

Agonist-specific coupling of G-protein-coupled receptors to second-messenger systems may be a general property shared by a range of different receptors. A cloned type 1 pituitary adenylyl cyclase-activating polypeptide (PACAP) receptor, and four spliced variant forms of the receptor, have been reported to be differentially coupled to

adenylate cyclase and phospholipase C by two naturally occurring forms of PACAP, namely PACAP-27 and PACAP-38 (Spengler et al., 1993). PACAP-27 was slightly more potent than PACAP-38 in stimulating cyclic AMP production when the receptor was transiently expressed in the LLC PK1 kidney cell line. However, when the ability of the two peptides to increase inositol phosphate production was assayed, PACAP-38 was found to be two orders of magnitude more potent than PACAP-27. The physiological significance of this observation is not yet clear. However, the basic message appears to be the same as for the cloned *Drosophila* receptor described above. In both cases the ability of a naturally

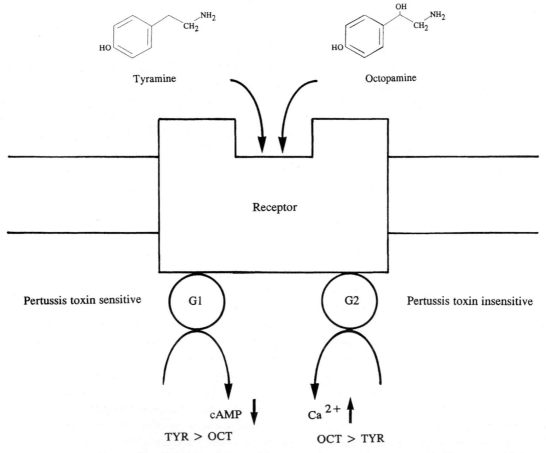

Fig. 3. Agonist-specific coupling of the cloned *Drosophila* octopamine/tyramine receptor to different second-messenger pathways.

occurring agonist to couple a receptor to one second-messenger system cannot necessarily predict its ability to couple the same receptor to a different second-messenger system. Equally, two naturally occurring agonists of a single receptor may couple the receptor differentially to multiple second-messenger systems.

Studies on several vertebrate cloned G-protein-coupled receptors have also demonstrated that a range of synthetic ligands which can act as agonists of these receptors may also be capable of coupling the receptors differentially to different second-messenger systems (Gurwitz et al., 1991, 1994; Eason et al., 1994). Thus, a range of muscarinic ligands can differentially couple the cloned M1-muscarinic cholinergic receptor (m1AChR) to different second-messenger systems when expressed in CHO cells (Gurwitz et al., 1991, 1994). Carbachol and pilocarpine are almost equipotent at coupling this receptor to inositol phosphate production and arachidonic acid release in CHO cells, whilst AF102B, a rigid M1-selective cholinergic agonist, only appears to be a partial agonist of these responses. However, whilst carbachol increases both basal and forskolin-stimulated cyclic AMP levels in the CHO cells transfected with the m1AChR, pilocarpine and AF102B have no effect on basal cyclic AMP levels and AF102B attenuates both forskolin- and carbachol-stimulated cyclic AMP accumulation. It is possible that a mechanism of ligand-induced conformational change in the expressed receptor, similar to those described above, may underlie the ability of the cloned muscarinic receptor to couple to different G-protein-mediated second-messenger systems. The design of muscarinic ligands which can selectively activate distinct second-messenger pathways may be important in cholinergic replacement therapy for treating Alzheimer's disease (Gurwitz et al., 1994).

A similar phenomenon has also been described recently for the coupling of α_2-adrenergic receptor subtypes to the activation of G_i and G_s-mediated effects on adenylate cyclase activity (Eason et al., 1994). When expressed in CHO cells the cloned human $\alpha_2 C10$, $\alpha_2 C4$ and $\alpha_2 C2$ adrenergic receptors can exert dual concentration dependent effects on adenylate cyclase activity. Low concentrations of both epinephrine and norepinephrine couple the three receptors to an inhibition of forskolin-stimulated adenylate cyclase activity via a G_i-type G-protein that can be inhibited by pertussis toxin. In contrast, at higher concentrations both these catecholamines couple the three receptors to a potentiation of forskolin-stimulated adenylate cyclase activity via a G_s-type G-protein. However, several synthetic agonists, including the imidazolines, UK14304 and oxymetazoline, and the azepines, BHT 920 and BHT 933, whilst being full agonists of the coupling of all three cloned receptors to the G_i-mediated inhibition of forskolin-stimulated adenylate cyclase activity, show a differential coupling of the G_s-mediated effects to these receptors. For example, oxymetazoline shows a reasonably strong coupling of the $\alpha_2 C2$ receptor subtype to G_s activation, but extremely poor coupling of the $\alpha_2 C10$ and $\alpha_2 C4$ receptor subtypes to this G-protein. The other agonists show a variety of different G_s coupling patterns for the three different receptor subtypes. A similar concept of the induction of differential conformational changes in the receptors by the different synthetic ligands has also been proposed to explain the ability of these receptors to couple differentially to different G-protein-mediated effects. Thus, not only can synthetic ligands specifically couple G-protein-coupled receptors to specific second-messenger systems, but it appears that the extent of this differential coupling can vary for closely related receptor subtypes.

We have recently examined the ability of a cloned α_{2A}-adrenergic receptor expressed in a CHO cell line (Fraser et al., 1989), to activate G_s-mediated stimulation and G_i-mediated inhibition of forskolin-stimulated adenylate cyclase activity when activated by either (−)-epinephrine or (±)-p-octopamine (Evans and Swales, in preparation). Fig. 4 shows that (−)-epinephrine produced an inhibition of forskolin-stimulated cyclic AMP levels at low concentrations and a stimulation at higher concentrations, as previously reported

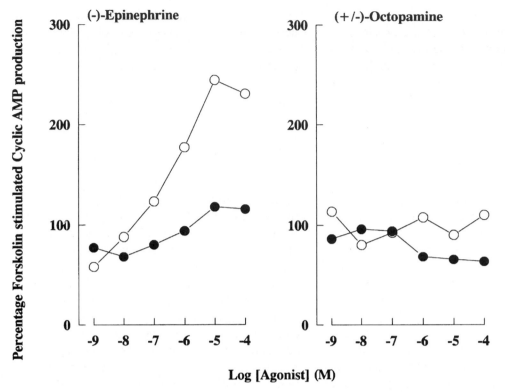

Fig. 4. The effect of (−)-epinephrine and (±)-*p*-octopamine on intracellular cyclic AMP concentrations in CHO cells transfected with a human α_{2A}-adrenergic receptor. Confluent cultures of transfected cells were incubated with 10 μM forskolin plus increasing concentrations of agonist for 20 min at 37°C, under control conditions (●) or after pretreatment with 200 ng/ml pertussis toxin at 37°C for 18 h (○) and processed for cyclic AMP determination as described previously (Robb et al., 1994).

(Fraser et al., 1989; Eason et al., 1994). The inhibition could be blocked by overnight pre-exposure of the cells to pertussis toxin (200 ng/ml at 37°C for 18 h), revealing a substantial concentration-dependent stimulation of forskolin-stimulated cyclic AMP levels in the transfected cells. In contrast, (±)-*p*-octopamine produced a dose-dependent inhibition of forskolin-induced cyclic AMP levels at a higher concentration than that induced by epinephrine. However, after the same pertussis toxin pretreatment, although the inhibitory effect of (±)-*p*-octopamine was blocked, no stimulatory effect was revealed. This suggests that octopamine may be capable of coupling the expressed α_{2A}-adrenergic receptor to G_i, but not to G_s, at any of the concentrations tested. Since octopamine is a naturally occurring agonist of

adrenergic receptors and can be co-released with norepinephrine from sympathetic neurones (Molinoff and Axelrod, 1969; Ibrahim et al., 1985), these findings could have important functional implications. It is possible that the octopamine co-released with norepinephrine could modulate, or bias, the responses of α-adrenergic receptors towards one particular second-messenger pathway rather than another. This possibility is currently being investigated. It is also possible that in future studies of α-adrenergic coupling to second messengers, systems could be found where octopamine shows an equal or even greater potency than the catecholamines, so that one would have to consider the possibility that α-adrenergic receptors could also function as octopamine receptors!

Conclusions

Agonist/ligand-specific coupling of G-protein-coupled receptors to different second-messenger systems appears to be a widespread phenomenon, since it has been demonstrated to occur in a range of receptors, including aminergic, muscarinic cholinergic and peptidergic receptors. The findings imply that single G-protein-coupled receptors may have different pharmacological profiles depending upon which second-messenger systems are used to assay them. This obviously has important implications for pharmacology in general. In the long term, it may be possible to develop drugs that have reduced side-effects by directing them to activate specific, desired G-protein-coupled receptor-activated second-messenger pathways and not others that produce unwanted side-effects.

Acknowledgements

We thank Drs. J. Craig Venter and Claire M. Fraser, The Institute for Genomic Research, for making the transfected CHO cell lines available to us. This work was in part funded by a project grant from the MRC (T.R.C.), by an AFRC/University Link Award (J.M.M. and P.D.E.), by a NATO grant (P.D.E. and L.M.H.) and by an NIH grant to L.M.H., who is a Jacob Javits Scholar in Neuroscience.

References

Abou-Samra, A.B., Juppner, H., Force, T., Freeman, M.W., Kong, X.F., Schipam, E., Ureva, P., Richards, J., Bonventre, J.V., Potts, J.T., Kronenberg, H.M. and Signe, G.V. (1992) Expression cloning of a common receptor for parathyroid hormone and parathyroid hormone-related peptide from rat osteoblast-like cells — a single receptor stimulates intracellular accumulation of both cAMP and inositol trisphosphate. *Proc. Natl. Acad. Sci. USA*, 89: 2732–2736.

Arakawa, S., Gocayne J.D., McCombie, W.R., Urquhart, D.A., Hall, L.M., Fraser, C.M. and Venter, J.C. (1990) Cloning, localization and permanent expression of a *Drosophila* octopamine receptor. *Neuron*, 2: 343–354.

Berridge, M.J. (1994) A tale of two messengers. *Nature*, 365: 388–389.

Brown, C.M., McGrath, J.C., Midgley, J.M., Muir, A.G.B., O'Brien, J.W., Thonoor, C.M., Williams, C.M. and Wilson, V.G. (1988) Activities of octopamine and synephrine stereoisomers on α-adrenoceptors. *Br. J. Pharmacol.*, 93: 417–429.

Bylund, D.B. (1992) Subtypes of alpha1 and alpha2 adrenergic receptors. *FASEB J.*, 6: 832–839.

Chabre, O., Conklin, B.R., Lin, H.Y., Lodish, H.F., Wilson, E., Ives, H.E., Catanzariti, L., Hemmings, B.A. and Bourne, H.R. (1992) A recombinant calcitonin receptor independently stimulates cAMP and Ca^{2+}/inositol phosphate signalling pathways. *Mol. Endocrinol.*, 6: 551–556.

Chakraborty, M., Chatterjee, D., Kellokumpu, S., Rasmussen, H. and Baron, R. (1991) Cell cycle-dependent coupling of the calcitonin receptor to different G proteins. *Science*, 251: 1078–1082.

Corps, A.N., Cheek, T.R., Moreton, R.B., Berridge, M.J. and Brown, K.D. (1989) Single-cell analysis of the mitogen-induced calcium responses of normal and protein kinase C-depleted Swiss 3T3 cells. *Cell Regulation*, 1: 75–86.

Cotecchia, S., Kobilka, B.K., Daniel, K.W., Nolan, R.D., Lapetina, E.Y., Caron, M.G., Lefkowitz, R.J. and Regan, J.W. (1990) Multiple second messenger pathways of alpha-adrenergic receptor subtypes expressed in eukaryotic cells. *J. Biol. Chem.*, 265: 63–69.

Crawford, K.W., Frey, E.A. and Cote, T.E. (1992) Angiotensin II receptor recognized by DuP753 regulates two distinct guanine nucleotide-binding protein signaling pathways. *Mol. Pharmacol.*, 41: 154–162.

Eason, M.G., Jacinto, M.T. and Liggett, S.B. (1994) Contribution of ligand structure to activation of α_2-adrenergic receptor subtype coupling to G_s. *Mol. Pharmacol.*, 45: 696–702.

Evans, P.D. (1980) Biogenic amines in the insect nervous system. *Adv. Insect Physiol.*, 15: 317–473.

Evans, P.D. (1981) Multiple receptor types for octopamine in the locust. *J. Physiol.*, 318: 99–122.

Evans, P.D. (1984a) A modulatory octopaminergic neurone increases cyclic nucleotide levels in locust skeletal muscle. *J. Physiol.*, 348: 307–324.

Evans, P.D. (1984b) Studies on the mode of action of octopamine, 5-hydroxytryptamine and proctolin on a myogenic rhythm in the locust. *J. Exp. Biol.*, 110: 231–251.

Evans, P.D. (1993) Molecular studies on insect octopamine receptors. In: Y. Pichon (Ed.), *Comparative Molecular Biology*, Birkauser Verlag AG, Basel, pp. 286–296.

Evans, P.D. and Robb, S. (1993) Octopamine receptor subtypes and their modes of action. *Neurochem. Res.*, 18: 869–874.

Evans, P.D., Thonoor, C.M. and Midgley, J.M. (1988) Activities of octopamine and synephrine stereoisomers on octopaminergic receptor subtypes in locust skeletal muscle. *J. Pharm. Pharmacol.*, 40: 855–861.

Fraser, C.M., Arakawa, S., McCombie, W.R. and Venter, J.C. (1989) Cloning, sequence analysis, and permanent expression of a human α_2-adrenergic receptor in Chinese Hamster Ovary cells. *J. Biol. Chem.*, 264: 11754–11761.

Gurwitz, D., Haring, R., Fraser, C.M., Heldman, E. and Fisher, A. (1991) Selective signal transduction by the M1 agonist, AF102B. *Soc. Neurosci. Abstr.*, 17: 388.

Gurwitz, D., Haring, H., Heldman, E., Fraser, C.M., Manor, D. and Fisher, A. (1994) Discrete activation of transduction pathways associated with acetylcholine m1 receptor by several muscarinic ligands. *Eur. J. Pharmacol.*, 267: 21–31.

Hosey, M.M. (1992) Diversity of structure, signalling and regulation within the family of muscarinic cholinergic receptors. *Faseb J.*, 6: 845–852.

Ibrahim, K.E., Couch, M.W., Williams, C.M., Fregly, M.J. and Midgley, J.M. (1985) *m*-Octopamine: Normal occurrence with *p*-octopamine in mammalian sympathetic nerves. *J.Neurochem.*, 44: 1862–1867.

Jordan, R., Midgley, J.M., Thonoor, C.M. and Williams, C.M. (1987) Beta-adrenergic activities of octopamine and synephrine stereoisomers on guinea-pig isolated atria and trachea. *J. Pharm. Pharmacol.*, 39: 752–754.

Lai, J., Waite, S.L., Bloom, J.W., Yamamura, H.I. and Roeske, W.R. (1991) The m2 muscarinic acetylcholine receptors are coupled to multiple signalling pathways via pertussis toxin-sensitive guanine nucleotide regulatory proteins. *J. Pharmacol. Exp. Ther.*, 258: 938–944.

Millard, P.J., Gross, D., Webb, W.W. and Fewtrell, C. (1988) Imaging asynchronous changes in intracellular Ca^{2+} in individual stimulated tumor mast cells. *Proc. Natl. Acad. Sci. USA*, 85: 1854–1858.

Milligan, G. (1993) Mechanisms of multifunctional signalling by G protein-linked receptors. *Trends Pharmacol. Sci.*, 14: 239–244.

Mitsuhashi, M., Ohashi, Y., Shichijo, S., Christian, C., Sudduth-Klinger, J., Harnowe, G. and Payan, D.G. (1992) Multiple intracellular signalling pathways of the neuropeptide Substance P receptor. *J. Neurosci. Res.*, 32: 437–443.

Molinoff, P.B. and Axelrod, J. (1969) Octopamine: normal occurrence in sympathetic nerves of rat. *Science.*, 164: 428–429.

Monck, J.R., Reynolds, E.E., Thomas, A.P. and Williamson, J.R. (1988) Novel kinetics of single cell Ca^{2+} transients in stimulated hepatocytes and A10 cells measured using Fura-2 and fluorescent videomicroscopy. *J. Biol. Chem.*, 263: 4569–4575.

Nakajima, Y., Tsuchida, K., Negishi, M., Ito, S. and Nakanishi, S. (1992) Direct linkage of three tachykinin receptors to stimulation of both phosphatidylinositol hydrolysis and cyclic AMP cascades in transfected Chinese Hamster Ovary cells. *J. Biol. Chem.*, 267: 2437–2442.

Raymond, J.R., Albers, F.J. and Middleton, J.P. (1992) Functional expression of human 5-HT$_{1A}$ receptors and differential coupling to second messengers in CHO cells. *N. S. Arch. Pharmacol.*, 346: 127–137.

Robb, S., Cheek, T.R., Venter, J.C., Midgley, J.M. and Evans, P.D. (1991) The mode of action and pharmacology of a cloned *Drosophila* phenolamine receptor. *Pest. Sci.*, 32: 369–371.

Robb, S., Cheek, T.R., Hannan, F.L., Hall, L.M., Midgley, J.M. and Evans, P.D. (1994) Agonist-specific coupling of a cloned *Drosophila* octopamine/tyramine receptor to multiple second messenger systems. *EMBO J.*, 13: 1325–1330.

Saudou, F., Amlaiky, N., Plassat, J.-L., Borrelli, E. and Hen, R. (1990) Cloning and characterization of a *Drosophila* tyramine receptor. *EMBO J.*, 9: 3611–3617.

Spengler, D., Waeber, C., Pantaloni, C., Holsboer, F., Bockaert, J., Seeburg, P.H. and Journot, L. (1993) Differential signal transduction by five splice variants of the PACAP receptor. *Nature*, 365: 170–175.

Taylor, C.W. (1990) The role of G proteins in transmembrane signalling. *Biochem. J.*, 272: 1–13.

Thompson, E.G. (1992) Comment: Single receptors, dual second messengers. *Mol. Endocrinol.*, 6: 501.

Van Sande, J., Raspe, E., Pernet, J., Lejeune, C., Maenhaut, C., Vassart, G. and Dumont, J.E. (1990) Thyrotropin activates both the cyclic AMP and the PIP2 cascades in CHO cells expressing the human cDNA of the TSH receptor. *Mol. Cell Endocrinol.*, 74: R1-R6.

Wolsing, D.H. and Rosenbaum, J.S. (1993) Bradykinin-stimulated inositol phosphate production in NG108-15 cells is mediated by a small population of binding sites which rapidly desensitize. *J. Pharm. Exp. Ther.*, 266: 253–261.

Peter M. Yu, Keith F. Tipton and Alan A. Boulton (Eds.)
Progress in Brain Research, Vol 106
© 1995 Elsevier Science BV. All rights reserved.

CHAPTER 27

Activation of brain 5-HT neurons by two alpha-methylated tryptamine derivatives

Y. Arai[1], T. Tadano[2], A. Yonezawa[2], T. Fujita[3], H. Kinemuchi[3] and K. Kisara[2]

[1]*Department of Pharmacology, School of Medicine, Showa University, Tokyo 142, Japan,* [2]*Department of Pharmacology, Tohoku College of Pharmacy, Sendai 983, Japan, and* [3]*Laboratory of Biological Chemistry, Faculty of Science and Engineering, Ishinomaki Senshu University, Ishinomaki 986, Japan*

Introduction

Changes in brain serotonergic function have been implicated in the mechanisms of action of hallucinogenic drugs of abuse such as LSD, mescaline and other similarly acting compounds. Among different serotonergic receptor subtypes, an interaction between brain serotonin ($5-HT_2$) receptors and hallucinogens has been shown to be necessary for the production of hallucination. Recently a highly significant correlation was demonstrated between the potencies of both phenylisopropylamines (α-methylated alkylamines) and indolealkylamines as either hallucinogens or behavioural cues (Leysen et al., 1978), and their high affinities for $5-HT_2$ receptors (Glennon et al., 1984; Peroutka and Snyder, 1979).

Many hallucinogens induce various abnormal behaviours in mice and among these behaviours, a rapid, discrete shaking movement of the head, referred to here as the head-twitch response (HTR), has long been regarded as an experimental model for hallucination in humans (Corne and Pickering, 1967; Teresa et al., 1975). Previous studies reported that, after systemic administration of amphetamine, its principal metabolite, *p*-hydroxyamphetamine (p-OHA), is formed (Cho et al., 1975) and distributed in various mouse brain regions (Jori and Caccia, 1974; Kuhn et al., 1978). When p-OHA is applied directly into mouse brain, it also induces HTR. The HTR induced by some compounds is greatly potentiated by a combined treatment with a non-selective form of a monoamine oxidase (MAO, EC 1.4.3.4) inhibitor (Corne et al., 1963; Sakurada, 1975). Thus, a mechanism for HTR production by p-OHA may be a result of an increased rate of interaction between brain 5-HT released by p-OHA into the synaptic cleft and postsynaptic $5-HT_2$ receptors following p-OHA uptake into the 5-HT nerve terminals. This was confirmed by showing that HTR can be similarly produced by intracerebral administration of 5-HT itself (Suchowsky et al., 1969) or after pheripheral administration of 5-hydroxytryptophan (Tadano et al., 1989).

Currently MAO is considered to exist in two functionally different forms, A (MAO-A) and B (MAO-B), each with particularly different substrate selectivities and inhibitor sensitivities. Distinct genes for human, bovine and rat MAO-A and MAO-B have been cloned and their nucleotide sequences analyzed (Hsu et al., 1989). The deduced amino acid sequences for MAO-A and MAO-B from each species display about 70% sequential homology, with different primary amino acid compositions (Weyler et al., 1990). In the CNS, the two forms of MAO are found both intra- and extra-neuronally in monoaminergic neurons with different A/B activity ratios (Oreland et al., 1983). With respect to p-OHA-induced

HTR, this effect is probably because of increased 5-HT levels in nerve terminals (Arai et al., 1990), This p-OHA-induced HTR is greatly reduced by inhibition of p-OHA uptake into 5-HT neurons by selective 5-HT blockers, probably since both p-OHA and 5-HT share the same uptake systems (Arai et al., 1990), or by inhibition of neuronal 5-HT biosynthesis, or by treatment with postsynaptic 5-HT$_2$ receptor antagonists. Thus, this HTR can serve as a useful measure of activities and functions of 5-HT neuronal systems. If a chlorine or fluorine atom is substituted into the phenyl ring of phenylethylamine (PEA) or tryptamine moieties, they are no longer MAO substrates, but rather change to inhibitors (Kinemuchi et al., 1986, 1988). Similarly the introduction of an α-methyl group into an MAO substrate causes them to become reversible MAO-A-selective inhibitors (Mantle et al., 1976; Fowler and Ross, 1982; Kinemuchi et al., 1986; Arai et al., 1986). For example α-methyltryptamine is a selective and reversible MAO-A inhibitor. The introduction of a methyl group into the β-position of the side chain of PEA, however, gives β-methylphenylethylamine; this derivative is, in contrast, a selective MAO-B inhibitor. Thus, MAO substrates can easily change to being either MAO-A- or MAO-B-selective inhibitors simply by introducing a methyl group into either the α- or β-carbon position of the primary amine chain.

In this study, we have examined the influence of both ring halogenation (5-F or 6-F atom on the phenyl ring) and α-methylation on the aliphatic side chain of tryptamine on brain MAO activity. Induction of HTR by these compounds in mice was also determined. Comparisons were made between four different tryptamine derivatives: 5- and 6-fluoro-α-methyltryptamine (5-FMT, 6-FMT) and 5- and 6-fluorotryptamine (5-FT, 6-FT).

Methods

Male ddY mice, weighing 22–25 g, were housed, with free access to food and water, under conditions of constant humidity (55 $\pm$ 5%), temperature (23 $\pm$ 1°C) and in a light/dark cycle (9:00 to 21:00 h). After administration (i.p.) of the compounds (HCl salts) the animals were immediately placed in individual plastic cages (25 $\times$ 18 $\times$ 13 cm) for HTR estimation.

Pretreatment with cyproheptadine (1 mg/kg) and fluoxetine (20 mg/kg) occurred 30 min before the tryptamine derivative injection. p-Chlorophenylalanine (p-CPA, 200 mg/kg) was administered twice in the same day with a 12 h interval before the administration of the tryptamine derivatives. 5,7-Dihydroxytryptamine (5,7-DHT; 0.1 mg per mouse) was injected intracerebroventricularly (i.c.v.) 5 days before either derivative was injected. The number of HTRs was counted for 2 min at 10 min intervals from 10 to 92 min following injection of either the tryptamine derivatives alone or in combination. Assessment of HTR was blind to treatment. All injected compounds were dissolved in 0.9% saline, except 5,7-DHT, which was dissolved in Ringer's solution and injected unilaterally as originally described by Brittain and Handley (1967), and mentioned in our previous study (Tadano et al., 1989; Arai et al., 1990).

5-HT and its main metabolite, 5-hydroxyindoleacetic acid (5-HIAA), in five different mouse brain regions (hypothalamus, hippocampus, brainstem, striatum and cortex) were assayed 30 min after injection of 5-FMT or 6-FMT. After dissection, the regions were homogenised in ice-cold 0.1 M perchloric acid containing 0.1 mM EDTA using an ultrasonic cell disruptor. The homogenates were then centrifuged at 12,000 $\times$ g for 10 min, and the supernatant was removed. 5-HT and 5-HIAA were assessed by high-performance liquid chromatography (HPLC) with electrochemical detection (Murai et al., 1988).

MAO-A and -B activity in mouse forebrain homogenates was measured using a radiochemical method, as reported earlier (Kinemuchi et al., 1985) with 0.1 mM [^{14}C]5-HT and 0.1 mM [^{14}C]benzylamine (BZ) as substrates.

Fluoxetine hydrochloride was provided by Eli Lilly & Co., USA. All other chemicals were of the highest grade commercially available. The data were analyzed by analysis of variance (ANOVA) and by Dunnett's test.

Results

The effects of tryptamine derivatives on HTR

HTRs in mice were rapidly and dose-relatedly induced by both 5- and 6-FMT (see Table 1 and Fig. 1), reaching a peak 10–40 min after injection. The duration of HTR was about 60 to 90 min but the frequency was greatest at the intermediate dose of 20–45 mg/kg. When HTR was expressed as cumulative numbers for 10 min intervals, the time courses for both 5- and 6-FMT-induced HTR were only linear for 40–50 min depending on dose. This linearity failed after 20 min at the highest dose probably because of the appearance of other 5-HT-induced behaviours, such as hindlimb abduction, head weaving etc. In contrast to the α-methylated derivatives, a variety of doses

of 5-FT and 6-FT induced a negligible frequency of HTR over a 90 min period (data not shown). Saline controls exhibited no effects on HTR.

Effects of drug pretreatment on tryptamine-derivative-induced HTR

The total number of HTRs induced by a dose of 45 mg/kg of 5- or 6-FMT was significantly reduced by intraperitoneal pretreatment with the selective 5-HT$_2$ receptor antagonist, cyproheptadine (1 mg/kg), the 5-HT reuptake blocker, fluoxetine (20 mg/kg) and by p-CPA (200 mg/kg), an inhibitor of 5-HT biosynthesis (Table 2). In contrast, pretreatment with 5,7-DHT (0.1 mg per mouse, i.c.v.), a serotonergic toxin, significantly increased the total number of HTRs induced by 5- and 6-FMT (Table 2).

The influence of tryptamine derivatives on MAO activity

Using 5-HT and Bz as substrates for MAO-A and MAO-B, respectively, all four tryptamine derivatives reversibly, competitively and differen-

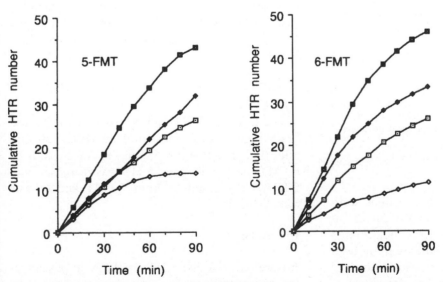

Fig. 1. Time course of 5-FMT- and 6-FMT-induced HTR in mice. Each point shows the number of cumulative head-twitches at various doses. Dose: □, 20 mg/kg; ◆, 30 mg/kg; ■, 45 mg/kg; ◇, 67.5 mg/kg.

TABLE 1

Influence of various doses of 5-FMT and 6-FMT on HTR in mice

Time (min)	0	10	20	30	40	50	60	70	80	90	Total
5-FMT											
20 mg/kg	0	3.8	3.6	3.4	3.4	2.2	3.0	3.0	2.1	1.7	26.2
30 mg/kg	0	4.1	3.9	3.5	2.8	3.4	4.1	3.4	3.0	3.8	32.0
45 mg/kg	0	6.0	6.3	6.0	6.2	5.0	4.3	4.3	3.4	1.5	43.0
67.5 mg/kg	0	3.2	3.3	2.2	1.8	1.7	1.0	0.3	0.2	0.2	13.9
6-FMT											
20 mg/kg	0	3.7	3.5	4.5	3.3	2.8	3.0	1.8	2.0	1.6	26.2
30 mg/kg	0	5.6	6.7	5.4	4.2	3.2	3.0	1.8	2.0	1.6	33.5
45 mg/kg	0	7.3	7.2	7.5	7.4	5.6	3.7	3.1	2.5	1.9	46.2
67.5 mg/kg	0	2.5	1.5	1.9	1.2	0.8	0.9	0.8	0.9	0.9	11.4

Total indicates total number of head twitches in 90 min.
Each value is expressed as the mean of head-twitches for 2 min. 5-FMT or 6-FMT was injected intraperitoneally at doses of 20, 30, 45, or 67.5 mg/kg. Total means the total number of head-twitches for 90 min. Time is expressed as min after i.p. injection of 5-FMT or 6-FMT.

TABLE 2

Influence of cyproheptadine, fluoxetine, p-chlorophenyl-alanine, and 5,7-dihydroxytryptamine on 5-FMT- and 6-FMT-induced HTR in mice

	5-FMT	6-FMT
Control	43 1 9	46 1 2
Cyproheptadine	3 1 1	0
Fluoxetine	14 1 2	9 1 3
p-CPA	17 1 2	17 1 1
5,7-DHT	123 1 30	1 54 1 33

Values are expressed as means ± 1 S.E.M. ($n = 10$) of total HTRs over a 90 min period. Both compounds were injected intraperitoneally at a dose of 45 mg/kg.
$*P < 0.05, **P < 0.01$ vs. control (Dunnett's test).

tially inhibited MAO activity. IC_{50} values were calculated graphically from inhibition curves; in addition, apparent K_i values were determined from linear slope replots of inhibition of both MAO forms against different concentrations of each derivative. IC_{50} values (i.e. the dose producing 50% inhibition of MAO activity) for 5-FT, 5-FMT, 6-FT and 6-FMT on MAO-A were 13,

0.2, 1.6 and 0.6 μM, and on MAO-B 53, 300, 6 and 250 μM, respectively. The K_i values of 5-FMT and 6-FMT on MAO-A were 0.03 and 1.6 μM, and those of 5-FMT and 6-FMT on MAO-B were 575 and 370 μM, respectively. The K_i values of 5- and 6-FT were not determined, since they did not induce HTR. It can be concluded that 5-FMT and 6-FMT are potent and highly selective MAO-A inhibitors with high potencies for HTR induction.

The effect of tryptamine derivatives on 5-HT and 5-HIAA levels

The levels of 5-HT and 5-HIAA in five mouse brain regions were measured by HPLC 30 min after i.p. injection of 45 mg/kg of 5-FMT or 6-FMT. As can be seen 5-HT was increased and 5-HIAA decreased by both 5-FMT and 6-FMT (see Table 3).

Discussion

It is well known that 5-HT and PEA, at physiological concentrations, are selectively catabolised by MAO-A and MAO-B respectively (for review, see Kinemuchi et al., 1984, 1987). Introduction of a

TABLE 3

Effect of 5-FMT and 6-FMT on 5-HT and 5-HIAA levels in five brain regions of the mouse

	5-HT			5-HIAA		
	Control	5FMT	6-FMT	Control	5FMT	6-FMT
Cortex	285 ± 23 (100%)	365 ± 34 (128%)	390 ± 21 (137%)	122 ± 12 (100%)	48 ± 3 (39%)	57 ± 4 (47%)
Striatum	429 ± 57 (100%)	611 ± 41 (142%)	614 ± 26 (143%)	351 ± 22 (100%)	252 ± 21 (72%)	286 ± 28 (81%)
Hippocampus	355 ± 52 (100%)	535 ± 50 (151%)	556 ± 39 (157%)	287 ± 27 (100%)	181 ± 16 (63%)	251 ± 26 (87%)
Hypothalamus	872 ± 73 (100%)	1265 ± 41 (145%)	1184 ± 148 (136%)	523 ± 47 (100%)	155 ± 10 (30%)	205 ± 26 (39%)
Brainstem	555 ± 31 (100%)	850 ± 80 (153%)	841 ± 62 (151%)	281 ± 15 (100%)	179 ± 11 (64%)	242 ± 40 (86%)

Values are expressed as means ± 1 S.E.M. of 5 g/mg tissue ($n = 10$).
Mice were killed 30 min after injection of 5-FMT or 6-FMT.
*$P < 0.05$, **$P < 0.01$ vs. control (Dunnett's test).

methyl group onto the α-carbon atom of the aliphatic carbon chains of MAO-B substrates (Satoh et al., 1985; Tadano et al., 1986, 1989) yields potent MAO-A-selective inhibitors; such compounds are also HTR inducers (Arai et al., 1990, 1991). In contrast, β-methylation, or chloride introduction into the *para*-position of the phenyl ring, yields potent MAO-B-selective inhibitors both in vitro and in vivo (Kinemuchi et al., 1986, 1988; Kim et al., 1991). The optical isomer (d-form) of another α-methylated MAO-B-selective substrate, namely α-methylbenzylamine, results in an MAO-A-selective inhibitor with a lower K_i value (24 μM) (Arai et al., 1986).

In confirming the earlier in vitro (Kinemuchi et al., 1988) and in vivo results (Kim et al., 1991), 5-HT, used here as an MAO-A substrate, was competitively and reversibly inhibited by 5-FMT and 6-FMT with K_i values of 0.03 μM and 1.6 μM, and 575 μM and 370 μM for MAO-B inhibition, respectively. The MAO-A selective inhibition by 5-FMT in rat brain was recently confirmed by May et al. (1991). It has also been shown in an in vitro study (Kinemuchi et al., 1988), that α-methyltryptamine strongly and selectively inhibits rat brain MAO-A activity with

K_i values of 0.82 μM for MAO-A, whilst the values for MAO-B were much lower (150μm) (Kinemuchi et al., 1986). These results indicate quite conclusively that the introduction of a fluorine atom into the 5 position of the phenyl ring contributes to selective MAO-A inhibition; in the 6 position, however, the effects are much lower. In addition, the introduction of a halogen atom into the phenyl ring in the absence of an α-methyl group (ie 5-FT and 6-FT) similarly inhibits both MAO-A and MAO-B activity, with 6-FT being slightly greater with respect to MAO-A selectivity than 5-FT.

The present findings show that in addition to being selective MAO-A inhibitors, 5- and 6-FMT markedly induce HTR; the two non-methylated derivatives, 5-FT and 6-FT, did not induce this response. These latter two non-methylated derivatives are also relatively weak MAO-A-selective inhibitors. From this, it seems reasonable to suggest that perhaps the induction of this animal behaviour may be because of selective, probably intraneuronal, MAO-A inhibition. In rat brain, the bulk of 5-HT oxidation is carried out within 5-HT synaptosomes (Oreland et al., 1983). This supports the hypothesis that HTR induced by the α-methylated amphetamine metabolite p-OHA, or by a 5-HT biosynthesis precursor, l-5-HTP, is greatly potentiated after high MAO-A-selective inhibition, but not MAO-B-selective inhibition (Tadano et al., 1989).

The HTR induced by many inducers is believed to be mediated by the activation of the interaction between neuronal 5-HT released into the synapse and the central post-synaptic 5-HT$_2$ receptor subtype (Lucki et al., 1984; Tadano et al., 1986). Some HTR inducers, on the other hand, act directly as post-synaptic 5-HT agonists (Anden et al., 1968; Yamamoto and Ueki, 1980; Lucki et al., 1984). An indirect action by 5- or 6-FMT is supported by the present findings, however, since the induced HTR is significantly suppressed by pretreatment with the 5-HT synthesis inhibitor, p-CPA. This suppression was also found after pretreatment with fluoxetine, a selective 5-HT reuptake blocker, and by cyproheptadine, a selective antagonist at post-synaptic 5-HT$_2$ receptors. Newly synthesized 5-HT is required for the production of HTR by 5- and 6-FMT, as well as by p-OHA (Tadano et al., 1986). This indicates that indirect, 5-HT-mediated HTR production by these two methylated derivatives results from active uptake of these derivatives into neurons by the 5-HT uptake system. It is possible therefore that similar mechanisms exist for the induction of HTR by p-OHA (Tadano et al., 1989; Arai et al., 1990).

The likely involvement of the releasing properties of 5- and 6-FMT on intraneuronally stored 5-HT is further supported by the increases seen in brain 5-HT levels in the five brain regions tested with the two compounds (Table 3). A decrease in 5-HIAA level in these brain regions was also caused by 5-FMT; 6-FMT, however, only caused a decrease in the hypothalamus and cortex. Fagervall and Ross's (1986) finding of predominant 5-HT oxidation by MAO-A in serotonergic synaptosomes in the rat hypothalamus supports this. 5-HT might mediate or be released in the presence of presynaptically stored 5-HT by accumulating 5- or 6-FMT. This hypothesis is supported by the HTR-blocking effect exhibited by fluoxetine and p-CPA. In contrast, 5- and

6-FMT-induced HTR was potentiated by 5,7-DHT, a 5-HT depletor, probably because of upregulation of post-synaptic 5-HT$_2$ receptors.

The findings discussed and presented here indicate that potentiation of HTR might be caused by increased intraneuronal 5-HT levels as a consequence of MAO-A inhibition. Such an increase in 5-HT results in an activation of post-synaptic 5-HT$_2$ receptors.

Acknowledgement

The authors are grateful to Eli Lilly & Co., Indianapolis, USA, for the gift of fluoxetine hydrochloride.

References

Anden, N.E., Corrodi, H., Fuxe, K. and Hokfelt, T. (1968) Evidence for a central 5-hydroxytryptamine receptor stimulation by lysergic acid diethylamide. Br. J. Pharmacol., 34: 1–7.

Arai, Y., Toyoshima, Y. and Kinemuchi, H. (1986) Studies on monoamine oxidase and semicarbazide-sensitive amine oxidase II. Inhibition by α-methylated substrate-analogue monoamines, α-methyltryptamine, α-methylbenzylamine and two enantiomers of α-methylbenzylamine. Japan. J. Pharmacol., 41: 191–197.

Arai, Y., Kim, S.K., Kinemuchi, H., Tadano, T., Satoh, S., Satoh, N.,Oyama, K. and Kisara, K. (1990) Selective inhibition of MAO-A in serotonergic synaptosomes by two amphetamine metabolites, p-hydroxyamphetamine and p-hydroxynorephedrine. Neurochem. Int., 17: 587–592.

Arai, Y., Kim, S.K., Kinemuchi, H., Tadano, T., Satoh, S., Satoh, N. and Kisara, K. (1990) Inhibition of brain type A monoamine oxidase and 5-hydroxytryptamine uptake by two amphetamine metabolites, p-hydroxyamphetamine and p-hydroxynorephedrine. J. Neurochem., 55: 403–408.

Arai, Y., Kim, S.K., Kinemuchi, H., Tadano, T., Oyama, K., Satoh, N. and Kisara, K. (1991) Inhibition of brain MAO-A and animal behaviour induced by p-hydroxyamphetamine. Brain Res. Bull., 27: 81–84.

Brittain, R.T. and Handley, S.L. (1967) Temperature changes produced by the injection of catecholamines and 5-hydroxytryptamine into the cerebral ventricules of the conscious mouse. J. Physiol. (Lond.) 192: 805–813.

Cho, A.K., Schaeffer, J.C. and Fischer, J.F. (1975) 4-Hydroxyamphetamine by rat striatal homogenates. Biochem. Pharmacol., 24: 1540–1542.

Corne, S.J., Pickering, R.W. and Warner, B.T. (1963) A method for assessing the effect of drugs on the central actions of 5-hydroxytryptamine. Br. J. Pharmacol., 20: 106–120.

Corne, S.J. and Pickering, R.W. (1967) A possible correlation between drug-induced hallucination in man and a behavioral response in mice. *Psychopharmacology* 211: 65–78.

Fagervall, I. and Ross, S.B. (1986) A and B forms of monoamine oxidase within the monoaminergic neurons of the rat. *J. Neurochem.*, 47: 569–576.

Fowler, C.J. and Ross, S.B. (1984) Selective inhibition of monoamine oxidase A and B: Biochemical, pharmacological, and clinical properties. *Med. Res. Rev.*, 4: 323–358.

Glennon, R.A, Titler, M. and McKenney, J.D. (1984) Evidence for 5-HT$_2$ receptor involvement in the mechanism of action of hallucinogen. *Life Sci.*, 35: 2205–2211.

Hsu, Y.P.P., Powell, J.F., Sims, K.B. and Breakefield, X.O. (1989) Molecular genetics of the monoamine oxidases. *J. Neurochem.*, 53: 12–18.

Jori, A. and Caccia, S. (1974) Distribution of amphetamine and its hydroxylated metabolites in various areas of the rat brain. *J. Pharm. Pharmacol.*, 26: 746–748.

Kim, S.K., Toyoshima, Y., Arai, Y., Kinemuchi, H., Tadano, T., Oyama, K., Satoh, N. and Kisara, K. (1991) Inhibition of monoamine oxidase by two substrate-analogues, with different preferences for 5-hydroxytryptamine neurons. *Neuropharmacology*, 30: 329–335.

Kinemuchi, H. and Arai, Y. (1986) Selective inhibition of monoamine oxidase A and B by two substrate-analogues, 5-fluoro-α-methyltryptamine and p-chloro-β-methylphenylethylamine. *Res. Commun. Chem. Pathol. Pharmacol.*, 54: 125–128.

Kinemuchi, H., Fowler, C.J. and Tipton, K.F. (1984) Substrate specificities of the two forms of monoamine oxidase. In: K.F. Tipton, P. Dostert and M. Strolin Benedetti (Eds.), *Monoamine Oxidase and Disease*, Academic Press, New York, pp. 53–62.

Kinemuchi, H., Arai, Y. and Toyoshima, Y. (1985) Participation of monoamine oxidase B form in the neurotoxicity of 1-methyl-4-phenyl-1,2,3,6-tetrahydropyridine: Relationship between the enzyme inhibition and the neurotoxicity. *Neurosci. Lett.*, 58: 195–200.

Kinemuchi, H., Fowler, C.J. and Tipton, K.F. (1987) The neurotoxicity of1-methyl-4-phenyl-1,2,3,6-tetrahydropyridine (MPTP) and its relevance to Parkinson's disease. *Neurochem. Int.*, 11: 359–373.

Kinemuchi, H., Arai, Y., Toyoshima, Y., Tadano, T. and Kisara, K. (1988) Studies on 5-fluoro-α-methyltryptamine and p-chloro-β-methylphenylamine: Determination of the MAO-A or MAO-B selective inhibition in vitro. *Japan. J. Pharmacol.*, 46: 197–199.

Kuhn, C.M., Schanberg, S.M. and Breese, G.R. (1978) Metabolism of amphetamine by rat brain tissue. *Biochem. Pharmacol.*, 27: 343–351.

Leysen, J.E., Niemegeers, C.J.E., Tollenaere, J.P. and Laudron, P.M. (1978) Serotonergic component of neuroleptic receptors. *Nature*, 272: 168–171.

Lucki, I., Nobler, M.S. and Frazer, A. (1984) Differential actions of serotonin antagonists on two behavioral models of serotonin receptor activation in the rat. *J. Pharmacol. Exp. Ther.*, 228: 133–139.

Mantle, T.J., Tipton, K.F. and Garrett, N.J. (1976) Inhibition of monoamine oxidase by amphetamine and related compounds. *Biochem. Pharmacol.*, 25: 2073–2077.

May, T., Rommelspacher, H. and Pawlik, M. (1991) [^{3}H] Harmine binding experiments. I. A reversible and selective radioligand for monoamine oxidase. *J. Neurochem.*, 56: 490–499.

Murai, S., Saito, H., Masuda, Y. and Itoh, T. (1988) Rapid determination of norepinephrine, dopamine, serotonin, their precursor amino acids, and related metabolites in discrete brain areas of mice within ten minutes by HPLC with electrochemical detection. *J. Neurochem.*, 50: 473–479.

Oreland, L., Arai, Y., Stenstrom, A. and Fowler.C.J. (1983) Monoamine oxidase activity and localisation in the brain and the activity in relation to psychiatric disorders. In: H. Beckmann and P. Riederer (Eds.), *Monoamine Oxidase and Its Selective Inhibitors*, Karger, Basel. pp. 246–254.

Peroutka, S.J. and Snyder, S.H. (1979) Multiple serotonin receptors: differential binding of [^{3}H]5-hydroxytryptamine, [^{3}H]lysergic acid diethylamine and [^{3}H]spiroperidol. *Mol. Pharmacol.*, 16: 687–699.

Sakurada, S. (1975) Central action of β-phenethylamine derivatives (6). Head-twitches induced by intracerebroventricularlly administered tyramine in isocarboxazide pretreated mice. *Folia Pharmacol. Japon.*, 71: 779–787.

Satoh, S., Satoh, N., Tadano, T. and Kisara, K. (1985) Enhancement of *para*-hydroxyamphetamine induced head-twitch response by catecholamine depletions. *Res. Commun. Sub. Abuse*, 6: 213–219.

Suchowsky, G.K., Pegrassi, L., Moretti, A. and Bonsignori, A. (1969) The effect of 4H-3-methylcarboxamide-1,3-benzoxazine-2-one (FI6654) on monoamine oxidase and cerebral 5-HT. *Archs. Int. Pharmacodyn. Ther.*, 182: 332–340.

Tadano, T., Satoh, S. and Kisara, K. (1986) Head-twiches induced by p- hydroxyamphetamine. *Japan. J. Pharmacol.*, 41: 519–523.

Tadano, T., Satoh, S., Satoh, N., Kisara, K., Arai, Y., Kim, S.K. and Kinemuchi, H. (1989) Potentiation of *para*-hydroxyamphetamine-induced head-twitch response by inhibition of monoamine oxidase type A in the brain. *J. Pharmacol. Exp. Ther.*, 250: 254–260.

Teresa, M., Silva, A. and Cali, H.M. (1975) Screening hallucinogenic drugs; Systemic study of three behavioural tests. *Psychopharmacology*, 42: 163–171.

Weyler, W., Hsu, Y.P.P. and Breakefield, X.O. (1990) Biochemistry and genetics of monoamine oxidase. *Pharmacol. Ther.*, 47: 391–417.

Yamamoto, T. and Ueki, S. (1990) The role of central serotonergic mechanisms on head-twitch and backward locomotion induced by hallucinogenic drugs. *Pharmacol. Biochem. Behav.*, 14: 89–95.

Peter M. Yu, Keith F. Tipton and Alan A. Boulton (Eds.)
Progress in Brain Research, Vol 106
© 1995 Elsevier Science BV. All rights reserved.

CHAPTER 28

Trace amines in hepatic encephalopathy

Darrell D. Mousseau and Roger F. Butterworth

Neuroscience Research Unit, St-Luc Hospital, University of Montreal, Montreal, Québec, Canada H2X 3J4

Liver failure is frequently accompanied by a neuropsychiatric syndrome generally referred to as hepatic encephalopathy. Portal-systemic encephalopathy (PSE), the most common form of HE, accompanies portal-systemic shunting which develops following portacaval anastomosis or spontaneously following portal hypertension most often due to cirrhosis. Neurologically, PSE develops slowly: symptoms, including a number of recognized components (e.g. changes in state of consciousness, intellectual function and personality/behavior, as well as motor and neuromuscular abnormalities), precede lethargy and ataxia, ultimately progressing to stupor and coma. The precise pathogenesis of this neuropsychiatric syndrome in humans remains unknown, although several mechanisms have been proposed (Mousseau and Butterworth, 1994a). One potential etiological candidate is an impairment of one or more of the neurotransmitter systems in brain resulting in altered synaptic availability of the transmitter(s) and a subsequent shift from excitation to inhibition. The most commonly studied transmitters in HE are the amino acids glutamate (Butterworth, 1992) and GABA (Schafer and Jones, 1982), although the study of the biogenic amines dopamine, serotonin and noradrenaline (Bengtsson et al., 1989; Bergeron et al., 1989) is being favoured by a resurgence in interest following a decade-long hiatus.

A "trace amine" hypothesis for HE was proposed by Fischer and Baldessarini (1971). Biogenic amines, metabolites of aromatic amino acids provided by protein catabolism, are normally produced by the bacteria of the gastrointestinal tract and subsequently catabolized by liver monoamine oxidase. Although normally cleared from the portal circulation, pathophysiological conditions leading to portal-systemic shunting could result in large quantities of the precursors reaching the CNS where they would be available for metabolism to their corresponding trace amines (see Fig. 1), each of which could be capable of replacing the true neurotransmitters (i.e. dopamine and noradrenaline) from the synaptosomes. Successful therapeutic trials using levodopa (L-DOPA, Fischer and Baldessarini, 1971; Lunzer et al., 1974; Loiudice et al., 1979), the immediate precursor to dopamine, and bromocriptine (Morgan et al., 1980), a specific dopamine receptor agonist, implied that a pathophysiological basis of PSE must include a disordered function of catecholamine synapses and thus further strengthened the "false-transmitter" hypothesis.

Additional evidence emerged from both the clinical and laboratory settings. As this has been discussed in great detail elsewhere (see Schenker et al., 1980), only the evidence most germane to this present discussion will be explored. Intestinal bacteria are presumed to play an integral role in the metabolism of precursor amino acids to their corresponding amines. It is, therefore, not surprising that protein loads from dietary sources or following ingestion of copious amounts of blood,

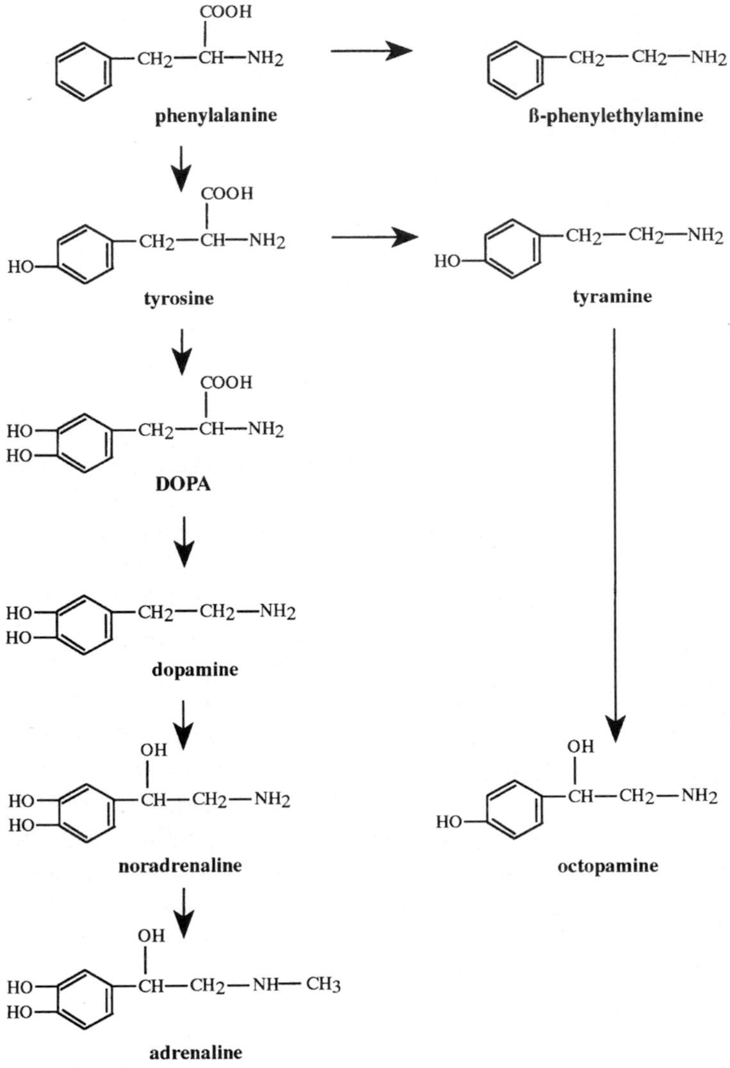

Fig. 1. Summary schematic of the synthetic pathways of catecholamine and related trace amines. Certain metabolites are omitted to simplify the diagram.

the latter being a common observation in patients with ruptured esophageal varicosities due to portal hypertension, should precipitate or exacerbate PSE. Conversely, controlling protein intake or using antibiotics to effectively rid the gastrointestinal tract of any bacteria has been shown to bring about clinical improvement of the patient's mental status (Fischer and Baldessarini, 1971; Fischer et al., 1972). By virtue of its structural similarity to both dopamine and noradrenaline and its known effects on catecholamine neurones,

octopamine was proposed as the most likely trace amine candidate in PSE, although tyramine, phenylethylamine and phenylethanolamine were also seriously considered (see Fig. 1 and Table 1). In fact, octopamine accumulates in the serum and urine of patients, correlating roughly with the grade of PSE (see Table 2; Fischer and Baldessarini, 1971; Lam et al., 1973; Manghani et al., 1975). A similar elevation in brain levels of octopamine (approximately a 4-fold increase) is observed in comatose rats having undergone hep-

TABLE 1

β-Hydroxylated phenylethylamines in experimental hepatic coma

Trace amine Treatment group (n)	Rat brain (ng/brain)
Octopamine	
Sham-operated (7)	6.0 ± 0.8
"Somnolent" (7)	$11.7 \pm 1.6**$
Severe coma (7)	$24.3 \pm 4.2**$
Phenylethanolamine	
Sham-operated (7)	23.2 ± 5.7
"Somnolent" (7)	35.3 ± 6.0
Severe coma (7)	$40.2 \pm 3.7*$

Results are the means $\pm$ S.E.M.: $*P < 0.05$; $**P < 0.01$, obtained with the Student's t test. Numbers in parentheses represent numbers of experimental subjects. Data adapted from Fischer and Baldessarini, 1971 (used with permission).

atic devascularization or in portacaval-shunted rats having been fed large quantities of aromatic amino acids (see Table 1; Fischer and

TABLE 2

24-hour urinary octopamine excretion in patients with asterixis and hepatic coma (top) and octopamine levels in post-mortem frontal cortex from cirrhotic patients with HE

Patient group	Octopamine
	Urinary excretions (μg/24 h)
Control (11)	1.07 ± 0.27
Cirrhotics	
Asterixis (5)	$2.57 \pm 0.47*$
Coma (6)	$4.99 \pm 1.23**$
	Frontal cortex (ng/g)
Control (5)	59.2 ± 13.3
Cirrhotics with HE (4)	$36.0 \pm 6.1**$

Results are the means $\pm$ S.E.M.: $*P < 0.02$; $**P < 0.01$. Numbers in parentheses represent number of experimental subjects. (Top) Data adapted from Fischer and Baldessarini, 1971 (used with permission) and (bottom) data adapted from Cuilleret et al., 1980 (used with permission).

Baldessarini, 1971; Fischer and James, 1971). Hepatic devascularization also diminishes the brain concentration of noradrenaline (Dodsworth et al., 1974). These same authors demonstrated that significant increases in brain octopamine preceded the increases in serum, thus suggesting a cerebral rather than a strictly intestinal source of this trace amine.

Several reports, however, have questioned the validity of this hypothesis. It was observed that intracerebroventricular injection of octopamine increased its concentration approx. 20,000-fold without altering the level of consciousness in rats (Zieve and Olsen, 1977). This is in contrast to the observed 4-fold increase which was previously thought to be sufficient to induce coma in the rat (see above; Fischer and Baldessarini, 1971). In addition, an almost complete depletion (to 10–15% of control levels) of whole brain dopamine and noradrenaline following administration of octopamine or the catecholamine neurotoxin 6-hydroxydopamine did not result in the expected loss of consciousness in rats (Krnjevic, 1974; Zieve and Olsen, 1977). Clinical data are just as equivocal. Besides the beneficial therapeutic trials using L-DOPA and bromocriptine, other clinical trials found that these compounds were ineffective in the treatment of patients with PSE (Uribe et al., 1979; Michel et al., 1980) and therefore indirectly questioned the catecholamine/octopamine hypothesis. Neurochemical analyses of post-mortem brain tissue appear as equivocal, given findings of no change in dopamine and noradrenaline levels (Cuilleret et al., 1980) or selective regional increases in the levels of noradrenaline and the dopamine metabolites homovanillic acid and 3-methoxytyramine (Bergeron et al., 1989). It is interesting and certainly relevant to the octopamine hypothesis of HE that Cuilleret et al. (1980) actually observed a decrease in the levels of octopamine in the frontal cortex of HE patients (see Table 2). Finally, in vitro binding analysis of dopamine receptors in post-mortem HE brain tissue revealed a significant decrease in dopamine D_2 receptor density in globus pallidus which could simply relate to the motor dysfunctions commonly encountered in human HE (Mousseau et al., 1993). It is obvious that beneficial catecholaminergic treatment in HE could be restricted to a subpopulation of patients with more pronounced motor dysfunctions or refractory to the more conventional treatments for HE (see below).

The presence of trace amines in the brain, and in the present context of hepatic encephalopathy and coma, obviously depends on the availability of the amino acid precursors. Coma can be induced in dogs by the co-infusion of large quantities of phenylalanine and tryptophan (Rossi-Fanelli et al., 1982). It appears that aromatic amino acids such as phenylalanine and tryptophan compete with each other and with branched-chain aliphatic amino acids (e.g. valine, leucine and isoleucine) at the cellular membrane for the transport carrier (Oldendorf, 1971; Young and Sourkes, 1977). It would also appear that the presence of branched-chain aliphatic amino acids is necessary for a balanced competition for the transport carrier. Indeed, treatment with these amino acids has therapeutic value in both the clinical (Smith et al., 1978) and laboratory (Rossi-Fanelli et al., 1982) settings, whereas the absence of these amino acids, as seen in patients with hepatic dysfunction, augments the transport of tryptophan, among others, into the brain (Müting, 1962; Fernstrom and Wurtman, 1972). The observation that oral administration of tryptophan to patients with hepatic dysfunction affected their mental status (Sherlock, 1975) led Sourkes (1978) to expand the scope of the "false-transmitter" hypothesis of HE to include trace amine metabolites of tryptophan. He suggested that a massive increase in brain tryptophan concentration, reflecting an abundance of free (i.e. non-albumin bound) plasma tryptophan during chronic liver failure, could promote the synthesis of alternative neuroactive tryptophan metabolites, besides the biogenic amine serotonin (5-hydroxytryptamine; 5-HT), including kynurenines, tryptamine and β-carbolines (see Fig. 2). A disruption of normal tryptophan metabolism in HE is indicated by several lines of evidence. An increase in 5-HT synthesis and turnover is observed in CSF samples (Knell et al., 1974) and necropsy material (Jellinger and Riederer, 1977; Bergeron et al., 1989) in human hepatic coma as well as in the brains of portacaval-shunted rats used as experimental models of HE (Baldessarini and Fischer, 1973; Bergeron et al., 1990). It has been suggested that increased 5-HT turnover in experimental portal-systemic encephalopathy could be related to early psychiatric symptoms such as altered sleep patterns and personality changes (Bergeron et al., 1990). However, evidence from other studies in humans argues against increased 5-HT turnover being a causative factor in HE (see Sourkes, 1978; Holm et al., 1988).

Most of the evidence regarding the involvement of the trace amine tryptamine in HE, as well as in other neuropsychiatric syndromes, is indirect given its post-mortem instability and the lack of sensitivity and specificity of most of the earlier methods of detection (see Mousseau, 1993). It has been suggested that the reduced brain respiration observed during hepatic insufficiency and coma (Wechsler et al., 1954; Fazekas et al., 1956) may be due to increased tryptamine content given that this indoleamine is able to inhibit cerebral oxidation in vitro by approx. 75% even in the presence of normal glucose and oxygen supplies (Walshe et al., 1958). Tryptamine metabolism is much more responsive than is 5-HT metabolism to tryptophan loading (Young et al., 1980a). These authors reported that CSF indoleacetic acid (IAA; the predominant tryptamine metabolite) levels increased 25-fold whereas CSF 5-hydroxyindoleacetic acid (5-HIAA; the predominant 5-HT metabolite) levels only doubled following a tryptophan load. This was interpreted as a result of tryptophan hydroxylase being much closer to saturation with tryptophan than is amino acid decarboxylase. In addition, given the relative proportions of CSF IAA and 5-HIAA levels in man and rat, it would appear that tryptamine metabolism is more important in human brain than in rat brain (Young et al., 1980b). Using CSF IAA concentrations as an index of central tryptamine turnover, it was observed that patients

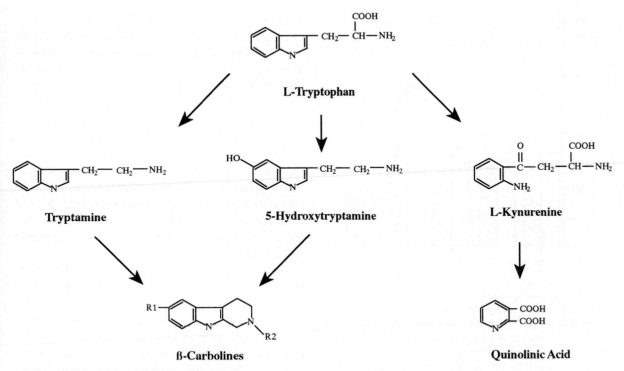

Fig. 2. Summary schematic of the synthetic pathways of serotonin (5-hydroxytryptamine; 5-HT) and related trace amines. Certain metabolites are omitted to simplify the diagram.

with hepatic coma had significantly higher brain tryptamine turnover when compared to cirrhotic patients not in coma (Young and Lal, 1980). Furthermore, the grade of coma was directly proportional to CSF IAA levels in these patients. A trend towards an increase in plasma IAA levels in patients with early HE was recently reported (Wiltfang et al., 1991).

A recent investigation (Mousseau and Butterworth, 1994b) demonstrated that [^{3}H]tryptamine binds in human frontal cortex with high affinity in a reversible and saturable manner. This binding site might perhaps be a species variant of the previously described rat [^{3}H]tryptamine binding site (see Mousseau, 1993). Although this remains to be determined, various lines of evidence including a heterogeneous distribution throughout human brain, in vitro stereospecific displacement (see Chapter 29, this volume) and linkage to a G protein (Ishitani et al., 1994) indicate that the human [^{3}H]tryptamine binding site might repre-

sent a functional receptor. Given the above mentioned evidence for increased CNS tryptamine concentrations in hepatic coma, a compensatory change (i.e. down-regulation) in [^{3}H]tryptamine binding site densities would be expected. In fact, regionally-specific decreases in human [^{3}H]tryptamine binding site densities were recently observed in post-mortem brain tissue from HE patients who died in hepatic coma (see Fig. 3; Mousseau et al., 1994). Tryptamine levels, however, were not significantly elevated in these regions (D.D. Mousseau, G.B. Baker and R.F. Butterworth, 1994; unpublished observations). This could be attributed to the post-mortem instability of this compound. On the other hand tryptophan levels, which had previously been shown to be directly correlated to levels of IAA in hepatic coma (Young and Lal, 1980), were significantly elevated in regions which had decreased [^{3}H]tryptamine binding density (D.D. Mousseau, G.B. Baker and R.F. Butterworth, 1994; unpub-

282

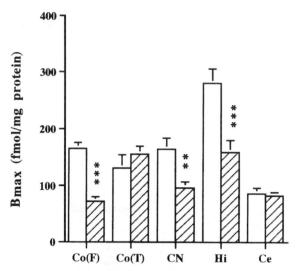

Fig. 3. Regional brain [^{3}H]tryptamine binding site densities in autopsied tissue from controls (open bars) and from cirrhotic patients with hepatic encephalopathy (hatched bars). Maximum binding site densities were determined by Scatchard analysis of saturation experiments (range 0.35–12 nM [^{3}H]tryptamine; $n = 6$–8 per group). Co(F), frontal cortex; Co(T), temporal cortex; CN, caudate nucleus; Hi, hippocampus; Ce, cerebellum. *$P < 0.01$; **$P < 0.001$. Taken from Mousseau et al., 1994 (used with permission).

lished observations). Whether the [^{3}H]tryptamine binding changes are purely the consequence of region-specific increases in the availability of tryptophan, and therefore tryptamine synthesis, or in region-specific increases in brain uptake of tryptamine resulting, for example, from decreased hepatic degradation of the amine in these patients, awaits further studies. Recent data indicate that the integrity of the [^{3}H]tryptamine receptor–G protein link (Mousseau and Butterworth, 1994b) is preserved in HE patient frontal cortical tissue (D.D. Mousseau and R.F. Butterworth, 1994; unpublished observations).

In addition to being the precursor for neuroactive monoamines such as 5-HT and tryptamine, tryptophan may be transformed in brain into other neuroactive and/or neurotoxic metabolites (see Fig. 2). One example involves the kynurenine pathway leading to the synthesis of quinolinic acid. Increased concentrations of quinolinic acid

have been described in the CSF of patients with PSE (Moroni et al. 1986a) and in the brains of portacaval-shunted rats (Moroni et al., 1986b). More recently, a preliminary report described increased levels of 3-hydroxykynurenine, a precursor along the quinolinic acid synthetic pathway, in post-mortem brain samples of patients with PSE (Pearson and Reynolds, 1991). The accumulation of these substances could result from decreased quinolinic acid degradation; the enzyme responsible for quinolinic acid metabolism, quinolinic acid phosphoribosyl transferase, is reportedly localized in astrocytes (Whetsell et al., 1988) whose integrity and function is lost in PSE (see Mousseau and Butterworth, 1994a).

Finally, Sourkes (1978) also suggested that β-carbolines might play a role in hepatic coma given their synthetic relation to both tryptamine and 5-HT. Preliminary studies indicate, however, that levels of the endogenous β-carboline 6-hydroxytetrahydro-β-carboline were not increased in the brain of HE patients having died in hepatic coma (D.D. Mousseau, G.B. Baker and R.F. Butterworth, 1994; unpublished observations).

Although the evidence for a direct involvement of trace amines in HE remains scarce, it would appear that increases in CNS concentrations of these amines as a result of increased amino acid precursor availability and/or diminished hepatic catabolism could well account for some of the neurological and neuropsychiatric manifestations commonly encountered in hepatic failure.

Summary

In 1971 Fischer and Baldessarini proposed the hypothesis that hepatic encephalopathy (HE), a neuropsychiatric syndrome associated with hepatic dysfunction, could result from the direct decarboxylation of amino acids leading to trace amines such as tyramine and octopamine which could then act as false neurotransmitters. This was supported by the observation that the clinical symptoms of HE appeared to improve following treatment with L-Dopa, which cannot be metabolized to either of these trace amines. In addition to serum and urine levels of octopamine correlating roughly with the grade of clinical HE, levels of octopamine were also significantly increased in rat brain following coma induced by hepatic devascularization and in portacaval-shunted rats fed high aromatic amino acid content diets. This hypothesis was questioned, however, given the lack of observable adverse behavioural effects following treatments with octopamine. Finally, the equivocal results of a limited number of clinical trials (using L-Dopa) argued against a direct intervention by catecholamine-like trace amines in HE. An alternative hypothesis was advanced by Sourkes in 1978 implicating increased tryptophan metabolism as a factor in the etiology of HE. Hepatic dysfunction in humans alters CNS concentrations of tryptophan which correlate well with levels of the tryptamine metabolite indoleacetic acid (IAA). Furthermore, regional densities of [^{3}H]tryptamine receptors in HE patient brain tissue are significantly decreased. These data support a pathophysiologic role for tryptophan and its neuroactive trace amine metabolite tryptamine in HE.

References

Baldessarini, R.J. and Fischer, J.E. (1973) Serotonin metabolism in rat brain after surgical diversion of the portal venous system. *Nature*, 245: 25–27.

Bengtsson, F., Bugge, M., Hall, H. and Nobin, A. (1989) Brain 5-HT$_1$ and 5-HT$_2$ binding sites following portacaval shunt in the rat. *Res. Exp. Med.*, 189: 249–256.

Bergeron, M., Reader, T.A., Pomier Layrargues, G. and Butterworth, R.F. (1989) Monoamines and metabolites in autopsied brain tissue from cirrhotic patients with hepatic encephalopathy. *Neurochem. Res.*, 14: 853–859.

Bergeron, M., Swain, M.S., Reader, T.A., Grondin, L. and Butterworth, R.F. (1990) Effect of ammonia on brain serotonin metabolism in relation to function in the portacaval shunted rat. *J. Neurochem.*, 55: 222–229.

Butterworth, R.F. (1992) Evidence that hepatic encephalopathy results from a defect of glutamatergic synaptic regulation. *Mol. Neuropharmacol.*, 2: 229–232.

Cuilleret, G., Pomier Layrargues, G., Pons, F., Cadilhac, J. and Michel, H. (1980) Changes in brain catecholamine levels in human cirrhotic hepatic encephalopathy. *Gut*, 21: 565–569.

Dodsworth, J.M., James, J.H., Cummings, M.C. and Fischer, J.E. (1974) Depletion of brain norepinephrine in acute hepatic coma. *Surgery*, 75: 811–820.

Fazekas, J.F., Ticktin, H.E., Ehrmantraut, W.R. and Alman, R.W. (1956) Cerebral metabolism in hepatic insufficiency. *Am. J. Med.*, 21: 843.

Fernstrom, J.D. and Wurtman, R.J. (1972) Brain serotonin content: physiological regulation by plasma neutral amino acids. *Science*, 178: 414–416.

Fischer, J.E. and Baldessarini, R.J. (1971) False neurotransmitters and hepatic failure. *Lancet*, 2: 75–80.

Fischer, J.E. and James, J.H. (1971) Mechanism of action of L-dopa in hepatic encephalopathy. *Surg. Forum*, 22: 347–349.

Fischer, J.E., James, J.H. and Baldessarini, R. (1972) Changes in brain amines following portal flow diversion and acute hepatic coma: effects of levodopa (L-dopa) and intestinal sterilization. *Surg. Forum*, 23: 348–350.

Holm, E., Jacob S., Kortsik C., Leweling H. and Fischer, B. (1988) Failure of selective serotonin re-uptake inhibition to worsen the mental state of patients with subclinical hepatic encephalopathy. In: P.B. Soeters, J.H.P. Wilson, A.J. Meijer and Holm E. (Eds.), *Advances in Ammonia Metabolism and Hepatic Encephalopathy*, Elsevier Scientific Publishers, Holland, pp. 474–486.

Ishitani, R., Kimura, M., Takeichi, M. and Chuang, D-M. (1994) Tryptamine induces phosphoinositide turnover and modulates adrenergic and muscarinic cholinergic receptor function in cultured cerebellar granule cells. *J. Neurochem.*, 63: 2080–2085

Jellinger, K. and Riederer, P. (1977) Brain monoamines in metabolic (endotoxic) coma: a preliminary biochemical study in human post-mortem material. *J. Neural Transm.*, 41: 275–286.

Knell, A.J., Davidson, A.R., Williams, R., Kantamanemi, B.D. and Curzon, G. (1974) Dopamine and serotonin metabolism in hepatic encephalopathy. *Br. Med. J.*, 1: 549–551.

Krnjevic, K. (1974) Chemical nature of synaptic transmission in vertebrates. *Physiol. Rev.*, 54: 418–505.

Lam, K.C., Tall, A.R., Goldstein, G.B. And Mistilis, S.P. (1973) Role of a false neurotransmitter, octopamine, in the pathogenesis of hepatic and renal encephalopathy. *Scand. J. Gastroenterol.*, 8: 465–472.

Loiudice, T.A., Tulman, A. and Buhac, I. (1979) L-Dopa and hepatic encephalopathy. *New York State J. Med.*, 3: 364–366.

Lunzer, M., James, I.M., Weinman, J. and Sherlock, S. (1974) Treatment of chronic hepatic encephalopathy with levodopa. *Gut*, 15: 555–561.

Manghani, K.K., Lunyer, M.R., Billing, B.H. and Sherlock, S. (1975) Urinary and serum octopamine in patients with portal-systemic encephalopathy. *Lancet*, 2: 943–946.

Michel, H., Solere, M., Granier, P., Cauvet, G., Bali, J.P. and Bellet-Hermann, H. (1980) Treatment of cirrhotic hepatic

284

encephalopathy with L-DOPA. A controlled trial. *Gastroenterology*, 79: 207–211.

Morgan, M.Y., Jakobovits, A.W., James, I.M. and Sherlock, S. (1980) Successful use of bromocriptine in the treatment of chronic hepatic encephalopathy. *Gastroenterology*, 78: 663–670.

Moroni, F., Lombardi, G., Carla, V., Lal, S., Etienne, P. and Nair, N.P.V. (1986a) Increase in the content of quinolinic acid in cerebrospinal fluid and frontal cortex of patients with hepatic failure. *J. Neurochem.*, 47: 1667–1671.

Moroni, F., Lombardi, G., Carla, V., Pellegrini, D., Carassale, G.L. and Cortesini, C. (1986b) Content of quinolinic acid and other tryptophan metabolites increases in brain regions of rats used as experimental models of hepatic encephalopathy. *J. Neurochem.*, 46: 869–874.

Mousseau, D.D. (1993) Tryptamine: A metabolite of tryptophan implicated in various neuropsychiatric disorders. *Metab. Brain Dis.*, 8: 1–44.

Mousseau, D.D. and Butterworth, R.F. (1994a) Current theories on the pathogenesis of hepatic encephalopathy. *Proc. Soc. Exp. Biol. Med.*, 206: 329–344.

Mousseau, D.D. and Butterworth, R.F. (1994b) The [^{3}H]tryptamine receptor in human brain: kinetics, distribution and pharmacologic profile. *J. Neurochem.*, 63: 1052–1059.

Mousseau, D.D., Perney, P., Pomier Layrargues, G. and Butterworth, R.F. (1993) Selective loss of pallidal dopamine D$_2$ receptor density in hepatic encephalopathy. *Neurosci. Lett.*, 162: 192–196.

Mousseau, D.D., Pomier Layrargues, G. and Butterworth, R.F. (1994) Region-selective decreases in densities of [^{3}H]tryptamine binding sites in autopsied brain tissue from cirrhotic patients with hepatic encephalopathy. *J. Neurochem.*, 62: 621–625.

Müting, D. (1962) Changes in the free amino acid composition of cerebrospinal fluid in liver disease. *Proc. Soc. Exp. Biol. Med.*, 110: 620–622.

Oldendorf, W.H. (1971) Brain uptake of radiolabeled amino acids, amines and hexoses after arterial injection. *Am. J. Physiol.*, 221: 1629–1639.

Pearson, S.J. and Reynolds G.P. (1991) Tryptophan metabolism in Huntington's disease and other neurodegenerative disorders. *J. Neurochem.*, 57 (Suppl. 1): S73B.

Rossi-Fanelli, F., Freund, H., Krause, R., Smith, A.R., James, J.H., Castorina-Ziparo, S. and Fischer, J.E. (1982) Induction of coma in normal dogs by the infusion of aromatic amino acids and its prevention by the addition of branched-chain amino acids. *Gastroenterology*, 83: 664–671.

Schafer, D.F. and Jones, E.A. (1982) Hepatic encephalopathy and the gamma-aminobutyric acid neurotransmitter system. *Lancet*, 2: 18–19.

Schenker, S., Desmond, P.V., Speeg, K.V. and Hoyumpa,

A.M., Jr. (1980) Cryptic nature of bromocriptine therapy in portal systemic encephalopathy. *Gastroenterology*, 78: 1094–1097.

Sherlock, S. (1975) *Diseases of the Liver and Biliary System*, 5th edn., Oxford, Blackwell.

Smith, A.R., Rossi-Fanelli, F., Ziparo, V., James, J.H., Prerelle, B.A. and Fischer, J.E. (1978) Alterations in plasma and CSF amino acids, amines and metabolites in hepatic coma. *Ann. Surg.*, 187: 343–350.

Sourkes, T.L. (1978) Tryptophan in hepatic coma. *J. Neural Transm.*, 14 (Suppl.): 79–86.

Uribe, M., Farca, A., Marquez, M.A., Garcia-Ramos, G. and Guevara, L. (1979) Treatment of chronic portal systemic encephalopathy with bromocriptine. *Gastroenterology*, 76: 1347–1351.

Walshe, J.M., De Carli, L. and Davidson, C.S. (1957) Some factors influencing cerebral ammonia production in relation to hepatic coma. *Clin. Sci.*, 17: 11–25.

Wechsler, R.L., Crum, W. and Roth, J.L.A. (1954) The blood flow and oxygen consumption of the human brain in hepatic coma. *Clin. Res. Proc.*, 2: 74.

Whetsell, W.O., Kohler, C. and Schwarz, R. (1988) Quinolinic acid: a glia-drived excitotoxin in the mammalian central neuron system. In: M.D. Norenberg (Ed.), *The Biochemical Pathology of Astrocytes*, Alan R. Liss, New York, pp. 1991–2002.

Wiltfang, J., Thiele, G., Weissenborn, K., Huther, G., Reimer, A., Pogeler, B., Kanzler, H., Schmidt, F.-W. and Wiltfang, A. (1991) Early hepatic encephalopathy, neurophysiological assessment and correlation with biochemical parameters. In: F. Bengtsson, B. Jeppson, T. Almdal and H. Vilstrup (Eds.), *Hepatic Encephalopathy and Metabolic Nitrogen Exchange*, CRC Press, Boca Raton, pp. 49–58.

Young, S.N., Anderson, G.M. and Purdy, W.C. (1980a) Indoleamine metabolism in rat brain studied through measurements of tryptophan, 5-hydroxyindoleacetic acid and indoleacetic acid in cerebrospinal fluid. *J. Neurochem.*, 34: 308–315.

Young, S.N., Anderson, G.M., Gauthier, S. and Purdy, W.C. (1980b) The origin of indoleacetic acid and indolepropionic acid in rat and human cerebrospinal fluid. *J. Neurochem.*, 34: 1087–1092.

Young, S.N. and Lal, S. (1980) CNS tryptamine metabolism in hepatic coma. *J. Neural Transm.*, 47: 153–161.

Young, S.N. and Sourkes, T.L. (1977) Tryptophan in the central nervous system: regulation and significance. *Adv. Neurochem.*, 2: 133–191.

Zieve, L. and Olsen, R.L. (1977) Can hepatic coma be caused by a reduction of brain noradrenaline ordopamine? *Gut*, 18: 688–691.

Peter M. Yu, Keith F. Tipton and Alan A. Boulton (Eds.)
Progress in Brain Research, Vol 106
© 1995 Elsevier Science BV. All rights reserved.

CHAPTER 29

A high-affinity [³H]tryptamine binding site in human brain

Darrell D. Mousseau and Roger F. Butterworth

Neuroscience Research Unit, St-Luc Hospital, University of Montreal, Montreal, Quebec, Canada H2X 3J4

Introduction

The trace amine tryptamine has been implicated in the etiology of numerous neuropsychiatric disorders (Dewhurst, 1968; see Mousseau, 1991 and 1993 for review). In vitro studies of rat brain [³H]tryptamine binding site parameters (Kellar and Cascio, 1982; Wood et al., 1984; Altar et al., 1986) and electrophysiological studies in rat cortical neurons (Jones and Boulton, 1981; Jones and Broadbent, 1982) support the suggested role of tryptamine in psychopathology (Dewhurst, 1968). Indeed, pharmacological manipulation of tryptamine synthesis either by neuronal ablation (Nguyen et al., 1989) or by chronic inhibition of monoamine oxidase, the major catabolic enzyme, (Graham and Langer, 1987; Martin et al., 1987; Nguyen and Juorio, 1989; Mousseau et al., 1993) induces changes in [³H]tryptamine binding site densities. Kellar and Cascio (1982) described a high-affinity binding site having a maximum density in the cerebral cortex of the rat of ~ 400 fmol/mg protein. In addition, [³H]tryptamine binding sites are heterogeneously distributed (exhibiting a rostral dominance) in rat brain (Cascio and Kellar, 1983; Wood et al., 1984). Descriptions of the parameters of a human tryptamine binding site are limited to a few preliminary reports (Cascio and Kellar, 1983; Kienzl et al., 1984) and a recent study done in our laboratory using postmortem tissue from patients with hepatic encephalopathy, a disorder whose symptomatology

includes neuropsychiatric manifestations (Mousseau et al., 1994). In view of these limited data we undertook to characterize more extensively the [³H]tryptamine binding site in human brain.

Materials and methods

Chemicals

[³H]Tryptamine (33.8–38.0 Ci/mmol) was purchased from New England Nuclear Research Products (Mississauga, ONT, Canada). Methysergide was a generous gift from Sandoz Canada Inc. (Whitby, ONT, Canada). Diazepam was a generous gift from Hoffmann LaRoche (Mississauga, ONT, Canada). (+)- and (−)-Amphetamine sulfate were generous gifts from Dr. R.D. Hossie of the Health Protection Branch of Health and Welfare, Ottawa, ONT, Canada. The remainder of the compounds needed for the present studies were purchased from either Sigma Chemical Co. (St. Louis, MO, USA), Research Biochemicals Inc. (Natick, MA, USA) or from Fisher Scientific Co. (Fairlawn, NJ, USA).

Tissue sampling

Postmortem human brains, obtained at autopsy from male subjects free from any neurological, neuropsychiatric or metabolic disorder, were dissected and the individual regions were manually chopped up and divided into aliquot parts (0.3–0.5 g wet weight tissue per vial) to ensure homogeneity in sampling. Each sample was frozen at $-80°C$ until time of assay. Mean age ($\pm$ SEM) for these subjects was 57.8 years ($\pm$ 2.7) (range: 49–75 years) whereas mean postmortem delay time ($\pm$ SEM) was 16.9 h ($\pm$ 3.0) (range: 7.15–28.5 h). No subjects had been exposed, in the 30 days prior to death, to drugs with known pharmacological effects on monoamine metabolism.

Radioligand binding assays

The assay method for [³H]tryptamine binding has been described elsewhere (Mousseau and Butterworth, 1994). Briefly, the tissue was mechanically suspended (five up-and-down strokes in a Teflon-glass motor-driven homogenizer) in approx. 10 vol. of ice-cold 50 mM Tris buffer (pH 7.4 at 25°C) and washed twice (40,000 $\times$ g for 10 min at 4°C). The final pellet was suspended in 10 vol. 50 mM Tris buffer containing pargyline (10 μM) and ascorbic acid (5.6 mM). This homogenate was preincubated at 37°C for 40 min. The kinetic (using 2.5 nM), saturation (using 0.35–12 nM) and displacement (using 3.0 nM) experiments to determine [³H]tryptamine binding parameters in human frontal cortex were done using standard experimental protocols. The nature of the [³H]tryptamine binding site (i.e. G protein-linked or not) was examined following the addition of the non-hydrolyzable guanosine 5′-triphosphate (GTP) analogue Gpp[NH]p (100 μM) (Gilman, 1987). In all experiments incubation was done at 4°C and specific binding was defined as the difference between total and non-specific binding using unlabelled tryptamine as a competing ligand. The data were determined and analyzed using commercially available computer programs. Protein determinations were carried out using the Folin phenol reagent procedure (Lowry et al., 1951).

Results

Kinetics of [³H]tryptamine binding

The association of [³H]tryptamine to the binding site was rapid, reaching steady state within approx. 20 min, and was stable for at least 120 min on ice. The K_{obs} (0.146 ± 0.022 min^{-1}) was used to calculate the rate constant of association K_1 (0.034 ± 0.004 min^{-1} nM^{-1}). The ratio of the dissociation (K_{-1}: 0.072 ± 0.014 min^{-1}) and association rate constants permitted the estimation of a dissociation constant (K_D) value of 2.14 ± 0.20 nM for [³H]tryptamine binding to human frontal cortex. The K_{-1} also allowed for estimation of the half-life of loss of specific binding ($t_{1/2}$: 9.625 min).

[³H]Tryptamine binding site distribution

Saturation and Scatchard (performed using least squares linear regression) analyses revealed saturable binding with a best-fit of the data to a single-site model with a Hill coefficient (n_H) of ~ 1.00 (see Table 1). The maximum binding site density (B_{max}) values were heterogeneous, ranging from 280 fmol/mg protein in hippocampus and thalamus to 90 fmol/mg protein in medulla oblongata and cerebellum (Fig. 1). No correlations were found between age or post-mortem interval and B_{max} or K_D values (data not shown).

Displacement studies

All of the cations tested, except for Cu^{2+}, inhibited [³H]tryptamine binding with K_i values in the low millimolar range (Na^+, 65 ± 28; K^+, 32 ± 6; Ca^{2+}, 18 ± 8; Mg^{2+}, 37 ± 8; Cu^{2+}, > 200). Certain of the following data have been presented elsewhere (Mousseau and Butterworth, 1994). The addition of 100 μM Gpp[NH]p to the incubation medium resulted in an average 41% shift towards a lower affinity ($1/K_D$) (Table 1). Effects of selected displacing compounds on cortical [³H]tryptamine binding are presented in Table 2. Tryptamine ($K_i = 6$ nM) was the most potent displacer of [³H]tryptamine. Of the remaining compounds investigated it would appear that sidechain-substitution of the parent (i.e. tryptamine or β-phenylethylamine) nucleus leads to a diminished potency to displace [³H]tryptamine from its binding site. Ring-substitution differentially altered the displacing potential of the parent nucleus depending on the position substituted (see p-tyramine versus dopamine) or the

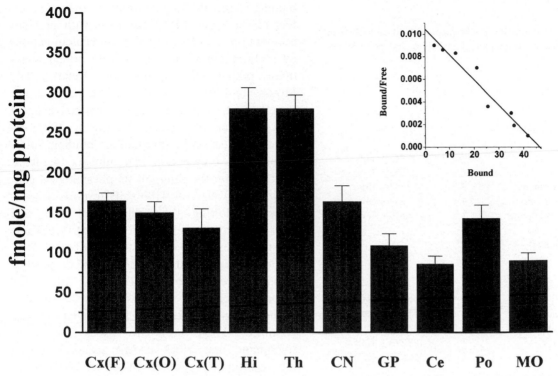

Fig. 1. Regional distribution of [^{3}H]tryptamine binding site densities in human brain. Scatchard analysis (insert), performed using least squares linear regression analysis, of the specific binding of [^{3}H]tryptamine to cortical homogenate preparations. Cx(F), frontal cortex; Cx(O), occipital cortex; Cx(T), temporal cortex; Hi, hippocampus; Th, thalamus; CN, caudate nucleus; GP, globus pallidus; Ce, cerebellum; Po, pons; MO, medulla oblongata; $n = 6-8$.

size of the substitution moeity itself (see 5-hydroxytryptamine versus 5-methoxytryptamine). Differences in displacing potencies of the enantiomers of amphetamine and deprenyl were also observed (Table 2).

TABLE 1

[^{3}H]Tryptamine binding parameters in human frontal cortex in the absence and presence of 100 μM Gpp[NH]p

	K_D	$1/K_D$	B_{max}	n_H
(−) Gpp[NH]	4.23 ± 0.25	0.24 ± 0.02	197 ± 9	0.99 ± 0.01
(+) Gpp[NH]	7.63 ± 1.06	0.14 ± 0.01	252 ± 17	1.00 ± 0.00
% Difference		40.5%		

K_D expressed in nM; B_{max} expressed in fmol/mg protein; $n = 6$.

Discussion

In vitro kinetic studies demonstrate specific high-affinity [^{3}H]tryptamine binding in human cerebral cortex. The K_D value of 2.14 nM estimated using the ratio of dissociation to association rate constants is consistent with previous K_D values for this site determined in rat cerebral cortex (Kellar and Cascio, 1982; Cascio and Kellar, 1983; Wood et al., 1984; Nguyen et al., 1989) and is in reasonable agreement with the K_D value determined by Scatchard analysis (see below).

The present cortical [^{3}H]tryptamine B_{max} and K_D values of 165 fmol/mg protein and 5.83 nM, respectively, confirm earlier estimates from preliminary studies using smaller sample sizes (Cascio and Kellar, 1983; Kienzl et al., 1984). A heterogeneous distribution for this binding site in human

TABLE 2

Displacement of specific [^{3}H]tryptamine binding to human frontal cortex by tryptophan metabolites and phenylethylamines

Drug	n	K_i
Tryptophan metabolites		
Tryptamine	5	6 ± 1
Kynuramine	7	116 ± 40
β-Carboline	5	332 ± 7
5-Methoxytryptamine	3	357 ± 101
5-Hydroxytryptamine	4	682 ± 187
Tetrahydro-β-carboline	5	$2,616 \pm 447$
Phenylethylamines		
β-Phenylethylamine	4	480 ± 18
p-Tyramine	3	315 ± 48
(+)-Amphetamine	3	966 ± 380
Dopamine	3	$7,953 \pm 355$
(−)-Amphetamine	3	$12,064 \pm 2,816$
(±)-Noradrenaline	3	$32,835 \pm 5,818$
DL-Octopamine	3	$182,373 \pm 87,054$
(+)-Deprenyl	3	$256,959 \pm 46,216$

The inhibitory constants (K_i; nM) were determined from the individual concentrations required to inhibit 50% of specific binding (IC$_{50}$). Tryptophan, methysergide, L-kynurenine, kynurenic acid, quinolinic acid, (−)-deprenyl, D- and L-tyrosine, GABA, diazepam, probenicid, reserpine, and *N*-methylamide and methyl ester congeners of β-carboline-3-carboxylic acid were not effective over the range tested. The K_i (nM) are reported as mean ± S.E.M. (Adapted from Mousseau and Butterworth, 1994.)

brain was also demonstrated (see Fig. 1). This observation is in good agreement with the regional [^{3}H]tryptamine binding site distribution determined for the rat brain using both filtration binding techniques (Cascio and Kellar, 1983; Wood et al., 1984) and quantitative receptor autoradiography (Kaulen et al., 1986; Perry, 1986). In addition, [^{3}H]tryptamine binding site density reflects the regional differences in concentrations of tryptamine previously observed in rat (Philips et al., 1974) and human brain (Philips et al., 1978).

Each of the cations studied (Na$^+$, K$^+$, Ca^{2+}, Mg^{2+}, but not Cu^{2+}) inhibited [^{3}H]tryptamine

binding within the low millimolar range. The effect of Ca^{2+} and Mg^{2+} contrasts with previous observations of a lack of effect of divalent cations on [^{3}H]tryptamine binding to rat cortical membrane preparations (Cascio and Kellar, 1983; Mousseau, 1991). This effect of cations was not an effect of osmolarity since a similar range of concentrations of sucrose (Mousseau, 1991) exerted no effect on [^{3}H]tryptamine binding. Interestingly, the only cation that appears to inhibit binding within the range of its physiological concentration is Na$^+$. A 41% shift towards a lower affinity following the addition of 100 μM Gpp[NH]p to the incubation medium (see Table 1) indicates an interaction between the [^{3}H]tryptamine binding site and a G protein. Given the recent proposal that Na$^+$ affects the affinity of receptors which are either dissociated from or negatively coupled to adenylate cyclase (Limbird, 1984) and the observation that tryptamine may block cAMP accumulation in mouse retina (Cohen and Blazinski, 1987), it appears that the present data support the possibility of a negative coupling of this trace indoleamine binding site/receptor to adenylate cyclase.

Tryptamine was the most potent inhibitor of [^{3}H]tryptamine binding to human cortical membrane preparations (see Table 2). Although ring-substitution of the tryptamine nucleus diminished the potency for competition at the site, 5-methoxy substitution imparted a greater potency at displacing [^{3}H]tryptamine binding than 5-hydroxy substitution. This had already been demonstrated for competition at the rat cortical [^{3}H]tryptamine binding site (Cascio and Kellar, 1983; Wood et al., 1984; Graham and Langer, 1987). In contrast, side-chain substitution, as seen with tryptophan (a carboxyl substitution at the α-carbon) and methysergide (whose indole nucleus is all but lost in extensive substitutions), appears to be important in diminishing the capacity for competing at the [^{3}H]tryptamine binding site. The activities of carboline and tetrahydro-β-carboline were unexpected given the respective 15-fold and 100-fold loss of potency at displacing [^{3}H]tryptamine in comparison to studies using rat cortical tissue (Cascio and Kellar, 1983; Wood et al., 1984; Graham and Langer, 1987). Substitution of the parent nucleus at the β-carboline position 3 (equivalent to the α-carbon in tryptamine) effectively eliminates the displacing capacity of β-carbolines (see Table 2), thus confirming previous findings concerning similar analogues (Wood et al., 1984). The moderate potency displayed by kynuramine fell between the high nanomolar affinity of the site previously reported for this compound (Charlton et al., 1984; Graham and Langer, 1987) and the total lack of activity reported by Wood et al. (1984).

β-Phenylethylamine was relatively effective at displacing [^{3}H]tryptamine in human brain tissue (Table 2) with a K_i value (480 nM) similar to those cited in the literature for the rat [^{3}H]tryptamine binding site (i.e. 87 to 486 nM) (Cascio and Kellar, 1983; Wood et al., 1984; Perry, 1986; Graham and Langer, 1987). Substitution of the phenylethylamine nucleus affects the displacing potency of these compounds in a manner similar to that observed with tryptamine. Indeed, the potency is increased with ring-hydroxylation of phenylethylamine but appears to be sensitive to side-chain substitution (see Table 2). Stereospecific displacement, which is an important indication of selectivity of the binding site, was observed with the enantiomers of amphetamine and deprenyl, with the [^{3}H]tryptamine binding site exhibiting a higher affinity for the (+)-enantiomer compared to the (−)-enantiomer. Cascio and Kellar (1983) and Wood et al. (1984) had previously suggested that the relatively high potency of amphetamine and the marked stereoselectivity of the binding site for the (+)-enantiomer compared to the (−)-enantiomer in rat brain may indicate that this binding site is responsible for certain of the pharmacological actions of amphetamine. The present data corroborate this suggestion. This argument may now be extended to include deprenyl and certain of its side-effects.

In comparing displacement potencies of the various tryptamines and β-phenylethylamines in the present study to literature values, it was interesting to note that the potencies of α-carboline, tetrahydro-β-carboline, kynuramine, p-tyramine and dopamine were significantly less than their respective potencies as displacers at the rat cortical [^{3}H]tryptamine binding site (Cascio and Kellar, 1983; see Mousseau, 1993). In contrast, the respective potencies of tryptamine itself, 5-hydroxy- and 5-methoxytryptamine, β-phenylethylamine, noradrenaline and the isomers of amphetamine were relatively similar to the potencies determined for the rat binding site.

Preliminary autoradiographic investigation of [^{3}H]tryptamine binding indicates a heterogeneous distribution in [^{3}H]tryptamine binding density throughout layers of the human frontal cortex. It appears that the distribution of these sites parallels the distribution of binding sites for [^{3}H]ketanserin (a radioligand for the serotoninergic 5-HT$_2$ receptors) but is independent of the distribution of binding sites for [^{3}H]8-OH-DPAT (a radioligand for the serotoninergic 5-HT$_{1A}$ receptors) (Mousseau and Butterworth, unpublished data).

In summary, we report evidence for the existence of high-affinity specific [^{3}H]tryptamine binding sites in human brain. These display a heterogeneous distribution which parallels documented regional endogenous brain tryptamine concentrations. These observations taken together with the observed stereoselectivity of the site (present study), the interaction of the site with a G protein (present study), the observed region-selective downregulation of the site in a human pathological condition, i.e. hepatic encephalopathy (Mousseau et al., 1994) and the documented tryptamine-induced electrophysiological and behavioural data derived from the rat (see Mousseau, 1993, for review) may be sufficient evidence to warrant calling the [^{3}H]tryptamine binding site a receptor. A similarity in kinetics and distribution of the [^{3}H]tryptamine receptor in human and rat brain indicates that these two entities represent homologous structures, although the difference in pharmacological profiles suggests species variants. One cannot exclude the possibility that the rat and human [3H]tryptamine receptors do, however, represent distinct subtypes. Finally, the suggested role for tryptamine in neuropsychiatric disorders as originally suggested by Dewhurst (1968) is supported by the present series of experiments.

Summary

In vitro filtration binding revealed high-affinity specific [3H]tryptamine binding sites in human brain. These binding sites are heterogeneously distributed throughout brain, ranging from 280 fmol/mg protein in hippocampus and thalamus to ~ 90 fmol/mg protein in medulla oblongata and cerebellum. Preliminary autoradiographic studies indicate a heterogeneous distribution within layers of the frontal cortex. The observed stereoselectivity of the site, the interaction of the site with a G protein and the observed region-selective downregulation of the site in a human pathological condition, i.e. hepatic encephalopathy (Mousseau et al., 1994), suggests that this binding site is a functional [3H]tryptamine receptor. A similarity in kinetics and distribution of the [3H]tryptamine receptor in human and rat brain indicates that these two entities represent homologous structures, although the difference in pharmacological profiles suggests species variants. One cannot exclude the possibility that the rat and human [3H]tryptamine receptors do represent distinct subtypes. Finally, the suggested role for tryptamine in neuropsychiatric disorders as originally suggested by Dewhurst (1968) is supported by the present series of experiments.

Acknowledgements

We thank the Medical Research Council of Canada for funding.

References

Altar, C.A., Wasley, A.M. and Martin, L.L. (1986) Autoradiographic localization and pharmacology of unique [3H]tryptamine binding sites in rat brain. Neuroscience, 17: 263–273.

Cascio, C.S. and Kellar, K.J. (1983) Characterization of [3H]tryptamine binding sites in brain. Eur. J. Pharmacol., 95: 31–39.

Charlton, K.G., Johnson, T.D., Maurice, R.W. and Clarke, D.E. (1984) Kynuramine: High affinity for [3H]tryptamine binding sites. Eur. J. Pharmacol., 106: 661–664.

Cohen, A.I. and Blazynski, C. (1987) Tryptamine and some related molecules block the accumulation of a light-sensitive pool of cyclic AMP in the dark-adapted, dark-incubated mouse retina. J. Neurochem., 48: 729–737.

Dewhurst, W.G. (1968) New theory of cerebral amine function and its clinical application. Nature (Lond.), 218: 1130–1133.

Gilman, A.G. (1987) G Proteins: Transducers of receptor-generated signals. Annu. Rev. Biochem., 56: 615–649.

Graham, D. and Langer, S.Z. (1987) [3H]Tryptamine binding sites of rat cerebral cortex: Pharmacological profile and plasticity. Neuropharmacology, 26: 1093–1097.

Jones, R.S.G. and Boulton, A.A. (1981) Tryptamine and 5-hydroxytryptamine's actions and interactions on cortical neurones in the rat. Life Sci., 27: 1849–1856.

Jones, R.S.G. and Broadbent, J. (1982) Further studies on the role of indoleamines in responses of cortical neurones evoked by stimulation of the nucleus raphé medianus: The effects of precursor loading. Neuropharmacology, 21: 1273–1278.

Kaulen, P., Brüning, G., Rommelspacher, H. and Baumgarten, H.G. (1986) Characterization and quantitative autoradiography of [3H]tryptamine binding sites in rat brain. Brain Res., 366: 72–88.

Kellar, K.J. and Cascio, C.S. (1982) [3H]Tryptamine: high affinity binding sites in rat brain. Eur. J. Pharmacol., 78: 475–478.

Kienzl, E., Riederer, P., Jellinger, K. and Noller, H. (1984) 14C-Tryptamine binding in Parkinson's disease and hepatic coma. In: A.A. Boulton, G.B. Baker, W.G. Dewhurst and M. Sandler M (Eds.), Neurobiology of the Trace Amines: Analytical, Physiological, Pharmacological, Behavioral and Clinical Aspects, Humana Press, Clifton, NJ, pp. 571–580.

Limbird, L.E. (1984) GTP and Na+ modulate receptor-adenyl cyclase coupling and receptor-mediated function. Am. J. Physiol., 247: E59–68.

Lowry, O.H., Rosebrough, N.J., Farr, A.L. and Randall, R.J. (1951) Protein measurements with the Folin phenol reagent. J. Biol. Chem., 193: 265–275.

Martin, L.L., Neale, R.F. and Wood, P.L. (1987) Down-regulation of tryptamine receptors following chronic administration of clorgyline. Brain Res., 419: 239–243.

Mousseau, D.D. (1991) Behavioural and neurochemical studies of tryptamine in the rat Ph.D. Thesis, University of Alberta, Edmonton, Canada.

Mousseau, D.D. (1993) Tryptamine: A metabolite of tryptophan implicated in various neuro-psychiatric disorders. Metab. Brain Dis., 8: 1–44.

Mousseau, D.D. and Butterworth, R.F. (1994) The

[^{3}H]tryptamine receptor in human brain: Kinetics, distribution and pharmacologic profile. *J. Neurochem.*, 63: 1052–1059.

Mousseau, D.D., McManus, D.J., Baker, G.B., Juorio, A.V., Dewhurst, W.G. and Greenshaw, A.J. (1993) Effects of age and of chronic antidepressant treatment on [^{3}H]-tryptamine binding to rat cortical membranes. *Cell. Mol. Neurobiol.*, 13: 3–13.

Mousseau, D.D., Pomier Layrargues, G. and Butterworth, R.F. (1994) Region-selective decreases in densities of [^{3}H]-tryptamine binding sites in autopsied brain tissue from cirrhotic patients with hepatic encephalopathy. *J. Neurochem.*, 62: 621–625.

Nguyen, T.V., Paterson, I.A., Juorio, A.V., Greenshaw, A.J. and Boulton, A.A. (1989) Tryptamine receptors: Neurochemical and electrophysiological evidence for postsynaptic and functional binding sites. *Brain Res.*, 476: 85–93.

Nguyen, T.V. and Juorio, A.V. (1989) Down-regulation of tryptamine binding sites following chronic molindone administration. *Naunyn-Schmiedeberg's Arch. Pharmacol.*, 340: 366–371.

Perry, D.C. (1986) [^{3}H]Tryptamine autoradiography in rat brain and choroid plexus reveals two distinct sites. *J. Pharmacol. Exp. Ther.*, 236: 548–559.

Philips, S.R., Durden, D.A. and Boulton, A.A. (1974) Identification and distribution of tryptamine in the rat. *Can. J. Biochem.*, 52: 447–451.

Philips, S.R., Rozdilsky, B. and Boulton, A.A. (1978) Evidence for the presence of *m*-tyramine, *p*-tyramine, tryptamine and phenylethylamine in the rat brain and several areas of human brain. *Biol. Psychiatry*, 13: 51–57.

Wood, P.L., Pilapil, C., LaFaille, F., Nair, N.P.V. and Glennon, R.A. (1984) Unique [^{3}H]tryptamine binding sites in rat brain: Distribution and pharmacology. *Arch. Int. Pharmacodyn.*, 268: 194–201.

Peter M. Yu, Keith F. Tipton and Alan A. Boulton (Eds.)
Progress in Brain Research, Vol 106
© 1995 Elsevier Science BV. All rights reserved.

CHAPTER 30

Substrate-specificity of mammalian tissue-bound semicarbazide-sensitive amine oxidase

G.A. Lyles

Department of Pharmacology and Clinical Pharmacology, University of Dundee, Ninewells Hospital and Medical School, Dundee DD1 9SY, UK

Introduction

The oxidative deamination of various endogenous and xenobiotic amines is catalyzed in mammalian tissues by a number of amine oxidase enzymes which exhibit different patterns of substrate specificity and inhibitor sensitivity, as well as differing in cellular and subcellular localization. These enzymes can be divided into two main groups by virtue of the chemical nature of their cofactors.

Flavin adenine dinucleotide is the prosthetic moiety within both the A and B forms of the outer mitochondrial membrane enzyme monoamine oxidase (MAO) and also in an intracellular polyamine oxidase which is largely found in peroxisomes (see Gorkin, 1983, for review). Other amine oxidases contain a cofactor possessing one or more carbonyl groups capable of reacting with semicarbazide and other "carbonyl reagents" which, therefore, act as inhibitors. There is continuing debate as to whether this cofactor is pyridoxal phosphate, pyroloquinoline quinone or 6-hydroxydopa (topa), whether or not the cofactor is the same in each enzyme, and also whether or not these particular enzymes are all copper-dependent (see Lyles, 1995, for review).

Within the category of carbonyl-containing amine oxidases are the intracellular diamine oxidases (or histaminases), the extracellular lysyl oxi-dases which participate in the formation of cross-linking between connective tissue proteins (collagen and elastin), and the various soluble amine oxidases of plasma which are capable of metabolizing monoamines, diamines and polyamines to varying extents in a species-dependent manner. The monoamine metabolizing plasma amine oxidases are particularly active against the synthetic amine benzylamine (BZ) as substrate, as also is a membrane-bound semicarbazide-sensitive amine oxidase (SSAO) found in high activity (although not exclusively) in the vasculature. These enzymes have, therefore, sometimes been called "benzyl-amine oxidases" (Lewinsohn, 1984) although it is not likely that BZ occurs physiologically as a natural substrate, and so they are increasingly being referred to nowadays as plasma and tissue-bound SSAOs.

While much still remains to be learned about the structure and function of all amine oxidases, the plasma and tissue-bound SSAOs are proving to be a particular challenge, since the demonstration of a convincing physiological role and the unequivocal identification of naturally occurring endogenous substrates continues to be elusive. Nevertheless, a variety of experimental approaches are beginning to provide a clearer perspective of the capability of these SSAOs to deaminate various aromatic and aliphatic monoamines, at least in vitro, and these findings have suggested possible physiological and/or toxicological influences which these enzymes may have upon tissue function in vivo. Although the plasma and tissue-bound SSAOs have many similar properties, this review focusses primarily upon the membrane-associated SSAO in mammalian tissues.

Cellular and subcellular localization of tissue-bound SSAO

The demonstration of SSAO activity in animal tissues has primarily depended upon two main criteria: (i) the ability to show that benzylamine is deaminated and (ii) being able to show that this metabolism is inhibited in vitro by semicarbazide concentrations around 0.1–1 mM. Since BZ is also a substrate for MAO, and especially for the B form of this enzyme, BZ metabolism by SSAO is often additionally confirmed by its insensitivity to inhibition by the MAO-selective (at 0.1–1 mM) acetylenic compounds clorgyline, deprenyl (selegiline) and pargyline. Semicarbazide is not an inhibitor of MAO at the concentrations used to define SSAO activity. Although semicarbazide and the acetylenic compounds have most frequently been the pharmacological tools used to distinguish between SSAO and MAO, an increasing number of other compounds have also been characterized as exhibiting varying degrees of selectivity with some usefulness for enzyme classification (see Lyles, 1984, 1995, for reviews).

A major focus of studies upon tissue-bound SSAO has been the vasculature, reflecting the discovery that enzyme activity is particularly high in blood vessels compared with other tissues. From studies to date, SSAO appears to exist as a vascular component of all mammalian species including man (Lewinsohn, 1984; Lyles, 1995). Histochemical staining for SSAO activity has revealed that the enzyme is associated with the smooth muscle layers of the tunica media of blood vessels (Lewinsohn, 1984; Lyles and Singh, 1985; Precious and Lyles, 1988). Cultured smooth muscle cells from pig and rat aorta express SSAO activity (Hysmith and Boor, 1987; Blicharski and

Lyles, 1990) whereas no detectable activity was found in pig or human endothelial cells (Hysmith and Boor, 1987; Yu and Zuo, 1993). SSAO also appears to be present in non-vascular smooth muscle in tissues such as the uterus, ureter and vas deferens (Lewinsohn, 1981; Lizcano et al., 1991). However, SSAO is not restricted solely to smooth muscle cells, since to date it has been demonstrated to occur in rat adipocytes (Barrand et al., 1984; Raimondi et al., 1991), rat chondrocytes (Lyles and Bertie, 1987) and pig odontoblasts (Norqvist and Oreland, 1989).

Subcellular fractionation techniques have indicated that a substantial proportion of SSAO appears as a membrane-bound enzyme in microsomal fractions, with a distribution when compared with various marker enzymes suggesting that it is associated at least in part with the plasma membrane of cells in blood vessels (Wibo et al., 1980), adipose tissue (Barrand and Callingham, 1982; Barrand et al., 1984) and dental pulp (Norqvist and Oreland, 1989). There is evidence that at least some of this SSAO activity may reside on the outer surface of the plasmalemma, suggesting that SSAO may be in a position to deaminate amines present in the extracellular compartment of tissues (Barrand et al., 1984; Holt and Callingham, 1994). In most studies of subcellular distribution, some SSAO activity is also found in mitochondrial and soluble fractions (e.g. Suzuki and Matsumoto, 1984) but it is unclear whether these represent genuine sites of SSAO potentially able to metabolize intracellular amines, or alternatively are due to plasmalemmal contamination of these fractions. In this respect, the plasma membrane SSAO presumably originates from intracellular synthesis before transport to and insertion into the plasma membrane although whether or not its catalytic properties are identical throughout these processes is unclear. Also, of possible relevance to these points is the existence of strong evidence for the presence of soluble forms of SSAO in bovine and porcine aorta, with properties very similar to those of the plasma SSAOs found in each particular species (Harris and O'Dell, 1972; Buffoni, 1980) and this has led to speculation that the vasculature may be the source of the soluble plasma enzyme. The latter is supported by findings that pig cultured aortic smooth muscle cells secrete a soluble SSAO activity into the culture medium, and this enzyme appears to be immunologically identical to the purified pig plasma SSAO (Hysmith and Boor, 1987, 1988a).

Substrate specificity of tissue-bound SSAO

Aromatic amines

SSAO activity has been studied in homogenates and cell fractions prepared from a variety of tissues, and it is now apparent that the substrate specificity determined in vitro can vary quite markedly in a species-dependent manner and this creates considerable difficulty when attempting to produce generalized hypotheses about the role of SSAO in mammalian amine metabolism.

As a starting point, it is generally accepted that SSAO only metabolizes primary amines. While the ability to deaminate the synthetic amine BZ is a common feature of the tissue-bound SSAO activities, there is a fairly wide range of K_m values reported for BZ as a substrate for SSAO in different species, with the human enzyme exhibiting a particularly high K_m (Table 1).

This theme of species-related differences in substrate affinity and metabolism is also evident in studies which have examined the in vitro metabolism by SSAO of a variety of biogenic amines which occur endogenously and/or are absorbed in the diet, although many of these studies only compare relative deaminating activities towards different amines at single concentrations without determinations of kinetic constants (K_m, V_{max}). Thus SSAO in rabbit aorta, heart and lung was fairly active against tyramine (Tyr), tryptamine (Tryp) and 2-phenylethylamine (PEA) (Rucker and Goettlich-Riemann, 1972; Buffoni et al., 1989). PEA is also metabolized by SSAO in pig aorta (Trevethick et al., 1981) and bovine lung, the latter also deaminating dopamine (DA), but apparently not Tyr or Tryp (Lizcano et al., 1990). Pig dental pulp is unique to date in ex-

pressing a 5-hydroxytryptamine (5-HT) metabolizing SSAO, which is also active towards Tyr, Tryp and PEA (Norqvist et al., 1981).

The most detailed perspective of substrate specificity currently available is for SSAO in rat tissues. Noradrenaline, octopamine and phenylethanolamine do not appear to be substrates for SSAO in rat vasculature (Coquil et al., 1973; Elliott et al., 1989a), suggesting that, in contrast to MAO, SSAO activities are virtually if not completely inactive against aromatic amines with a hydroxyl substituent on the β-carbon of the side chain. However, rat SSAO is capable of deaminating physiological aromatic monoamines (Tyr, Tryp, PEA and DA) having unsubstituted ethylamine side chains, with representative K_m values shown in Table 2, which are in fact fairly similar to K_m values for metabolism of these substrates by mitochondrial MAO activities (Strolin Benedetti and Dostert, 1985). There is some evidence that kynuramine (Kyn), which contains its ethylamine side chain linked to its aromatic ring through an additional carbonyl (C = O) group is also a substrate for SSAO in rat aorta

TABLE 1

K_m values for benzylamine metabolism by tissue-bound SSAO in various species

SPECIES/tissue	K_m (μM)
Rat skull[a], brown fat[b], cartilage[c], aorta[d]	3[a,b,c], 6[d]
Pig dental pulp	2[e]
Cat uterine artery	7[f]
Sheep femoral artery	11[g]
Rabbit heart[h], lung[i]	10[h], 13[i]
Bovine lung	40[j]
Human aorta[k], umbilical artery[l,m]	110[k], 155[l], 222[m]

[a]Andree and Clarke, 1982b; [b]Barrand and Callingham, 1982; [c]Lyles and Bertie, 1987; [d]Clarke et al. 1982; [e]Norqvist et al., 1982; [f]Callingham et al., 1988; [g]Elliott et al., 1992; [h,i]Buffoni et al., 1989; [j]Lizcano et al., 1994; [k]Lewinsohn, 1984; [l]Yu et al., 1994; [m]Lyles et al., 1990.

TABLE 2

K_m values (μM) for aromatic amine substrates of SSAO in some rat and human tissues

Substrate	Rat	Human
Benzylamine	3[abc], 6[d]	110[k], 161[l]
2-Phenylethylamine	10[b], 15[ae], 44[c]	7900[l]
Tyramine	40[b], 52[e]	10500[l]
Tryptamine	54[a], 67[f]	(1%[m], 7%[n])
Dopamine	130[g], 270[a], 1058[h]	(5%[n])
Histamine	320[i], 583[j]	(0%[m])

Where K_m values have not been determined, percentages in parentheses show amine metabolism relative to benzylamine, each at 500 μM.
[a]Skull (Andree and Clarke, 1982b); [b]brown fat (Barrand and Callingham, 1982); [c]cartilage (Lyles and Bertie, 1987); [d]aorta (Clarke et al., 1982); [e]aorta (Guffroy et al., 1985); [f]aorta (Lyles and Taneja, 1987); [g]aorta (Yu, 1988); [h]vas deferens (Lizcano et al., 1991); [i]white adipocytes (Raimondi et al., 1993); [j]aorta (Yu, 1990); [k]aorta (Lewinsohn, 1984); [l]umbilical artery (Precious and Lyles, 1988); [m]aorta (Suzuki and Matsumoto, 1984); [n]aorta (Hayes et al., 1983).

(Dial and Clarke, 1977), and although a K_m has not been reported, it is notable that Kyn exhibited a very low K_i (5 μM) compared with other amines as a competitive inhibitor of BZ metabolism in rat aorta (Elliott et al., 1989a). Rat tissue-bound SSAO is also reported to deaminate histamine (Hist) with a fairly high K_m (Table 2), although Hist metabolism by SSAO has not been detected in all tissues examined (e.g. rat lung: Ueda and Kinemuchi, 1984).

Table 2 also compares K_m values where available for amines as substrates of the rat and human enzyme. Here it is apparent that PEA and Tyr have considerably higher K_m values in man, and comparisons of relative deaminating activity of DA, Tryp and Hist with that of BZ in human tissues suggested that these also were poor substrates (if at all) for the human enzyme. These results cast some doubt upon the probability that aromatic amines represent significant physiological substrates for SSAO in man, although it is of interest that patients with Norrie's Disease, char-

acterized by a genetic absence of MAO activity, still excrete normal urinary amounts of deaminated metabolites of 5-HT and DA. This has led to some speculation, albeit with no direct proof yet, that enzymes such as SSAO could be involved in metabolite formation (Murphy et al., 1991).

Other differences between rat and human SSAO have been detected in studies upon the mechanisms of catalysis of amine oxidation. Thus rat aorta SSAO preferentially abstracts the pro-S hydrogen from the α-carbon atom in amine substrates (BZ, DA) so far examined, whereas no such stereospecificity (with BZ) was exhibited by the human umbilical artery SSAO (Yu and Davis, 1988; Yu et al., 1994). As a whole, therefore, these species-related variations in substrate metabolism suggest that considerable caution has to be exercised when attempting to use experiments with laboratory animals as possible models of SSAO function in man.

Does SSAO play a role in degrading aromatic amines in vivo in some species, perhaps modifying the pharmacological effects of amines upon target tissues? This idea is supported by evidence that MAO and SSAO activities can contribute to the formation of deaminated metabolites of PEA and Tyr when these amines are perfused through rabbit and rat vascular beds (Roth and Gillis, 1975; Elliott et al., 1989b). Furthermore, administration to rats of semicarbazide or the MAO inhibitor tranylcypromine slowed the disappearance of ^{14}C-PEA (and also the appearance of PEA metabolites) in plasma, with even greater effects if the inhibitors were given together (Guffroy et al., 1985). The direct contractile effects of Tryp upon rat aortic smooth muscle, and the indirect sympathomimetic effects of Tyr to increase perfusion pressure in the rat mesenteric arterial bed, were potentiated by a combination of MAO and SSAO inhibition, suggesting that these enzymes may act in concert to regulate vascular effects of some amines (Taneja and Lyles, 1988; Elliott et al., 1989c). In contrast, evidence that MAO inhibition but not SSAO inhibition could potentiate vasoconstrictor effects of Tryp on human umbilical artery (Johnson et al., 1986) is consistent with evidence that SSAO has little if any activity towards Tryp in this tissue (Precious and Lyles, 1988). More recently, Raimondi et al. (1993) showed that lipolysis induced by Hist in rat white adipocytes was enhanced after inhibition of the SSAO activity associated with these cells.

While there remains considerable interest in whether or not SSAO can metabolize endogenously occurring physiological aromatic amines, it should be noted that xenobiotic agents or synthetic drug molecules which are aromatic compounds containing primary amine functions on their alkyl side chains may also potentially be metabolised by SSAO. For instance, there is evidence that the GABA mimetic compound kojic amine (Ferkany et al., 1981) and the MAO inhibitor MD 220661 (Dostert et al., 1984) are both substrates. In addition, it appears that the slow reversal of the inhibitory actions of the hydrazine derivative, phenelzine, upon SSAO may be as a result of its slow metabolism by the enzyme (Andree and Clarke, 1982a).

Aliphatic amines

Considerable interest has followed from the discovery that tissue-bound SSAO from various species has significant deaminating activity against a number of aliphatic amines, some of which occur endogenously or exist as xenobiotic agents. In 1965, McEwen first showed that human plasma SSAO was able to metabolize several short-chain aliphatic amines, with particularly good activity against methylamine (MA), although no suggestion was made at the time that MA might be a physiological substrate for the enzyme. However, MA can be absorbed as a component of foodstuffs (Neurath et al., 1977), or can be produced and absorbed as a consequence of the metabolism of dietary choline, lecithin and creatinine by intestinal bacteria (Zeisel et al.,1983; Lowis et al., 1985). MA may also be generated endogenously by mammalian degradation of sarcosine and creatinine (Davis and De Ropp, 1961) and by the oxidative deamination of adrenaline by MAO (Schayer et al., 1952).

Our laboratory originally became interested in the possible role of tissue-bound SSAOs in the metabolism of MA since this amine is not a substrate for MAO (Blaschko, 1952). We developed assay methods which provided the first direct demonstration that MA is metabolized by SSAO in homogenates of rat and human vasculature (Precious et al., 1988; Precious and Lyles, 1988; Lyles et al., 1990). It was later confirmed that formaldehyde could be detected as the deaminated aldehyde product of MA metabolism (Boor et al., 1992). More recently, it has been shown that MA is a substrate for adipose tissue SSAO in man, pig, rabbit, mouse and rat (Raimondi et al., 1992; Conforti et al., 1993), and is also deaminated by SSAO in bovine lung and aorta (Lizcano et al., 1994; Yu et al., 1994), as well as in rat brain microvessels and in retina and sclera from the eye (Zuo and Yu, 1994). Consequently, this ability of SSAO to metabolize MA appears to be widespread among mammals. However, it should be noted again that there are species-related variations in substrate metabolism. For example, Table 3 shows some comparative K_m values obtained for MA in rat, bovine and human tissues. Although MA was a fairly high K_m substrate for human SSAO compared with BZ, we also found that the rate of MA turnover, represented by the V_{max} for metabolism, was 70%

TABLE 3

Comparison of K_m (μM) values for benzylamine, methylamine and aminoacetone as SSAO substrates in different species

Source	Benzylamine	Methylamine	Aminoacetone
Rat aorta	6[ab]	247[b], 182[c]	19[d]
Bovine lung	40[e]	340[e]	94[e]
Human umbilical artery	222[c], 155[f]	832[c]	92[g]

[a]Clarke et al., 1982; [b]Yu, 1990; [c]Lyles et al., 1990; [d]Lyles and Chalmers, unpublished; [e]Lizcano et al., 1994; [f]Yu et al., 1994; [g]Lyles and Chalmers, 1992.

greater for MA than for BZ (Precious et al., 1988).

There is some experimental evidence that the tissue (and plasma) SSAOs may contribute to MA metabolism in vivo. In several studies in which amine oxidase inhibitors have been administered either to rats or mice, it has been found that a number of drugs which share the common feature of being able to inhibit SSAO can increase the levels of urinary MA excretion, and decrease the appearance of $^{14}CO_2$ in expired air arising from ^{14}C-MA metabolism in vivo (Davis and De Ropp, 1961; Werner et al., 1961; Dar et al., 1985; Lyles and McDougall, 1989).

While MA has provided an initial focus of attention among saturated aliphatic amines as potential endogenous substrates of SSAO, Guffroy et al. (1983) and Yu (1990) have shown that certain other straight-chain aliphatic primary amines, some of which may also occur naturally (e.g. ethylamine, n-butylamine) are also substrates for SSAO (at least in the rat). It appears that SSAO can also metabolize some branched-chain aliphatic amines (e.g. isoamylamine and 2-propylaminopentane) which contain a primary amino function linked to an unsubstituted methylene group (Elliott et al., 1989a; Yu and Davis, 1991; Elliott et al., 1992).

Another endogenously occurring aliphatic amine which has been investigated recently as a potential substrate of tissue-bound SSAO is aminoacetone (AA). This amine, which is detectable in urine (Marver et al., 1966), can be formed endogenously as a result of mitochondrial metabolism of threonine by the enzyme threonine dehydrogenase, or from glycine via the enzyme aminoacetone synthetase. Metabolism of glycine to AA is favoured by high acetyl CoA/low CoA levels, whereas, conversely, glycine formation from AA occurs at low acetyl CoA/high CoA levels (Urata and Granick, 1963; Bird et al., 1984; Tressel et al., 1986). Following from studies showing that AA is a substrate for plasma SSAO from the ox, goat, sheep and horse (but not in pig) (Elliott, 1960; Buffoni and Blaschko, 1963; Ray and Ray, 1983) as well as for an amine oxidase purified from goat liver (Ray and Ray, 1987), we have recently demonstrated that AA is deaminated by SSAO to methylglyoxal in tissue fractions of rat aorta, human umbilical artery and bovine lung. K_m values for AA obtained in these studies are shown in Table 3 in comparison with BZ and MA. It is of interest that AA has a K_m for human SSAO which is much lower not only than that of BZ and MA, but also than those of the aromatic amines shown in Table 2. Whether or not these in vitro findings result eventually in the confirmation that AA is indeed an endogenous substrate for SSAO remains to be seen.

At present there have been no obvious physiological properties ascribed to endogenous MA or AA and thus it is unclear whether these amines are important regulators of cellular function. However, some attention has been focussed upon the aldehydes, formaldehyde and methylglyoxal, which result from the deamination of these amines by SSAO, and which are well-known potentially cytotoxic agents (Heck et al., 1990; Thornalley, 1990). This interest in the deamination of aliphatic amines to produce cytotoxic aldehydes has received considerable impetus from studies with the industrial unsaturated amine allylamine. This compound can induce cardiovascular lesions when administered to various laboratory species, producing pathological characteristics which, under some circumstances, mimic certain features of atherosclerosis (Boor and Hysmith, 1987). These effects have been ascribed to the ability of SSAO, especially in the vascular wall, to metabolize allylamine to the highly toxic aldehyde acrolein (Nelson and Boor, 1982; Boor et al., 1990). Cytotoxic effects of allylamine can also be demonstrated in cultured vascular smooth muscle cells from the pig and rat, and these actions can be prevented by inhibitors of SSAO (but not of MAO) activity (Hysmith and Boor, 1988b; Ramos et al., 1988). Similar results have recently been obtained with rat cardiac myocytes, even though the existence of SSAO in this type of cell has not previously been demonstrated (Toraason et al., 1989).

Is it possible that the deamination of endogenously occurring aliphatic amines may initiate mechanisms of cellular dysfunction? Support for this has come from studies by Yu and Zuo (1993), demonstrating that MA is cytotoxic towards human cultured endothelial cells (which themselves do not contain SSAO) when incubated in the presence of exogenous sources of SSAO (e.g. human plasma or umbilical artery homogenates) capable of converting MA to formaldehyde. Of course, metabolism of amines by SSAO also produces hydrogen peroxide as another agent capable of producing cellular damage, although upon exposure of endothelial cells directly to added formaldehyde or hydrogen peroxide, the aldehyde proved to be the more potent cytotoxic agent (Yu and Zuo, 1993).

The intracellular and extracellular levels of reduced glutathione (GSH) may be important factors in determining the likelihood of toxicity arising from aliphatic aldehyde and hydrogen peroxide generation. For example, conjugation with GSH is involved in the detoxification and excretion of allylamine as a mercapturic acid derivative (Boor et al., 1987), and in relation to this we have shown that depletion of GSH from rat aortic cultured smooth muscle cells, by treatment with the GSH synthesis inhibitor buthionine sulphoximine, can enhance the cytotoxic effects of allylamine upon these cells (Blicharski and Lyles, 1991). Conjugation of formaldehyde and methylglyoxal with GSH is also a prerequisite for metabolism of these aldehydes by the enzymes formaldehyde dehydrogenase and glyoxalase (I and II), which convert the aldehydes to formate and D-lactate, respectively (Uotila and Koivusalo, 1989; Thornalley, 1990). GSH is also important in the degradation of hydrogen peroxide by glutathione peroxidase (Shan et al., 1990). However, in addition to helping in the removal of toxic agents, GSH could also be involved in producing biologically active molecules. For example, after conjugation of methylglyoxal with GSH, the adduct is metabolized by glyoxalase I to produce S-D-lactoyl GSH, which has been implicated as a possible physiological regulator of cellular cytoskeletal function (Thornalley, 1990).

Conclusions

The ability of SSAO to deaminate various aromatic and aliphatic primary monoamines differs in a species-related fashion. Those aromatic amines studied so far as potential physiological substrates were metabolized quite well in vitro in some species, suggesting that SSAO could be involved in regulating cellular actions of such amines, for example in the vasculature. However, these same aromatic amines were very poorly metabolized by the human enzyme. In contrast, the endogenously occurring aliphatic amines methylamine and aminoacetone appear to be better candidates as physiological substrates for SSAO in man and other species. However, the possibility that deamination of aliphatic amines to generate potentially cytotoxic products which could contribute to cellular (especially cardiovascular) dysfunction remains to be explored further.

Summary

Although the existence of a membrane-bound (probably plasmalemmal) semicarbazide-sensitive amine oxidase (SSAO) is well established in various mammalian tissues, and especially within vascular smooth muscle, its importance and the possible consequences of its metabolism of certain physiological and xenobiotic amines in vivo are under continuing investigation. In this respect, there are major species-related differences in substrate specificity determined in vitro, not only towards the synthetic amine benzylamine, but also towards some other aromatic amines (e.g. tyramine, tryptamine, 2-phenylethylamine, dopamine, histamine) which are possible endogenous substrates. Inhibition of SSAO can potentiate the pharmacological activity of some amines in isolated tissue (e.g. blood vessel) preparations from some species. Recent evidence has accumulated that SSAO may also be involved in metabolizing endogenous aliphatic amines such as methylamine and aminoacetone, focussing attention on the fact that the aldehyde products (formaldehyde and methylglyoxal, respectively) are potentially cytotoxic agents. Indeed, SSAO has been implicated in experimental models of cardiovascular toxicity involving conversion of the industrial aliphatic amine allylamine to acrolein. In summary, metabolism by SSAO may reduce the physiological/pharmacological effects of some amines, but the resulting metabolites (aldehydes, H_2O_2) may also have important actions.

Acknowledgement

Work in the author's laboratory is currently supported by European Economic Community Research Contract (CHRX-CT93-0256) under the Human Capital and Mobility Programme.

References

Andree, T.H. and Clarke, D.E. (1982a) Characteristics and specificity of phenelzine and benserazide as inhibitors of benzylamine oxidase and monoamine oxidase. *Biochem. Pharmacol.*, 31: 825–830.

Andree, T.H. and Clarke, D.E. (1982b) Characteristics of rat skull benzylamine oxidase. *Proc. Soc. Exp. Biol. Med.*, 171: 298–305.

Barrand, M.A. and Callingham, B.A. (1982) Monoamine oxidase activities in brown adipose tissue of the rat: some properties and subcellular distribution. *Biochem. Pharmacol.*, 31: 2177–2184.

Barrand, M.A., Callingham, B.A. and Fox, S.A. (1984) Amine oxidase activities in brown adipose tissue of the rat: identification of semicarbazide-sensitive (clorgyline-resistant) activity at the fat cell membrane. *J. Pharm. Pharmacol.*, 36: 652–658.

Bird, M.I., Nunn, P.B. and Lord, L. (1984) Formation of glycine and aminoacetone from L-threonine by rat liver mitochondria. *Biochim. Biophys. Acta*, 802: 229–236.

Blaschko, H. (1952) Amine oxidase and amine metabolism. *Pharmacol. Rev.*, 4: 415–458.

Blicharski, J.R.D. and Lyles, G.A. (1990) Semicarbazide-sensitive amine oxidase activity in rat aortic cultured smooth muscle cells. *J. Neural Transm.*, (Suppl.) 32: 337–339.

Blicharski, J.R.D. and Lyles, G.A. (1991) D,L-Buthionine sulphoximine, a glutathione-depleting agent potentiates allylamine-induced cytotoxicity in rat aortic smooth muscle cultures. *Br. J. Pharmacol.*, 102: 184P.

Boor, P.J. and Hysmith, R.M. (1987) Allylamine cardiovascular toxicity. *Toxicology*, 44: 129–145.

Boor, P.J., Sanduja, R., Nelson, T.J. and Ansari, G.A.S. (1987) In vivo metabolism of the cardiovascular toxin, allylamine. *Biochem. Pharmacol.*, 36: 4347–4353.

Boor, P.J., Hysmith, R.M. and Sanduja, R. (1990) A role for a new vascular enzyme in the metabolism of xenobiotic amines. *Circ. Res.*, 66: 249–252.

Boor, P.J., Trent, M.B., Lyles, G.A., Tao, M. and Ansari, G.A.S. (1992) Methylamine metabolism to formaldehyde by vascular semicarbazide-sensitive amine oxidase. *Toxicology*, 73: 251–258.

Buffoni, F. (1980) Some contributions to the problem of amine oxidases. *Pharmacol. Res. Commun.*, 12: 101–114.

Buffoni, F. and Blaschko, H. (1963) Enzymic oxidation of aminoketones in mammalian blood plasma. *Experientia*, 14: 1–2.

Buffoni, F., Banchelli, G., Bertocci, B. and Raimondi, L. (1989) Effect of pyridoxamine on semicarbazide-sensitive amine oxidase activity of rabbit lung and heart. *J. Pharm. Pharmacol.*, 41: 469–473.

Callingham, B.A., Elliott, J. and Williams, R.B. (1988) Amine oxidase interactions in the cardiovascular system. In: *Progress in Catecholamine Research Neurology and Neurobiology*, Vol. 42A, Alan R. Liss, New York, pp. 109–113.

Clarke, D.E., Lyles, G.A. and Callingham, B.A. (1982) A comparison of cardiac and vascular clorgyline-resistant amine oxidase and monoamine oxidase. *Biochem Pharmacol.*, 31: 27–35.

Conforti, L., Raimondi, L. and Lyles, G.A. (1993) Metabolism of methylamine by semicarbazide-sensitive amine oxidase in white and brown adipose tissue of the rat. *Biochem. Pharmacol.*, 46: 603–607.

Coquil, J.F., Goridis, C., Mack, G. and Neff, N.H. (1973) Monoamine oxidase in rat arteries: evidence for different forms and selective localization. *Br. J. Pharmacol.*, 148: 590–599.

Dar, M.S., Morselli, P.L. and Bowman, E.R. (1985) The enzymatic systems involved in the mammalian metabolism of methylamine. *Gen. Pharmacol.*, 16: 557–560.

Davis, J.E. and De Ropp, R.S. (1961) Metabolic origin of urinary methylamine in the rat. *Nature*, 190: 636–637.

Dial, E.J. and Clarke, D.E. (1977) Observations on the monoamine oxidase activity of rat vasa deferentia, major blood vessels and human saphenous vein. *Res. Commun. Chem. Pathol. Pharmacol.*, 17: 145–156.

Dostert, P., Guffroy, C., Strolin Benedetti, M. and Boucher, T. (1984) Inhibition of semicarbazide-sensitive amine oxidase by monoamine oxidase inhibitors from the oxazolidinone series. *J. Pharm. Pharmacol.*, 36: 782–785.

Elliott, J., Callingham, B.A. and Sharman, D.F. (1989a) Semicarbazide-sensitive amine oxidase (SSAO) of the rat aorta. Interactions with some naturally occurring amines and their structural analogues. *Biochem. Pharmacol.*, 38: 1507–1515.

Elliott, J., Callingham, B.A. and Sharman, D.F. (1989b) Metabolism of amines in the isolated perfused mesenteric arterial bed of the rat. *Br. J. Pharmacol.*, 98: 507–514.

Elliott, J., Callingham, B.A. and Sharman, D.F. (1989c) The influence of amine metabolizing enzymes on the pharmacology of tyramine in the isolated perfused mesenteric arterial bed of the rat. *Br. J. Pharmacol.*, 98: 515–522.

Elliott, J., Callingham, B.A. and Sharman, D.F. (1992) Amine oxidase enzymes of sheep blood vessels and blood plasma: a comparison of their properties. *Comp. Biochem. Physiol.*, 102C: 83–89.

Elliott, W.H. (1960) Methylglyoxal formation from aminoacetone by ox plasma. *Nature*, 185: 467–468.

Ferkany, J.W., Andree, T.H., Clarke, D.E. and Enna, S.J. (1981) Neurochemical effects of kojic amine, a gabamimetic, and its interaction with benzylamine oxidase. *Neuropharmacology*, 20: 1177–1182.

Gorkin, V.Z. (1983) *Amine Oxidases in Clinical Research*, Pergamon Press, Oxford, UK.

Guffroy, C., Fowler, C.J. and Strolin Benedetti, M. (1983) The deamination of *n*-pentylamine by monoamine oxidase and a semicarbazide-sensitive amine oxidase of rat heart. *J. Pharm. Pharmacol.*, 35: 416–420.

Guffroy, C., Boucher, T. and Strolin Benedetti, M. (1985) Further investigations of the metabolism of two trace amines, β-phenylethylamine and *p*-tyramine by rat aorta semicarbazide-sensitive amine oxidase. In: A.A. Boulton, L.L. Maitre, P.R. Bieck and P. Riederer (Eds.), *Neuropharmacology of the Trace Amines*, Humana Press, Clifton, NJ, pp. 39–50.

Harris, E.D. and O'Dell, B.L. (1972) Comparison of soluble and particulate amine oxidases from bovine aorta. *Biochem. Biophys. Res. Commun.*, 48: 1173–1178.

Hayes, B.E., Ostrow, P.T. and Clarke, D.E. (1983) Benzylamine oxidase in normal and atherosclerotic human aortae. *Exp. Mol. Pathol.*, 38: 243–254.

Heck, H.d'A., Casanova, M. and Starr, T.B. (1990) Formaldehyde toxicity - new understanding. *Crit. Rev. Toxicol.*, 20: 397–426.

Holt, A. and Callingham, B.A. (1994) Location of the active site of rat vascular semicarbazide-sensitive amine oxidase. *J. Neural. Transm.*, (Suppl.) 41: 433–437.

Hysmith, R.M. and Boor, P.J. (1987) In vitro expression of benzylamine oxidase activity in cultured porcine smooth muscle cells. *J. Cardiovasc. Pharmacol.*, 9: 668–674.

Hysmith, R.M. and Boor, P.J. (1988a) Purification of benzylamine oxidase from cultured porcine aortic smooth muscle cells. *Biochem. Cell. Biol.*, 66: 821–829.

Hysmith, R.M. and Boor, P.J. (1988b) Role of benzylamine oxidase in the cytotoxicity of allylamine toward aortic smooth muscle cells. *Toxicology*, 51: 133–145.

Johnson, T.D., Takebayashi, D.T., Forster, R.M. and Clarke, D.E. (1986) Monoamine oxidase inhibition but not inhibi-

tion of semicarbazide sensitive amine oxidase potentiates responses in the human umbilical artery: a comparison with 5-hydroxytryptamine. *Proc. West. Pharmacol. Soc.*, 29: 109–112.

Lewinsohn, R. (1981) Amine oxidase in human blood vessels and non-vascular smooth muscle. *J. Pharm. Pharmacol.*, 33: 569–575.

Lewinsohn, R. (1984) Mammalian monoamine-oxidizing enzymes, with special reference to benzylamine oxidase in human tissues. *Braz. J. Med. Biol. Res.*, 17: 223–256.

Lizcano, J.M., Balsa, D., Tipton, K.F. and Unzeta, M. (1990) Amine oxidase activities in bovine lung. *J. Neural Transm.*, (Suppl.) 32: 341–344.

Lizcano, J.M., Balsa, D., Tipton, K.F. and Unzeta, M. (1991) The oxidation of dopamine by the semicarbazide-sensitive amine oxidase (SSAO) from rat vas deferens. *Biochem. Pharmacol.*, 41: 1107–1110.

Lizcano, J.M., Fernandez de Arriba, A., Lyles, G.A. and Unzeta, M. (1994) Several aspects on the amine oxidation by semicarbazide-sensitive amine oxidase (SSAO) from bovine lung. *J. Neural Transm.*, (Suppl.) 41, 415–420.

Lowis, S., Eastwood, M.A. and Brydon, W.G. (1985) The influence of creatinine, lecithin and choline feeding on aliphatic amine production and excretion in the rat. *Br. J. Nutr.*, 54: 43–51.

Lyles, G.A. (1984) The interaction of semicarbazide-sensitive amine oxidase with MAO inhibitors. In: K.F. Tipton, P. Dostert and M. Strolin Benedetti (Eds.), *Monoamine Oxidase and Disease*, Academic Press, London, pp. 547–556.

Lyles, G.A. (1995) Mammalian plasma and tissue-bound semicarbazide-sensitive amine oxidases: biochemical, pharmacological and toxicological aspects. *Int. J. Biochem.*, in press.

Lyles, G.A. and Bertie, K.H. (1987) Properties of a semicarbazide sensitive amine oxidase in rat articular cartilage. *Pharmacol. Toxicol.*, 60 (Suppl.): 33.

Lyles, G.A. and Chalmers, J. (1992) The metabolism of aminoacetone to methylglyoxal by semicarbazide-sensitive amine oxidase in human umbilical artery. *Biochem. Pharmacol.*, 43: 1409–1414.

Lyles, G.A. and McDougall, S.A. (1989) The enhanced daily excretion of urinary methylamine in rats treated with semicarbazide or hydralazine may be related to the inhibition of semicarbazide-sensitive amine oxidase. *J. Pharm. Pharmacol.*, 41: 97–100.

Lyles, G.A. and Singh, I. (1985) Vascular smooth muscle cells: a major source of the semicarbazide-sensitive amine oxidase of the rat aorta. *J. Pharm. Pharmacol.*, 37: 637–643.

Lyles, G.A. and Taneja, D.T. (1987) Effects of amine oxidase inhibitors upon tryptamine metabolism and tryptamine-induced contractions of rat aorta. *Br. J. Pharmacol.*, 90: 16P.

Lyles, G.A., Holt, A. and Marshall, C.M.S. (1990) Further studies on the metabolism of methylamine by semicarbazide-sensitive amine oxidase activities in human plasma,

302

umbilical artery and rat aorta. *J. Pharm. Pharmacol.*, 42: 332–338.

Marver, H.S., Tschudy, D.P., Perlroth, M.G., Collins, A. and Hunter, G. (1966) The determination of aminoketones in biological fluids. *Anal. Biochem.*, 14: 53–60.

McEwen, C.M. (1965) Human plasma monoamine oxidase. *J. Biol. Chem.*, 240: 2003–2010.

Murphy, D.L., Sims, K.B., Karoum, F., Garrick, N.A., de la Chapelle, A., Sankila, E.M., Norio, R. and Breakefield, X.O. (1991) Plasma amine oxidase activities in Norrie disease patients with an X-chromosomal deletion affecting monoamine oxidase. *J. Neural Transm.*, (Gen. Sect.) 83: 1–12.

Nelson, T.J. and Boor, P.J. (1982) Allylamine cardiotoxicity - IV. Metabolism to acrolein by cardiovascular tissues. *Biochem. Pharmacol.*, 31: 509–514.

Neurath, G.B., Dunger, M., Pein, F.G., Ambrosius, D. and Schreiber, O. (1977) Primary and secondary amines in the human environment. *Fd. Cosmet. Toxicol.*, 15: 275–282.

Norqvist, A. and Oreland, L. (1989) Localization of a semicarbazide-sensitive serotonin-oxidizing enzyme from porcine dental pulp. *Biogenic Amines*, 6: 65–74.

Norqvist, A., Fowler, C.J. and Oreland, L. (1981) The deamination of monoamines by pig dental pulp. *Biochem. Pharmacol.*, 30: 403–409.

Norqvist, A., Oreland, L. and Fowler, C.J. (1982) Some properties of monoamine oxidase and a semicarbazide-sensitive amine oxidase capable of the deamination of 5-hydroxytryptamine from porcine dental pulp. *Biochem. Pharmacol.*, 31: 2739–2744.

Precious, E. and Lyles, G.A. (1988) Properties of a semicarbazide-sensitive amine oxidase in human umbilical artery. *J. Pharm. Pharmacol.*, 40: 627–633.

Precious, E., Gunn, C.E. and Lyles, G.A. (1988) Deamination of methylamine by semicarbazide-sensitive amine oxidase in human umbilical artery and rat aorta. *Biochem. Pharmacol.*, 37: 707–713.

Raimondi, L., Pirisino, R., Ignesti, G., Capecchi, S., Banchelli, G. and Buffoni, F. (1991) Semicarbazide-sensitive amine oxidase activity (SSAO) of rat epididymal white adipose tissue. *Biochem. Pharmacol.*, 41: 467–470.

Raimondi, L., Pirisino, R., Banchelli, G., Ignesti, G., Conforti, L., Romanelli, E. and Buffoni, F. (1992) Further studies on semicarbazide-sensitive amine oxidase activity (SSAO) of white adipose tissue. *Comp. Biochem. Physiol.*, 102B: 953–960.

Raimondi, L., Conforti, L., Ignesti, G., Pirisino, R. and Buffoni, F. (1993) Histamine lipolytic activity and semicarbazide-sensitive amine oxidase activity (SSAO) of rat white adipose tissue (WAT). *Biochem. Pharmacol.*, 46: 1369–1376.

Ramos, K., Grossman, S.L. and Cox, L.R. (1988) Allylamine-induced vascular toxicity in vitro: prevention by semicarbazide-sensitive amine oxidase inhibitors. *Toxicol. Appl. Pharmacol.*, 95: 61–71.

Ray, S. and Ray, M. (1983) Formation of methylglyoxal from aminoacetone by goat plasma. *J. Biol. Chem.*, 258: 3461–3462.

Ray, M and Ray, S. (1987) Aminoacetone oxidase from goat liver. Formation of methylglyoxal from aminoacetone. *J. Biol. Chem.*, 262: 5974–5977.

Roth, J.A. and Gillis, C.N. (1975) Multiple forms of amine oxidase in perfused rabbit lung. *J. Pharmacol. Exp. Ther.*, 194: 537–544.

Rucker, R.B. and Goettlich-Riemann, W. (1972) Properties of rabbit aorta amine oxidases. *Proc. Soc. Exp. Biol. Med.*, 139: 286–289.

Schayer, R.W., Smiley, L.R. and Kaplan, H.E. (1952) The metabolism of epinephrine containing isotopic carbon. *J. Biol. Chem.*, 198: 545–551.

Shan, X., Aw, T.Y. and Jones, D.P. (1990) Glutathione-dependent protection against oxidative injury. *Pharmacol. Ther.*, 47: 61–71.

Strolin Benedetti, M. and Dostert, P. (1985) Stereochemical aspects of MAO interactions: reversible and selective inhibitors of monoamine oxidase. *Trends Pharmacol. Sci.*, 6: 246–251.

Suzuki, O. and Matsumoto, T. (1984) Some properties of benzylamine oxidase in human aorta. *Biogenic Amines*, 1: 249–257.

Taneja, D.T. and Lyles, G.A. (1988) Use of an oil immersion technique to study the role of amine oxidase inhibition in potentiating tryptamine-induced contractions of rat aorta. *Pharmacol. Res. Commun.*, 20 (Suppl. 4): 127–128.

Thornalley, P.J. (1990) The glyoxalase system: new developments towards functional characterization of a metabolic pathway fundamental to biological life. *Biochem. J.*, 269: 1–11.

Toraason, M., Luken, M.E., Breitenstein, M., Krueger, J.A. and Biagini, R.E. (1989) Comparative toxicity of allylamine and acrolein in cultured myocytes and fibroblasts from neonatal rat heart. *Toxicology*, 56: 107–117.

Tressel, T., Thompson, R., Zieske, L.R., Menendez, M.I.T.S. and Davis, L. (1986) Interaction between L-threonine dehydrogenase and aminoacetone synthetase and mechanism of aminoacetone production. *J. Biol. Chem.*, 261: 16428–16437.

Trevethick, M.A., Olverman, H.J., Pearson, J.D., Gordon, J.L., Lyles, G.A. and Callingham, B.A. (1981) Monoamine oxidase activities of porcine vascular endothelial and smooth muscle cells. *Biochem. Pharmacol.*, 30: 2209–2216.

Ueda, T. and Kinemuchi, H. (1984) Deamination of some biogenic monoamines in rat lung by monoamine oxidase and benzylamine oxidase. *Biogenic Amines*, 1: 179–182.

Uotila, L. and Koivusalo, M. (1989) Glutathione-dependent oxido-reductases: formaldehyde dehydrogenase. In: D. Dolphin, R. Poulson and O. Avramovic (Eds.), *Glutathione: Chemical, Biochemical and Medical Aspects - Part A*. J. Wiley and Sons, pp. 518–551.

Urata, G. and Granick, S. (1963) Biosynthesis of α-aminoketones and the metabolism of aminoacetone. *J. Biol. Chem.,* 238, 811–820.

Werner, C.G., Seiler, N. and Schmidt, H.-L. (1961) Über die wirkung von monoaminoxydase-hemmern und anderen psychotropen substanzen auf den oxydativen abbau von methylamin bei einigen säugetieren. *Med. Exp.,* 5, 151–159.

Wibo, M., Duong, A.T. and Godfraind, T. (1980) Subcellular location of semicarbazide-sensitive amine oxidase in rat aorta. *Eur. J. Biochem.,* 112: 87–94.

Yu, P.H. (1988) Three types of stereospecificity and the kinetic deuterium isotope effect in the oxidative deamination of dopamine as catalyzed by different amine oxidases. *Biochem. Cell. Biol.,* 66, 853–861.

Yu, P.H. (1990) Oxidative deamination of aliphatic amines by rat aorta semicarbazide-sensitive amine oxidase. *J. Pharm. Pharmacol.,* 42: 882–884.

Yu, P.H. and Davis B.A. (1988) Stereospecific deamination of benzylamine catalyzed by different amine oxidases. *Int. J. Biochem.,* 20: 1197–1201.

Yu, P.H. and Davis, B.A. (1991) 2-Propyl-1-aminopentane, its deamination by monoamine oxidase and semicarbazide-sensitive amine oxidase, conversion to valproic acid and behavioral effects. *Neuropharmacology,* 30: 507–515.

Yu, P.H. and Zuo, D.-M. (1993) Oxidative deamination of methylamine by semicarbazide-sensitive amine oxidase leads to cytotoxic damage in endothelial cells. *Diabetes,* 42: 594–603.

Yu, P.H., Zuo, D.-M. and Davis, B.A. (1994) Characterization of human serum and umbilical artery semicarbazide-sensitive amine oxidase (SSAO). *Biochem. Pharmacol.,* 47: 1055–1059.

Zeisel, S.H., Wishnok, J.S. and Blusztajn, J.K. (1983) Formation of methylamines from ingested choline and lecithin. *J. Pharmacol. Exp. Ther.,* 225: 320–324.

Zuo, D.-M. and Yu, P.H. (1994) Semicarbazide-sensitive amine oxidase and monoamine oxidase in rat brain microvessels, meninges, retina and eye sclera. *Brain Res. Bull.,* 33: 307–311.

Peter M. Yu, Keith F. Tipton and Alan A. Boulton (Eds.)
Progress in Brain Research, Vol 106
© 1995 Elsevier Science BV. All rights reserved.

CHAPTER 31

Some aspects of the pathophysiology of semicarbazide-sensitive amine oxidase enzymes

Brian A. Callingham, Alan E. Crosbie and Brian A. Rous

*Veterinary Pharmacology Unit, Department of Pharmacology, University of Cambridge Tennis Court Road,
Cambridge CB2 1QJ, UK*

Introduction

Although the history of amine oxidases, whose actions are inhibited by the hydrazine, semicarbazide and other so-called carbonyl reagents (see Kapeller-Adler, 1970; Blaschko, 1974; Lewinsohn, 1984; Lyles, 1994) is almost as long as that of monoamine oxidase, they have, until recently, attracted far less attention. The probable reason is that, unlike the traditional FAD-dependent monoamine oxidases (MAO), little has been known about the importance of these so-called, "semicarbazide-sensitive amine oxidases" (SSAO enzymes) in health or disease. Perhaps there are two long-standing exceptions that should be mentioned. One is diamine oxidase (histaminase; DAO), which was the first member of the group classed as amine:oxidoreductase (deaminating)(copper containing); EC 1.4.3.6 (see Dixon and Webb, 1979) and the enzyme lysyl oxidase, which, although inhibited by semicarbazide, is classified as protein-lysine 6-oxidase; EC 1.4.3.13. (Buffoni, 1966; Blaschko, 1974; Levene and Carrington, 1985; Levene et al., 1992). Here we use SSAO to describe a somewhat amorphous and growing group of enzymes, inhibited by semicarbazide and other carbonyl reagents and which deaminate, often as their preferred substrate, the monoamine benzylamine.

In general, SSAO enzymes (except DAO and lysyl oxidase) appear to deaminate only aromatic and aliphatic primary amines (unlike MAO), many showing a preference for the aromatic amine benzylamine, although it has not been identified as a physiologically significant amine.

SSAO, like MAO, catalyses a double-displacement or ping-pong reaction, although it would appear to be of the aminotransferase type to produce an aldehyde and hydrogen peroxide:

$$E\text{-}CHO + R\text{-}CH_2\text{-}NH_2 \rightarrow$$
$$E\text{-}CH_2\text{-}NH_2 + R\text{-}CHO$$
$$E\text{-}CH_2\text{-}NH_2 + O_2 + H_2O \rightarrow$$
$$E\text{-}CHO + NH_3 + H_2O_2$$

The wide distribution of SSAO enzymes across eukaryotic (and many prokaryotic) organisms (Blaschko, 1974) would suggest important physiological functions. In man and other animals, SSAO specific activity is highest in highly vascularized tissues and some other tissues composed of smooth muscle (Coquil et al., 1973; Lewinsohn et al., 1978; Lewinsohn, 1984). While much SSAO activity is located in vascular smooth muscle, non-vascular articular cartilage, for example, contains SSAO distinct from lysyl oxidase (Lyles and Bertie, 1987). Adipose tissues of the rat, both brown (Barrand and Callingham, 1984) and white (Raimondi et al., 1991, 1992), are excellent sources of enzyme activity, as are various parts of the bovine eye (retina, optic nerve, iris and epithelium; Fernandez de Arriba et al., 1990).

Various workers have demonstrated a subcellular association of these tissue-bound SSAO activities with the membrane fractions of cells, particularly the plasmalemma (Wibo et al., 1980), where, in the rat aorta, it is distributed like 5'-nucleotidase and Mg^{2+}-ATPase. Similar results have been obtained with rat brown adipose tissue, where activity was also seen in microsomal fractions (Barrand and Callingham, 1982, 1984). Affinity chromatography with concanavalin and *Lens culinaris* lectin has shown a plasmalemmal glycoprotein element in SSAO, although at a distance from the active site, since the activity of the concanavalin-bound enzyme remains (Yasunobu et al., 1976; Falk et al., 1983). Although it is generally accepted that protein-bound carbohydrates in animal cells face outwards (Rothman and Lenard, 1977), the uncertainty concerning how large a proportion of the active centres face outwards from the cell surface (see Barrand and Callingham, 1984) is not fully resolved, although recent evidence from the use of non-penetrating inhibitors supports the view that it is an ectoenzyme (Holt and Callingham, 1994).

Another important tissue containing substantial amounts of SSAO activities is blood plasma. Indeed, activity of what we would now refer to as SSAO, in ovine and bovine serum, which deaminated the polyamines, spermine and spermidine, was discovered by Hirsch in 1953, who called it "spermine oxidase".

This was followed by the discovery by Bergeret et al. (1957) of an amine oxidase in horse serum, with an inhibitor profile similar to that of spermine oxidase, but without activity on spermine. They called this enzyme "benzylamine oxidase" because this substrate was most rapidly oxidised. This name has received some recognition and has been used by some other authors (see for example, Lewinsohn, 1984), but as benzylamine has not been shown to be an endogenous substrate and is also a substrate for both MAO-A and MAO-B, the term "SSAO" has recently become more popular, although it is still inadequate.

Later, McEwen and Cohen (1963) identified a similar amine oxidase activity in human plasma.

Plasma amine oxidases have since been identified in many other vertebrates, although, in the rat, the activity is low (Obata and Yamanaka, 1990). However, the substrate selectivity of the various enzyme activities is highly species-dependent, with pig plasma amine oxidase highly active against histamine (Kolb, 1956), while only ruminant enzymes have activity against the polyamines. Elliott et al. (1992) found two plasma SSAO enzymes in sheep, with DAO activity being very low when measured with putrescine as substrate. Here, the two ruminant SSAO enzymes will be called "low K_m" and "high K_m" SSAO enzymes, from their relative K_m values towards benzylamine as substrate. (Alternatively, they could be called "high affinity" and "low affinity" enzymes.)

A requirement for copper has been demonstrated for many but not all SSAO enzymes and the term "copper-containing amine oxidases" has been used in the past to describe them. Bovine serum amine oxidase has been reported to contain two tightly bound copper atoms per dimeric unit (Yasunobu et al., 1976). Experiments with copper-depleted enzyme indicate that the metal centre is necessary for enzyme activity in bovine serum amine oxidase (Suzuki et al., 1986).

Possible pathophysiological roles for SSAO enzymes

Instead of helping attempts to understand the pathophysiology of SSAO enzymes, this multiplicity of enzymes and locations has made the task much harder. The problem is compounded further by the lack of specific, or even selective, inhibitors of individual SSAO enzymes. Many of the compounds used previously as inhibitors of SSAO have activities on other enzymes. For example, studies of SSAO inhibition by phenelzine, an irreversible inhibitor of MAO (Andree and Clarke, 1982), hydrallazine, a reversible inhibitor of MAO, although it is an irreversible inhibitor of SSAO (Lyles and Callingham, 1982a; Barrand and Callingham, 1985) and benserazide, an inhibitor of DOPA-decarboxylase (Lyles and Callingham, 1982b) have all been complicated by lack of specificity. MDL 72145 ((E)-2-(3′,4′-dimetho-xyphenyl)-3-fluoroallylamine) was shown to be a potent and selective inhibitor of SSAO in the rat aorta (Lyles and Fitzpatrick, 1985) and in the rat mesenteric arterial bed (Elliott et al., 1989b,c). However, it also irreversibly inhibits MAO-B in tissues containing MAO-B (Zreika et al., 1984b,c) and competitively inhibits MAO-A (Elliott, 1989). The 4-picolylamine derivative B24 (3,5-ethoxy-4-aminomethylpyridine) is a highly selective reversible inhibitor of SSAO (Banchelli et al., 1990). It is a substrate for the plasma-borne but not the tissue-bound SSAO, and has little or no action on MAO. Lewinsohn et al. (1978) first demonstrated that procarbazine (N-isopropyl-α-(2-methyl hydrazino)-p-toluamide hydrochloride), a carcinostatic agent used in the treatment of Hodgkin's disease, inhibited benzylamine oxidation by SSAO in homogenates of various human tissues and rat lung. It was later shown that procarbazine is a potent inhibitor of SSAO in the intrascapular brown adipose tissue of the rat but has very little effect on MAO-A and MAO-B in rat liver (Holt et al., 1992).

At present, however, although some compounds have been found that have some selectivity between the SSAO activities of sheep plasma SSAO, such as MDL 72145 (Elliott, 1989; Elliott et al., 1989a), we still seem a long way away from being able to inhibit selectively SSAO enzymes in vivo and both to observe physiological parameters and to measure changes in substrates and products in any reliable way.

The importance of being able to measure changes in putative substrates in vivo cannot be overestimated, since, at present, much uncertainty surrounds even the physiological substrate or, more likely, substrates of these enzymes. A proper knowledge of the relative amounts and locations of possible substrates and the contribution made by the SSAO enzymes is an important prerequisite to any reliable identification of a pathophysiological role. There is only limited physiological value in measuring, in vitro, the substrate selectivity of SSAO enzymes in tissue homogenates although, clearly, there is a substan-

tial contribution to their enzymology. In addition, the fact that SSAO enzymes are either soluble and freely circulating or face outwards from the surface of cells does enhance the relevance of homogenate experiments, provided, of course, that possible changes in availability of cofactors is not forgotten. In the end, it is the presence and availability of a particular substrate to a particular site of SSAO that really matters.

It has been suggested that the function of plasma SSAO in the ruminant is to serve a protective role (see Callingham and Barrand, 1987) in a similar manner to the way MAO, in the gastro-intestinal tract, protects animals from potentially harmful amines, such as tyramine. For example, polyamines, such as spermine, which are growth factors for most living cells (Tabor and Tabor, 1984), are produced by fermentation in the divided stomachs of ruminants and are metabolized by SSAO in the plasma of these species. Ruminants, unlike other species, have large amounts of dopamine in their mast cells (Falck et al., 1964). Sharman et al. (1983) have suggested that a function of ruminant plasma SSAO is to metabolize this dopamine released from mast cells. It has also been suggested that the function of SSAO could be to metabolize some aromatic biogenic amines, such as tryptamine and tyramine. Indeed, Lyles and Taneja (1987) showed that inhibition of the SSAO of the rat aorta in vitro caused significant potentiation of the contractions produced by tryptamine but only after concomitant inhibition of MAO activity. This observation was confirmed by use of the isolated perfused mesenteric arterial bed of the rat where again SSAO could be shown to deaminate tyramine in the perfusing medium but that potentiation of the tyramine pressor effect could only be seen if the MAO had been inhibited as well (Elliott et al., 1989c). However, although these amines are metabolized by SSAO in the rat (Elliott et al., 1989d), they are weak substrates ($K_m > 1$ mM) for human SSAO, so this particular scavenging role seems unlikely in human subjects (see Lewinsohn, 1984).

A pharmacological clue suggesting a possible role for SSAO enzymes as scavengers was first found when plasma SSAO was shown to deaminate the hallucinogen mescaline and the antimalarial agent primaquine (8-(4-amino-1-methylbutylamino)-6-methoxyquinoline; Blaschko et al., 1959). However, mescaline does not appear to be a substrate for the human enzyme. Other pharmacological agents reported to be metabolized by SSAO include the GABA-mimetic agent, kojic amine (Ferkany et al., 1981) and the MAO inhibitor, MD220661 (Dostert et al., 1984). SSAO enzymes, by this scavenging action, may also protect against the cardiovascular actions of vasoactive amines produced in response to lipopolysaccharides released on the death of pathogenic bacteria (Garner et al., 1978; Moore et al., 1981) and, by inference, have some role to play in the events that unfold in toxaemia and septic shock. However, deamination to aldehydes and hydrogen peroxide may well not be a protective mechanism as some of these aldehyde metabolites could be more toxic than their parent compounds, either directly (Morgan, 1987) or via an effect on the immune system (Byrd et al., 1977), although Henle et al. (1986) have suggested that the main toxic agent is peroxide. Thus, inhibition of SSAO activity in conditions associated with excessive liberation of amines might lead to a happier outcome.

While a clear consensus view is still lacking about which amine or amines are realistic substrates for SSAO, speculation must develop along other lines. What, for example, if these enzymes can use any available amine, without the need for any selective uptake process preceding deamination, simply as a source of hydrogen peroxide and an aldehyde? Particularly in the case of SSAO enzymes facing outwards at selected locations on smooth muscle and adipose tissue cells, it could be that the hydrogen peroxide is the more important, owing to its production taking place closer to its point of use than in the case of that produced by other H_2O_2-producing enzymes. This locally formed peroxide could then have a physiological role in its own right. Seregi et al. (1982, 1983) showed that the deamination of dopamine in the brain by MAO yielded H_2O_2, which stimulated $PGF_{2\alpha}$ formation. It is possible that hydrogen peroxide produced from SSAO activity may also have a role in eicosanoid synthesis.

H_2O_2 action has been implicated in the cardiovascular system; for example it induces relaxation of isolated rabbit aorta (Mittal and Murad, 1977), vasodilatation of rat cremasteric arterioles (Wolin et al., 1986) and vasoconstriction in the isolated perfused rabbit lung (via thromboxane production; Tate et al., 1984). Burke and Wolin (1987) demonstrated that peroxide causes pulmonary arterial relaxation via activation of soluble guanylate cyclase, resulting in formation of cGMP, causing smooth muscle relaxation. This peroxide-dependent activation of guanylate cyclase appears to involve metabolism of peroxide by catalase. Peroxide probably activates guanylate cyclase by oxidising sulphydryl groups. This suggests that peroxide could have an influence on the activities of many other enzymes and receptors which have sulphydryl groups and even have a regulatory role on some. In white adipose tissue, for example, it has been suggested that peroxide could be involved in transmembrane signalling (Mukherjee and Mukherjee, 1982). It has been demonstrated that the effects of insulin on glucose transport in fat cells can be mimicked by H_2O_2 as it can stimulate the insulin receptor kinase and thus enhance tyrosine phosphorylation, suggesting a possible regulatory effect of peroxide on metabolism in the absence of insulin (Yu et al., 1987).

Toxicology of three SSAO substrates, allylamine, methylamine and aminoacetone

Allylamine

An observation of fundamental importance to the quest to assign some function to SSAO enzymes was made by Boor and Nelson (1980), who showed that administration of the unsaturated aliphatic amine, allylamine, to rats caused serious cardiovascular lesions. The pathological effects involve predominantly the heart, aorta and coronary arteries and are typically necrotic lesions of the myocardium and arterial smooth muscle and smooth muscle cell proliferation in the intima of damaged vessels (Boor and Hysmith, 1987; Hysmith and Boor, 1987).

There is now strong evidence from in vitro and in vivo studies that allylamine itself is not the causative agent, but that it is metabolized by SSAO to the highly toxic α,β-unsaturated aldehyde, acrolein, in vascular smooth muscle (Boor et al., 1990). Ramos et al. (1988) showed that the addition of catalase to cultures afforded some protection from allylamine, suggesting that peroxide produced during amine oxidation may contribute to the cytotoxicity. Acrolein is able to alkylate the thiol group on glutathione transferase, thereby depleting glutathione (Haenen et al., 1988), which is necessary for acrolein detoxification. Glutathione-dependent mechanisms are also involved in peroxide breakdown. Thus, inhibition of γ-glutamylcysteine synthetase, which is responsible for glutathione synthesis, in cultured smooth muscle cells by pre-treatment with buthionine sulphoximine increased the cytotoxicity of allylamine (Blicharski and Lyles, 1991).

If SSAO could produce toxic products from a foreign amine, such as allylamine, would similar products be possible from an endogenous amine? First identify your endogenous amine and prove that realistic conditions can occur in vivo to produce it in adequate amounts for its products to produce measurable effects. Just two prime candidates will be considered, methylamine and aminoacetone.

Methylamine

Methylamine is a substrate for SSAO, with Michaelis-Menten constants of the same order of magnitude as for benzylamine, in the rat aorta and human umbilical artery and human plasma (Precious et al., 1988; Lyles et al., 1990). It is known to be cytotoxic, to inhibit the release of insulin from pancreatic cells and to disrupt intracellular processing of certain plasma membrane receptors (see Precious et al., 1988). It is possible that both tissue-bound and plasma SSAO might act to maintain circulating levels of methylamine

at an acceptably low level. Methylamine is known to occur endogenously as a product of various metabolic pathways for the degradation of creatinine, sarcosine (Davis and De Ropp, 1961) and adrenaline (Schayer et al., 1952). In the rat, its urinary excretion can be increased by the in vivo administration of semicarbazide or hydrallazine (Lyles and McDougall, 1989). Plasma methylamine levels are increased substantially above normal levels in patients with uraemia (Simenhoff et al., 1963; Baba et al., 1984), although it is unclear whether or not SSAO activity is reduced in these subjects. Two of the products of the oxidation of methylamine are formaldehyde and hydrogen peroxide (Boor et al., 1992). Both formaldehyde and peroxide are cytotoxic (Ramos et al., 1988; Yu and Zuo, 1993). Yu and Zuo (1993) have suggested that the formaldehyde formed from the oxidative deamination of methylamine may contribute to the pathogenicity of diabetes. This evidence, taken together with evidence showing methylamine deamination in many blood vessels, for example, in the rat (Zuo and Yu, 1994), supports a pathophysiological function for SSAO in the production of toxic metabolites from methylamine. But is methylamine the only possible substrate, particularly in view of the comparative lack of precise substrate selectivity of SSAO?

Aminoacetone

Aminoacetone has been shown to be formed in significant quantities by the catabolism of glycine, by the addition of glycine and acetyl-CoA to extracts of chicken erythrocytes (Gibson et al., 1958), by certain bacteria such as *Staphylococcus aureus* (Elliott, 1960) and by guinea pig liver mitochondria (Urata and Granick, 1963). These last authors also observed that aminoacetone could be formed from malonyl-CoA instead of acetyl-CoA (presumably by decarboxylation of malonyl-CoA to acetyl-CoA).

Elliott (1960) also demonstrated that as well as being produced from glycine, aminoacetone could be formed by the catabolism of L-threonine. In *Rhodopseudomonas spheroides*, L-threonine dehydrogenase (which converts L-threonine to aminoacetone) was specific for L-threonine, and required the presence of NAD$^+$, which cannot be replaced by NADP$^+$ (Neuberger and Tait, 1962).

L-Threonine dehydrogenase was present in such large quantities in the liver of various mammals that Green and Elliott (1964) claimed it must be of metabolic significance and suggested an "aminoacetone cycle" with 2-amino-3-oxobutyrate as an intermediary, common to both substrates in the production of aminoacetone. Soon afterwards, Marver et al. (1966) demonstrated that aminoacetone made up a significant proportion (about 20–60%) of the aminoketones in normal rat urine, and that, in rats given 2 mmoles/100 g body weight of L-threonine, about 10–15-times greater urinary excretion of aminoacetone can be measured.

It has also been shown that L-threonine dehydrogenase can produce acetyl-CoA and glycine (Dale, 1978; Bird and Nunn, 1979; Aoyama and Motokawa, 1981). It has been proposed that L-threonine dehydrogenase could, under physiological conditions, produce either acetyl-CoA and glycine or aminoacetone, and that the ratio of mitochondrial CoA to acetyl-CoA controlled which route was taken (Bird and Nunn, 1979; Bird et al., 1984). A two-stage reaction was envisaged, with 2-amino-3-oxobutyrate as an intermediate. However, Tressel et al. (1986) pointed out that the production of 2-amino-3-oxobutyrate had not been demonstrated and showed that L-threonine dehydrogenase and aminoacetone synthase were associated in a soluble form (with an apparent stoichiometry of 2 aminoacetone synthase dimers for every L-threonine dehydrogenase) and that 2-amino-3-oxobutyrate was not a dissociable product. Tressel and co-workers proposed that, when the ratio of CoA to acetyl-CoA was high, L-threonine was metabolized by threonine dehydrogenase to glycine with the production of acetyl-CoA but, when the ratio of CoA to acetyl-CoA was low, L-threonine was converted to aminoacetone.

Elliott (1960) had earlier demonstrated the decomposition of aminoacetone to methylglyoxal (2-oxopropanal), but could not be sure whether this was part of a transamination or an oxidation reaction. Urata and Granick (1963) showed that various guinea pig tissues deaminated aminoacetone and suggested that MAO could be involved in the conversion of aminoacetone to methylglyoxal as the process was inhibited by benzylamine, phenylethylamine and isoniazid. However, these compounds are now known to be substrates or inhibitors of SSAO activity. In addition, Ray and Ray (1982, 1983) demonstrated that an enzyme that deaminated benzylamine in goat plasma also deaminated aminoacetone to methylglyoxal. Here then, was the clue that SSAO could have a role in aminoacetone deamination.

An increase in methylglyoxal concentration, in response to pathophysiological changes or through ingestion, could be of significance as methylglyoxal is cytotoxic, as are the aldehyde products of methylamine and allylamine, although, at present, the precise mechanisms by which methylglyoxal causes cytotoxicity in vivo have not been fully clarified (Kalapos et al., 1992). Several possible methods including the generation of superoxide anions and hydroxyl radicals (Fazal et al., 1994) have been proposed. Methylglyoxal may damage protein structure, as it binds to, and modifies, arginine residues in proteins (Takahashi, 1977) producing crosslinks (Lee et al., 1989). In this regard, aminoguanidine, which prevents diabetes-induced arterial wall protein crosslinking (Brownlee et al., 1986), is an efficient scavenger of methylglyoxal (Selwood and Thornalley, 1993) and may exert its therapeutic effect by preventing methylglyoxal-induced cytotoxicity. Methyglyoxal can bind to guanine and guanyl nucleoside and nucleotides of DNA and tRNA and induces crosslinking in DNA (Krymkiewicz, 1973; Marinari et al., 1984). Under normal levels of methylglyoxal production it would be expected that DNA repair mechanisms could counter effectively the mutagenicity of methylglyoxal, which would explain how we can consume significant amounts of methylglyoxal in ingested foodstuffs such as toast (3.47 μmoles per 100 g) and decaffeinated coffee (1.95 μmoles per 100 ml) (Thornalley, 1993). Indeed, coffee and caffeine have been shown to be mutagenic to bacteria and fungi, and in high concentrations they are also mutagenic to mammalian cells in culture (see Nehlig and Debry, 1994). The mutagenicity of caffeine and coffee is mainly attributed to chemically reactive components, including methylglyoxal, produced by the roasting process. Concomitant production of hydrogen peroxide, while not very active alone, appears to enhance substantially the mutagenic effects of methylglyoxal. However, the reviewers (Nehlig and Debry, 1994) conclude that the chances that coffee and caffeine consumption in moderate to normal amounts (sic!) could lead to mutagenic effects in humans are almost non-existent.

Glutathione-dependent mechanisms are involved in peroxide breakdown, so a shortage in cellular glutathione as a result of methylglyoxal metabolism may result in peroxide toxicity. S-D-Lactoylglutathione is also cytotoxic, and induces growth arrest and toxicity in proliferating HL-60 cells (Thornalley and Tisdale, 1988), which has been suggested to contribute to the dysfunction of endothelial cells in diabetes mellitus (McLellan et al., 1993).

From what has gone before, it seems a reasonable premise that the endothelial and smooth muscle cells of blood vessels are prime targets for the toxic actions of both peroxide and aldehydes. While toxic aldehydes can be produced by processes independent of SSAO, pathophysiological conditions could increase the risk of toxicity to a point where it is important due to increased production of an endogenous substrate or an increase in either tissue-bound or plasma SSAO. Alternatively, it is possible that some protection may be afforded by a rise in substrate being accompanied by a decrease in SSAO activity through down-regulation or by increased product inhibition or an increase in concentration of an endogenous inhibitor.

In view of the potential importance of SSAO in diabetes mellitus in the vascular and other damage seen in this disease (see Yu and Zuo, 1993), it may be possible to suggest that the deamination

of aminoacetone by plasma SSAO is involved. In addition, this reaction may be involved in the development of some of the manifestations of other conditions, such as starvation and toxaemia of pregnancy, with their attendant rise in ketone bodies.

Conditions that alter SSAO specific activity in vivo

An alternative approach to the understanding of the importance of SSAO enzymes is to look for changes in SSAO activities that can be reliably correlated with changes in physiological or pathological state. In experimental animals, SSAO activities have been made to change experimentally or in association with genetic differences. As an example of the latter, SSAO activities were found to be increased in the brown adipose tissue of the obese Zucker rat when compared with litter mate controls (Barrand and Callingham, 1982). However, this observation was not extended to identifying the real cause of this increase. Increases in plasma SSAO activity have been identified in many clinical conditions, including chronic congestive heart failure (McEwen and Harrison, 1965), liver cirrhosis (McEwen and Castell, 1967) and in diabetes mellitus in human subjects (Nilsson et al., 1968; Tryding et al., 1969) and in alloxan-treated ewes (Elliott et al., 1991). A decreased plasma SSAO activity has been associated with various solid tumours and severe burns (Lewinsohn, 1977) as well as in patients receiving corticosteroids (Tryding et al., 1969). Indeed, Lewinsohn, as a result of her extensive work in the clinic, was able to suggest that measurement of plasma SSAO activity, towards benzylamine as substrate, could have important prognostic value in these conditions. In pregnant women, it had been reported that plasma SSAO activity did not change (McEwen, 1964) but, in a more detailed study, Lewinsohn and Sandler (1982) showed that plasma SSAO activity increased at parturition and declined 6–72 h post partum. In ewes, however, it was reported to remain stable for the first 100 days of pregnancy but declined by 50% in the last month of pregnancy (Elliott et al., 1991).

Although, in ewes, toxaemia of pregnancy (twin lamb disease) is now less common, due to improvements in husbandry, the sheep is an ideal animal for studies of both the enzymology of the SSAO enzymes in blood plasma and the changes in these and other relevant enzymes that take place during pregnancy. The same flock is available over several years and pregnancy is an entirely natural event, which, nonetheless, leads to profound changes in the physiological condition of the ewes. Sheep, besides tissue-bound SSAO activities in blood vessels, for example, also possess two, and possibly more, plasma SSAO enzymes. When benzylamine is used as a substrate, two kinetically separable enzyme activities have been identified (a "low K_m" and a "high K_m" enzyme; Elliott et al., 1992). When the deamination of certain other substrates is measured, two enzyme activities are also seen (Crosbie and Callingham, 1994). However, with some amines, for example, spermidine, allylamine and octylamine, only one enzyme activity seems to be responsible for their deamination. From evidence such as this, the suspicion is growing that these enzymes have preferred physiological (or endogenous) substrates and may, thus, subserve different functions both from the tissue-bound enzyme and from each other, adding to the overall complexity of the picture.

Our own experiments have been planned to extend the original observations of Elliott et al. (1991) that showed changes in SSAO activity in pregnancy and to see whether aminoacetone could be a candidate endogenous substrate for ovine plasma and tissue-bound SSAO. Plasma for these experiments was prepared from blood obtained by routine venepuncture from a flock of mixed breed (mainly Clun-Suffolk crosses) ewes, together with their attendant rams under the care of Dr. Roger Connan, Department of Clinical Veterinary Medicine, University of Cambridge. Plasma was also prepared from blood obtained at slaughter from fallow deer (*Dama dama*). Sheep femoral arteries were obtained from sheep killed

with intravenous overdose of pentobarbitone. Amine oxidase activities were measured either fluorimetrically by a method described by Crosbie and Callingham (1994) based on the method of Guilbault et al. (1968), but with adrenaline as a proton donor rather than homovanillic acid, or by a radiochemical assay (based on Lyles and Callingham, 1982b), except when methylamine was the substrate, activity in this case being assayed by the method of Tipton and Youdim (1976).

Fluorimetric assay of sheep plasma revealed that aminoacetone was deaminated by a single enzyme activity, K_m and V_{max} values of 6.6 μM and 1991 nmoles h^{-1} ml^{-1}. Similar experiments, with plasma SSAO from Fallow Deer, also revealed a single enzyme activity with K_m and V_{max} values of 13 μM and 1094 nmoles h^{-1} ml^{-1}, respectively. Aminoacetone was then used as a possible inhibitor in radiochemical assays with [^{14}C]benzylamine used as a substrate. Aminoacetone reduced the deamination of benzylamine at both low (2.5–25 μM) and high (400–1000 μM) concentrations, which corresponded to the "low K_m" and "high K_m" enzyme activities towards benzylamine. Aminoacetone appeared to be a competitive inhibitor of benzylamine oxidation by the "low K_m" sheep plasma SSAO enzyme, with a K_i value of 8.9 μM. However, it appeared to be a non-competitive inhibitor of the "high K_m" sheep plasma SSAO enzyme, with a K_i value of about 32.4 μM. This observation indicates that the enzyme responsible for deamination of aminoacetone is the so-called "low K_m" plasma SSAO. Aminoacetone (50–500 μM) was also deaminated by sheep femoral arterial SSAO, with a K_m value of 72.4 μM and a V_{max} of 17.1 $\pm$ 0.5 nmoles h^{-1} per mg protein. Aminoacetone was a competitive inhibitor of benzylamine oxidation by sheep femoral artery SSAO. The apparent K_i value was 48.7 μM.

The deamination of aminoacetone was greatly inhibited by 10^{-4} M semicarbazide, insensitive to 10^{-4} M clorgyline and completely abolished by 10^{-4} M MDL 72145. The small residual deamination of aminoacetone in the presence of 10^{-4} M semicarbazide is consistent with previous experimental results. For example, Hirsch (1953) found that 5×10^{-4} M semicarbazide did not completely inhibit SSAO activity. There was also a slight increase in the metabolism of high concentrations (> 100 μM) of aminoacetone in the presence of 5×10^{-4} M clorgyline. There is no apparent explanation for the mechanism of this increase, but it has been previously reported by several authors for other substrates (see, for example, Elliott, 1989). In any event, the evidence all points towards the fact that aminoacetone in the sheep is exclusively a substrate for SSAO.

Deamination of aminoacetone by sheep and deer plasma SSAO takes place with lower K_m values (7 and 13 μM respectively) than those reported for other tissues (human umbilical artery 92 μM, Lyles and Chalmers, 1992; rat aorta 19 μM, Lyles, 1994; bovine lung 94 μM, Lizcano et al., 1994).

Aminoacetone is not a substrate for MAO-A or MAO-B in either rat or deer liver or sheep blood vessels and no other mechanism is currently known by which aminoacetone is metabolized. It is therefore proposed that aminoacetone is an endogenous substrate for plasma SSAO and that SSAO plays an essential role in the deamination of aminoacetone.

Experiments undertaken, over two successive breeding seasons with our flock of ewes, partially confirmed our earlier observations (Elliott et al., 1991) that changes in plasma SSAO activities take place but also have highlighted some differences (Crosbie et al., 1994).

Preparative isoelectric focusing with sheep plasma, after ammonium sulphate fractionation and extraction (see Rucker and Goettlich-Riemann, 1972) failed to resolve the enzyme activities. Attempts to find inhibitors highly selective for one or other form were also unsuccessful, although tranylcypromine was about 100-times more potent against the "high K_m" enzyme. Again, while two enzyme activities were clearly at work with benzylamine as substrate, only a single enzyme could be revealed kinetically, as in the case of aminoacetone, that deaminated methylamine and spermidine.

Measurements, undertaken in two successive years with the same flock of ewes, of the activities of the "low" and "high" K_m enzyme activities towards benzylamine during pregnancy revealed that the "low K_m" enzyme activity fell significantly with time, only recovering at the end of lactation (see Fig. 1). However, the "high K_m" activity only fell significantly after parturition in one year and just before parturition in the second year, with little or no change in the metabolism of spermidine being observed. A possible explanation, which will need further study, is that the quality of husbandry in these present experiments was superior, with better control to ensure adequate nutrition, including copper, of the ewes.

The fact that the different SSAO enzymes appear to respond differently to the changing state of the pregnant ewe may suggest that separate roles for these plasma enzymes exist. While it cannot be ruled out that such changes could be caused by changes in nutrition or competition for

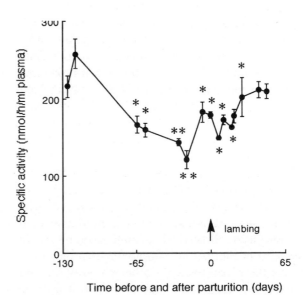

Fig. 1. Specific activity of "low K_m" sheep plasma SSAO against benzylamine (5 μM), as substrate, during pregnancy, parturition and lactation in mixed breed ewes. Each point is the mean $\pm$s.e.m. of 3–10 ewes; *, $P < 0.05$; **, $P < 0.01$, compared with the mean enzyme activity measured at 126 and 90 days before parturition, i.e. at the period when pregnancy could be confirmed.

essential nutrients and co-factors, such as copper, the possibility exists that these changes may be caused by a basic modification of the ewes' metabolism, in response to the growing lambs in utero. Indeed, this decrease in the activity in the "low K_m" enzyme may be to reduce the production of methylglyoxal from aminoacetone generated along with other ketone bodies in pregnancy and in excess in the very serious twin lamb disease.

Pathophysiological implications of aminoacetone metabolism by SSAO

Figure 2 summarises the metabolic pathways in aminoacetone production and metabolism. The evidence that aminoacetone is an endogenous substrate for SSAO is overwhelming. Aminoacetone has been shown to be formed in significant quantities, by the addition of glycine and acetyl-CoA to chicken erythrocytes (Gibson et al., 1958), certain bacteria (Elliott, 1960) and in guinea pig liver mitochondria (Urata and Granick, 1963). However, these were in vitro experiments and it seems more likely that aminoacetone is formed from the metabolism of L-threonine at physiological substrate concentrations (Elliott, 1960; Neuberger and Tait, 1962; Tressel et al., 1986). Aminoacetone is present in rat urine under normal feeding conditions as it constitutes a significant proportion of the aminoketones in normal rat urine (Marver et al., 1966), consistent with the lack of plasma SSAO activity in the rat. In support of the hypothesis that aminoacetone originates from L-threonine metabolism, Marver et al. (1966) also showed that aminoacetone is increased in rats fed an L-threonine-rich diet.

As there has been no other pathway for aminoacetone degradation yet described, it must be assumed that the metabolism by SSAO and excretion are the only methods for lowering its concentration in the plasma. This is of particular importance, since very little SSAO activity can be found in the liver where it is confined solely to the blood vessels in the organ (Parkinson et al., 1980).

The observation that aminoacetone production is sensitive to the ratio of acetyl-CoA and CoA in the mitochondria (Bird and Nunn, 1979; Bird et al., 1984; Tressel et al., 1986) suggests that aminoacetone production may be linked to the metabolic state of the cell. In states of starvation, the ratio of acetyl-CoA to CoA increases, and this would cause an increase in aminoacetone production and a concurrent decrease in glycine and L-threonine (Bird and Nunn, 1979; Bird et al., 1984). Aminoacetone is metabolized to methylglyoxal and then by various routes to pyruvate (Higgins et al., 1967):

(i) Methylglyoxal forms a hemithioacetal non-enzymatically with reduced glutathione and this is then converted to S-D-lactoylglutathione, a reaction catalysed by glyoxalase I (EC 4.4.1.5, lactoylglutathione lyase; see Thornalley, 1993). Glyoxalase II (EC 3.1.2.6, hydroxyacylglutathione hydrolase) then catalyses the hydrolysis of S-D-lactoylglutathione to D-lactate, reforming the glutathione used up in the glyoxalase I catalysed reaction (see Thornalley, 1993). This glyoxalase system is ubiquitous, being found in the cytosol of all cells. The D-lactate formed by the action of glyoxalase II is then converted to pyruvate by 2-hydroxyacid dehydrogenase (EC 1.1.99.6), an FAD-linked mitochondrial enzyme (Cammack, 1969).

(ii) In addition, methylglyoxal dehydrogenase converts methylglyoxal directly to pyruvate. Two such enzymes have been isolated and purified from goat liver: one requiring NAD^+ and the other $NADP^+$ as cofactor.

Pyruvate may then be converted to oxaloacetate, and can participate in the citric acid cycle or can be involved in gluconeogenesis, by well established metabolic routes. Thus, increased aminoacetone production during nutritional deficiency may play a role in providing substrates for the citric acid cycle or gluconeogenesis.

Several amino acids are actively metabolized during exercise and nutritional deprivation in animals and man (see Greenberg, 1969) so the suggestion that L-threonine could be involved in such a mechanism is not an unusual concept.

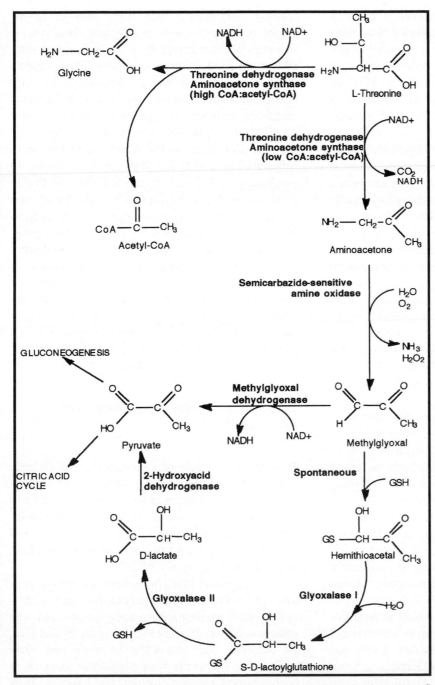

Fig. 2. Possible metabolic pathways for the production and catabolism of aminoacetone (based on Tressel et al., 1986; Thornalley, 1993).

A number of in vivo experiments in diabetes and exercise support the hypothesis that aminoacetone may be increased in nutritional deprivation. Methylglyoxal and its metabolites have previously been found to be raised in diabetes and have been implicated in the pathogenicity of diabetes mellitus (Thornalley et al., 1989; McLellan et al., 1993; Thornalley, 1994) but it was assumed that the increased methylglyoxal came from the same source as it does under normal metabolic conditions, i.e. the non-enzymatic elimination of glyceraldehyde 3-phosphate via its phospho-enediolate intermediate (Thornalley, 1993).

Activities of some of the enzymes in the proposed aminoacetone pathway have been reported to change in diabetic animals, with glyoxalase I and glyoxalase II activities increased in the liver and decreased in the muscles of streptozotocin-induced diabetic rats (Phillips et al., 1993). SSAO activity is increased in the serum of streptozotocin-induced diabetic rats (Hayes and Clarke, 1990) and plasma of alloxan-induced diabetic ewes (Elliott et al., 1991).

Human studies have also shown that the activity of glyoxalase I and glyoxalase II in red blood cells is altered relative to normal controls (McLellan et al., 1993) and that SSAO activity increased in diabetic patients (Nilsson et al., 1968; Tryding et al., 1969). Similarly, the substrates of the aminoacetone pathway (methylglyoxal, D-lactate and S-D-lactoylglutathione) are increased in blood samples from diabetic patients (McLellan et al., 1993). These results all support the proposal that a change in activity in this system occurs in diabetes.

Strenuous exercise may also result in nutritional deprivation, and an increase in glyoxalase I activity, methylglyoxal and D-lactate levels has been found in blood taken from German national team cyclists, after exercise (Haralambie and Mössinger, 1980).

Metabolic demand is also increased in pregnancy, which may result in nutritional deprivation if adequate food is not available. If the increased metabolic demand of pregnancy is met by increased food intake, then there may be no increase in aminoacetone production. However, if this demand is not met then an increase in aminoacetone production could follow. If the activity of SSAO in the plasma is determined by aminoacetone concentrations (as the activity of many metabolic enzymes is dependent on the amount of substrate present), then it is not unrealistic that the differences in the results recorded above reflected the nutritional state of the females. In pregnancy, SSAO activity may also be sensitive to copper availability. Malinowska (1986) found that levels of copper and caeruloplasmin (a copper-containing enzyme) were highest in late pregnancy in sows and suggested that caeruloplasmin was transported across the placental barrier. If this does occur, it could mean that copper is channelled across the placental barrier to the fetus, leaving less available for SSAO synthesis in the mother (Elliott et al., 1991). But we may not exclude the possibility that SSAO activity is controlled by a factor that still remains to be found.

Contribution of aminoacetone deamination to pathological states

In support of a role of aminoacetone in diabetic complications it has been shown that the activities of various enzymes in the aminoacetone pathway (glyoxalase I and glyoxalase II) are significantly altered in diabetic patients suffering from retinopathy compared to those without complications (Thornalley et al., 1989).

It is suggested that the aminoacetone pathway may be involved in diabetic complications such as neuropathy, nephropathy, retinopathy and the changes seen in the microcirculation in diabetes. In addition, early lactation in dairy cows and pregnancy, especially twin pregnancy in ewes, is accompanied by negative energy balance. It is suggested that these conditions may be associated with increased aminoacetone production. The metabolism of this aminoacetone could have the same consequences as are described above for diabetes.

Conclusion

Although this has not been a comprehensive and totally objective review, it does seem that the overall impression is one of optimism that these enzymes have roles to play in the pathophysiology and toxicology of certain endogenous and xenobiotic amines. As for a truly important physiological function, the remaining sum of uncertainty is still very large. However, with the advent of inhibitors that can distinguish between the different enzymes and the growing use of cell and molecular biological techniques, it should not be too long before the physiological importance (if any!) of the SSAO enzymes, both soluble and tissue-bound, will be unravelled.

Summary

The widespread distribution of enzymes classed as semicarbazide-sensitive amine oxidases (SSAO enzymes) throughout a very wide range of eukaryotic as well as prokaryotic organisms encourages the aspirations of those who wish to demonstrate physiological, pathological or pharmacological importance. Such enzymes are found in several tissues of mammals, both freely soluble, as in blood plasma, and membrane-bound, for example, in smooth muscle and adipose tissue. While they are capable of deaminating many amines with the production of an aldehyde and hydrogen peroxide, doubt still surrounds the identity of the most important endogenous substrates for these enzymes. At present, methylamine and aminoacetone appear to head the list of candidates. The possibility that SSAO enzymes can convert amine substrates to highly toxic metabolites is illustrated by the production of acrolein from the xenobiotic amine, allylamine and formaldehyde and methylglyoxal from methylamine and aminoacetone, respectively. Activities of SSAO enzymes may be influenced by physiological changes, such as pregnancy or pathologically by disease states, including diabetes, tumours and burns. Increased deamination of aminoacetone by tissue and plasma SSAO enzymes as a result of its increased production from L-threonine in conditions such as exhaustion, starvation and diabetes mellitus may be harmful. Such dangers could be mitigated either physiologically by a compensatory reduction in SSAO activity or pharmacologically by treatment with inhibitors of SSAO.

Acknowledgements

A.E.C. is a Medical Research Council Scholar. We are grateful for support from the European Union Human Capital and Mobility Programme, Contract No. ERBCHRXCT930256.

References

Andree, T.H. and Clarke, D.E. (1982) Characteristics and specificity of phenelzine and benserazide as inhibitors of benzylamine oxidase and monoamine oxidase. *Biochem. Pharmacol.*, 31: 825–830.

Aoyama, Y. and Motokawa, Y. (1981) L-Threonine dehydrogenase of chicken liver: purification, characterisation and physiological significance. *J. Biol. Chem.*, 256: 12367–12371.

Baba, S., Watanabe, Y., Gejyo, F. and Arakawa, M. (1984) High-performance liquid chromatographic determination of serum aliphatic amines in chronic renal failure. *Clin. Chim. Acta*, 136: 49–56.

Banchelli, G., Buffoni, F., Elliott, J. and Callingham, B.A. (1990) A study of the biochemical pharmacology of 3,5-ethoxy-4-aminomethylpyridine (B24), a novel amine oxidase inhibitor with selectivity for tissue bound semicarbazide-sensitive amine oxidase enzymes. *Neurochem. Int.*, 17: 215–221.

Barrand, M.A. and Callingham, B.A. (1982) Monoamine oxidase activities in brown adipose tissues of the rat: some properties and subcellular distribution. *Biochem. Pharmacol.*, 31: 2177–2184.

Barrand, M.A. and Callingham, B.A. (1984) Solubilization and some properties of a semicarbazide-sensitive amine oxidase in brown adipose tissue of the rat. *Biochem. J.*, 222: 467–475.

Barrand, M.A. and Callingham, B.A. (1985) The interaction of hydralazine with a semicarbazide-sensitive amine oxidase in brown adipose tissue of the rat. *Biochem. J.*, 232: 415–423.

Bergeret, B., Blaschko, H. and Hawes, R. (1957) Occurrence of an amine oxidase in horse serum. *Nature (Lond.)*, 180: 1127–1128.

Bird, M.I. and Nunn, P.B. (1979) Glycine formation from L-threonine in intact isolated rat liver mitochondria. *Biochem. Soc. Trans.*, 7: 1276–1277.

Bird, M.I., Nunn, P.B. and Lord, L. (1984) Formation of glycine and aminoacetone from L-threonine by rat liver mitochondria. *Biochim. Biophys. Acta*, 802: 229–236.

Blaschko, H. (1974) The natural history of amine oxidases. *Rev. Physiol. Biochem. Pharmacol.*, 70: 84–128.

Blaschko, H., Friedman P.J., Hawes, R. and Nilsson, K. (1959) The amine oxidases of mammalian plasma. *J. Physiol. (Lond.)*, 145: 384–404.

Blicharski, J.R.D. and Lyles, G.A. (1991) D,L-Buthionine sulphoximine, a glutathione-depleting agent, potentiates allylamine-induced cytotoxicity in rat aortic smooth muscle cell cultures. *Br. J. Pharmacol.*, 102: 184P.

Boor, P.J. and Hysmith, R.M. (1987) Allylamine cardiovascular toxicity. *Toxicology*, 44: 129–145.

Boor, P.J. and Nelson, T.J. (1980) Allylamine cardiotoxicity: III. Protection by semicarbazide and in vivo derangements of monoamine oxidase. *Toxicology*, 18: 87–102.

Boor, P.J., Hysmith, R.M. and Sanduja, R. (1990) A role for a new vascular enzyme in the metabolism of xenobiotic amines. *Circ. Res.*, 66: 249–252.

Boor, P.J., Trent, M.B., Lyles, G.A., Tao, M. and Ansari, G.A.S. (1992) Methylamine metabolism to formaldehyde by vascular semicarbazide-sensitive amine oxidase. *Toxicology*, 73: 251–258.

Brownlee, M., Vlassara, H., Kooney, A., Ulrich, P. and Cerami, A. (1986) Aminoguanidine prevents diabetes-induced arterial wall protein cross-linking. *Science*, 232: 1629–1632.

Buffoni, F. (1966) Histaminase and related amine oxidases. *Pharmacol. Rev.* 18: 1163–1199.

Burke, T.M. and Wolin, S. (1987) Hydrogen peroxide elicits pulmonary arterial relaxation and guanylate cyclase activation. *Am. J. Physiol.*, 252: H721-H732.

Byrd, W.J., Jacobs, D.M. and Amoss, M.S. (1977) Synthetic polyamines added to cultures containing bovine sera reversibly inhibit in vitro parameters of immunity. *Nature*, 267: 621–623.

Callingham, B.A. and Barrand, M.A. (1987) Some properties of semicarbazide-sensitive amine oxidases. *J. Neural Transm. [Suppl.]*, 23: 37–54.

Cammack, R.C. (1969) Assay, purification and properties of mammalian D-2-hydroxyacid dehydrogenase. *Biochem. J.*, 115: 5–64.

Coquil, J.F., Goridis, C., Mack, G. and Neff, N.H. (1973) Monoamine oxidase in rat arteries: evidence for different forms and selective localisation. *Br. J. Pharmacol.*, 48: 590–599.

Crosbie, A.E. and Callingham, B.A. (1994) Semicarbazide-sensitive amine oxidase in sheep plasma: interactions with some substrates and inhibitors. *J. Neural Transm. [Suppl.]*, 41: 427–432.

Crosbie, A.E., Callingham, B.A. and Connan, R.M. (1994) Changes in plasma semicarbazide-sensitive amine oxidase activities during pregnancy in mixed breed ewes. *J. Auton. Pharmacol.*, 14: 15P.

Dale, R.A. (1978) Catabolism of threonine in mammals by coupling of L-threonine 3-dehydrogenase with 2-amino-3-oxobutyrate-CoA ligase. *Biochim. Biophys. Acta*, 544: 496–503.

Davis, E.J. and De Ropp, R.S. (1961) Metabolic origin of urinary methylamine in the rat. *Nature*, 190: 636–637.

Dixon, M. and Webb, E.C. (1979) *Enzymes*, 2nd edn., Longmans, London.

Dostert, P., Guffroy, C., Strolin Benedetti, M. and Boucher, T. (1984) Inhibition of semicarbazide-sensitive amine oxidase by monoamine oxidase B inhibitors from the oxazolidinone series. *J. Pharm. Pharmacol.*, 36: 782–785.

Elliott, J. (1989) Semicarbazide-sensitive amine oxidase of blood vessels: a functional study. (PhD Thesis, University of Cambridge).

Elliott, J., Callingham, B.A. and Barrand, M.A. (1989a) In vivo effects of (E)-2-(3′,4′-dimethoxyphenyl)-3-fluorallylamine (MDL 72145) on amine oxidase activities in the rat. Selective inhibition of semicarbazide-sensitive amine oxidase in vascular and brown adipose tissues. *J. Pharm. Pharmacol.*, 41: 37–41.

Elliott, J., Callingham, B.A. and Sharman, D.F. (1989b) Metabolism of amines in the isolated perfused mesenteric arterial bed of the rat. *Br. J. Pharmacol.*, 98: 507–514.

Elliott, J., Callingham, B.A. and Sharman, D.F. (1989c) The influence of amine metabolizing enzymes on the pharmacology of tyramine in the isolated perfused mesenteric bed of the rat. *Br. J. Pharmacol.*, 98: 515–522.

Elliott, J., Callingham, B.A. and Sharman, D.F. (1989d) Semicarbazide-resistive amine oxidase (SSAO) of the rat aorta. *Biochem. Pharmacol.*, 30: 1507–1515.

Elliott, J., Fowden, A.L., Callingham, B.A., Sharman, D.F. and Silver, M. (1991) Physiological and pathological influences on sheep blood plasma amine oxidase: effect of pregnancy and experimental alloxan-induced diabetes mellitus. *Res. Vet. Sci.*, 50: 334–339.

Elliott, J., Callingham, B.A. and Sharman, D.F. (1992) Amine oxidase enzymes of sheep blood vessels and blood plasma: a comparison of their properties. *Comp. Biochem. Physiol.*, 102C: 83–89.

Elliott, W.H. (1960) Aminoacetone formation by *Staphylococcus aureus*. *Biochem. J.*, 74: 478–485.

Falck, B., Nystedt, T., Rosengren, E. and Stenlo, J. (1964) Dopamine and mast cells in ruminants. *Acta Pharmacol. Toxicol.*, 21: 51–58.

Falk, M.C., Staton, A.J. and Williams, T.J. (1983) Heterogeneity of pig plasma amine oxidase: molecular and catalytic properties of chromatographically isolated forms. *Biochemistry*, 22: 3746–3751.

Fazal, F., Ahmed, M.S., Rahman, A. and Hadi, S.M. (1994) Generation of superoxide anion and hydroxyl radical by methylglyoxal. *Med. Sci. Res.*, 22: 21–22.

Ferkany, J.W., Andree, T.H., Clarke, D.E. and Enna, S.J. (1981) Neurochemical effects of kojic amine, a

GABAmimetic and its interaction with benzylamine oxidase. *Neuropharmacology,* 20: 1177–1182.

Fernandez de Arriba, A., Balsa, D., Tipton, K.F. and Unzeta, M. (1990) Monoamine oxidase and semicarbazide-sensitive amine oxidase activities in bovine eye. *J. Neural Transm. [Suppl.],* 32: 327–330.

Garner, H.E., Moore, J.N., Johnson, J.H., Clarke, L., Amend, J.F., Tritschler, L.G., Coffman, J.R., Sprouse, P.E., Hutcheson, D.P. and Salem, C.A. (1978) Changes in the caecal flora associated with the onset of laminitis. *Equine Vet. J.,* 10: 249–252.

Gibson, K.D., Layer, W.G. and Neuberger, A. (1958) Initial stages in the biosynthesis of porphyrins. *Biochem. J.,* 70: 71–81.

Green, M.L. and Elliott, W.H. (1964) The enzymic formation of aminoacetone and its further metabolism. *Biochem. J.,* 92: 537–549.

Greenberg, D.M. (1969) Carbon catabolism of aminoacids. In: D.M. Greenway (Ed.), *Metabolic Pathways,* Vol. 2, 3rd edn., Academic Press, New York, pp. 126–128.

Guilbault, G., Brignac, P.J. Jr. and Juneau, M. (1968) New substrates for the fluorimetric determination of oxidative enzymes. *Anal. Chem.,* 40, 1256–1263.

Haenen, G.R.M.M., Vermeulen, N.P.E., Tai Tin Tsoi, J.N.L., Ragetli, H.M.N.,Timmerman, H., and Bast, A. (1988) Activation of the microsomal glutathione-S-transferase and reduction of the glutathione dependent protection against lipid peroxidation by acrolein. *Biochem. Pharmacol.,* 37: 1933–1938.

Haralambie, G. and Mössinger, M. (1980) Metabolites of aminoacetone pathway in blood after exercise. *Metabolism,* 29: 1258–1261.

Hayes, B.E. and Clarke, D.E. (1990) Semicarbazide-sensitive amine oxidase activity in streptozotocin diabetic rats. *Res. Commun. Chem. Path. Pharm.,* 69: 71–83.

Henle, K.J., Moss, A.J. and Nagel, W.A. (1986) Mechanism of spermidine cytotoxicity at 37° and 43° in Chinese hamster ovary cells. *Cancer Res.,* 46: 175–182.

Higgins, I.J., Turner, J.M. and Willetts, A.J. (1967) Enzyme mechanism of aminoacetone metabolism by micro-organisms. *Nature,* 215: 887–888.

Hirsch, J.G. (1953) Spermine oxidase: an amine oxidase with specificity for spermine and spermidine. *J. Exp. Med.,* 97: 345–355.

Holt, A. and Callingham, B.A. (1994) Location of the active site of rat vascular semicarbazide-sensitive amine oxidase. *J. Neural Transm. [Suppl.],* 41: 433–437.

Holt, A., Sharman, D.F., Callingham, B.A. and Kettler, R. (1992) Characteristics of procarbazine as an inhibitor in vitro of rat semicarbazide-sensitive amine oxidase. *J. Pharm. Pharmacol.,* 44: 487–493.

Hysmith, R.M. and Boor, P.J. (1987) In vitro expression of benzylamine oxidase activity in cultured porcine smooth muscle cells. *J. Cardiovasc. Pharmacol.,* 9: 668–674.

Kalapos, N.P., Garzo, T., Antoni, F. and Mardl, S. (1992) Accumulation of *S*-D-lactoylglutathione and transient decrease of glutathione level caused by methylglyoxal load in isolated hepatocytes. *Biochim. Biophys. Acta,* 1135: 159–164.

Kapeller-Adler, R. (1970) *Amine Oxidases and Methods for their Study,* Wiley Interscience, New York.

Kolb, E. (1956) Histaminase and diamine oxidase in the serum of domestic animals (ruminants, pig, horse) and in *Escherichia coli* and *Streptococcus faecalis. Z. Veterinärmed.,* 3: 570–591.

Krymkiewicz, N. (1973) Reactions of methylglyoxal with nucleic acids. *FEBS Lett.,* 29: 511–554.

Lee, T.H., Park, J.B., Han, H.J. and Lee, J.Y. (1989) Methylglyoxal induces crosslinking of protein in vitro. *Korean J. Biochem.,* 21: 75–80.

Levene, C.I. and Carrington, M.J. (1985) The inhibition of protein-lysine 6-oxidase by various lathyrogens. Evidence for two different mechanisms. *Biochem. J.,* 232: 293–296.

Levene, C.I., Sharman, D.F. and Callingham, B.A. (1992) Inhibition of chick embryo lysyl oxidase by various lathyrogens and the antagonistic effect of pyridoxal. *Int. J. Exp. Pathol.,* 73: 613–624.

Lewinsohn, R. (1977) Human serum amine oxidase. Enzyme activity in severely burnt patients and in patients with cancer. *Clin. Chim. Acta,* 81: 247–256.

Lewinsohn, R. (1984) Mammalian monoamine-oxidizing enzymes, with special reference to benzylamine oxidase in human tissues. *Braz. J. Med. Biol. Res.,* 17: 223–256.

Lewinsohn, R. and Sandler, M. (1982) Monoamine-oxidizing enzymes in human pregnancy. *Clin. Chim. Acta,* 120: 301–312.

Lewinsohn, R., Böhm, K.-H., Glover, V. and Sandler, M. (1978) A benzylamine oxidase distinct from monoamine oxidase B — widespread distribution in man and rat. *Biochem. Pharmacol.,* 27, 1857–1863.

Lizcano, J.M., Fernandez de Arriba, A., Lyles, G.A. and Unzeta, M. (1994) Several aspects on the amine oxidation by the semicarbazide-sensitive amine oxidase (SSAO) from bovine lung. *J. Neural Transm. [Suppl].* 41: 415–420.

Lyles, G.A. (1994) Properties of mammalian tissue-bound semicarbazide-sensitive amine oxidase: possible clues to its physiological function? *J. Neural Transm. [Suppl].* 41: 387–396.

Lyles, G.A. and Bertie, K.H. (1987) Properties of a semicarbazide-sensitive amine oxidase in rat articular cartilage. *Pharmacol. Toxicol.,* 60 (Suppl. 1): 33.

Lyles, G.A. and Callingham, B.A. (1982a) Hydralazine is an irreversible inhibitor of the semicarbazide-sensitive, clorgyline-resistant amine oxidase in rat aorta homogenates. *J. Pharm. Pharmacol.,* 34: 139–140.

Lyles, G.A. and Callingham, B.A. (1982b) In vitro and in vivo inhibition by benserazide of clorgyline-resistant amine oxidases in rat cardiovascular tissues. *Biochem. Pharmacol.,* 31: 1417–1424.

Lyles, G.A. and Chalmers, J. (1992) The metabolism of aminoacetone to methylglyoxal by semicarbazide-sensitive amine oxidase in human umbilical artery. *Biochem. Pharmacol.*, 43: 1409–1414.

Lyles, G.A. and Fitzpatrick, C.M.S. (1985) An allylamine derivative (MDL 72145) with potent irreversible inhibitory actions on rat aorta semicarbazide-sensitive amine oxidase. *J. Pharm. Pharmacol.*, 37: 329–335.

Lyles, G.A. and McDougall, S.A. (1989) The enhanced daily excretion of urinary methylamine in rats treated with semicarbazide or hydralazine may be related to the inhibition of semicarbazide-sensitive amine oxidase activities. *J. Pharm. Pharmacol.*, 41: 97–100.

Lyles, G.A. and Taneja, D.T. (1987) Effects of amine oxidase inhibitors upon tryptamine metabolism and tryptamine-induced contractions of rat aorta. *Br. J. Pharmacol.*, 90: 16P.

Lyles, G.A., Holt, A. and Marshall, C.M.S. (1990) Further studies on the metabolism of methylamine by semicarbazide-sensitive amine oxidase in human plasma, umbilical artery and rat aorta. *J. Pharm. Pharmacol.*, 42: 332–338.

Malinowska, A. (1986) Zmiany zawartosci cynku, miedzi i ceruloplazminy w plynah biologicnych i tkanach macior i ich plodow podczas ciqzy. *Med. Weteryn.*, 42: 368–372.

Marinari, U.M., Ferro, M., Sciabi, L., Finolli, R., Bassi, A.M. and Brambilla, G. (1984) DNA-damaging activity of biotic and xenobiotic aldehydes in Chinese hamster ovary cells. *Cell Biochem. Funct.*, 2: 243–248.

Marver, H.S., Tschudy, D.P., Pelroth, M.G., Collins, A. and Hunter, G. (1966) The determination of aminoketones in biological fluids. *Anal. Biochem.*, 14: 53–60.

McEwen, C.M. Jr. (1964) Serum amine oxidases in pregnancy. *J. Lab. Clin. Med.*, 64: 540–547.

McEwen, C.M. Jr. and Castell, D.O. (1967) Abnormalities of serum monoamine oxidase in chronic liver disease. *J. Lab. Clin. Med.*, 70: 36–47.

McEwen, C.M. Jr. and Cohen, J.D. (1963) An amine oxidase in normal human serum. *J. Lab. Clin. Med.*, 62: 766–776.

McEwen, C.M. Jr. and Harrison, D.C. (1965) Abnormalities of serum monoamine oxidase in chronic congestive heart failure. *J. Lab. Clin. Med.*, 65: 546–559.

McLellan, A.C., Thornalley, P.J., Benn, J. and Sonksen, P.H. (1993) Modification of the glyoxalase system in clinical diabetes mellitus. *Biochem. Soc. Trans.*, 21: 158S.

Mittal, C.K. and Murad, F. (1977) Activation of guanylate cyclase by superoxide dismutase and hydroxyl radical: a physiological regulator of guanosine $3',5'$-monophosphate formation. *Proc. Natl. Acad. Sci. USA*, 74: 4360–4364.

Moore, J.N., Garner, H.E. and Coffman, J.R. (1981) Haematological changes during development of acute laminitis hypertension. *Equine Vet. J.*, 13: 240–242.

Morgan, D.M.L. (1987) Oxidized polyamines and the growth of human vascular endothelial cells. Prevention of cytotoxic effects by acetylation. *Biochem. J.*, 242: 347–352.

Mukherjee, S.P. and Mukherjee, C. (1982). Similar activities of nerve growth factor and its homologue proinsulin in intracellular hydrogen peroxide production and metabolism in adipocytes. Transmembrane signalling relative to insulin-mimicking cellular effects. *Biochem. Pharmacol.*, 31: 3163–3172.

Nehlig, A. and Debry, G. (1994) Potential genotoxic, mutagenic and antimutagenic effects of coffee: A review. *Rev. Gen. Toxicol.*, 317: 145–162.

Neuberger, A. and Tait, G.H. (1962) Production of aminoacetone by *Rhodopseudomonas spheroides*. *Biochem. J.*, 84: 317–328.

Nilsson, S.E., Tryding, N. and Tufvesson, G. (1968) Serum monoamine oxidase (MAO) in diabetes mellitus and some other internal diseases. *Acta Med. Scand.*, 184: 105–108.

Obata, T. and Yamanaka, Y. (1990) Comparative studies on semicarbazide-sensitive amine oxidase in heart and plasma of rats treated with hepatotoxin allyl formate. *Int. J. Biochem.*, 22: 837–839.

Parkinson, D., Lyles, G.A., Browne, B.J. and Callingham, B.A. (1980) Some factors influencing the metabolism of benzylamine by type A and B monoamine oxidase in rat heart and liver. *J. Pharm. Pharmacol.*, 32: 844–850.

Phillips, S.A., Mirrlees, D. and Thornalley, P.J. (1993) Modification of the glyoxalase system in streptozotocin-induced diabetic rats. Effect of the aldose reductase inhibitor Statil. *Biochem. Pharmacol.*, 46: 805–811.

Precious, E., Gunn, C.E. and Lyles, G.A. (1988) Deamination of methylamine by semicarbazide-sensitive amine oxidase in human umbilical artery and rat aorta. *Biochem. Pharmacol.*, 37: 707–713.

Raimondi, L., Banchelli, G., Pirisino, R., Capecchi, S. and Buffoni, F. (1991) Semicarbazide-sensitive amine oxidase activity (SSAO) of rat epididymal white adipose tissue. *Biochem. Pharmacol.*, 41: 467–470.

Raimondi, L., Pirisino, R., Banchelli, G., Ignesti, G., Conforti, L., Romanelli, E. and Buffoni, F. (1992) Further studies on semicarbazide-sensitive amine oxidase activities (SSAO) of white adipose tissue. *Comp. Biochem. Physiol.*, 102B: 953–960.

Ramos, K., Grossman, S.L. and Cox, L.R. (1988) Allylamine-induced vascular toxicity in vitro: prevention by semicarbazide sensititve amine oxidase inhibitors. *Toxicol. Appl. Pharmacol.*, 95: 61–71.

Ray, S. and Ray, M. (1982) Purification and characterisation of NAD and NADP-linked α-ketoaldehyde dehydrogenase involved in catalyzing the oxidation of methylglyoxal to pyruvate. *J. Biol. Chem.*, 257: 10566–10570.

Ray, S. and Ray, M. (1983) Formation of methylglyoxal from aminoacetone by amine oxidase from goat plasma. *J. Biol. Chem.*, 258: 3461–3462.

Rothman, J.E. and Lenard, J. (1977) Membrane asymmetry. *Science*, 195: 743–753.

Rucker, R.B. and Goettlich-Riemann, W. (1972) Purification

and properties of sheep plasma amine oxidase. *Enzymologia,* 43: 33–44.

Schayer, R.W., Smiley, L.R. and Kaplan, H.E. (1952) The metabolism of epinephrine containing isotopic carbon. *J. Biol. Chem.,* 198: 545–551.

Selwood, T.W. and Thornalley, P.J. (1993) Binding of methylglyoxal to albumin and formation of fluorescent adducts. Inhibition by arginine, Nα-acetyl-arginine and aminoguanidine. *Biochem. Soc. Trans.,* 21: 170S.

Seregi, A., Serfözö, P., Mergl, Z. and Schaefer, A. (1982) On the mechanism of the involvement of monoamine oxidase in catecholamine-stimulated prostaglandin biosynthesis in particulate fraction of rat brain homogenates: role of hydrogen peroxide. *J. Neurochem.,* 38: 20–27.

Seregi, A., Serfözö, P. and Mergl, Z. (1983) Evidence for the localization of hydrogen peroxide-stimulated cyclooxygenase activity in rat brain mitochondria: a possible coupling with monoamine oxidase. *J. Neurochem.,* 40: 407–413.

Sharman, D.F., Kelly, M.J. and Loncar-Stevanovic, H. (1983) The metabolism of dopamine in the blood of ruminant animals: an enzyme system to metabolize dopamine released from mast cells in these species? *Comp. Biochem. Physiol.,* 75C: 217–222.

Simenhoff, M.L., Asatoor, A.M., Milne, M.D. and Zilva, J.F. (1963) Retention of aliphatic amines in uræmia. *Clin. Sci.,* 25: 65–77.

Suzuki, S., Sakurai, T., Nakahara, A., Manabe, T. and Okuyama, T. (1986) Role of the two copper ions in bovine serum amine oxidase. *Biochemistry,* 25: 338–341.

Tabor, C.W. and Tabor, H. (1984) Polyamines. *Annu. Rev. Biochem.,* 53: 749–790.

Takahashi, K. (1977) Further studies of phenylglyoxal and related reagents with proteins. *J. Biochem.,* 81: 403–414.

Tate, R.M., Morris, H.G., Schroeder, W.R. and Repine, J.E. (1984) Oxygen metabolites stimulate thromboxane production in isolated saline-perfused lungs. *J. Clin. Invest.,* 74: 608–613.

Thornalley, P.J. (1993) The glyoxalase system in health and disease. *Mol. Asp. Med.,* 14: 287–371.

Thornalley, P.J. (1994) Methylglyoxal, glyoxalases and the development of diabetic complications. *Amino Acids,* 6: 15–23.

Thornalley, P.J. and Tisdale M.J. (1988) Inhibition of proliferation of human promyelocytic leukaemia HL60 cells by S-D-lactoylglutathione in vitro. *Leuk. Res.,* 12: 897–904.

Thornalley, P.J., Hooper, N.I., Jennings, P.E., Florkowski,

C.M., Jones, A.F., Lunec, J. and Barnett, A.H. (1989) The human red blood cell glyoxalase system in diabetes mellitus. *Diab. Res. Clin. Pract.,* 7: 115–120.

Tipton, K.F. and Youdim, M.B.H. (1976) Assay of monoamine oxidase. In: G.E.W. Wolstonholme and J. Knight (Eds.), *Monoamine Oxidase and its Inhibition,* Ciba Foundation Symposium, 39, Appendix 1, Elsevier Excerpta Medica, Amsterdam, pp. 393–403.

Tressel, T., Thompson, R., Zieske, L.R., Menendez, M.I.T.S. and Davis, L. (1986) Interaction between L-threonine dehydrogenase and aminoacetone synthetase and mechanism of aminoacetone production. *J. Biol. Chem.,* 261: 16428–16437.

Tryding, N., Nilsson, S.E., Tufvesson, G., Berg, R., Carlström, S., Elmfors, B. and Nilsson, J.E. (1969) Physiological and pathological influences on serum monoamine oxidase levels. *Scand. J. Clin. Lab. Invest.,* 23: 79–84.

Urata, G. and Granick, S. (1963) Biosynthesis of α-aminoketones and the metabolism of aminoacetone. *J. Biol. Chem.,* 238: 811–820.

Wibo, M., Duong, A.T. and Godfraind, T. (1980) Subcellular location of semicarbazide-sensitive amine oxidase in rat aorta. *Eur. J. Biochem.,* 112: 87–94.

Wolin, M.S., Rodenberg, J.M., Messina, E.J. and Kaley, G. (1986) Hydrogen peroxide elicits vasodilation of rat cremasteric arterioles. *Fed. Proc.,* 45: 1157.

Yasunobu, K.T., Ishizaki, H. and Minamiura, N. (1976) The molecular, mechanistic and immunological properties of amine oxidases. *Mol. Cell. Biochem.,* 13: 3–19.

Yu, K.T., Khalaf, N. and Czech, M.P. (1987) Insulin stimulates the tyrosine phosphorylation of a $M_r = 160,000$ glycoprotein in rat adipocyte plasma membranes. *J. Biol. Chem.,* 262: 7865–7873.

Yu, P.H. and Zuo, D.-M. (1993) Oxidative deamination of methylamine by semicarbazide-sensitive amine oxidase leads to cytotoxic damage in endothelial cells. *Diabetes,* 42: 594–603.

Zreika, M., McDonald, I.A., Bey, P. and Palfreyman, M.G. (1984) MDL 72145, an enzyme-activated irreversible inhibitor with selectivity for monoamine oxidase type B. *J. Neurochem.,* 43: 448–454.

Zuo, D.-M. and Yu, P.H. (1994) Semicarbazide-sensitive amine oxidase and monoamine oxidase in rat brain microvessels, meninges, retina and eye sclera. *Brain Res. Bull.,* 33: 307–311.

Peter M. Yu, Keith F. Tipton and Alan A. Boulton (Eds.)
Progress in Brain Research, Vol 106

CHAPTER 32

Semicarbazide-sensitive amine oxidases: some biochemical properties and general considerations

F. Buffoni

Department of Preclinical and Clinical Pharmacology, University of Florence, Italy

Introduction

Many enzymes which are present in nature catalyze the general reaction:

$$RCH_2NH_2 + O_2 + H_2O ---> $$
$$RCOH + H_2O_2 + NH_3 (*)$$

where the amines may be primary, secondary and even tertiary. The semicarbazide-sensitive amine oxidases (SSAO) belong to the large class of enzymes for which a common feature of the amines to be substrates is that the α-carbon atom needs to be unsubstituted.

Some enzymes of this class in microorganisms produce nitrogen when amines are the only source of nitrogen (Yamada et al., 1965), produce aldehydes in plants (Tabor and Tabor, 1964) and also in animals (Siegel, 1979) as precursors of heterocyclic ring compounds (alkaloids, desmosine and isodesmosine) or produce aldehydes as precursors of alcohols and acids.

Amines are generally messengers for cells and the messages are terminated by the amine oxidase reaction. The biochemical elements at the basis of cellular communications are found to be very close to the base of the evolutionary tree. This means that ancestral molecular messages have changed very little with evolution even if the communicative function has become differentiated evolutionarily in diverse directions. This

process explains the presence of amine oxidases which are widespread in nature and their evolutionarily different substrate specificity and rate of oxidation.

Some of these enzymes act on primary, secondary and tertiary amines (Blaschko, 1989), others only on primary amines. This simple division is biologically very important because it reflects different recognition sites on the enzymes and different mechanisms of reaction.

FAD-containing enzymes (E.C. 1.4.3.4) are able to oxidize primary, secondary and tertiary amines and are largely diffused in nature: mitochondrial monoamine oxidase, aminoacetone oxidase (Ray and Ray, 1987), pyridoxamine-phosphate oxidase (Horiike et al., 1979), polyamine oxidase (Seiler et al., 1980) and many other enzymes discovered in microorganisms such as tyramine oxidase of *Sarcina lutea* (Kumagai et al., 1968), putrescine oxidase of *Micrococcus rubens* (Okada et al., 1979), spermidine oxidase of *Serratia marcescens* (Bachrach, 1962), etc.

The enzymes which oxidize only primary amines are inhibited by carbonyl reagents including semicarbazide, and all may be called SSAO (E.C. 1.4.3.6).

A characteristic feature of these enzymes is that they contain a carbonyl group which is part of their recognition site and which determines their biological property of acting only on primary amines. They are widespread in nature: in Gram-negative bacteria (Cooper et al., 1992), in many fungi, in plants and mammals (see Buffoni, 1993).

These enzymes differ in their substrate specificity but seem to differ very little in the mechanism of reaction and show a high degree of homology, which suggests evolutionary differentiation to cope with the diversity of the cellular messages (see Buffoni, 1993).

Recent discoveries indicate that nature has solved the problem of the carbonyl cofactor, which is involved in different types of enzymatic reactions, in many ways: in fact, it may be pyridoxal phosphate (PLP) (Dunathan, 1971), pyrroloquinoline quinone (PQQ) (see Duine, 1991), tryptophan tryptophylquinone (TTQ) (McIntire et al., 1991), TOPA-quinone derived from trihydroxyphenylalanine (Janes et al., 1990) or pyruvate (Riley and Snell, 1963; Demetriou et al., 1978; Yang and Abeles, 1987).

A completely new point of view derives from some recent observations that show that cofactors are not necessarily preformed substances such as vitamins but may be formed post-translationally by a modification of the apoenzyme (Yang and Abeles, 1987), for example by a process of auto-oxidation which is catalyzed by the presence of copper as in the case of phenylethylamine oxidase (Tanizawa et al., 1994).

In addition, different cofactors may catalyze the same enzymatic reaction: l-serine dehydratase from *Peptostreptococcus asaccharolyticum* may be either a PLP or an iron-sulfur-containing enzyme (Grabowski and Buckel, 1991). The iron-sulfur enzymes may represent more primitive forms than those containing pyridoxal phosphate (Grabowski and Buckel, 1991). Analogously quinoproteins may represent more primitive forms than those containing pyridoxal phosphate.

Evolution might have required a more selective substrate specificity and therefore different prosthetic groups to better cope with biological needs.

All the reactions catalyzed by a carbonyl group have the common property of starting with the formation of a Schiff's base. The nature of substrate and the influence of the apoenzyme dictate which of the bonds in α-carbon (see reaction *) is broken and controls the further reaction step.

Snell (1972) has clearly shown that structural requirements for enzymatic reaction are more demanding than for non-enzymatic reactions: in PLP, unmodified groupings at positions 1, 3 and 4 are required for enzymatic activity and the phosphate residue at position 5' is also required for high activity.

Semicarbazide-sensitive amine oxidases are a class of enzymes which differ mainly in the substrate specificity; therefore it may not be surprising if they also differ in the nature of their organic prosthetic group, as is seen in the literature (see Beinert, 1991).

Most SSAO are copper-enzymes that might catalyze the formation of their own prosthetic group. On the other hand the role of copper in copper-containing amine oxidase has long been a source of debate and uncertainty. Numerous experiments have failed to detect changes in the copper oxidation state in the presence of substrate amines. Recently Dooley et al. (1991) presented evidence for the generation of a Cu(I)-semiquinone state by substrate reduction of several amine oxidases under anaerobic conditions and suggested that Cu(I)-semiquinone may be the catalytic intermediate that reacts with oxygen.

It thus appears that much has to be learned about the biochemistry of SSAO enzymes and even more about the physiological role of some of them.

Tissue-bound semicarbazide-sensitive amine oxidases: distribution and biochemical properties

Distribution

Early studies on the immunological reactivity of various pig tissues with rabbit antibodies raised to pig plasma benzylamine oxidase (Bz.SSAO) have shown the presence of a protein possessing the same immunological determinants as pig plasma amine oxidase in the connective tissue of all organs (Buffoni et al., 1977). Blood vessels appeared to be particularly rich, as did brain meninges. Histochemical studies have shown that

TABLE 1

Tissues in which Bz.SSAO activities have been described

Chick	aorta, femurs
Mouse	white adipose tissue
Rat	aorta, mesenteric artery, heart, lung, vas deferens, anococcygeus muscle, liver, brown and white adipose tissue, retina, sclera, meninges, skin
Guinea pig	longitudinal smooth muscle of ileum, skin
Rabbit	heart, lung, cornea
Sheep	arterial wall
Ox	aorta, lung, retina, dental pulp
Pig	aorta
Human	blood vessels, white adipose tissue, placenta, liver, skin

(see Buffoni, 1993)

TABLE 2

Kinetic constants for the oxidation of benzylamine by some tissue Bz.SSAO

	K_m (μM)	V_{max} (nmoles/mg/min)
Mouse: WAT (1)	12.5 ± 3.0	0.77 ± 0.17
Rat: heart (2)	5.6 ± 0.8	0.09 ± 0.008
lung (2)	4.0 ± 0.5	0.18 ± 0.008
aorta (3)	6.8 ± 2.6	4.00 ± 0.66
adipocytes (4)	11.3 ± 1.7	15.30 ± 2.80
Guinea pig skin (5)	5.3 ± 1.4	0.015 ± 0.001
Rabbit: heart (6)	10.3 ± 3.0	0.15 ± 0.015
lung (6)	12.7 ± 4.0	0.36 ± 0.030
WAT (1)	8.0 ± 1.5	0.42 ± 0.060
Ox: dental pulp (7)	2.0 ± 0.3	11.0 ± 0.30
Pig: aorta (2)	4.3 ± 1.0	0.07 ± 0.006
Mini pig: skin (2)	12.8 ± 5.4	0.14 ± 0.024

WAT = white adipose tissue.
(1) Raimondi et al., 1992; (2) Buffoni, unpublished results; (3) Precious et al., 1988; (4) Raimondi et al., 1991; (5) Buffoni et al., 1994a; (6) Buffoni et al., 1989; (7) Norquist et al., 1982.

SSAO is localized in vascular smooth muscle cells of the aorta (Lyles and Singh, 1985), in adipocytes (Raimondi et al., 1990) and in fibroblasts of guinea pig skin (Buffoni et al., 1992). Rat aorta fibroblasts express Bz.SSAO activity, which is also present in the culture medium. Fibroblasts of guinea pig aorta express very little Bz.SSAO activity and then only after many doublings in culture, but they express good diamine oxidase (DAO) activity which decreases with doublings in culture. Fibroblasts of guinea pig skin express both Bz.SSAO and DAO activities (Buffoni,unpublished). An increased expression of Bz.SSAO in cultured cells with population doublings has also been described by Hysmith and Boor (1987) in pig aorta smooth muscle cells.

It has also been shown that the enzyme is mainly localized on plasma membrane (Wibo et al., 1980; Barrand and Callingham, 1984; Raimondi et al., 1991).

The presence of Bz.SSAO activity has been described in many tissues of different animals which are summarized in Table 1.

Biochemical properties

Few tissue-bound semicarbazide-sensitive amine oxidases have been fully purified and char-

acterized. As far as we know, they show a high affinity for benzylamine (Table 2) and therefore may be called Bz.SSAO to better differentiate them from the other SSAOs. They show many similarities to other SSAOs in their molecular weight (Table 3) and in their inhibitor sensitivity patterns (see Buffoni, 1993).

Elliott et al. (1992) have recently observed the presence of two different SSAO enzymes in sheep blood plasma, one with a high affinity for benzylamine and one with a low affinity for benzylamine. The activity showing lower affinity for benzylamine was able to oxidize spermine and spermidine whereas a single component metabolized benzylamine in arterial homogenates and spermidine at a very slow rate.

This interesting observation that in ruminants two different amine oxidases might exist in blood plasma, a benzylamine oxidase and a spermine oxidase, raises the question regarding which of these two enzymes has been fully purified and studied in previous work.

TABLE 3

Molecular weight and copper content of some purified SSAO enzymes

	m.w. (kDa)	Subunits number	Copper (atom/mole)
Bovine plasma (1)	180	2	2
Pig plasma (2)	194	2	2
Pig kidney DAO (3)	185	2	2
Human placental DAO (4)	235	3	3
Rat BAT (5)	183	–	–
Rat WAT (6)	175	2	–
Guinea pig skin (7)	194	2	–
Pig aorta (7)	194	2	–

BAT = brown adipose tissue; WAT = white adipose tissue. (1) Turini et al., 1982; (2) Buffoni et al., 1968; 1994a; (3) Yamada et al., 1967; (4) Crabbe et al., 1976; (5) Barrand and Callingham, 1984; (6) Raimondi et al., 1992; (7) Buffoni, unpublished results.
–, not determined.

Little is known for the moment about the nature of the carbonyl cofactor of tissue-bound SSAO. If the plasma enzymes are secreted by the blood vessel wall, blood vessel SSAOs should have the same carbonyl cofactor as the plasma enzymes, which is now considered to be TOPA-quinone (Janes et al., 1992).

In 1990 a method was described which permitted the release of pyridoxal from enzymes containing PLP and its identification by gas-chromatography—mass spectrometry (GC-MS) (Buffoni and Cambi, 1990). This procedure has recently been applied to pig kidney diamine oxidase and has shown that this enzyme contains PLP (Buffoni, 1994). Similar results have been previously obtained with pig plasma benzylamine oxidase (Buffoni, 1990). The presence of PLP in pig plasma benzylamine oxidase has also been recently observed with a different procedure in which a very selective site-directed inhibitor of this enzyme was used to label the carbonyl cofactor, 3,5-diethoxy-4-aminomethylpyridine (B24) (Buffoni et al., unpublished results). B24 is a more selective label than is phenylhydrazine for the active site of the enzyme. It reacted with pig plasma benzylamine oxidase and was stably linked to the enzyme by reduction in the proportion of 1 mole/mole of enzyme. Chemical hydrolysis of the B24-labeled enzyme permitted the isolation of B24-pyridoxamine, which was identified by GC-MS.

These results are in net contrast with the observations of the presence of TOPA-quinone in pig plasma benzylamine oxidase and in pig kidney diamine oxidase (Janes et al., 1992).

A procedure similar to those described by Janes et al. (1990) has recently been applied to purified pig kidney diamine oxidase. After inactivation of DAO with ^{14}C-phenylhydrazine, incubation of the enzyme with the proteolytic enzymes under alkaline (7.5) conditions split the incorporated radioactivity into different peptides. Bovine albumin was also found to bind some ^{14}C-phenylhydrazine, as has been previously described by Riley and Snell (1963).

Chemical hydrolysis of the largest peptide derived from DAO, in the presence of excess unlabelled phenylhydrazine, permitted the observation, by HPLC, of an adduct which had the same retention time as the phenylhydrazone of pyridoxal, some radioactivity and an absorbance in methanol at 370 nm, which is the maximal absorbance of pyridoxal phenylhydrazone.

This sample was treated with a large excess of benzaldehyde as described by Buffoni and Cambi (1990). It lost radioactivity and the formed substance gave the same HPLC retention time as free pyridoxal. No further experiments were carried out. However, the formation of many labeled peptides obtained with this procedure is in agreement with the results obtained by Janes et al. (1990).

Mechanism of reaction

The reaction catalyzed by SSAOs proceeds through a ping-pong mechanism in which 1 mole of benzaldehyde is formed anaerobically per mole of enzyme when benzylamine is used as substrate (Oi et al., 1970; Lindstrom et al., 1974).

The results reported in the literature are in good agreement regarding the fact that a proton is removed from the α-carbon atom (Olsson et al., 1976; Buffoni et al., 1981; Farnum et al., 1986) and that this is the rate-limiting step.

SSAOs are also characterized by unusual stereochemical patterns in their reactions: the porcine plasma enzyme is pro-R-specific for tyramine and dopamine (Coleman et al., 1991), whereas the bovine plasma enzyme is an example of mirror-image binding and catalysis (Summers et al., 1979). The purified bovine and porcine aorta SSAO are pro-S-specific but with solvent exchange into C-2, a pattern which has not been observed for any other copper amine oxidases (Scaman and Palcic, 1992). Therefore, although Bz.SSAO enzymes show a high degree of homology (Janes et al., 1992), which is also supported by some immunological cross-reactivity (see Buffoni, 1993), evolutionary pressures and the underlying chemistry of the transformation have changed the substrate orientation, which is generally conserved for the same class of enzymes (Coleman et al., 1991). SSAOs are probably a multigenic class of enzymes which share some properties, for instance, some amino acid sequences, but differ in the shape of the active site and may differ in the nature of their cofactor. For instance, antibodies raised against pure pig kidney diamine oxidase do not cross-react with pure pig plasma benzylamine oxidase and vice versa. This shows that these two SSAOs have different antigenic determinants.

Physiological role of Bz.SSAO in mammals

Benzylamine, which is the best substrate of these enzymes, is not a physiologically endogenous substance. Therefore, the nature of the physiological substrate and the possible physiological role of these enzymes have been the subject of much discussion (see Callingham and Barrand, 1987; Lyles, 1994).

SSAOs are able to oxidize many aromatic and aliphatic amines of which some, such as dopamine (Lizcano et al., 1991) and 5-hydroxytryptamine (Elliott et al., 1989; see Buffoni, 1993),

are of physiological interest. Deamination of methylamine and aminoacetone is particularly interesting because both these amines are readily deaminated by tissue Bz.SSAOs and they are normally present in the organism (Lyles et al., 1990; Lyles and Chalmers, 1992). On the other hand there are some species differences in the oxidation of these substances, for instance the K_m for methylamine is high in the human umbilical artery (Precious et al., 1988) and aminoacetone is not oxidized by some plasma amine oxidases (Buffoni and Blaschko, 1963).

Coming back to the points raised in the introduction of this paper we may say that if the physiological role of blood and tissue Bz.SSAO in mammals is a degradative role of cell messengers, localization of these enzymes should reflect localization of messengers receptors. The fact that these enzymic activities are not present in neurons but are mainly localized in mesenchymal cells suggests that the physiological role of these enzymes might be the metabolism of autacoids acting on these cells. The localization of Bz.SSAO in the meninges (Buffoni et al., 1977; Zuo and Yu, 1994) may suggest a role for these enzymes in the brain blood barrier.

One of the most important autacoids is histamine, which has been known to be a substrate of a Bz.SSAO for over 30 years (Blaschko et al., 1959; Buffoni and Blaschko, 1964).

Bz.SSAO with histaminase activity has been described in plasma of different animals and in different tissues (Table 4). The only enzyme in the rat mesenteric arterial bed that is able to catabolize histamine appears to be Bz.SSAO (Buffoni et al., 1994c).

The localization of "classical DAO", which is also an important enzyme for the oxidative deamination of histamine, is completely different from that of Bz.SSAO. DAO is largely present in the intestinal walls, placenta and kidney and it circulates in blood only during pregnancy or some pathological conditions (see Buffoni, 1993). Bz.SSAO activity is present in blood and blood vessels where histamine may be released. Therefore these two enzymes appear to have different

TABLE 4

Bz.SSAO with histaminase activity

Source	Oxidation ratio histamine/ benzylamine	Reference
Human plasma	0.019	McEwen, 1965
Horse plasma	0.23	Blaschko, 1959
Ox plasma	0.06	Blaschko, 1959
Pig plasma	0.35	Buffoni and Blaschko, 1964
Sheep plasma	0.09	Blaschko, 1959
Goat plasma	0.06	Blaschko, 1959
Dog plasma a	0.23	Blaschko, 1959
Dog plasma b	0.28	Blaschko, 1959
Rabbit plasma	0.13	McEwen et al., 1966
Pig aorta a	6.0	Buffoni et al., 1994b
Pig aorta b	2.3	Buffoni et al., 1994b
Pig WAT	0.43	Raimondi et al., 1992
Rabbit lung	0.62*	Buffoni et al., 1989
Guinea pig skin	0.09	Buffoni et al., 1994a
Rat aorta	0.73	Yu, 1990
Rat mes.art. bed	0.83*	Banchelli et al., 1994
Rat lung	0.47	Ignesti et al., 1992
Rat WAT	1.40	Raimondi et al., 1991
Mouse WAT	0.27	Raimondi et al., 1992

WAT = white adipose tissue; mes.art. = mesenteric arterial bed.
* ratio obtained at different substrate concentrations.
a and b indicate values obtained in different strains of dogs and values of two enzymes which were isolated from pig aorta.

roles: DAO might act on exogenous histamine or diamines, whereas Bz.SSAO may oxidize endogenous histamine. The fact that Bz.SSAO generally shows a low affinity for histamine suggests that this enzyme may have only a role in the oxidation of high concentrations of histamine such as those which are obtained in blood vessels by a sudden release from mast cells. We do not know whether the rate of oxidation of histamine and of its metabolite, N-tele-methylhistamine, may have a physiological role under physiological conditions. On the basis of these considerations one might expect tissue Bz.SSAOs from different species to have varying substrate specificity, as a consequence of the evolutionary adaptive role to various autacoids.

Histamine may not necessarily be one of the most important physiological substrates in every species. For example, rats are generally very resistant to histamine and have high Bz.SSAO activity in their blood vessels, whereas guinea pigs, which are very sensitive to histamine, have low levels of this activity in their blood vessels.

It is also important to point out that both DAO, which oxidizes putrescine and histamine, and Bz.SSAO, which oxidizes histamine, may also help regulate cell reproduction. Polyamines and histamine are in fact growth factors. Adipocytes express Bz.SSAO when they express their phenotype (Raimondi et al., 1990). This might suggest that Bz.SSAO is present in adipocyte membranes to reduce the stimulating effects of histamine on these cells.

Concluding remarks

There has been much speculation regarding the physiological role of Bz.SSAO in mammalian. General conclusions must await further experimental results.

The biochemistry of these enzymes also reveals discrepancies on many points which need clarification. Recently new specific and selective inhibitors of Bz.SSAO have been described, which will help to differentiate the role of these enzymes from that of DAO, enzymes which until recently were inhibited by the same inhibitors.

Variations in the blood and tissue levels of Bz.SSAO have been described in some pathological conditions such as diabetes (Yu and Zuo, 1993), skin healing (Buffoni et al., 1992) and some tumors (Lewinsohn, 1977). Specific inhibitors may therefore become useful drugs.

Summary

Semicarbazide-sensitive amine oxidases with a high affinity for benzylamine (Bz.SSAO) (E.C.1.4.3.6) have been biochemically described in many mammalian tissues (adipose tissue, lung, heart, blood vessels). The enzymic activity appears to be expressed by mesenchymal cells (fibroblasts, adipocytes, smooth muscles). Although the physiological role of this enzymic activity is still unclear, some possible physiological substrates such as histamine are discussed. Some enzymes of this class (SSAO) have been purified. They share many similarities, among which are that they contain copper and a carbonyl active site. The nature of the organic cofactor of these enzymes is discussed and data are presented which have identified pyridoxal in pig kidney diamine oxidase and in pig plasma benzylamine oxidase by gas chromatography-mass spectrometry.

Acknowledgement

This paper was supported by a grant from the European Community (Human Capital and Mobility).

References

Bachrach, U. (1962) Spermidine oxidase from *Serratia marcescens. J. Biol. Chem.*, 237: 3434–3448.

Banchelli, G., Ignesti, G., Pirisino, R., Raimondi, L. and Buffoni, F. (1994) Histaminase activity of mesenteric artery of the rat. *J. Neural. Transm.*, (Suppl.), 41: 445–448.

Barrand, M.A. and Callingham, B.A. (1984) Solubilization and some properties of a semicarbazide-sensitive amine oxidase in brown adipose tissue of the rat. *Biochem. J.*, 222: 467–475.

Beinert, E. (1991) Copper in biological system. A report from the 6th Manziana Conference, September 23–27, 1990. *J. Inorg. Chem.*, 44: 173–218.

Blaschko, H. (1959) The oxidation of 1,4-methylhistamine by mammalian plasma. *J. Physiol.*, 148: 570–573.

Blaschko, H. (1989) Oxidation of tertiary amines by monoamine oxidases. *J. Pharm. Pharmacol.*, , 41: 664.

Blaschko, H., Friedman, P.J., Hawes, R. and Nilsson, K. (1959) The amine oxidases of mammalian plasma. *J. Physiol.*, 145: 384–404.

Buffoni, F. (1990) Nature of the organic cofactor of pig plasma benzylamine oxidase. *Biochim. Biophys. Acta*, 1040: 77–83.

Buffoni, F. (1993) Properties, distribution and physiological role of semicarbazide-sensitive amine oxidases. *Curr. Topics Pharmacol.*, 2: 33–50.

Buffoni, F. (1994) Isolation and identification by gas chromatographic mass spectrometry of the carbonyl-active site of pig kidney diamine oxidase. *Anal. Biochem.*, 220: 185–191.

Buffoni, F. and Blaschko, H. (1963) Enzymic oxidation of aminoketones in mammalian blood plasma. *Experientia*, 19: 1–2.

Buffoni, F. and Blaschko, H. (1964) Benzylamine oxidase and histaminase: purification and crystallization of an enzyme from pig plasma. *Proc. R. Soc.*, B 161: 153–167.

Buffoni, F.and Cambi, S. (1990) A method for isolation and identification of pyridoxal phosphate in proteins. *Anal. Biochem.*, 187: 44–50.

Buffoni, F., Della Corte, L. and Knowles, P.F. (1968) The nature of copper in pig plasma benzylamine oxidase. *Biochem. J.*, 106: 575–576.

Buffoni, F., Della Corte, L. and Hope, D.B. (1977) Immunofluorescence histochemistry of porcine tissue using antibodies to pig plasma amine oxidase. *Proc. R. Soc.*, B 195: 417–423.

Buffoni, F., Coppi, C., Ignesti, G. and Waight, R.D. (1981) pH variation of isotope effect on the catalytic activity of pig plasma benzylamine oxidase. *Biochem. Int.*, 3: 391–397.

Buffoni, F., Banchelli, G., Bertocci, B. and Raimondi, L. (1989) Effect of pyridoxamine on semicarbazide-sensitive amine oxidase activity of rabbit lung and heart. *J. Pharm. Pharmacol.*, 41: 469–473.

Buffoni, F., Banchelli, G., Cambi, S., Ignesti, G., Pirisino, R., Raimondi, L. and Vannelli, G. (1992) Skin wound healing: some biochemical parameters in guinea pig. *J. Pharm. Pharmacol.*, 45: 784–790.

Buffoni, F., Cambi, S., Banchelli, G., Ignesti, G., Pirisino, R. and Raimondi, L. (1994a) Semicarbazide-sensitive amine oxidase activity of guinea pig dorsal skin. *J. Neural Transm. (Suppl.)*, 41: 421–426.

Buffoni, F., Banchelli, G., Ignesti, G., Pirisino, R. and Raimondi, L. (1994b) Histaminase activity of some tissue-bound semicarbazide-sensitive amine oxidase (SSAO) activities. *Br. J. Pharmacol.*, 111: 85P

Buffoni, F., Banchelli, G., Ignesti, G., Pirisino, R. and Raimondi, L. (1994c) The role of semicarbazide-sensitive amine oxidase with high affinity for benzylamine (Bz.SSAO) in the catabolism of histamine in arterial bed of the rat. *Agents Actions*, 42: 1–6.

Callingham, B.A. and Barrand, M.A. (1987) Some properties of semicarbazide-sensitive amine oxidases. *J. Neural Transm. (Suppl.)*, 23: 37–54.

Coleman, A.A., Scaman, C.H., Kang, Y.J. and Palcic, M.M. (1991) Stereochemical trends in copper amine oxidase reactions. *J. Biol. Chem.*, 266: 6795–6800.

Cooper, R.A., Knowles, P.F., Brown, D.E., McGuirl, M.A. and Dooley, D.M. (1992) Evidence for copper and 3,4,6-trihydroxyphenylalanine quinone cofactors in an amine oxidase from Gram-negative bacterium *Escherichia coli* K-12. *Biochem. J.*, 288: 337–340.

Crabbe, M.J.C., Waight, R.D., Bardsley, W.G., Barker,R. W., Kelly, I.D. and Knowles, P.F. (1976) Human placental diamine oxidase. Improved purification and characterization of a copper and manganese containing amine oxidase with a novel substrate specificity. *Biochem. J.*, 155: 679–687.

Demetriou, A.A., Cohn, M.S., Tabor, C.W. and Tabor, H. (1978) Identification of pyruvate in S-adenosylmethionine decarboxylase from rat liver. *J. Biol. Chem.*, 253: 1684–1686.

Dooley, D.M., McGuirl, M.A., Brown, D.E., Turowski, P.N., McIntire, W.S. and Knowles. P.F. (1991) A Cu(I)-semi-quinone state in substrate-reduced amine oxidases. *Nature*, 349: 262–264.

Duine, A. (1991) Quinoproteins:enzymes containing the quinoid cofactor pyrroloquinoline quinone, topaquinone or tryptophan-tryptophan quinone. *Eur. J. Biochem.*, 200: 271–284.

Dunathan, H.C. (1971) Stereochemical aspects of pyridoxal phosphate catalysis. *Adv. Enzymol.*, 35: 79–134.

Elliott, J., Callingham, B.A. and Sharman, D.F. (1989) Semi-carbazide-sensitive amine oxidase (SSAO) of the rat aorta. Interactions with some naturally occurring amines and their structural analogues. *Biochem. Pharmacol.*, 38: 1507–1515.

Elliott, J., Callingham,B.A. and Sharman, D.F. (1992) Amine oxidase enzymes of sheep blood vessels and blood plasma: a comparison of their properties. *Comp. Biochem. Physiol.*, 102C: 83–89.

Farnum, M., Palcic, M. and Klinman, J.P. (1986) pH dependence of deuterium isotope effects and tritium exchange in the bovine plasma amine oxidase reaction: a role for single-base catalysis in amine oxidation and imine exchange. *Biochemistry*, 25: 1898–1904.

Grabowski, R. and Buckel, W. (1991) Purification and properties of an iron-sulphur containing and pyridoxal phosphate independent l-serine dehydratase from *Peptostreptococcus asaccharolyticus*. *Eur. J. Biochem.*, 199: 89–94.

Horiike, K., Tsuge, H. and McCormick, D.B. (1979) Evidence for an essential histidyl residue at the active site of pyridoxamine (pyridoxine)-5'-phosphate oxidase from rabbit liver. *J. Biol. Chem.*, 254: 6638–6643.

Hysmith, R.M. and Boor, P.J. (1987) In vitro expression of benzylamine oxidase activity in cultured porcine smooth muscle cells. *J. Cardiovasc. Pharmacol.*, 9: 668–674.

Ignesti, G., Banchelli, G., Raimondi, L., Pirisino, R. and Buffoni, F. (1992) Histaminase activity in rat lung and its comparison with intestinal mucosal diamine oxidase. *Agents Actions*, 35: 192–199.

Janes, S.M., Mu, D., Wenner, D., Smith, A.J., Kaur, S., Maltby, D., Burlingame, A.L. and Klinman, J.P. (1990) A new redox cofactor in eukaryotic enzymes: 6-hydroxydopa at the active site of bovine serum amine oxidase. *Science*, 248: 981–987.

Janes, S.M., Palcic, M.M., Scaman, C.H., Smith, A.J., Brown, D.E., Dooley, D.M., Mure, M. and Klinman, J.P. (1992) Identification of topaquinone and its consensus sequence in copper amine oxidase. *Biochemistry*, 31: 12147–12154.

Kumagai, H., Matsui, H. and Ogata, K. (1968) Oxidation of dopamine by crystalline tyramine oxidase from *Sarcinea lutea*. *Mem. Res. Inst. Food Sci. Kyoto Univ.*, 29: 69–71.

Lewinsohn, R. (1977) Human serum amine oxidase, enzyme activity in severely burnt patients and in patients with cancer. *Clin. Chim. Acta*, 81: 247–256.

Lindstrom, A., Olsson, B. and Pettersson, G. (1974) Transient kinetics of benzaldehyde formation during the catalytic action of pig plasma benzylamine oxidase. *Eur. J. Biochem.*, 42: 377–381.

Lizcano, J.M., Belsa, D., Tipton, K.F. and Unzeta, M (1991) The oxidation of dopamine by the semicarbazide-sensitive amine oxidase (SSAO) from rat vas deferens. *Biochem. Pharmacol.*, 41: 1107–1110.

Lyles G. (1994) Properties of mammalian tissue-bound semi-carbazide-sensitive amine oxidase: possible clues to its physiological function? *J. Neural Transm. (Suppl.)*, 41: 287–396.

Lyles, G. and Chalmers, J. (1992) The metabolism of aminoacetone to methylglyoxal by semicarbazide-sensitive amine oxidase in human umbilical artery. *Biochem. Pharmacol.*, 43: 1409–1414.

Lyles, G.A. and Singh, I. (1985) Vascular smooth muscle cells a major source of the semicarbazide-sensitive amine oxidase of the rat aorta. *J. Pharm. Pharmacol.*, 37: 637–643.

Lyles, G.A., Holt, A. and Marshall, C.M.S. (1990) Further studies on the metabolism of methylamine by semicarbazide-sensitive amine oxidase activities in human plasma, umbilical artery and rat aorta. *J. Pharm. Pharmacol.*, 42: 332–338.

McEwen, M. Jr. (1965) Human plasma monoamine oxidase. *J. Biol. Chem.*, 240: 2003–2010.

McEwen, M. Jr., Kenneth, T.C. and Sober, A.J. (1966) Rabbit serum monoamine oxidase. *J. Biol. Chem.*, 241: 4544–4556.

McIntire, W.S., Wenner, D.E., Chistoserdov, A. and Lindstrom, M.E. (1991) A new cofactor in prokaryotic enzyme:tryptophan tryptophylquinone as the redox prosthetic group in methylamine dehydrogenase. *Science*, 252: 817–824.

Norquist, A., Oreland, L. and Fowler, C.J. (1982) Some properties of monoamine oxidase and a semicarbazide-sensitive amine oxidase capable of the deamination of 5-hydroxytryptamine from porcine dental pulp. *Biochem. Pharmacol.*, 31: 2739–2744.

Oi, S., Melvin, I. and Yasunobu, K.T. (1970) Mechanistic studies of beef plasma amine oxidase. *Biochemistry*, 9: 3378–3383.

Okada, M., Kawashima, S. and Imahori, K. (1979) Affinity chromatography of putrescine oxidase from *Micrococcus rubens* and spermidine dehydrogenase from *Serratia marcescens*. *J. Biochem.*, 85: 1225–1233.

Olsson, B., Olsson, J. and Pettersson, G. (1976) Kinetic isotope effects on the catalytic activity of pig plasma benzylamine oxidase. *Eur. J. Biochem.*, 64: 327–331.

Precious, E., Gunn, C.E. and Lyles, G.A. (1988) Deamination of methylamine by semicarbazide-sensitive amine oxidase in human umbilical artery and rat aorta. *Biochem. Pharmacol.*, 37: 707–713.

Raimondi, L., Pirisino, R., Banchelli, G., Ignesti, G., Conforti, L. and Buffoni, F.(1990) Cultured preadipocytes produce a semicarbazide-sensitive amine oxidase (SSAO) activity. *J. Neural Transm. (Suppl.)*, 32: 331–336.

Raimondi, L., Pirisino, R., Ignesti, G., Capecchi, S., Banchelli, G. and Buffoni, F. (1991) Semicarbazide-sensitive amine oxidase activity (SSAO) of rat epididymal white adipose tissue. *Biochem. Pharmacol.*, 41: 467–470.

Raimondi, L., Pirisino, R., Banchelli, G., Ignesti, G., Conforti, L. and Buffoni, F. (1992) Further studies on semicarbazide-sensitive amine oxidase activities (SSAO) of white adipose tissue. *Comp. Biochem. Physiol.*, 102B: 953–960.

Ray, M. and Ray, S. (1987) Aminoacetone oxidase from goat liver. *J. Biol. Chem.*, 262: 5974–5977.

Riley, W.D. and Snell, E.E. (1963) Histidine decarboxylase of *Lactobacillus* 30a. IV. The presence of covalently bound pyruvate as the prosthetic group. *Proc. Natl. Acad. Sci. USA*, 50: 3520–3528.

Scaman, C.H. and Palcic, M.M. (1992) Stereochemical course of tyramine oxidation by semicarbazide-sensitive amine oxidase. *Biochemistry*, 31: 6829–6841.

Seiler, N., Bolkenius, F.N. and Mamont, P. (1980) Polyamine oxidase in rat tissues. *Biochim. Biophys. Acta*, 615: 480–488.

Siegel, R.C. (1979) Lysyl oxidase. *Int. Rev. Connect. Tissue Res.*, 8: 73–118.

Snell, E.E. (1972) Relation of chemical structure to metabolic activity of vitamin B6. *Adv. Biochem. Psychopharmacol.*, 4: 1–22.

Summers, M.C., Markovic, R. and Klinman, J.P. (1979) Stereochemistry and kinetic isotope effects in the bovine plasma amine oxidase catalyzed oxidation of dopamine. *Biochemistry*, 18: 1969–1979.

Tabor, H. and Tabor, C.W. (1964) Spermidine, spermine and related amines. *Pharmacol. Rev.*, 16: 245–300.

Tanizawa, K., Matsuzaki, R., Shimizu, E., Yorifuji, T. and Fukui, T. (1994) Cloning and sequencing of phenylethylamine oxidase from *Arthrobacter globiformis* and implication of tyr.-382 as the precursor to its covalently bound quinone cofactor. *Biochem. Biophys. Res. Commun.*, 199: 1096–1102.

Turini, P., Sabatini, S., Befani, F., Chimenti, F., Casanova, C., Riccio, P.L. and Mondovi, B. (1982) Purification of bovine plasma amine oxidase. *Anal. Biochem.*, 125: 294–298.

Wibo, M., Duong, A.T. and Godfraind, T. (1980) Subcellular location of semicarbazide-sensitive amine oxidase in rat aorta. *Eur. J. Biochem.*, 112: 87–94.

Yamada, Y., Adachi, O. and Ogata, K. (1965) Amine oxidases of Microrganisms Part. I. Formation of amine oxidase by fungi. *Agr. Biol. Chem.*, 29: 117–123.

Yamada, H., Kumagai, H., Kawasaki, H., Matsui, H. and Ogata, T. (1967) Crystallization and properties of diamine oxidase from pig kidney. *Biochem. Biophys. Res. Commun.*, 29: 723–727.

Yang, H. and Abeles, R.H. (1987) Purification and properties of *Escherichia coli* 4′-phosphopantothenoylcysteine decarboxylase. Presence of covalently bound pyruvate. *Biochemistry*, 26: 4076–4081.

Yu, P.H. (1990) Oxidative deamination of aliphatic amines by rat aorta semicarbazide-sensitive amine oxidase. *Biochem. Pharmacol.*, 42: 882–884.

Yu, P.H. and Zuo, D.-M. (1993) Oxidative deamination of methylamine by semicarbazide-sensitive amine oxidase leads to cytotoxic damage in endothelial cells. *Diabetes*, 42: 594–603.

Zuo, D.-M. and Yu, P.H. (1994) Semicarbazide-sensitive amine oxidase and monoamine oxidase in rat brain microvessels, meninges, retina and eye sclera. *Brain Res. Bull.*, 33: 307–311.

Peter M. Yu, Keith F. Tipton and Alan A. Boulton (Eds.)
Progress in Brain Research, Vol 106
© 1995 Elsevier Science BV. All rights reserved.

CHAPTER 33

Polyamine oxidase, properties and functions

N. Seiler

Groupe de Recherche en Thérapeutique Anticancéreuse, Laboratoire de Biologie Cellulaire, Faculté de Médecine, Université de Rennes 1, 2 Avenue du Professeur Léon Bernard, 35043 Rennes, Cédex, France

Introduction

The lack of a rational nomenclature for the enzymes that oxidize the natural polyamines, spermidine and spermine, has considerably contributed to the confusion which exists in the pertinent literature. Basically two types of oxidase are involved in eukaryotic polyamine metabolism (Seiler, 1990, 1992).

(a) Copper-containing amine oxidases (CuAO) deaminate oxidatively the primary amino groups of the polyamines to the corresponding aldehydes. To this type of enzyme belong serum amine oxidase (SAO) and diamine oxidase (DAO). SAO, which is especially rich in ruminant serum, was the first polyamine-selective oxidase (Hirsch, 1953) to be described. Since ruminant serum is a component of many tissue culture media, oxidative deamination of the polyamines by SAO was a frequent source of erroneous interpretation of experiments with cultured cells. CuAOs possess 6-hydroxydopa as cofactor, which is integrated into the peptide chain within the active site of the enzyme, with the following amino acid sequence around the 6-hydroxydopa site (X): Leu-Asn-X-Asp-Tyr (Janes et al., 1990; Brown et al., 1991).

(b) A flavin adenine dinucleotide (FAD)-dependent oxidase has been isolated from liver, for which the designation polyamine oxidase (PAO) has been suggested (Hölttä, 1977). Subsequently it was shown that this enzyme is involved in most tissues in the oxidative splitting of the monoacetyl derivatives of spermidine and spermine, thus catalyzing a reaction sequence which, in reverse of the biosynthetic route, forms spermidine from spermine, and putrescine from spermidine (see Fig. 1) (Seiler, 1987). This enzyme is the topic of the present review.

In addition to PAO, polyamine-oxidizing activities which show properties of the tissue-type PAO have been demonstrated in sera (McGowan et al., 1987; Morgan, 1985a,b), but these enzymes have not yet been fully characterized.

Purification and properties of PAO

(a) Purification

PAO has been purified from rat and porcine liver by a series of chromatographic steps (Hölttä, 1977, 1983), and by affinity chromatography (Tsukada et al., 1988). The liver enzyme has a molecular mass of 62 kDa and an isoelectric point at pH 4.5.

From L1210 cells a PAO has been separated into two isozymes on the basis of chromatography on hydroxyapatite. Each had different elution characteristics from MGBG Sepharose; the molecular masses were estimated to be 260 kDa and 200 kDa. The isozymes showed differences in their kinetics with several substrates (Libby and Porter, 1987).

PAO possesses several properties in common

with MAO. Both enzymes are present in excess and are not rapidly inducible; both enzymes use O_2 as substrate, and have tightly bound FAD, and there is evidence for Fe^{2+} as cofactor. The optimal pH for catalytic activity is close to pH 10. PAO is sensitive to sulfhydryl reagents (Hölttä, 1977).

(b) Activity and subcellular localization

PAO is found in virtually all vertebrate tissues, though with different activities (Seiler et al., 1980; Pavlov et al., 1991), as is shown in Table 1. As a rule PAO activity seems to be higher in differentiated than in non-differentiated or de-differentiated cells: Quash et al. (1987) observed an increase of PAO activity after differentiation of Friend erythroleukemia cells, but lower activities in transformed than in normal cells of several cell lines (Quash et al., 1979). Likewise PAO activity was lower in tumors of the mammary gland, and in oesophageal carcinoma than in the normal tissue (Quash et al., 1979; Romano and Bonelli, 1986). In agreement with this notion PAO activity is low in brain and liver of rats at the time of

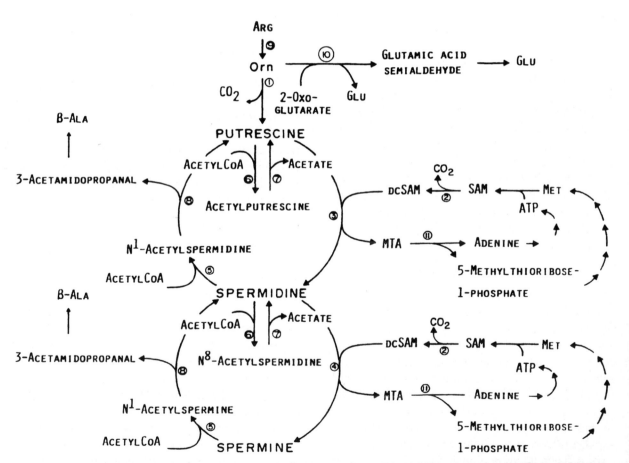

Fig. 1. Polyamine metabolic cycle. Enzymes: (1) L-ornithine decarboxylase (ODC); (2) S-adenosyl-L-methionine decarboxylase (AdoMetDC); (3) spermidine synthase; (4) spermine synthase; (5) acetylCoA:spermidine/spermine N^1-acetyltransferase (cytosolic); (6) acetylCoA:spermidine N^8-acetyltransferase (nuclear); (7) N^8-acetylspermidine deacetylase (cytosolic); (8) polyamine oxidase (PAO); (9) arginase; (10) L-ornithine:2-oxoglutarate aminotransferase; (11) 5′-methylthioadenosine (MTA) phosphorylase.

335

birth. It increases rather dramatically, however, during postnatal development, as is shown in Fig. 2. Surprisingly brain, in contrast with liver PAO activity, seems not to approach plateau levels in 2-month-old rats (Bolkenius and Seiler, 1986).

PAO has been localized using centrifugation methods both in peroxisomes and in the cytoplasm of rat liver (Hölttä, 1977). Since peroxisome-like structures are also found in brain, with the highest activity of peroxysomal enzymes being in non-neuronal cells (oligodendrocytes) (Holtzman, 1982), it is likely that the subcellular distribution of PAO in brain is similar to that in liver. Initiation of peroxisome proliferation by clofibrate or L-thyroxine causes an increase in PAO activity in liver. The increase in PAO activity roughly parallels the increase in catalase, a marker of peroxisomes (Beard et al., 1978; Just et al., 1984). Oxidation of spermine by peroxisome-

containing structures has also been demonstrated histochemically (Beard et al., 1985).

Substrates

Spermine and spermidine were originally considered to be the natural substrates of PAO, although it had been recognized that spermidine was rather poorly metabolized by the purified enzyme (Hölttä, 1977). From the fact that the rate of oxidation of spermidine and spermine was enhanced in the presence of certain aldehydes (Hölttä, 1977), it was concluded that the Schiff's bases formed from the polyamines and the aldehydes were better substrates than the non-derivatized amines. It was also presumed that the positive charge located on the primary amino groups of the aminopropyl moieties of spermidine and spermine was counterproductive to the enzyme reaction. In agreement with this notion,

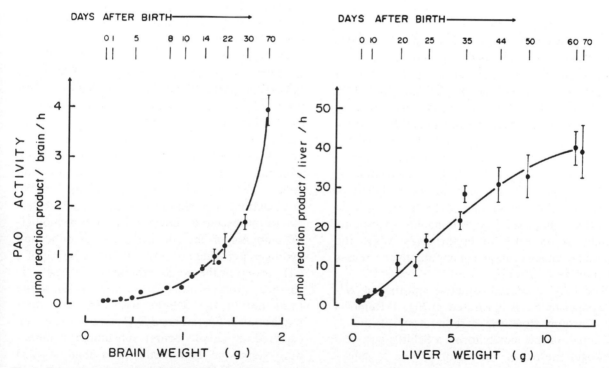

Fig. 2. Polyamine oxidase (PAO) activity in rat brain and liver during post-natal development. (Each point represents the mean value ± S.D. of five Sprague-Dawley rats). From Bolkenius, F.N. and Seiler, N. (1986) *Int. J. Dev. Neurosci.*, 4: 217–224.

TABLE 1

Polyamine oxidase activity in rat tissues

Organ	μmol g^{-1} h^{-1}
Pancreas	22.9 ± 2.2 (3)[a]
Liver	12.1 ± 1.7 (14)
Spleen	9.1 ± 1.6 (7)
Kidney	8.9 ± 1.3 (6)
Small intestine	6.5 ± 0.9 (6)
Testes	5.9 ± 0.2 (5)
Thymus	5.6 ± 1.2 (3)
Ventral prostate	4.1 ± 0.2 (3)
Brain	3.7 ± 1.3 (6)
Lung	2.6 ± 1.1 (4)
Heart	1.2 ± 0.2 (3)
Skeletal muscle	0.6 ± 0.2 (1)

[a] Number of animals in parentheses.
PAO activity was assayed in tissue homogenates at 37°C by determination of the rate of N^1-acetylspermidine formation from N^1,N^{12}-diacetylspermine in borate buffer, pH 9.0.
Data from Seiler et al., 1980.

evidence was presented in 1979 that N^1-acetylspermidine, N^1-acetylspermine and N^1, N^{12}-diacetylspermine were natural substrates of PAO (Seiler, 1981; Bolkenius and Seiler, 1981). Our observations led Pegg and collaborators to study polyamine N^1-acetylation (Matsui and Pegg, 1980; Della Ragione and Pegg, 1983). Recent findings have proved that spermine is also metabolized in vivo by PAO: long-term selective inactivation of PAO in mice causes a gradual accumulation of spermine in red blood cells. If the treatment with the PAO inactivator is terminated, spermidine rapidly accumulates in erythrocytes, while the spermine concentration concomitantly decreases (Sarhan et al., 1991a).

The PAO catalyzed oxidative splitting of N^1-acetylspermidine is illustrated in Fig. 3. Removal of a proton from the carbon atom of the 3-acetamidopropyl moiety forms a Schiff's base and hydrogen peroxide. The Schiff's base is subsequently hydrolyzed to putrescine and an aldehyde, 3-acetamidopropanal. (From spermine 3-aminopropanal and spermidine is formed.) The reaction is selective for the 3-aminopropyl moieties of spermine, and the 3-acetamidopropyl moieties of the N^1-acetylpolyamines. The 4-acetamidobutyl moiety of N^8-acetylspermidine is not attacked by PAO. By analogy with the reaction scheme in Fig. 3, N^1-acetylspermine is oxidatively split by PAO into spermidine and 3-acetamidopropanal. From N^1, N^{12}-diacetylspermine, N^1-acetylspermidine and the above-mentioned aldehyde is formed (Bolkenius and Seiler, 1981; Seiler, 1987). The final product of the aldehyde is β-alanine, which may accumulate in tissues, if polyamine degradation is induced (Seiler, et al., 1985a). According to Quash et al. (1987) malondialdehyde may be formed from 3-aminopropanal by a DAO-catalyzed oxidative deamination.

For the natural substrates of PAO the following K_m (μM) values and relative reaction rates (in parentheses) were observed: N^1, N^{12}-diacetylspermine 5.0 (1.0); N^1-acetylspermine 0.6 (0.7); N^1-acetylspermidine 14 (0.6); spermine 40 (0.02) (Bolkenius and Seiler, 1981).

During the evaluation of N-substituted putrescines as potential inhibitors of PAO (see below) the partial dealkylation by PAO of N-(2-propenyl)putrescine to putrescine was observed (Bolkenius and Seiler, 1989a). This reaction was further explored, mostly at the hand of the N-benzyl- and N,N'-bisbenzyl derivatives of the homologous aliphatic diamines (Bolkenius and Seiler, 1989b). The reaction scheme for the dealkylation of a mono-substituted alkyl derivative of putrescine is shown in Fig. 4. Stoichiometric amounts of the aldehyde, the diamine and hydrogen peroxide are formed. The presence of a CH_2 group in the neighborhood of the positively charged nitrogen atom is essential to allow the formation of the Schiff's base. The structural requirements for the residue R have not yet been explored in detail. Benzyl substituted diamines were somewhat better substrates than N-alkyl derivatives. N-Benzyl-1,4-butanediamine (K_m 28 μM) was dealkylated at the highest rate among

N^1-Acetylspermidine

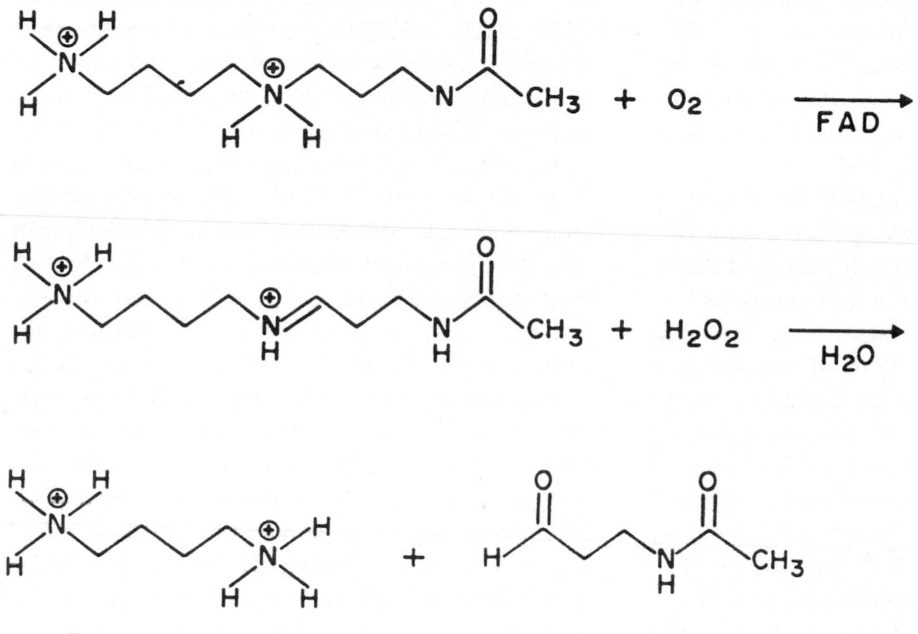

Putrescine

3-Acetamidopropanal

Fig. 3. Oxidative splitting of N^1-acetylspermidine by polyamine oxidase (PAO) to putrescine and 3-acetamidopropanal.

the alkylation products of the homologous diamines studied so far, although N^1, N^4-bisbenzyl-1,4-butanediamine (K_m 11 μM) possessed a higher affinity for the enzyme. Our observations were confirmed (Bitonti et al., 1990) for bisbenzylpolyamine analogs of the general formula

$$Ph\text{-}CH_2\text{-}NH\text{-}(CH_2)_x\text{-}NH\text{-}(CH_2)_y\text{-}NH\text{-}(CH_2)_x\text{-}NH\text{-}CH_2\text{-}Ph$$

In accordance with the above-defined struc-

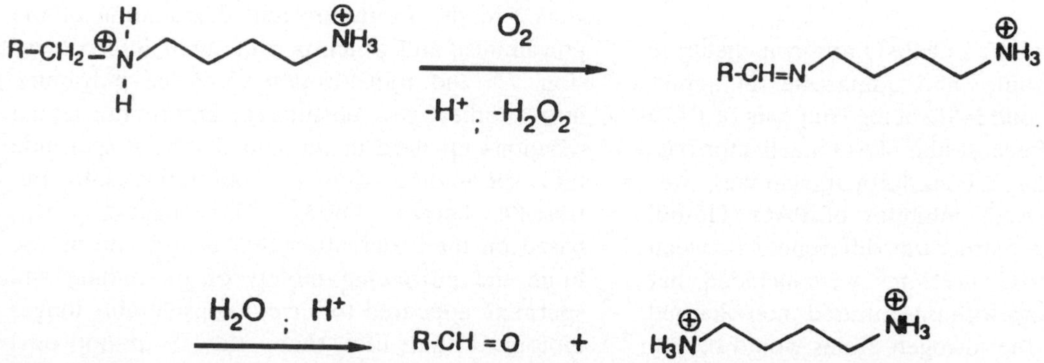

Fig. 4. Oxidative splitting of an N-alkyl derivative of putrescine by polyamine oxidase (PAO).

tural requirements for PAO substrates is the observation that N,N'-bis(3-(ethylamino)propyl)-1,7-heptanediamine, a homolog of N^1, N^{12}-bis(ethyl)spermine, is a substrate of PAO. Therefore, it is not surprising that the antitumoral effect of this compound is potentiated by inactivation of PAO (Prakash et al., 1990).

From the available information, the following minimal structural requirements for a substrate of PAO have been deduced (Bolkenius and Seiler, 1989b): two positively charged amino groups separated by a short carbon chain with one alkyl substituent on one or on both of the nitrogen atoms. Tertiary amines (two alkyl residues on the same nitrogen atom of the diamine) have not yet been studied. More recently it has been reported that milacemide (2-(n-pentylamino)-acetamide), an anticonvulsant drug, is metabolized by PAO (Strolin Benedetti et al., 1992). This observation indicates that the second positive charge is not an absolute requirement for PAO substrates. The previously mentioned relationship between PAO and MAO B is further documented by the fact that milacemide is also a substrate for MAO B (Janssens de Varebeke et al., 1988).

From the known structural requirements of PAO substrates it is evident that the aliphatic residue and the acetamidopropyl moiety, respectively, have to fit into a lipophilic pocket of the enzyme.

Inhibitors

Non-specific inhibitors of PAO are iron chelators (e.g. phenanthroline) and quinacrine, in agreement with Fe^{2+} and FAD being cofactors of PAO (Hölttä, 1977). Because the MAO inactivator pargyline (N-methyl-N-benzylpropargylamine) was found to be a weak inhibitor of PAO (Hölttä, 1977), despite the structural differences between pargyline and PAO substrates, we concluded that putrescine analogs with unsaturated, non-charged substituents on the nitrogen atoms would be potential inactivators of PAO. Among the compounds synthesized (Bey et al., 1985; Bolkenius and Seiler, 1989a) N^1-methyl-N^4-(2,3-butadi-

enyl)-1,4-butanediamine · 2HCl (MDL 72521) and N^1, N^4-bis(2,3-butadienyl)-1,4-butanediamine · 2HCl (MDL 72527) (Fig. 5) proved to be the most potent irreversible and selective inhibitors of PAO. They inactivate PAO in a time-dependent manner. Although the precise mechanism of the inactivation has not yet been elucidated, there is little doubt that N-(2,3-butadienyl)-1,4-butanediamines are enzyme-activated ("mechanism based") inactivators (Bolkenius and Seiler, 1989a). In order to inactivate PAO in cells, low concentrations (1–10 μM) in the culture medium are sufficient (Seiler et al., 1985a), and at an intraperitoneal dose > 20 mg/kg, PAO is completely inactivated in virtually all tissues of mice (Bolkenius et al., 1985; Seiler et al., 1985a). The compounds are also orally active. The N-2,3-butadienyl derivatives of putrescine do not affect any other tissue enzyme involved in polyamine metabolism, except that the deacetylase, which hydrolyzes N^8-acetylspermidine and N-acetylputrescine (Fig. 1), is competitively inhibited (Bolkenius and Seiler, 1989a). This effect is, however, too weak to possess observable consequences in in vivo experiments. These compounds, therefore, have become the most important tools in the elucidation of the functions of PAO.

Functions of PAO

(a) Polyamine interconversion

The existence of a reaction cycle which is involved in the formation and degradation of the polyamines, and which permits their interconversion, i.e. the transformation of one polyamine into another, was postulated, before the actual reactions involved in the conversion of spermine into spermidine, and of spermidine into putrescine, became known. This suggestion was based on the observation that in fish and mouse brain the putrescine moiety of spermidine and spermine appeared to have a considerably longer biological half-life than the 3-aminopropyl moieties; i.e. the putrescine moiety of the polyamines was reutilized in the formation of spermidine, whereas the 3-aminopropyl residue

	K_i (μM)	$\tau_{1/2}$ (min)
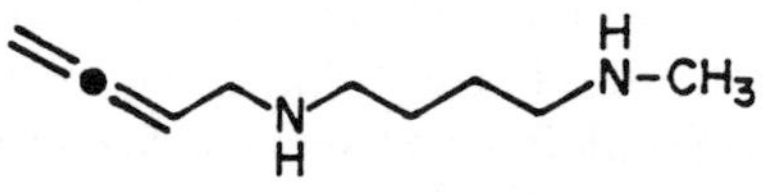 MDL 72521	0.3	0.5
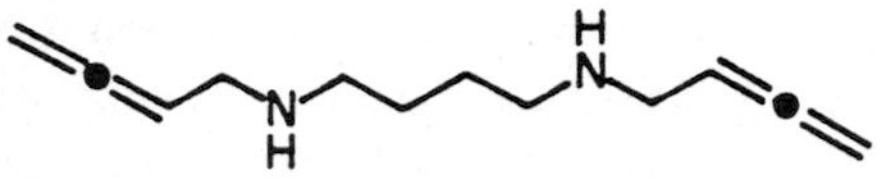 MDL 72527	0.1	2.2

Fig. 5. Inactivators of polyamine oxidase N^1-methyl-N^4-(2,3-butadienyl)-1,4-butanediamine (MDL 72521) and N^1,N^4-bis(2,3-buta-dienyl)-1,4-butanediamine (MDL 72527).

was metabolically eliminated (Seiler et al., 1979; Antrup and Seiler, 1980). Fig. 1 is the current scheme of the polyamine interconversion cycle. PAO, according to this scheme, forms spermidine from N^1-acetylspermine and putrescine from N^1-acetylspermidine. The importance and approximate rate of formation of putrescine from N^1-acetylspermidine has been demonstrated in the brain of experimental animals by inactivating PAO, using MDL 72527. Since the vertebrate brain is a nearly closed system for the polyamines and many of their derivatives, it permits the determination of (minimum) reaction rates from concentration changes. In agreement with expectations, N^1-acetylspermidine accumulated in mouse brain, linearly with time, at a rate of 1.1 nmol g^{-1} h^{-1}; whereas the putrescine concentration decreased concomitantly at the same rate (Fig. 6). It was calculated from these results that about 70% of the putrescine in adult mouse brain is formed by PAO-catalyzed degradation of spermidine, while only 30% is formed by de novo synthesis from ornithine (Seiler and Bolkenius,

1985). In early postnatal development, when cell proliferation is still active, the amount of putrescine formed in brain via the interconversion reactions is negligible compared with its formation from ornithine by decarboxylation (Bolkenius and Seiler, 1986). This is indicative of the fact that in embryonal and tumor cells, mainly de novo formation of the polyamines is required, not their precise regulation. In mature, non-dividing cells the maintenance of polyamine homeostasis is the major requirement. This is achieved, among other mechanisms, by regulation of the polyamines via the interconversion cycle.

The rate of PAO-catalyzed reactions is limited by the availability of the substrates, N^1-acetylspermidine and N^1-acetylspermine. Their concentration is regulated by the activity of the inducible acetylCoA:spermidine/spermine N^1-acetyltransferase, and by the rate of polyamine excretion. (For more details of polyamine regulation and the potential roles of the polyamine interconversion cycle, see Seiler, 1987, 1988; Seiler and Heby, 1988; Pegg, 1989).

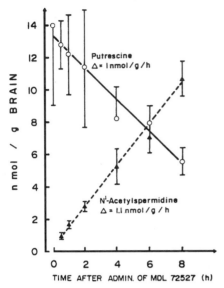

Fig. 6. N^1-Acetylspermidine accumulation and putrescine depletion in mouse brain after a single intraperitoneal dose of 50 mg/kg N^1,N^4-bis(2,3-butadienyl)-1,4-butanediamine (MDL 72527); mean values of three mice ± S.D. Data from Seiler, N. and Bolkenius, F.N. (1985) *Neurochem. Res.*, 4: 529–544.

(b) In vivo effects of PAO inactivation

PAO is presumably not of vital importance. Although long-term inactivation by MDL 72527 of the enzyme in experimental animals causes the accumulation of N^1-acetylspermidine and N^1-acetylspermine in tissues, the elevation of spermine concentration in red blood cells and plasma, and a limited depletion of tissue putrescine and spermidine concentrations, causes no apparent toxic effects or behavioral changes (Bolkenius and Seiler, 1987; Bolkenius et al., 1985; Sarhan et al., 1991a). However, because in these animals putrescine re-utilization is prevented, they excrete considerably more polyamines (in the form of acetyl derivatives) in urine than untreated rats (Seiler et al., 1985b). This fact was used by Hessels et al. (1990) to improve the assay for cell death by determining N^1, N^{12}-diacetylspermine in urine.

The reason for a lack of pathophysiological effects following PAO inactivation relates pre-sumably to the ability of healthy animals to compensate for polyamine losses, which are caused by the prevention of putrescine re-utilization, by enhanced de novo putrescine formation from ornithine (see Fig. 1), or by uptake from the gastrointestinal tract. In tumor-bearing animals, with an enhanced demand for polyamines, however, PAO inactivation may become apparent. Thus, for example, the colonic tumor burden produced by 1,2-dimethylhydrazine in rats became smaller if PAO was inactivated by MDL 72527 (Halline et al., 1990). The effect of PAO inhibition is even more accentuated if putrescine formation from ornithine is inhibited: combined treatment with MDL 72527 and 2-(difluoromethyl)ornithine, or a different inactivator of ornithine decarboxylase, is the most effective method for depleting tissue putrescine and spermidine concentrations. This treatment reduces the growth rate of tumors, including brain tumors (Claverie et al., 1987; Sarhan et al.,1989; 1991b; Moulinoux et al., 1991). Since, however, polyamine depletion stimulates immune defense (Chamaillard et al., 1993), and PAO inactivation by MDL 72527 is known to enhance interleukin-2 production by monocytes (Flescher et al., 1989), the observed effects on tumor growth are most probably not exclusively due to limited access to polyamines, but also to an effect of the immune-stimulating effect of polyamine depletion (Seiler and Atanassov, 1994).

If cell death is increased above physiological levels (i.e. if spermine is liberated in excess from cells of animals which have been treated with MDL 72527, and at the same time with either a cytotoxic agent, or an inhibitor of ornithine decarboxylase (Fig. 7), and especially if such treatment is applied to tumor-bearing animals) spermine dramatically accumulates in blood, and lethal toxic effects develop in about 4 weeks of treatment (Sarhan et al., 1991a). If in the above-mentioned treatments of tumor-bearing animals the administration of MDL 72527 is interrupted for 1 or 2 days per week (i.e. if accumulation of spermine in blood is limited by periodically allowing its PAO-catalyzed degradation to spermidine) the development of lethal toxicity is prevented (Quemener et al., 1992). These observations indicate that the excessive accumulation of spermine in blood is basically the reason for the development of the toxic effects following treatment with the PAO inactivator, although the mechanisms underlying this toxicity of spermine are still obscure. The presence of PAO in red blood cells, and its function there to eliminate spermine (which is not well excreted in urine), became known from these experiments.

Conclusions

PAO is a ubiquitous enzyme of vertebrate tissues. It is intimately involved in intracellular polyamine metabolism. The occurrence of PAO in animals of low evolutionary status, plants and bacteria has not yet been systematically studied, although it is known that several oxidases exist which in one way or another metabolize the natural polyamines (Morgan, 1985). The basic functional role of PAO appears to be the same in all vertebrate tissues, namely to participate in the transformation of spermine into spermidine, and of spermidine into putrescine. The exchange of polyamines between brain and the periphery is limited (Shin et al., 1985). This implies that the brain, in contrast with peripheral organs, cannot efficiently utilize exogenous (e.g. gastrointestinal) polyamines. It is, therefore, more dependent on putrescine re-utilization and de novo synthesis than other tissues in the vertebrate organism. This may imply a greater importance of PAO-catalyzed reactions in the brain than in other organs. Since it is difficult to obtain sufficiently precise quantitative data on the dynamics of polyamine metabolism, this type of consideration must remain at the present at a qualitative level.

It is not only the derivatives of the natural polyamines that are substrates for PAO and so it is important to explore whether PAO plays a role in the metabolism of biogenic amines, especially the secondary amines with structural features similar to known PAO substrates. Furthermore,

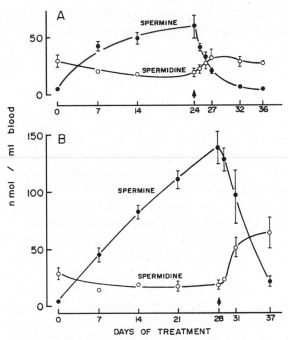

Fig. 7. Effect of treatment with the polyamine oxidase inhibitor MDL 72527 alone (A) or in combination with 2-(di fluoromethyl)ornithine (B) on whole blood spermidine and spermine concentrations of mice. C57BL mice received standard rodent chow which contained either 0.05% MDL 72527 (A) or 0.05% MDL 72527 and 3% 2-(difluoromethyl)ornithine (B). At certain intervals blood polyamines were analyzed . The arrow indicates the time when treatment was discontinued and drug-containing chow was exchanged against standard rodent chow. From Sarhan et al. (1991) *Int. J. Biochem.*, 23: 617–626.

the metabolism of milacemide (Strolin Benedetti et al., 1992) indicates the possibility that PAO may be involved in the metabolism of certain drugs.

The PAO inactivator MDL 72527 possesses important effects on the function of peripheral blood monocytes: it enhances interleukin-2 production, and it prevents the formation of lymphocytotoxic amounts of ammonia (Flescher et al., 1989, 1991). Should it turn out that the enzyme involved in these processes is identical with PAO, then it becomes possible to predict a rather general function for PAO in cellular immune defense mechanisms, not only in peripheral tissues, but also in activated microglia in the brain.

Summary

Polyamine oxidase (PAO) is a FAD-dependent enzyme with a molecular mass of about 62 kDa, present with high activity in most tissues of vertebrates. Structural requirements of a substrate for PAO are two positively charged amino groups, separated by a short carbon chain and an alkyl substituent on one or both nitrogen atoms. Spermine and the monoacetyl derivatives N^1-acetylspermine and N^1-acetylspermidine appear to be the natural substrates. Spermidine is only poorly oxidized by PAO. Using O_2, the substrates are oxidatively cleaved by PAO to form equimolar amounts of an amine, an aldehyde and hydrogen peroxide. PAO is an integral part of the polyamine interconversion cycle, a major intracellular regulatory system, which contributes to the maintenance of polyamine homeostasis in non-proliferating cells, including brain cells. Selective inactivators were used as tools in the elucidation of the functions of PAO. Interestingly, even long-term inactivation of PAO did not provoke behavioral changes in experimental animals, despite considerable changes in polyamine metabolism. PAO inactivation, however, improves the growth-inhibitory effects of inhibitors of polyamine biosynthetic enzymes and the antitumoral effects of some structural analogs of the polyamines.

References

Antrup, H. and Seiler, N. (1980) On the turnover of polyamines spermidine and spermine in mouse brain and other organs. *Neurochem. Res.*, 5: 123–143.

Beard, M.E., Edmonson, G. and Harrelson, A. (1978) Polyamine oxidase, clofibrate and peroxisomes. *J. Cell Biol.*, 79: Abstr. No. 214A.

Beard, M.E., Baker, R., Conomos, P., Pugatch, D. and Holtzman, E. (1985) Oxidation of oxalate and polyamines by rat peroxisomes. *J. Histochem. Cytochem.*, 33: 460–464.

Bey, P., Bolkenius, F.N., Seiler, N. and Casara, P. (1985) N-2,3-Butadienyl-1,4-butanediamine derivatives: Potent ir-

reversible inactivators of mammalian polyamine oxidase. *J. Med. Chem.*, 28: 1–2.

Bitonti, A.J., Dumont, J.A., Bush, T.L., Stemerick, D.M., Edwards, M.L. and McCann, P.P. (1990) Bis(benzyl)polyamine analogs as novel substrates for polyamine oxidase. *J. Biol. Chem.*, 265: 382–388.

Bolkenius, F.N. and Seiler, N. (1981) Acetylderivatives as intermediates in polyamine catabolism. *Int. J. Biochem.*, 13: 287–292.

Bolkenius, F.N. and Seiler, N. (1986) Developmental aspects of polyamine interconversion in rat brain. *Int. J. Dev. Neurosci.*, 4: 217–224.

Bolkenius, F.N. and Seiler, N. (1987) The role of polyamine reutilization in depletion of cellular stores of polyamines in non-proliferating tissues. *Biochim. Biophys. Acta*, 923: 125–135.

Bolkenius, F.N. and Seiler, N. (1989a) Polyamine oxidase inhibitors. In: M. Sandler and H.J. Smith (Eds.), *Design of Enzyme Inhibitors as Drugs*, Oxford Science Publications, Oxford, pp. 245–256.

Bolkenius, F.N. and Seiler, N. (1989b) New substrates of polyamine oxidase. *Biol. Chem. Hoppe Seyler*, 370: 525–531.

Bolkenius, F.N., Bey, P. and Seiler, N. (1985) Specific inhibition of polyamine oxidase in vivo is a method for the elucidation of its physiological role. *Biochim. Biophys. Acta*, 838: 69–76.

Brown, D.E., McGuire, M.A., Dooley, D.M., Janes, S.M., Mu, D. and Klinman, J.P. (1991) The organic functional group in copper-containing amine oxidases. *J. Biol. Chem.*, 266: 4049–4051.

Chamaillard, L., Quemener, V., Havouis, R. and Moulinoux, J.P. (1993) Polyamine depletion stimulates natural killer cell activity in cancerous mice. *Anticancer Res.*, 13: 1027–1033.

Claverie, N., Wagner, J., Knödgen, B. and Seiler, N. (1987) Inhibition of polyamine oxidase improves the antitumoral effects of ornithine decarboxylase inhibitors. *Anticancer Res.*, 7: 765–772.

Della Ragione, F. and Pegg, A.E. (1983) Studies of the specificity and kinetics of rat liver spermidine/spermine N^1-acetyltransferase. *Biochem. J.*, 213: 701–706.

Flescher, E., Bowlin, T.L. and Talal, N. (1989) Polyamine oxidation downregulates IL-2 production by human peripheral blood mononuclear cells. *J. Immunol.*, 142: 907–912.

Flescher, E., Fossum, D. and Talal, N. (1991) Polyamine-dependent production of lymphocytotoxic levels of ammonia by human peripheral blood monocytes. *Immunol. Lett.*, 28: 85–95.

Halline, A.G., Dudeja, P.K., Jacoby, R.F., Llor, X., Teng, B.B., Chowdhury, L.N., Davidson, N.O. and Brasitus, T.A. (1990) Effect of polyamine oxidase inhibition on the colonic malignant transformation process induced by 1,2-dimethylhydrazine. *Carcinogenesis*, 11: 2127–2132.

Hessels, J., Ferwerda, H., Kingma, A.W. and Muskiet, F.A.J. (1990) Inhibition of polyamine oxidase in rats improves the sensitivity of urinary polyamines as markers for cell death. *Biochem. J.*, 266: 843–851.

Hirsch, J.G. (1953) Spermine oxidase: An amine oxidase with specificity for spermine and spermidine. *J. Exp. Med.*, 97: 345–355.

Hölttä, E. (1977) Oxidation of spermidine and spermine in rat liver: Purification and properties of polyamine oxidase. *Biochemistry*, 16: 91–100.

Hölttä, E. (1983) Polyamine oxidase (rat liver). *Methods Enzymol.*, 94: 306–311.

Holtzman, E. (1982) Peroxisomes in nervous tissue. *Ann. N.Y. Acad. Sci. USA*, 386: 523–525.

Janes, S.M., Mu, D., Wemmer, D., Smith, A.J., Swinder, K., Maltby, D., Burlingame, A.L. and Klinman, J.P. (1990) A new redox cofactor in eukaryotic enzymes: 6-Hydroxydopa at the active site of bovine serum amine oxidase. *Science*, 248: 981–987.

Janssens de Varebeke, P., Cavalier, R., David-Remacle, M. and Youdim, M.B.H. (1988) Formation of neurotransmitter glycine from the anticonvulsant milacemide is mediated by brain monoamine oxidase B. *J. Neurochem.*, 50: 1011–1016.

Just, W.W., Hartl, F.U., Schimassek, H., Bolkenius, F.N. and Seiler, N. (1984) Polyamines and polyamine oxidase (PAO) in rat liver peroxisomes in response to peroxisomal proliferation. *Int. Conf. on Polyamines, Budapest*, Abstr. No. 106.

Libby, R.P. and Porter, C.W. (1987) Separation of two isozymes of polyamine oxidase from murine L1210 leukemia cells. *Biochem. Biophys. Res. Commun.*, 144: 528–535.

Matsui, I. and Pegg, A.E. (1980) Increase in acetylation of spermidine in rat liver extracts brought about by treatment with carbon tetrachloride. *Biochem. Biophys. Res. Commun.*, 92: 1009–1015.

McGowan, S.H., Keir, H.M. and Wallace, H.M. (1987) Presence of tissue-type polyamine oxidase activity in mammalian serum. *Med. Sci. R.B.*, 15: 687.

Morgan, D.M.L. (1985a) Polyamine oxidases. *Biochem. Soc. Trans.*, 13: 322–326.

Morgan, D.M.L. (1985b) Human pregnancy-associated polyamine oxidase: partial purification and properties. *Biochem. Soc. Trans.*, 13: 351–352.

Moulinoux, J.P., Darcel, F., Quemener, V., Havouis, R. and Seiler, N. (1991) Inhibition of the growth of U-251 human glioblastoma in nude mice by polyamine deprivation. *Anticancer Res.*, 11: 175–180.

Pavlov, V., Nikolov, I., Damjanov, D. and Dimitrov, O. (1991) Distribution of polyamine oxidase activity in rat tissues and subcellular fractions. *Experientia*, 47: 1209–1211.

Pegg, A.E. (1989) Polyamine metabolism and its importance in neoplastic growth and as a target for chemotherapy. *Cancer Res.*, 48: 759–774.

Prakash, N.J., Bowlin, T.L., Edwards, M.L., Sunkara, P.S., and Sjoerdsma, A. (1990) Antitumor activity of a novel synthetic polyamine analogue, N,N'-bis(3-(ethylamino)-propyl)1,7-heptanediamine: Potentiation by polyamine oxidase inhibitors. *Anticancer Res.*, 10: 1281–1288.

Quash, G., Keolouangkhot, T., Gazzolo, L., Ripoll, H. and Saez, S. (1979) Diamine oxidase and polyamine oxidase activities in normal and transformed cells. *Biochem. J.*, 177: 275–282.

Quash, G., Ripoll, H., Gazzolo, L., Doutheau, A., Saba, A. and Gore, J. (1987) Malondialdehyde production from spermine by homogenates of normal and transformed cells. *Biochimie*, 69: 101–108.

Quemener, V., Moulinoux, J.P., Havouis, R. and Seiler, N. (1992) Polyamine deprivation enhances antitumoral efficacy of chemotherapy. *Anticancer Res.*, 12: 1447–1454.

Romano, M. and Bonelli, P. (1986) Polyamine oxidase activity in carcinoma-bearing human breast: significant decreased activity in carcinomatous tissue. *Tumori*, 72: 31–33.

Sarhan, S., Knödgen, B. and Seiler, N. (1989) The gastrointestinal tract as polyamine source for tumor growth. *Anticancer Res.*, 9: 215–224.

Sarhan, S., Quemener, V., Moulinoux, J.P., Knödgen, B. and Seiler, N. (1991a) On the degradation and elimination of spermine by the vertebrate organism. *Int. J. Biochem.*, 23: 617–626.

Sarhan, S., Weibel, M. and Seiler, N. (1991b) Effect of polyamine deprivation on the survival of intracranial glioblastoma bearing rats. *Anticancer Res.*, 11: 987–992.

Seiler, N. (1981) Amide bond-forming reactions of polyamines. In: D.R. Morris and L.J. Marton (Eds.), *Polyamines in Biology and Medicine*, Marcel Dekker, New York, pp. 127–149.

Seiler, N. (1987) Functions of polyamine acetylation. *Can. J. Physiol. Pharmacol.*, 65: 2024–2035.

Seiler, N. (1988) Potential roles of polyamine interconversion in the mammalian organism. In: V. Zappia and A.E. Pegg (Eds.), *Progress in Polyamine Research*, Plenum, New York, pp. 127–145.

Seiler, N. (1990) Polyamine metabolism. *Digestion*, 46: (Suppl. 2) 319–330.

Seiler, N. (1992) Polyamine catabolism and elimination by the vertebrate organism. In: R.H. Dowling, U.R. Fölsch and C. Löser (Eds.), *Polyamines in the Gastrointestinal Tract*, FALK Symposium 62, Kluwer, Dordrecht, pp. 65–85.

Seiler, N. and Atanassov, C. (1994) The natural polyamines and the immune system. *Progr. Drug Res.*, 43: 87–141.

Seiler, N. and Bolkenius, F.N. (1985) Polyamine reutilization and turnover in brain. *Neurochem. Res.*, 10: 529–544.

Seiler, N. and Heby, O. (1988) Regulation of cellular polyamines in mammals. *Acta Biochim. Biophys. Hung.*, 23: 1–36.

344

Seiler, N., Al-Therib, M.J., Fischer, H.A. and Erdmann, G. (1979) Dynamic and regional aspects of polyamine metabolism in the brain of trout (*Salmo irideus* Gibb.) *Int. J. Biochem.,* 10: 961–974.

Seiler, N., Bolkenius, F.N., Knödgen, B. and Mamont, P. (1980) Polyamine oxidase in rat tissues. *Biochim. Biophys. Acta,* 615: 480–488.

Seiler, N., Bolkenius, F.N., Bey, P., Mamont, P.S. and Danzin, C. (1985a) Biochemical significance of inhibition of polyamine oxidase. In: L. Selmeci, M.E. Brosnan and N. Seiler (Eds.), *Recent Progress in Polyamine Research*, Akademiai Kiado, Budapest, pp. 305–319.

Seiler, N., Bolkenius, F.N. and Knödgen, B. (1985b) The influence of catabolic reactions on polyamine excretion. *Biochem. J.,* 225: 219–226.

Shin, W.W., Fong, W.F., Pang, S.F. and Wong, P.C.L (1985) Limited blood-brain barrier transport of polyamines. *J. Neurochem.,* 44: 1056–1059.

Strolin Benedetti, M., Allievi, C., Cocchiara, G., Pevarello, P. and Dostert, P. (1992) Involvement of FAD-dependent polyamine oxidase in the metabolism of milacemide in the rat. *Xenobiotica,* 22: 191–197.

Tsukada, T., Furusako, S., Maekawa, S., Hibasami, H. and Nakashima, K. (1988) Purification by affinity chromatography and characterization of porcine liver cytoplasmic polyamine oxidase. *Int. J. Biochem.,* 20: 695–702.

Peter M. Yu, Keith F. Tipton and Alan A. Boulton (Eds.)
Progress in Brain Research, Vol 106
© 1995 Elsevier Science BV. All rights reserved.

CHAPTER 34

Role of aldehyde oxidase in biogenic amine metabolism

Christine Beedham, Caroline F. Peet, Georgious I. Panoutsopoulos, Helen Carter and John A. Smith

Pharmaceutical Chemistry, School of Pharmacy, University of Bradford, Bradford BD7 1DP, UK

Introduction

Oxidative deamination of biogenic amines, catalysed either by monoamine oxidase A or B (EC 1.4.3.4 monoamine:oxygen oxidoreductase) generates reactive intermediate aldehydes which in vivo are immediately transformed to either alcohol or acid metabolites (Tabakoff et al., 1973). In the brain glycolic aldehydes, formed by monoamine oxidase A from noradrenaline and adrenaline, are principally reduced to their corresponding alcohol by either alcohol dehydrogenase (EC 1.1.1.1) or aldehyde reductase (EC 1.1.1.2) whereas in the periphery acid metabolites are formed (Callingham and Barrand, 1979; Tipton et al., 1977). In contrast, aldehydes produced via monoamine oxidase B from 2-phenylethylamine or monoamine oxidase A from 5-hydroxytryptamine (5-HT) are rapidly converted in liver and brain to their respective acids. Aldehyde metabolites of biogenic amines are not detected in plasma or urine; they are rapidly metabolized in vitro (Helander and Tottmar, 1987b). However, even in vitro, monoamine oxidase activity is rarely investigated using a direct measurement of aldehyde production as these are usually unstable (Nilsson and Tottmar, 1987) and preparations often contain the aldehyde-oxidising enzymes. Thus when the aldehyde metabolites are incubated with intact erythrocytes only acid metabolites are formed

(Helander and Tottmar, 1987a). Furthermore, levels of acid metabolites in both plasma and brain are often used as markers of central neurone activity (Lambert et al., 1993; Palmer et al., 1987) or as indicators of monoamine oxidase dysfunction (Abeling et al., 1994).

The oxidation of biogenic aldehydes is generally attributed to NAD-dependent aldehyde dehydrogenase (ALDH) (Tabakoff et al., 1973; Pettersson and Tottmar, 1982b). This enzyme is universally distributed throughout all mammalian tissues with maximum activity in the liver but lower levels are found in other organs, brain and blood (Deitrich, 1966; Helander, 1989; Tottmar, 1986). Within the liver cell aldehyde dehydrogenase is distributed in all compartments, with different isozymes present in mitochondria (Han and Joo, 1991), cytosol (Vallari and Pietruszko, 1982) and microsomes (Cho and Joo, 1990). Aldehyde dehydrogenase isozymes catalyse the irreversible oxidation of a broad range of aldehydes to acids in an NAD^+-dependent reaction.

$$RCHO + NAD^+ + H_2O \rightarrow RCOOH + NADH + H^+$$

These include 5-hydroxy-3-indoleacetaldehyde and 3,4-dihydroxyphenylacetaldehyde, the aldehyde metabolites of the neurotransmitters 5-HT and dopamine which have K_m values in the μmolar range (Ambroziak and Pietruszko, 1991; Erwin and Deitrich, 1966).

However, there are two other enzymes which catalyse aldehyde oxidation; the molybdenum-hydroxylases, aldehyde oxidase (EC 1.2.3.1) and xanthine oxidase (EC 1.2.3.2) (Palmer, 1962; Pelsy and Klibanov, 1983). The molybdenum hydroxylases are more widely known for their role in the metabolism of heterocyclic compounds, such as purines, pteridines and iminium ions (Beedham, 1987). In fact aliphatic aldehydes, particularly acetaldehyde, have a weak affinity towards either aldehyde or xanthine oxidase, giving K_m values from 1–100 mM (Rajagopalan et al., 1962; Johns, 1967; Morpeth, 1983). Consequently, the contribution of these enzymes to the metabolism of other aldehydes has largely been ignored. Nevertheless, aromatic aldehydes are excellent substrates of hepatic aldehyde oxidase with lower activities towards xanthine oxidase (Rajagolapan et al., 1962; Morpeth, 1983; Panoutsopoulos, 1994). Vanillin (4-hydroxy-3-methoxybenzaldehyde) is rapidly oxidized by guinea pig liver aldehyde oxidase whereas its structural isomer, isovanillin (3-hydroxy-4-methoxy-benzaldehyde), is a potent competitive inhibitor (Panoutsopoulos, 1994).

Aldehyde oxidase activity can be detected in most mammalian tissues and, like aldehyde dehydrogenase, is mainly found in the liver with different isozymes present in cytosol and mitochondria (Beedham et al., 1987a; Critchley et al., 1992). Minimal activity has been found in brain (Krenitsky et al., 1974; Holmes and Vandeberg, 1986). In addition to two molybdenum atoms, each molecule of aldehyde oxidase contains four non-haem iron-sulphur centres and two flavin adenine dinucleotide molecules, each of which can function as redox centres in the intra-molecular transfer of electrons from reducing to oxidizing substrates. The reaction, illustrated below, involves nucleophilic attack at an electropositive carbon whereby the oxygen incorporated into the substrate is derived from water and not molecular oxygen.

$$RCHO + OH^- ----> RCOOH + 2e^- + H^+$$

As we have shown that vanillin and indole-3-acetaldehyde, stable analogues of 4-hydroxy-3-methoxyphenylacetaldehyde (homovanillyl aldehyde) and 5-hydroxyindoleacetaldehyde are excellent substrates for guinea pig liver aldehyde oxidase, we thought it likely that this enzyme may be important in peripheral 5-HT and homovanillamine metabolism. Guinea pig is a good model for in vivo and in vitro screening of human aldehyde oxidase activity (Beedham et al., 1987b; Beedham et al., 1990). The major metabolite of 5-HT in plasma, urine and brain is 5-hydroxyindoleacetic acid (5-HIAA) whereas homovanillic acid accounts for a significant proportion of dopamine excretion. Preliminary studies, using isovanillin as an in vitro inhibitor, have implicated aldehyde oxidase in 5-HIAA formation in both guinea pig liver and brain (Peet et al., 1993). In the present investigation the involvement of aldehyde oxidase in the production of homovanillic acid (HVA) and 5-HIAA has been investigated using precision-cut liver slices and brain homogenates from Dunkin-Hartley guinea pigs.

Homovanillyl aldehyde and 5-hydroxy-3-indoleacetaldehyde as substrates of guinea pig liver aldehyde oxidase

Homovanillyl aldehyde and 5-hydroxyindole-3-acetaldehyde can be prepared enzymatically from the parent amines as bisulphite complexes using rat liver monoamine oxidase (Pettersson and Tottmar, 1982b). Subsequent extraction with ether yields the free aldehydes. However, these aldehydes are relatively unstable and we have found that bisulphite has an inhibitory effect on aldehyde oxidase. Consequently, homovanillyl aldehyde and 5-hydroxyindole-3-acetaldehyde have been generated in situ from homovanillamine (HV) and 5-HT with guinea pig liver monoamine oxidase in the presence of aldehyde oxidase. Disrupted mitochondrial membranes were used as source of guinea pig liver monoamine oxidase. Partially purified aldehyde oxidase was prepared by heating guinea pig liver homogenates for 10 min at 55–60°C, centrifugation and precipitation of the enzyme from supernatant with $(NH_4)_2SO_4$ (Beedham et al., 1990). HV (2 mM) or 5-HT (1 mM) was incubated with guinea pig liver monoamine oxidase and aldehyde oxidase in oxygenated Krebs-Henseleit buffer pH 7.4 at 37°C. Aliquots (0.2 ml) were removed periodically, added to 0.1 ml 3.6% (v/v) perchloric acid and centrifuged for 2 min prior to HPLC analysis for comparison with authentic standards. HV and 5-HT incubations were analysed with a C18 Hypersil column coupled to UV detector set at 280 nm. The mobile phase was acetonitrile/tetrahydrofuran/0.22 M orthophosphoric acid containing 0.11 M diethylamine at pH 2.9 (8.5%/1%/90.5%) at flow rate of 1.5 ml/min for HV incubations and acetonitrile/0.22 M orthophosphoric acid containing 0.11 M diethylamine at pH 2.9 (7.5%/92.5%) at a flow rate of 2 ml/min for 5-HT incubations.

In the presence of both monoamine oxidase and aldehyde oxidase about 50% HV was converted to HVA within 90 min (Fig. 1). Similarly, 5-HIAA was the major metabolite formed from 5-HT with lower concentrations of 5-hydroxytryptophol also produced (Fig. 2). This shows that 4-hydroxy-3-methoxyphenylacetaldehyde and 5-

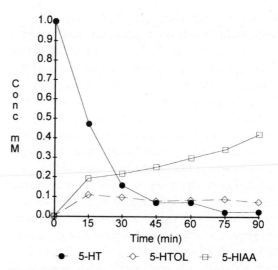

Fig. 2. Metabolite formation from 1 mM 5-hydroxytryptamine (5-HT) with guinea pig liver MAO (0.75 ml) and AO (0.1 ml) in 3 ml Krebs-Henseleit buffer pH 7.4 at 37°C. 5-HTOL, 5-hydroxytryptophol; 5-HIAA, 5-hydroxyindoleacetic acid.

hydroxy-3-indoleacetaldehyde are oxidized to their corresponding acids by aldehyde oxidase. The partially purified enzyme preparation would not contain contaminating aldehyde dehydrogenase, as the mitochondrial isozyme would be removed by the centrifugation and both cytosolic and mitochondrial isozymes are heat labile. Furthermore NAD^+ is required as a cofactor for aldehyde dehydrogenase, but was not added to these incubations as aldehyde oxidase utilizes molecular oxygen as an electron acceptor (Beedham, 1987).

Oxidation of homovanillyl aldehyde and 5-hydroxy-3-indoleacetaldehyde in guinea pig liver slices

The ability of partially purified aldehyde oxidase to catalyse homovanillyl aldehyde and 5-hydroxy-indoleacetaldehyde oxidation does not necessarily imply that this enzyme will play a major role in vivo when other aldehyde oxidizing enzymes are also present. Thus 5-hydroxy-3-indoleacetaldehyde is also a substrate of cytosolic and mitochondrial ALDH isozymes with K_m values of 2.4 and 0.8 μM, respectively (Ambroziak and Pietruszko,

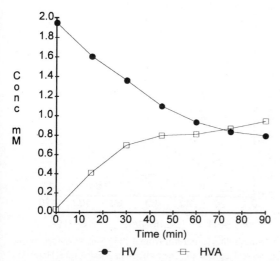

Fig. 1. Formation of homovanillic acid (HVA) from 2 mM homovanillamine (HV) with guinea pig liver MAO (0.4ml) and AO (0.1ml) in 2 ml Krebs-Henseleit buffer pH 7.4 at 37°C.

1991; Erwin and Deitrich, 1966) and indole-3-acetaldehyde is a less efficient substrate of xanthine oxidase (Morpeth, 1983). The contribution of each oxidizing enzyme towards aldehyde metabolism will depend on the comparative affinity of an aldehyde for each enzyme, their relative oxidation rates and the concentration of the enzymes within a particular tissue. Consequently, the oxidation of homovanillyl aldehyde and 5-hydroxy-3-indoleacetaldehyde has been studied using precision-cut liver slices, an integrated in vitro system, in which a high degree of hepatic lobular architecture of the tissue and intercellular communication are maintained, giving similar conditions to those in vivo (Smith et al., 1987a). In liver slices, activities of endobiotic and xenobiotic-metabolising enzymes are retained for many hours in addition to normal physiological and biochemical functions (Smith et al., 1987a; Barr et al., 1991).

HV (0.5 mM) or 5-HT (1 mM) was incubated with four precision-cut liver slices in 3 ml oxygenated Krebs-Henseleit buffer pH 7.4 at 37°C, aliquots were removed and analysed as described above. The major metabolites formed in HV and 5-HT incubations with guinea pig liver slices were HVA (Fig. 3) and 5-HIAA (Fig. 4), respectively, with lower amounts of homovanillyl alcohol (HVOL) and 5-hydroxytryptophol (5-HTOL) also being produced.

Inhibition of homovanillic acid and 5-hydroxyindoleacetic acid formation in guinea pig liver slices

We have investigated further the involvement of aldehyde oxidase in HV and 5-HT metabolism using in vitro and in vivo enzyme inhibitors. Allopurinol and disulfiram are used clinically to treat gout-associated hyperuricaemia and alcoholism as they are potent inhibitors of xanthine oxidase and aldehyde dehydrogenase, respectively (Massey et al., 1970; Deitrich and Erwin, 1971; Yourick and Faiman, 1991; Peterson et al., 1990). In vitro less than 10% aldehyde dehydrogenase activity remains when 25 μM disulfiram is present

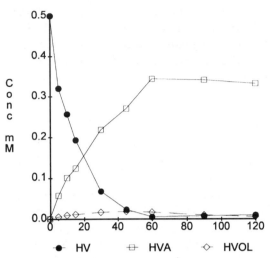

Fig. 3. Metabolite formation from 0.5 mM homovanillamine (HV) with two guinea pig liver slices in 2 ml Krebs-Henseleit buffer pH 7.4 at 37°C. HVOL, homovanillyl alcohol; HVA, homovanillic acid. Each point is the mean of four determinations.

in the assay (Berger and Weiner, 1977) and 1 mM allopurinol is sufficient to reduce the oxidation of 1 mM xanthine by 90% (Tweedie et al., 1991).

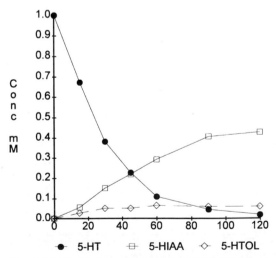

Fig. 4. Metabolite formation from 1 mM 5-hydroxytryptamine (5-HT) with 4 guinea pig liver slices in 3 ml Krebs-Henseleit buffer pH 7.4 at 37°C. 5-HTOL, 5-hydroxy-tryptophol; 5-HIAA, 5-hydroxyindoleacetic acid. Each point is the mean of 10 determinations.

Menadione is a selective inhibitor of aldehyde oxidase in vitro but acts as an efficient electron acceptor of xanthine oxidase. Rajagopalan and Handler (1964) achieved 85% inhibition of rabbit liver aldehyde oxidase with concentrations as low as 0.1 μM. We have inhibited aldehyde oxidase in vivo by administration of either hydralazine or tungsten to guinea pigs. Hydralazine is a potent, progressive inhibitor of hepatic aldehyde oxidase, both in vitro and in vivo with no effect on xanthine oxidase (Johnson et al., 1985; Critchley et al., 1994) whereas a diet supplemented with tungsten reduces the levels of both molybdenum hydroxylases (Shaw and Jayatilleke, 1992; Smith et al., 1987b).

In vitro inhibition

Menadione (0.1 mM), disulfiram (0.1 mM) and allopurinol (1 mM) were added to liver slice incubations as specific inhibitors of aldehyde oxidase, aldehyde dehydrogenase and xanthine oxidase, respectively. In the presence of menadione, HVA (Fig. 5) and 5-HIAA (Fig. 6) production after 60 min was inhibited by 75–85%, whereas amine breakdown was not affected in either case. Disulfiram did not significantly reduce acid pro-

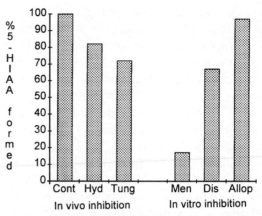

Fig. 6. Effect of inhibitors, in vivo (Hyd, hydralazine; Tung, tungsten) and in vitro (Men, menadione; Dis, disulfiram; Allop, allopurinol) on 5-hydroxyindole acetic acid (5-HIAA) formation from 1 mM 5-hydroxytryptamine with guinea pig liver slices; results are expressed as % formation of 5-HIAA in 60 min compared to each respective control, $n = 2–6$.

duction and allopurinol had no effect on the formation of either acid. It is, therefore, concluded from these experiments that aldehyde oxidase is the predominant enzyme in the oxidation of homovanillyl aldehyde and 5-hydroxy-3-indoleacetaldehyde in guinea pig liver slices. Xanthine oxidase would appear to have negligible activity towards these aldehydes, whereas the weak inhibition observed with disulfiram may indicate that aldehyde dehydrogenase may also be important. On the other hand, we have shown (Panoutsopoulos, 1994) that 0.1 mM disulfiram inhibits the oxidation of vanillin by guinea pig liver aldehyde oxidase by about 18%; thus it is not entirely specific towards aldehyde dehydrogenase. The importance of aldehyde oxidase in the metabolism of HV and 5-HT has been confirmed using in vivo inhibitors.

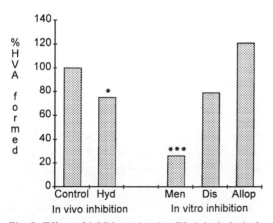

Fig. 5. Effect of inhibitors, in vivo (Hyd, hydralazine) and in vitro (Men, menadione; Dis, disulfiram; Allop, allopurinol), on homovanillic acid (HVA) formation from 2 mM homovanillamine with guinea pig liver slices; results are expressed as % formation of HVA in 60 min compared to each respective control. *$P < 0.05$, $n = 4$; ***$p < 0.001$, $n = 4$.

In vivo inhibition of aldehyde oxidase activity with hydralazine

When guinea pigs were given hydralazine HCl (10 mg/kg/day) in 5 mM phosphate buffer pH 6 to drink for 7–8 days, hepatic aldehyde oxidase activity towards a specific heterocyclic aldehyde oxidase substrate (a substituted purine) was reduced by 35%, $P < 0.05$, $n = 4$ (S. Oldfield and C. Beedham, personal communication). Control animals received phosphate buffer for 7–8 days. We found that the formation of HVA in guinea pig liver slices from hydralazine-treated guinea pigs was significantly decreased. Production of 5-HIAA was also reduced (17% against phosphate controls in 60 min, 46% against untreated guinea pigs) in slices from hydralazine-treated animals (Fig. 6). Hepatic aldehyde oxidase activity in these animals was monitored using phthalazine as a substrate and was ound to be reduced by approx. 65%.

In vivo inhibition of aldehyde oxidase activity with tungsten

5-HT metabolism was also studied in guinea pig liver slices from tungsten-treated guinea pigs which contain reduced aldehyde oxidase and xanthine oxidase activity. Guinea pigs were given sodium tungstate (100 ppm) in 29 mM sucrose to drink for 24–29 days and control animals received 29 mM sucrose for the same time period. Hepatic aldehyde oxidase activity was reduced by 40% with respect to phthalazine as a substrate in these animals. By comparison, tungsten treatment caused a 28% reduction in the formation of 5-HIAA from 5-HT in guinea pig liver slices (Fig. 6).

Metabolism of homovanillamine and 5-HT in guinea pig cortex

Kinetic and electrophoretic studies indicate a multiplicity of aldehyde dehydrogenase isozymes in mammalian brain (Pettersson and Tottmar, 1982a; Holmes and Vandeberg, 1986). There is also some evidence for cranial xanthine oxidase activity (for reviews see Parks and Granger, 1986; Beedham, 1987). Betz (1985) has proposed that brain capillaries may be susceptible to damage from xanthine-oxidase-derived oxygen radicals during re-perfusion injury although this hypothesis has been challenged by Wajner and Harkness (1989), who found that human and rabbit brain

enzyme predominantly uses NAD^+ rather than O_2 as an electron acceptor. However, aldehyde oxidase activity has not been detected in brain using either electrophoretic or relatively insensitive kinetic techniques (Krenitsky et al., 1974; Holmes and Vandeberg, 1986). In contrast, using a highly sensitive HPLC-EC assay for HVA and 5-HT we hoped to establish the presence of brain aldehyde oxidase. Guinea pig cortex homogenates (10%, w/v) were prepared in 0.25 M sucrose, 0.75 ml aliquots were incubated with either HV and 5-HT (30 μM) and analysed by HPLC. Peaks were detected using an electrochemical detector set at 1.05 V and 0.65 V for HV and 5-HT, respectively.

Almost complete conversion of homovanillamine to homovanillic acid occurred within 60 min in cortex homogenates with low levels of homovanillyl alcohol also produced. In homogenates from hydralazine-treated guinea pigs there was a significant reduction in HVA formation with a slight decrease in homovanillamine breakdown compared to phosphate controls (Fig. 7). HVA production in cortex homogenates from

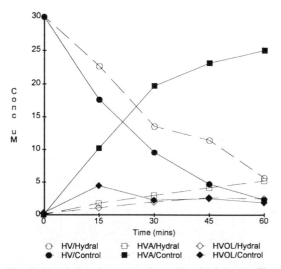

Fig. 7. Metabolite formation from 30 μM homovanillamine (HV) with cortex homogenates (0.75 ml), from hydralazine-treated and control guinea pigs, in 1.5 ml Krebs-Henseleit buffer pH 7.4 at 37°C. HVOL, homovanillyl alcohol; HVA, homovanillic acid. HVA formation was significantly reduced; at 30 min $P < 0.002$, $n = 4$.

tungsten-treated guinea pigs was also reduced over sucrose controls (Fig. 8). These results strongly indicate the involvement of brain aldehyde oxidase in homovanillamine metabolism.

The formation of 5-HIAA from 5-HT in guinea pig cortex homogenates was about 50% the rate of homovanillic acid production although 5-HT breakdown was similar to that of homovanillamine. Tungsten treatment did inhibit 5-HIAA production in cortex homogenates although the effect was less marked than that on homovanillic acid production (Fig. 8). Hydralazine administration apparently increased 5-HIAA formation in guinea pig cortex.

In vitro inhibition of 5-HIAA formation was studied using low concentrations (3 μM) of menadione and disulfiram (Fig. 9). Under these conditions disulfiram had no effect whereas similar disulfiram concentrations cause a marked inhibitory effect ($\sim$ 50%) on acetaldehyde and DOPAL oxidation by aldehyde dehydrogenase in rat brain mitochondria (Pettersson and Tottmar, 1982b). Menadione only reduced 5-HIAA production by about 15% although isovanillin (30 μM), another potent aldehyde oxidase inhibitor, had a marked inhibitory effect (70%) on the conversion of 5-HT to 5-HIAA. In contrast, the xanthine oxidase in-

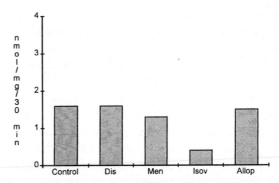

Fig. 9. Effect of in vitro inhibitors (Dis, disulfiram; Men, menadione; Isov, isovanillin; Allop, allopurinol) on 5-hydroxyindoleactic acid (5-HIAA) formation in 30 min by guinea pig cortex homogenates.

hibitor, allopurinol (100 μM), did not reduce 5-HIAA formation in guinea pig homogenates.

Conclusions

It has been proposed that aldehyde dehydrogenase is the only enzyme, or rather group of isozymes, in human liver that metabolize biogenic aldehydes and neurotransmitters (Pietruszko et al., 1991). Nevertheless, we have shown that both homovanillyl aldehyde and 5-hydroxy-3-indoleacetaldehyde are substrates for guinea pig liver aldehyde oxidase. Furthermore, the results obtained with both in vivo and in vitro inhibitors indicate that aldehyde oxidase plays a major role in HV and 5-HT metabolism in guinea pig liver. In view of the similarity between guinea pig and human liver aldehyde oxidase (Beedham et al., 1987b; Critchley, 1989) it is likely that human hepatic aldehyde oxidase may also be important in biogenic amine metabolism. Helander et al. (1994) have recently examined the urinary metabolites of 5-HT in Oriental subjects but were unable to find any correlation between 5-HIAA production and mitochondrial aldehyde dehydrogenase genotype. They suggested that cytosolic aldehyde dehydrogenase could oxidize physiological concentrations of 5-hydroxyindoleacetaldehyde when the mitochondrial isozyme is absent. However, this oxidation could equally well be

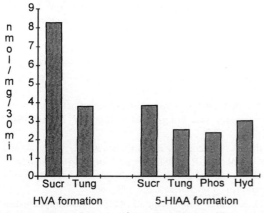

Fig. 8. Effect of in vivo (Hyd, hydralazine; Tung, tungsten) inhibitors on homovanillic acid (HVA) and 5-hydroxyindoleacetic acid (5-HIAA) formation in 30 min by guinea pig cortex homogenates. Sucr, sucrose control; phosphate, phosphate control.

carried out by aldehyde oxidase. Although peripheral plasma levels of HVA, the deaminated and O-methylated metabolite of dopamine, are often used as an indicator of central dopaminergic activity, Lambert et al. (1993) have shown that HVA is produced locally, perhaps from circulating DOPA. HVA and vanillylmandelic acid, another dopamine metabolite, are excreted in excessive amounts in the urine of children with neuroblastomas (Candito et al., 1992). Aldehyde oxidase may be the enzyme responsible for the peripheral formation of HVA which occurs during dopamine metabolism. Furthermore, brain aldehyde oxidase is strongly implicated in the metabolism of aldehydes derived from biogenic amines, particularly HV. This is consistent with the finding of Deitrich (1966) that brain oxidation of indole-3-acetaldehyde is not entirely dependent on the presence of NAD^+.

References

Abeling, N.G.G.M., Vangennip, A.H., Overmars, H., Vanoost, B.A. and Brunner, H.G. (1994) Biogenic amine metabolite patterns in urine of MAO-A deficient patients — a possible tool for diagnosis. *J. Inher. Met. Disease*, 17: 339–341

Ambroziak, W. and Pietruszko, R. (1991) Human aldehyde dehydrogenase activity with aldehyde metabolites of monoamine, diamines and polyamines. *J. Biol. Chem.*, 266: 13011–13018.

Barr, J., Weir, A.J., Brendel, K. and Sipes, I.G. (1991) Liver slices in dynamic organ culture. I. An alternative in vitro technique for the study of rat hepatic drug metabolism. *Xenobiotica*, 21: 331–339.

Beedham, C. (1987) Molybdenum hydroxylases: Biological distribution and substrate-inhibitor specificity. In: G.P. Ellis and G.B. West (Eds.), *Progress in Medicinal Chemistry*, Vol. 24, Elsevier, Amsterdam, New York, Oxford, pp. 85–127.

Beedham, C., Bruce, S.E. and Rance, D.J. (1987a) Tissue distribution of the molybdenum hydroxylases, aldehyde oxidase and xanthine oxidase, in male and female guinea pigs. *Eur. J. Drug Met. Pharmacokin.*, 12: 303–306.

Beedham, C., Bruce, S.E., Critchley, D.J., Al-Tayib, Y. and Rance, D.J. (1987b) Species variation in hepatic aldehyde oxidase. *Eur. J. Drug Met. Pharmacokin.*, 12: 307–310.

Beedham, C., Bruce, S.E., Critchley, D.J. and Rance, D.J. (1990) 1-Substituted phthalazines as probes of the substrate-binding site of mammalian molybdenum hydroxylases. *Biochem. Pharmacol.*, 39: 1213–1221.

Berger, D. and Weiner, H. (1977) Effects of disulfiram and chloral hydrate on the metabolism of catecholamines in rat liver and brain. *Biochem. Pharmacol.*, 26: 741- 747.

Betz, A.L. (1985) Identification of hypoxanthine transport and xanthine oxidase activity in brain capillaries. *J. Neurochem.*, 44: 574–579.

Callingham, B.A. and Barrand, M.A. (1979) The catecholamines: noradrenaline and adrenaline. In: C.H. Gray and V.H.T. James (Eds.), *Hormones in the Blood*, Vol. 2, 3rd Edn., Academic Press, London, pp. 143–207.

Candito, M., Thyss, A., Albertini, M., Deville, A., Politano, S., Mariani, R. and Chambon, P. (1992) Methylated catecholamine metabolites for diagnosis of neuroblastoma. *Med. Paed. Oncol.*, 20: 215–220.

Cho, E.-W. and Joo, J.N. (1990) Probable function of rat liver microsomal aldehyde dehydrogenase. *Korean Biochem. J.*, 23: 528–534.

Critchley, D.J.P. (1989) Diazanaphthalenes as probes of molybdenum hydroxylase activity. Ph.D. Thesis, University of Bradford.

Critchley, D.J.P., Rance, D.J. and Beedham, C. (1994) Biotransformation of carbazeran in guinea pig: effect of hydralazine pre-treatment. *Xenobiotica*, 24: 37–47.

Deitrich, R.A. (1966) Tissue and subcellular distribution of mammalian aldehyde-oxidising activity. *Biochem Pharmacol.*, 15: 1911–1922.

Deitrich, R.A. and Erwin, V.G. (1971) Mechanism of the inhibition of aldehyde dehydrogenase in vivo by disulfiram and diethyldithiocarbamate. *Mol. Pharmacol.*, 7: 301–307.

Erwin, V.G. and Dietrich, R.A. (1966) Brain aldehyde dehydrogenase — localization, purification and properties. *J. Biol. Chem.*, 241: 3533–3539.

Han, I.O. and Joo, C.N. (1991) Purification and characterization of the rat liver mitochondrial aldehyde dehydrogenases. *Korean Biochem. J.*, 24:353–360.

Helander, A. and Tottmar, O. (1987a) Metabolism of biogenic aldehydes in isolated human blood cells, platelets and in plasma. *Biochem. Pharmacol.*, 36: 1077–1082.

Helander, A. and Tottmar, O. (1987b) Effects of ethanol, acetaldehyde and disulfiram on the metabolism of biogenic aldehydes in isolated human blood cells and platelets. *Biochem. Pharmacol.*, 36: 3981–3985.

Helander, A. (1989) Aldehyde dehydrogenase activity in blood from various vertebrates. *Comp. Biochem. Physiol.*, 94B: 461–464.

Helander, A., Walzer, C., Beck, O., Balant, L., Borg, S. and von Warburg, J.-P. (1994) Influence of genetic variation in alcohol and aldehyde dehydrogenase on serotonin metabolism. *Life Sciences*, 55: 359–366.

Holmes, R.S. and Vandeberg, J.L. (1986) Aldehyde dehydrogenases, aldehyde oxidase and xanthine oxidase from baboon tissues: phenotypic variability and subcellular distribution in liver and brain. *Alcohol*, 3: 205–214.

Johns, D.G. (1967) Human liver aldehyde oxidase. *J. Clin. Invest.*, 46: 1492–1505.

Johnson, C. Stubley-Beedham, C. and Stell, J.G.P. (1985) Hydralazine: a potent inhibitor of aldehyde oxidase activity in vitro and in vivo. *Biochem. Pharmacol.*, 34: 4251–4256.

Krenitsky, T.A., Tuttle, J.V., Cattau, E.L. and Wang, P. (1974) A comparison of the distribution and electron acceptor specificities of xanthine oxidase and aldehyde oxidase. *Comp. Biochem. Physiol.*, 49B: 687.

Lambert, G.W., Eisenhofer, G., Jennings, G.L. and Esler, M D. (1993) Regional homovanillic acid production in humans. *Life Sci.*, 53: 63–75.

Massey, V., Komai, H., Palmer, G. and Elion, G.B. (1970) On the mechanism of inactivation of xanthine oxidase by allopurinol and other pyrazolo[3,4-d]pyrimidines. *J. Biol. Chem.*, 245: 2837–2844.

Morpeth, F. (1983) Studies on the specificity towards aldehyde substrates and steady-state kinetics of xanthine oxidase. *Biochim. Biophys. Acta*, 744: 328–333.

Nilsson, G.E. and Tottmar, O. (1987) Biogenic aldehydes in brain; on their properties and reactions with rat brain tissue. *J. Neurochem.*, 48: 1566–1572.

Palmer, G. (1962) Purification and properties of aldehyde oxidase. *Biochim. Biophys. Acta*, 56: 444–459.

Palmer, A.M, Wilcock, G.K., Esiri, M.M., Francis, P.T. and Bowen, D.M. (1987) Monoaminergic innervation of the frontal and temporal lobes in Alzheimer's disease. *Brain Res.*, 401: 231–238.

Parks, D.A. and Granger, D.N. (1986) Xanthine oxidase: biochemistry, distribution and physiology. *Acta Physiol. Scand. Suppl.*, 548: 87–99.

Panoutsopoulos, G.I. (1994) Hepatic oxidation of aromatic aldehydes. Ph.D. Thesis, University of Bradford.

Pelsy, G. and Klibanov, A.M. (1983) Remarkable regional specificity of xanthine oxidase and some dehydrogenases in the reactions with substituted benzaldehydes. *Biochim. Biophys. Acta*, 742: 352–357.

Peet, C.F., Smith, J.A. and Beedham, C. (1993) Aldehyde oxidase catalysed formation of 5-hydroxy-indoleacetic acid in guinea pig liver and brain. *Br. J Pharmacol.*, 110S: 191.

Peterson, G.M., Boyle, R.R., Francis, H.W., Oliver, N.W.J., Paterson, J., Von Witt, R.J. and Taylor, G.R. (1990) Dosage prescribing and plasma oxipurinol levels in patients receiving oxipurinol therapy. *Eur. J. Clin. Pharmacol.*, 39: 419–421.

Pettersson, H. and Tottmar, O. (1982a) Aldehyde dehydrogenases in rat brain: Subcellular distribution and properties. *J. Neurochem.*, 38: 477–487.

Pettersson, H. and Tottmar, O. (1982b) Inhibition of aldehyde dehydrogenases in rat brain and liver by disulfiram and coprine. *J. Neurochem.*, 39: 628–634.

Pietruszko, R., Kurys, G. and Ambroziak, A. (1991) Physiological role of aldehyde dehydrogenase (EC 1.2.1.3). *Alcoholism*, 206: 101–106.

Rajagopalan, K. V., Fridovich, I. and Handler, P. (1962) Hepatic aldehyde oxidase I: Purification and properties. *J. Biol. Chem.*, 237: 922–928.

Rajagopalan, K. V. and Handler, P. (1964) Hepatic aldehyde oxidase III: The substrate binding site. *J. Biol. Chem.*, 239: 2027–2035.

Shaw, S. and Jayatilleke, E. (1992) The role of cellular oxidase and catalytic iron in the pathogenesis of ethanol-induced liver injury. *Life Sci.*, 50: 2045–2052.

Smith, P.F., Fisher, R., Shubat, P.J., Gandolfi, A.J., Krumdieck, C.L. and Brendel, K. (1987a) In vitro cytotoxicity of allyl alcohol and bromobenzene in a novel organ culture system. *Toxicol. Appl. Pharmacol.*, 87: 509–522.

Smith, S.M., Grisham, M.B., Manci, E.A., Granger, D.N. and Kvietys, P.R. (1987b) Gastric mucosal injury in the rat. Role of iron and xanthine oxidase. *Gastroenterology*, 92: 950–956.

Tabakoff, B., Anderson, R. and Alivisatos, S.G.A. (1973) Enzymic reduction of "biogenic" aldehydes in brain. *Mol. Pharmacol.*, 9: 428–437.

Tipton, K., Houselay, M.D. and Turner, A.J. (1977) Metabolism in brain. In: M.B.H. Youdim, G. Lovenberg, G. F. Sharman and J. R. Lagnado (Eds.), *Essays in Neurochemistry and Neuropharmacology*, Vol. 1, Wiley, London, pp. 103–138.

Tottmar, O. (1986) Assay of brain aldehyde dehydrogenase activity using high-performance liquid chromatography with electrochemical detection. *Anal. Biochem.*, 158: 6–11.

Tweedie, D.J., Fernandez, D., Spearman, M.E., Feldhoff, R.C. and Prough, R.A. (1991) Metabolism of azoxy derivatives of procarbazine by aldehyde dehydrogenase and xanthine oxidase. *Drug Metab. Disp.*, 19: 793–803.

Vallari, R.C. and Pietruszko, R. (1982) Human aldehyde dehydrogenase; mechanism of inhibition by disulfiram. *Science*, 216: 637–639.

Wajner, M. and Harkness, R.A. (1989) Distribution of xanthine dehydrogenase and oxidase activities in human and rabbit tissues. *Biochim. Biophys. Acta*, 991: 79–84.

Yourick, J.J. and Faiman, M.D. (1991) Disulfiram metabolism as a requirement for the inhibition of rat liver mitochondrial low K_m aldehyde dehydrogenase. *Biochem. Pharmacol.*, 42: 1361–1366.

Subject Index